Estimated Safe and Adequate Daily Dietary Intakes of Additional Selected Vitamins and Minerals (United States)[a]

Age (years)	Vitamins: Biotin (μg)	Vitamins: Pantothenic Acid (mg)
Infants		
0–0.5	10	2
0.5–1	15	3
Children		
1–3	20	3
4–6	25	3–4
7–10	30	4–5
11 +	30–100	4–7
Adults	30–100	4–7

Age (years)	Trace Elements[b]: Chromium (μg)	Molybdenum (μg)	Copper (mg)	Manganese (mg)	Fluoride (mg)
Infants					
0–0.5	10–40	15–30	0.4–0.6	0.3–0.6	0.1–0.5
0.5–1	20–60	20–40	0.6–0.7	0.6–1.0	0.2–1.0
Children					
1–3	20–80	25–50	0.7–1.0	1.0–1.5	0.5–1.5
4–6	30–120	30–75	1.0–1.5	1.5–2.0	1.0–2.5
7–10	50–200	50–150	1.0–2.0	2.0–3.0	1.5–2.5
11 +	50–200	75–250	1.5–2.5	2.0–5.0	1.5–2.5
Adults	50–200	75–250	1.5–3.0	2.0–5.0	1.5–4.0

[a]Because there is less information on which to base allowances, these figures are not given in the main table of the RDA and are provided here in the form of ranges of recommended intakes.
[b]Because the toxic levels for many trace elements may be only several times usual intakes, the upper levels for the trace elements given in this table should not be habitually exceeded.

Source: *Recommended Dietary Allowances*, © 1989 by the National Academy of Sciences, National Academy Press, Washington, D.C.

Estimated Minimum Requirements of Sodium, Chloride, and Potassium

Age (years)	Sodium[a] (mg)	Chloride (mg)	Potassium[b] (mg)
Infants			
0.0–0.5	120	180	500
0.5–1.0	200	300	700
Children			
1	225	350	1000
2–5	300	500	1400
6–9	400	600	1600
Adolescents	500	750	2000
Adults	500	750	2000

[a]Sodium requirements are based on estimates of needs for growth and for replacement of obligatory losses. They cover a wide variation of physical activity patterns and climatic exposure but do not provide for large, prolonged losses from the skin through sweat.
[b]Dietary potassium may benefit the prevention and treatment of hypertension and recommendations to include many servings of fruits and vegetables would raise potassium intakes to about 3500 mg/day.

Source: *Recommended Dietary Allowances*, © 1989 by the National Academy of Sciences, National Academy Press, Washington, D.C.

Median Heights and Weights and Recommended Energy Intakes (United States)

Age (years)	Weight (kg)	Weight (lb)	Height (cm)	Height (inches)	Average Energy Allowance: REE[a] (cal/day)	Multiples of REE[b]	cal per kg	cal per day[c]
Infants								
0.0–0.5	6	13	60	24	320		108	650
0.5–1.0	9	20	71	28	500		98	850
Children								
1–3	13	29	90	35	740		102	1300
4–6	20	44	112	44	950		90	1800
7–10	28	62	132	52	1130		70	2000
Males								
11–14	45	99	157	62	1440	1.70	55	2500
15–18	66	145	176	69	1760	1.67	45	3000
19–24	72	160	177	70	1780	1.67	40	2900
25–50	79	174	176	70	1800	1.60	37	2900
51 +	77	170	173	68	1530	1.50	30	2300
Females								
11–14	46	101	157	62	1310	1.67	47	2200
15–18	55	120	163	64	1370	1.60	40	2200
19–24	58	128	164	65	1350	1.60	38	2200
25–50	63	138	163	64	1380	1.55	36	2200
51 +	65	143	160	63	1280	1.50	30	1900
Pregnant (2nd and 3rd trimesters)								+300
Lactating								+500

[a]REE (resting energy expenditure) represents the energy expended by a person at rest under normal conditions.
[b]Recommended energy allowances assume light to moderate activity and were calculated by multiplying the REE by an activity factor.
[c]Average energy allowances have been rounded.

Source: *Recommended Dietary Allowances*, © 1989 by the National Academy of Sciences, National Academy Press, Washington, D.C.

U.S. RDA (used on food labels)

Nutrient	RDA for an Adult Man (1968)	RDA for an Adult Woman (1968)	U.S. RDA
Nutrients that *must* appear on the label[a]			
Protein (g), PER ⋅ casein[b]	45	—	45
Protein (g), PER < casein	65	55	65
Vitamin A (RE)	1,000	800	1,000
Vitamin C (ascorbic acid) (mg)	60	55	60
Thiamin (vitamin B_1) (mg)	1.4	1.0	1.5
Riboflavin (vitamin B_2) (mg)	1.7	1.5	1.7
Niacin (mg)	18	13	20
Calcium (g)	0.8	0.8	1.0
Iron (mg)	10	18	18
Nutrients that *may* appear on the label			
Vitamin D (IU)	—	—	400
Vitamin E (IU)	30	25	30
Vitamin B_6 (mg)	2.0	2.0	2.0
Folate (folic acid, folacin) (mg)	0.4	0.4	0.4
Vitamin B_{12} (μg)	6	6	6
Phosphorus (g)	0.8	0.8	1.0
Iodine (μg)	120	100	150
Magnesium (mg)	350	300	400
Zinc (mg)	—	—	15
Copper (mg)	—	—	2
Biotin (mg)	—	—	0.3
Pantothenic acid (mg)	—	—	10

[a]Whenever nutrition labeling is required. [b]PER is an index of protein quality. Source: Adapted from *Food Technology* 28, no. 7 (1974): 5.

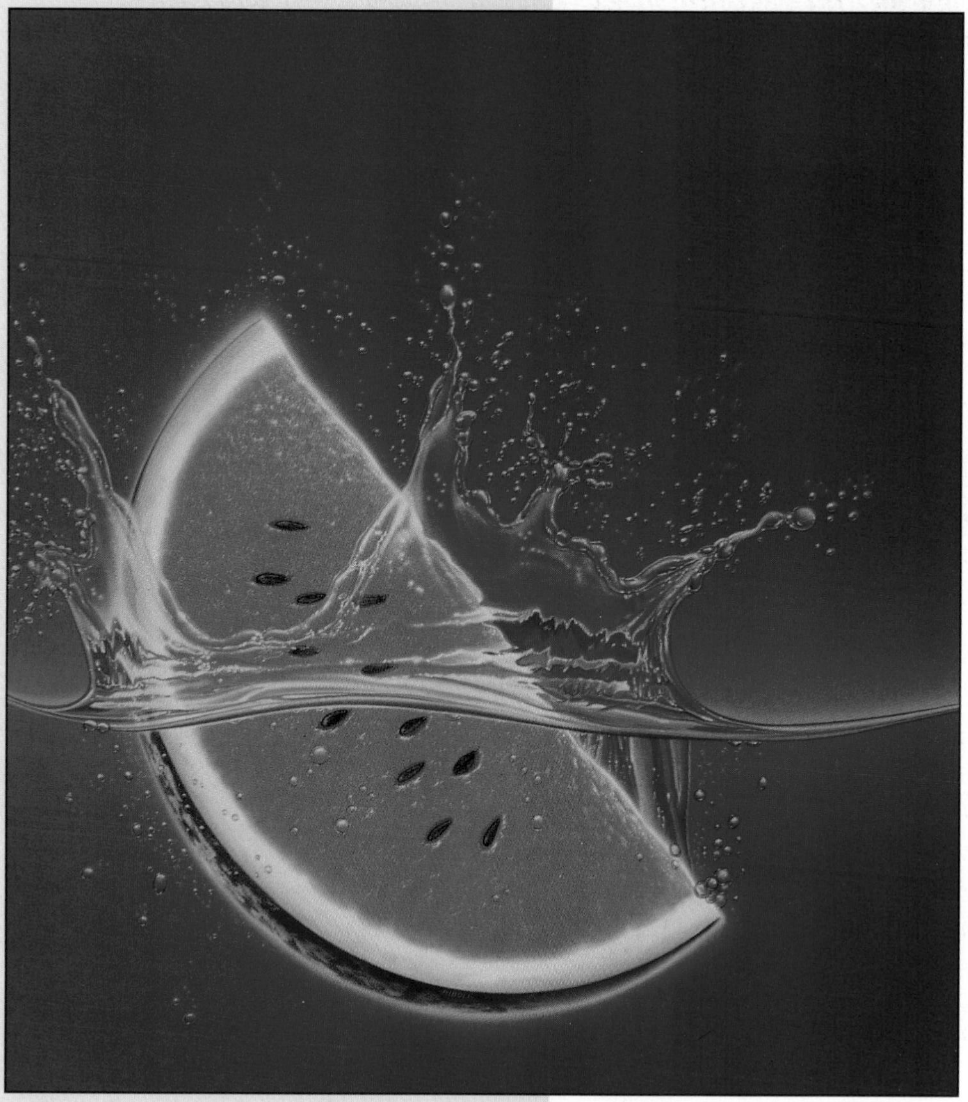

Personal Nutrition

SECOND EDITION

Marie A. Boyle
University of Florida

Gail Zyla

WEST PUBLISHING COMPANY
ST. PAUL • NEW YORK • LOS ANGELES • SAN FRANCISCO

WEST'S COMMITMENT TO THE ENVIRONMENT

In 1906, West Publishing Company began recycling materials left over from the production of books. This began a tradition of efficient and responsible use of resources. Today, up to 95 percent of our legal books and 70 percent of our college texts are printed on recycled, acid-free stock. West also recycles nearly 22 million pounds of scrap paper annually—the equivalent of 181,717 trees. Since the 1960s, West has devised ways to capture and recycle waste inks, solvents, oils, and vapors created in the printing process. We also recycle plastics of all kinds, wood, glass, corrugated cardboard, and batteries, and have eliminated the use of styrofoam book packaging. We at West are proud of the longevity and the scope of our commitment to our environment.

Copyediting: Deborah Cady
Composition: Carlisle Communications
Artwork: Miyake Illustration, Sandra McMahon
Text design and dummy: Roslyn Stendahl, Dapper Design
Cover image: "Watermelon in Water" by Stefano Riboli
Cover design: Roslyn Stendahl, Dapper Design
Indexing: Pat Lewis

Production, Prepress, Printing and Binding by West Publishing Company.

610 Opperman Drive
P.O. Box 64526
St. Paul, MN 55164-0526

Printed in the United States of America

99 98 97 96 95 94 93 8 7 6 5 4 3 2

Library of Congress Cataloging-in-Publication Data

Boyle, Marie A. (Marie Ann)
Personal nutrition / Marie Boyle, Gail Zyla. — 2nd ed.
p. cm.
Includes index.
ISBN 0-314-93333-6 (soft)
1. Nutrition/ I. Zyla, Gail. II. Title.
RA784.B65 1992
613.2—dc20 91–43360
CIP

Photo Credits

Chapter 1 **4** © Mary Kate Denny/Photo Edit; **13** © Williams & Edwards/The Image Bank; **18** Marilyn Herbert; **Chapter 2** **23** © 1990 Robert Brenner/PhotoEdit; **26** Felicia Martinez/Photo Edit; **34** Felicia Martinez-/Photo Edit; **48** (Meats) Ray Stanyard; (all others) The International Diabetes Center, MN; **49** (Legumes) The International Diabetes Center, MN; (all others) Ray Stanyard; **Chapter 3** **58**© Tony Freeman/Photo Edit; **60** © Felicia Martinez/Photo Edit; **68** Ray Stanyard; **70** © Felicia Martinez/Photo Edit; **71** Alan Oddie/Photo Edit; **73** © Juan-Pablo Lira/The Image Bank, Courtesy of USDA; **83** Ray Stanyard; **Chapter 4** **91** Ray Stanyard; **103** © Felicia Martinez/Photo Edit; **104** Ray Stanyard; **106** Felicia Martinez/Photo Edit; **118** Ray Stanyard; **Chapter 5** **126** © Tony Freeman/Photo Edit; **135** Courtesy of Dr. Robert S. Goodhard, M.D.; **136** ©David Young-Wolff/Photo Edit; **139** Ray Stanyard; **140** Felicia Martinez/ Photo Edit; **146** (top three photographs) Tony Freeman/Photo Edit; (bottom left) Leslye Borden/Photo Edit; (bottom middle and right) Tony Freeman/Photo Edit; **Chapter 6** **151** Courtesy of Parke-Davis and Company; **154** © Tony Freeman/Photo Edit; **159** Ray Stanyard; **160** Ray Stanyard;

Continued on last page of index

To our parents

David and Marie Boyle
and
Edward and June Zyla

About the Authors

Marie Ann Boyle, Ph.D., R.D., received her B.A. in psychology from the University of Maine in 1975, her M.S. in nutrition from Florida State University in 1985, and her Ph.D. in nutrition, food, and movement science from Florida State University in 1992. Currently she teaches undergraduate and graduate nutrition and health-related courses at the University of Florida, and supervises students' clinical and community rotations in the American Dietetic Association's Approved Preprofessional Practice Program (AP4). In the past, she has taught nutrition courses at Tallahassee Community College and at Florida State University, and a Culinary Hearts course for the American Heart Association. She also acts as a consultant dietitian and continues to write nutrition literature. She assisted in revising and preparing the third and fourth editions of *Understanding Nutrition,* and continues to update and revise a chapter on Domestic and World Hunger for *Understanding Nutrition.* She has also worked in the outpatient and dietetics departments of the Maine Medical Center in Portland and as a nutritionist for a children's weight-loss camp in Florida.

Gail Zyla, M.S., R.D., received her B.S. in home economics from Valparaiso University, Valparaiso, Indiana, in 1985 and completed her dietetic internship at Massachusetts General Hospital, Boston, in 1986. She received her M.S. in nutrition and communications from Boston University in 1988. Currently she serves as senior editor of the *Tufts University Diet & Nutrition Letter* in Boston. She also writes about nutrition for a variety of consumer publications. Her articles have appeared in magazines including *American Health, McCall's, Reader's Digest,* and *Redbook.*

Contents in Brief

Contents

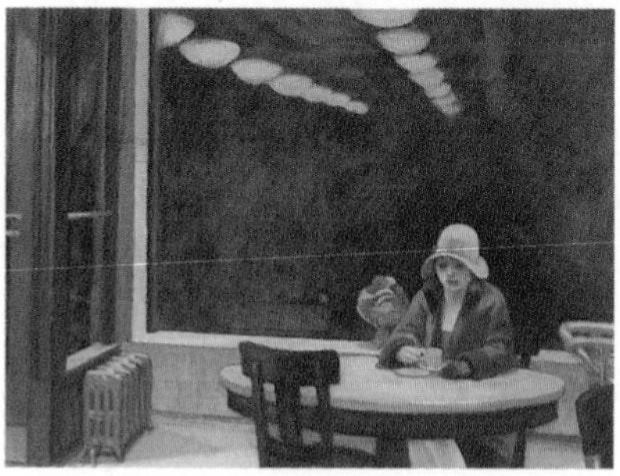

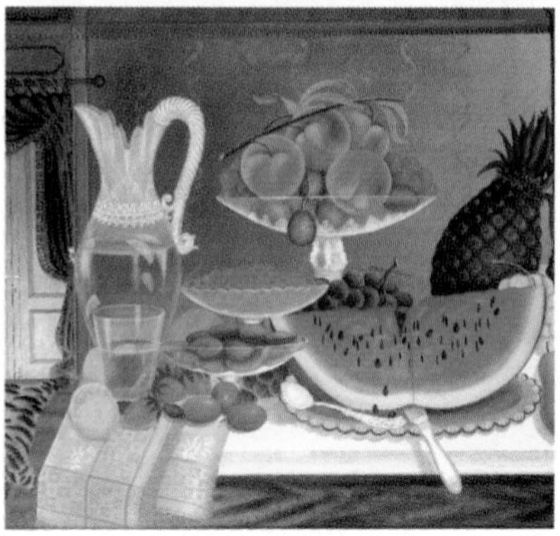

CHAPTER 7

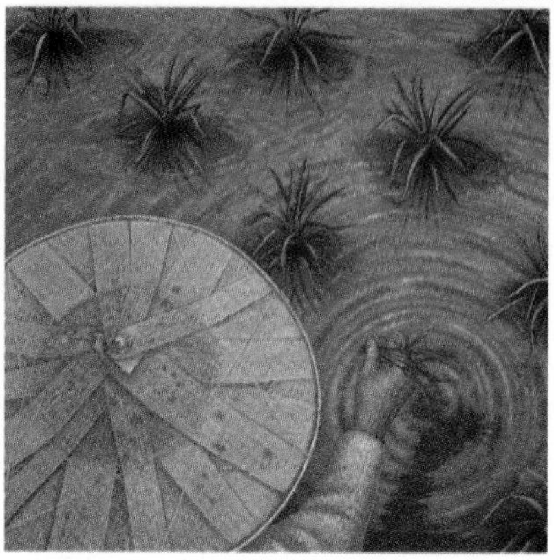

CHAPTER 8

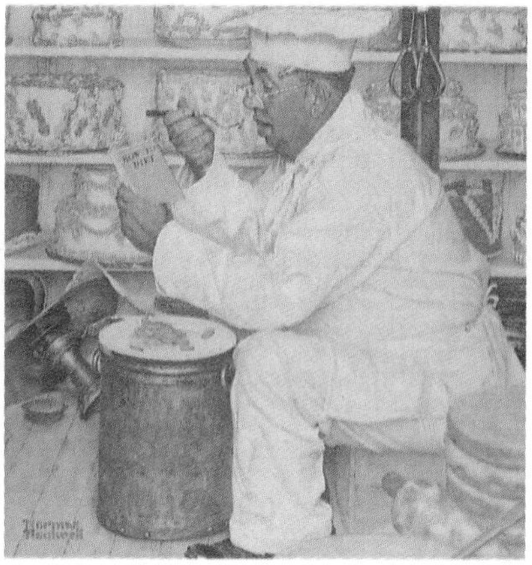

CHAPTER 9

Nutrition and Fitness 241

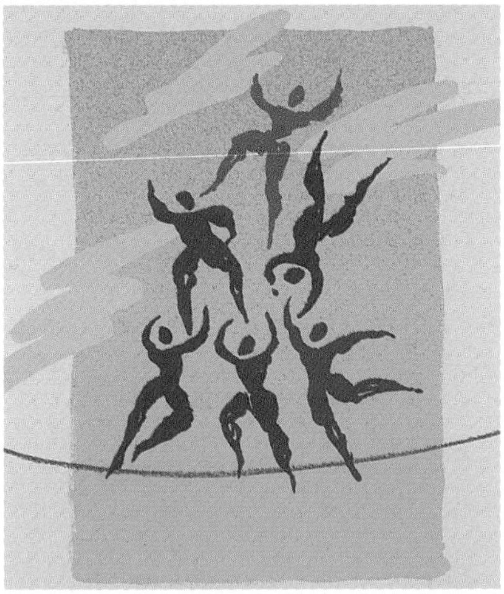

CHAPTER 10

The Life Cycle: Conception Through Adulthood 277

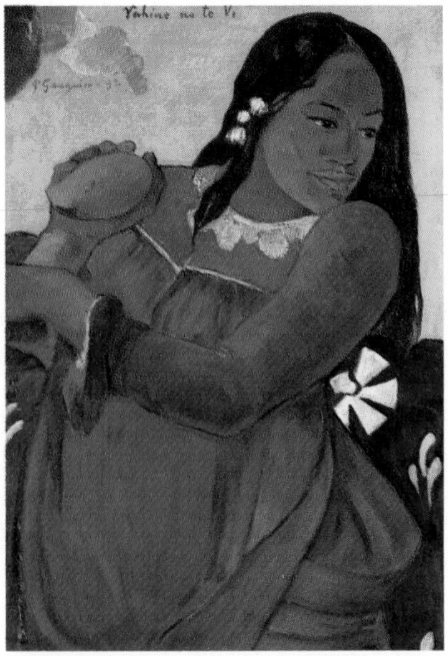

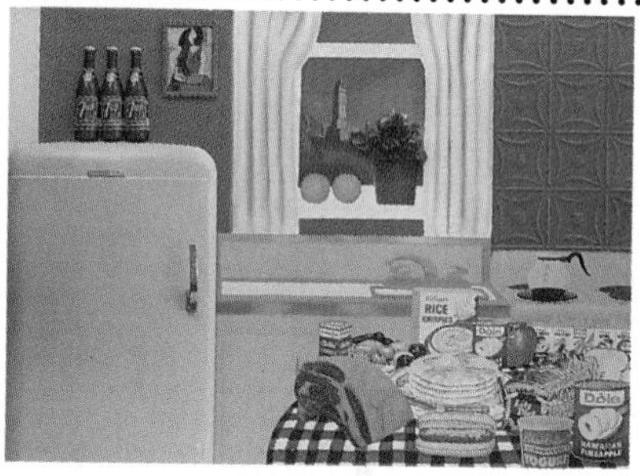

To The Reader

With this edition of *Personal Nutrition,* we have enjoyed monitoring the changes that have taken place in the field of nutrition and in our readers' needs. Our challenges have been to teach not only the facts about nutrition but also how to evaluate them and, most importantly, to motivate readers to apply what they learn in daily life. It is our hope that you will enjoy the new information and the new features of this text in its new full-color format.

Nutrition is a subject that is forever changing, and it is important that you, as a consumer of nutrition information, have the knowledge to evaluate the nutrition issues and controversies that confront you, both today and tomorrow. Newspapers are quick to print nutrition breakthroughs, new fad diets appear monthly on the magazine racks, and television advertising extols the wonders of products of questionable value. These are examples of the nutrition claims that bombard us and that we must evaluate and assess. This edition of *Personal Nutrition* continues to provide a sieve through which to separate the valid nutrition claims from the rest.

Chapter 1 provides a personal invitation to eat well for optimum health and assists the reader in becoming a sophisticated consumer of new nutrition information. Chapter 2 introduces the basic nutrients the body needs along with the nutrition tools and most recent guidelines needed to help make sound food choices. Chapters 3 through 7 present the nutrients and show how they all work together to nourish the body. Chapter 8 discusses weight control and offers nutrition and behavior modification principles for weight loss and weight gain. Chapter 9 addresses the relationships between nutrition and personal fitness. Chapter 10 describes the special nutrition needs and concerns of the various stages of the life cycle from conception through old age. Chapter 11 looks at foods, themselves, and offers perspective on our food supply and food safety, as well as a glimpse at food and nutrition in the twenty-first century.

The *Nutrition Action* features that appear in every chapter are new to this edition, and keep you abreast of current topics important to the nutrition-conscious consumer. The *Nutrition Action* features address topics such as fast foods, smart snacking, sweet alternatives to sugar, fat substitutes, amino acid supplements, vitamin-mineral supplements, diet and blood pressure, yo-yo dieting, behavior modification, fitness aids and supplements, dental health, caffeine, and food and the environment.

Each chapter also offers a practical *Consumer Tips* feature to provide strategies for a nutritionally sound lifestyle. They include stocking your cupboards with nutritious staple goods, supermarketing, adding fiber to the diet, recipe modification, choosing healthful ethnic foods, preserving vitamins in foods, seasoning foods without excess salt, defensive dining, packing healthful bag lunches, making meals for one, and food safety for microwave oven users.

Scorecards are a hands-on feature included in every chapter. *Scorecards* allow readers to evaluate their own nutrition behaviors and knowledge in many areas. Some of the *Scorecards* assess readers' longevity, their application of the current dietary guidelines, their food label literacy, the amounts of carbohydrate, fat, and protein in their diets, their own appropriate weight and level of physical activity, their aging I.Q., and the safety of their own kitchens.

The final special feature of each chapter is the *Spotlight*—many are brand new to this edition, and the others have been updated. Each addresses a common concern people have about nutrition. *Spotlight* topics include nutrition and the media, food labels, nutrition and cancer, diet and heart disease, the vegetarian diet, nutrition savvy in cooking to preserve nutrients, water, eating disorders, nutrition and stress, and alcohol and nutrition. The final *Spotlight* presents the many factors that influence nutrition and hunger among the people of the world and concludes that the practical suggestions offered throughout this book for attaining the ideals of personal nutrition are the very suggestions that best support the health of the whole earth as well. The *Spotlights* continue in their question and answer format to encourage the reader to ask further questions about nutrition issues. We encourage you to ask us questions, too, in care of the publisher.

We are pleased that you desire to learn about the fascinating subject of nutrition. We hope that the book speaks to you personally, and that you find it practical for your everyday use. We hope, too, that by reading it, you may enhance your own personal nutrition and health.

Marie Boyle
Gail Zyla
February 1992

Acknowledgments

We are grateful to the many individuals who have made contributions to this second edition of *Personal Nutrition*. We thank Diane H. Morris, Ph.D., R.D., of Mainstream Nutrition, for her revisions to Chapters 6, 7, and 11, her work on the *Spotlights* that accompany Chapters 3, 4, and 10, and her tireless enthusiasm and support throughout this project. We thank Susan Sewell-Fenbers, M.S., R.D., for her update of Chapter 9, and her contributions to the *Spotlight* features in Chapters 2, 6, 8, and 9. We thank Felicia Busch, M.S., R.D., for her work on specific pieces on snacking, recipe modification, and supermarketing. Thanks also to Bob Geltz and Betty Hands and their staff at ESHA research for creating the food composition table (Appendix F), and the computerized diet analysis program that accompanies this book. We also wish to thank Eleanor Whitney, Ph.D., R.D., from whose original work on this book we continue to draw inspiration. We appreciate the artwork of Randy Miyake and Sandra McMahon.

We are grateful to our editors Peter Marshall, Jayne Lindesmith, and Becky Tollerson whose efforts have greatly enhanced the quality of this book. We also owe much to those who provided expert reviews of the manuscript:

Ellen Brennan
San Antonio College

Susan J. Cooper
Glendale Community College

Donald W. Janes
University of Southern Colorado

Rita Johnson
Indiana University of Pennsylvania

Noelle Kehrberg
Western Carolina University

Gregg Kloss
Anoka-Ramsey Community College

Carolyn Knutson
Clackamas Community College

Ann P. Leftwich
University of Central Oklahoma

Shortie McKinney
Drexel University

John Milner
Pennsylvania State University

Connie Mueller
Illinois State University

Anne Murphy
University of Michigan–Flint

Elizabeth Randall
SUNY–University of Buffalo

Carol Reynolds
Rancho Santiago College

Joyce Rizzo
Indiana University of Pennsylvania

Kathy Sielski
Erie Community College–North Campus

Linda Vaughan
Arizona State University

Finally, we thank the instructors and students who first wanted this book for telling us what they needed to know and for their interest in personal nutrition.

Personal Nutrition

SECOND EDITION

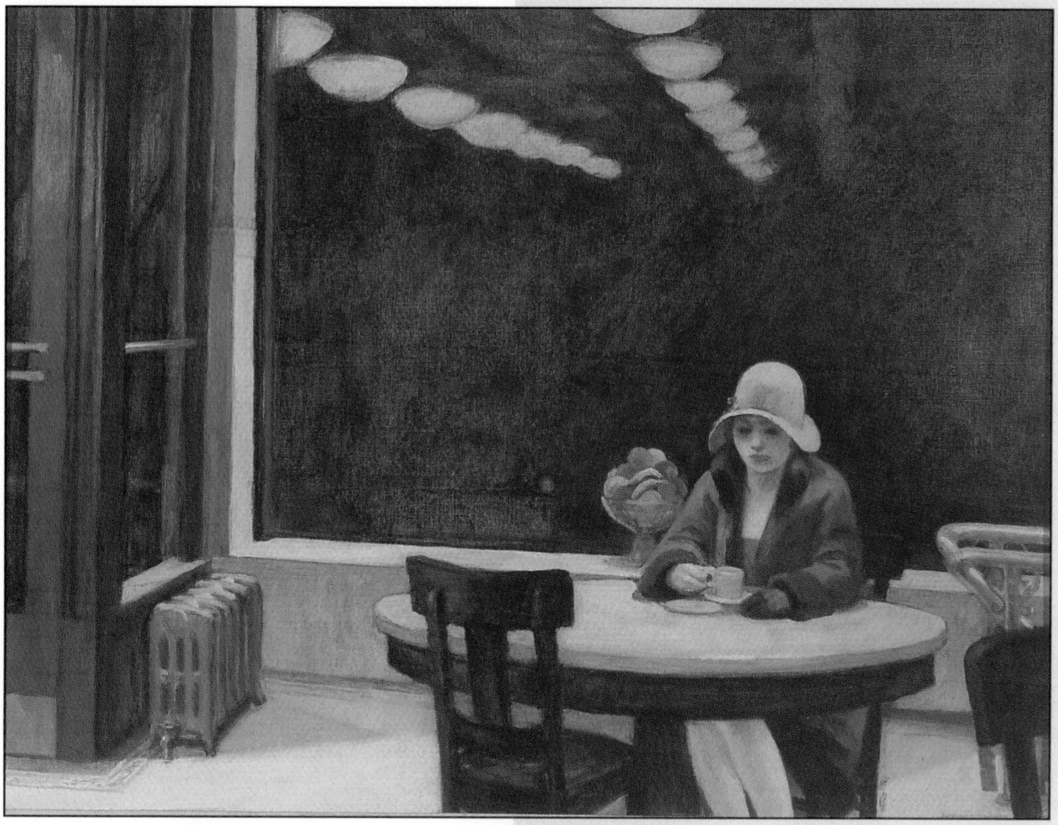

Edward Hopper, Automat, Des Moines Art Center Permanent Collection, purchased with funds from the Edmundson Art Foundation, Inc., 1958. 2.

CHAPTER 1
The Art of Understanding Nutrition

> *Tell me what you eat, and I will tell you what you are.*
> *—Anthelme Brillat-Savarin*

Contents

Ask Yourself . . . ?

Which of these statements about nutrition are true, and which are false? For the false statements, what *is* true?

1. The way people choose to live and eat can affect their health and quality of life as they age.
2. Dieting can be more hazardous to health than remaining overweight.
3. It is wise to pick out certain fruits, vegetables, grains, meats, and dairy products that you like and then eat those same foods pretty much every day.
4. You can order a low-fat, balanced meal at a fast-food outlet.
5. A nutritionist is a professional certified to advise people on nutrition.
6. The more current a dietary claim, the more you can trust its accuracy and reliability.
7. Milk is such a perfect food that it alone can provide all the nutrients a person needs.
8. An author who makes a statement about nutrition in a published book has a legal obligation to tell the truth.
9. Dietary excesses have been linked to five of the ten leading causes of death in the United States.
10. Certain foods, such as cookies and candy, are bad for you and cannot be included in a healthful diet.

Answers: 1. True. 2. True. 3. False. It is unwise to eat the same foods day in and day out; your diet will lack variety and probably will not supply all the dietary constituents your body needs. 4. True. 5. False. A nutritionist is a person who claims to specialize in the study of nutrition, but some are self-described experts whose training is questionable. 6. False. If a nutrition claim is too new, it may not have been tested adequately. Findings must be confirmed many times over by experiment and considered in light of other knowledge before they can be translated into recommendations for the public. 7. False. Milk rates as an excellent source of nutrients such as calcium and protein, but it contains only very small amounts of iron and several other nutrients. 8. False. Authors who write about nutrition are morally, but not legally, obligated to tell the truth. 9. True. 10. False. Any food can be fit into a healthful eating plan. It's the total diet, not individual foods, that can be either good or bad for health.

Stroll down the aisle of any supermarket and you'll see all manner of foods touted as "low in cholesterol," "fat-free," "reduced-calorie," and "made with oat bran," to name just a few claims. Flip through the pages of just about any magazine and you're likely to find advice on how to lose weight as well as advertisements for vitamin and mineral supplements boasted as remedies for everything from arthritis to premenstrual syndrome. Walk into any gym and you'll probably hear an athlete or two discussing the merits of one or another performance-enhancing food or diet. Pick up a newspaper and you might notice headlines here and there regarding the federal government's ongoing debate with industry over how to label foods. What it all boils down to is that nutrition has become part and parcel of the American lifestyle.

It wasn't always that way, however. The field of nutrition is a relative newcomer on the scientific block. Although Hippocrates recognized diet as a component of health back in 400 B.C., it has been only a hundred years or so since researchers have begun to understand that carbohydrates, fats, and proteins are needed for normal growth. The next nutrition breakthrough—the discovery of the first vitamin—occurred in the early 1900s. And it wasn't until 1934, when an organization called the American Institute of Nutrition was formed, that nutrition was officially looked upon as a distinct field of study.[1*] It took several more decades before nutrition achieved its current status as one of the most talked about scientific disciplines around.

*Reference notes for each chapter are found in Appendix E.

Today we spend billions of dollars each year to investigate the many aspects of nutrition, a science that encompasses the study of not only vitamins, minerals, and the like but also subjects as diverse as alcohol, caffeine, and pesticides. In addition, nutrition scientists continually add to our understanding of the impact food has on our bodies by examining research in chemistry, physics, biology, biochemistry, immunology, and other nutrition-related fields.

A number of disciplines have made contributions to the study of nutrition. Related fields include psychology, anthropology, geography, ethics, economics, sociology, aesthetics, and philosophy.

At the same time that science has shown that to some extent we really are what we eat, so to speak, many consumers are more confused than ever about how to translate the steady stream of new findings about nutrition into healthful eating. As Table 1–1 illustrates, people's priorities regarding diet have changed dramatically over the past decade. Each additional nugget of nutrition news that comes along raises new concerns: Is caffeine bad for me? Does oat bran reduce cholesterol? Should I take vitamin supplements? Will diet pills work? Can a sports drink improve my performance? Are pesticides posing a hazard?

Some manufacturers of food and nutrition-related products as well as many members of the media feed into the confusion by offering a myriad of unreliable products and misleading dietary advice targeted to health-

Table 1–1

Nature of Shoppers' Concerns about Diet

While consumers have long placed importance on the nutritional profile of their diets, the nature of those concerns has changed over the years. The figures below show how respondents to a national survey answered this question in 1983 and 1991:

What is it about the nutritional content of what you eat that concerns you and your family most?

	1983 Total %	1991 Total %	Percentage Point Change
Fat content, low fat	9	42	+33
Cholesterol levels	5	37	+32
Salt content, less salt	18	22	+ 4
Calories, low calories	6	12	+ 6
Sugar content, less sugar	21	12	− 9
Vitamin/mineral content	24	15	− 9
Preservatives	22	8	−14
Making sure we get a balanced diet	10	5	− 5
Chemical additives	27	8	−19
Freshness, purity, no spoilage	14	4	−10
As natural as possible, not overly processed	12	3	− 9
No harmful ingredients, nothing that causes illness/cancer	10	2	− 8
Desire to be healthy, eat what's good for us	0	8	+ 8
Ingredients/content	0	6	+ 6
Excess food coloring, dyes	6	1	− 5

Source: The Food Marketing Institute, *Trends: Consumer Attitudes and the Supermarket,* 1990 and 1991 editions (Washington, D.C.: The Research Department, Food Marketing Institute).

Health fraud conscious deceit, practiced for profit, such as the promotion of a false or unproven product or therapy.
Quackery fraud. A **quack** is a person who practices health fraud.
quack = to boast loudly

conscious consumers. Unfortunately, many consumers fall prey to this vast array of information. Americans spend some $25 billion annually on medical and nutritional **health fraud** and **quackery**, up from only $1 billion to $2 billion in the early 1960s.[2] The problem is so widespread that the U.S. Food and Drug Administration (FDA) ranked false nutritional schemes and food products such as bee pollen, over-the-counter herbal remedies, and wheat germ capsules among its list of top ten health frauds in 1989. In addition, weight-loss gimmicks—skin patches, herbal capsules, grapefruit diet pills, and even magic weight-loss earrings—made the FDA's list, leaving no doubt that nutrition-related quackery is big business.[3] Even more disturbing is that such misinformation can be harmful. One survey of 29,000 claims, treatments, and theories for losing weight found fewer than 6 percent of them effective—and 13 percent dangerous.[4]

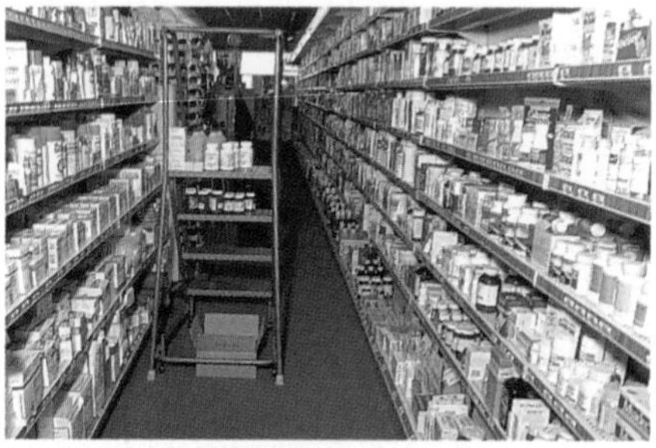

Some stores sell pills and potions to treat "whatever ails you." Vitamins and other supplements are estimated to account for more than 40 percent of total sales in health food stores.[5]

To be sure, the widespread interest in nutrition has generated some positive changes in the marketplace as well. Consider that whereas the sale of low-fat, low-sodium items such as salads in fast-food restaurants was virtually unheard of ten years ago, those eateries can't survive in the current nutrition-conscious environment without offering such healthful fare. (See the Nutrition Action feature later in the chapter for tips on eating healthfully at fast-food outlets.) By the same token, food manufacturers have responded to consumer concern about diet by developing new technologies, such as the creation of fat substitutes, to provide shoppers with an unprecedented number of choices at the supermarket. In 1969 the average grocery store carried only 8,000 items. In 1990, more than 1,000 low-fat and fat-free foods alone were introduced into supermarkets, which now typically stock in the neighborhood of 25,000 products.[6]

Nevertheless, with the amount of nutrition information and the number of food alternatives ever on the rise, it's easy to see why choosing a healthful diet can seem like a daunting task. Fortunately, you don't need a degree in nutrition to put the principles of the science to use in your own life. A basic understanding of nutrition can go a long way in helping you protect your health (and your wallet). This book will lay the foundation you need to take the science out of the laboratory and move it into your kitchen, both today and tomorrow. It provides a sieve through which you can separate valid nutrition information from the rest as you confront the new issues and controversies that are sure to arise. The first step is exploring the current thrust of the field of nutrition.

Nutrition and Health Promotion

Time was when scientists investigating the role diet plays in health zeroed in on the consequences of getting too little of one or another nutrient. Until the end of World War II, in fact, nutrition researchers concentrated on eliminating deficiency diseases such as **goiter**, a condition in which the thyroid gland swells as a result of a lack of the mineral iodine, and **pellagra**, inflammation of the skin due to deficiency of the B vitamin niacin.

Goiter (GOY-ter) enlargement of the thyroid gland due to iodine deficiency.
Pellagra (pell-AY-gra) niacin deficiency characterized by diarrhea, inflammation of the skin, and, in severe cases, mental disorders.

These days, however, the focus is just the opposite. While deficiency diseases have been virtually eliminated in America because of our country's abundant food supply and the practice of fortifying foods with essential nutrients (adding iodine to salt, for example), diseases related to dietary excess and imbalance run rampant. Five of the ten leading causes of death—namely heart disease, cancer, stroke, diabetes, and atherosclerosis (hardening of the arteries)—have been linked to diet. Another three are associated with excessive alcohol consumption—liver disease, accidents, and suicides. Together these eight problems account for more than 70 percent of the two million deaths that occur each year, not to mention hospitalizations, lost time on the job, and poor quality of life among many Americans. Dietary excesses and imbalances contribute to other ills as well, including high blood pressure, dental disease, and osteoporosis.[7]

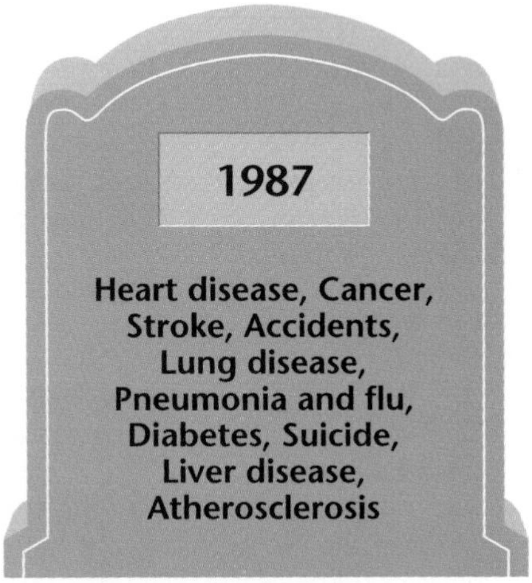

The Ten Leading Causes of Death

That's not to say that diet is the sole culprit responsible for those conditions. A number of environmental, behavioral, social, and genetic factors work together to determine a person's likelihood of falling victim to a disease. Diet notwithstanding, someone who smokes, doesn't exercise regularly, and has a parent who suffered a heart attack, for example, is more likely to end up with heart disease than a nonsmoker who works out habitually and does not have a close relative with heart disease. The way to alter disease risk is to concentrate on changing the day-to-day habits that can be controlled. The results can be significant.

Consider that when researchers looked at the habits of a group of nearly 7,000 Californians, they were able to pinpoint six common lifestyle elements among those who were particularly healthy for their age. Adequate sleep, consistent eating patterns, regular exercise, abstinence from smoking, little or no alcohol use, and weight control all made an impact on the adults' **physiological age.** The effects of these factors were cumulative. That is, the more of those six positive health practices the adults followed, the better their health, regardless of their age in calendar years. In fact, the physical well-being of those who reported adhering to all six positive health practices was consistently about the same as that of people *30 years younger* who followed few or none of them.[8] The six health practices recommended follow:

Physiological age age as estimated from the body's health and probable life expectancy. **Chronological age** is measured in years from birth.

1. *Get adequate sleep.* People who typically sleep about 8 hours a night are physiologically younger.
2. *Eat regular meals.* People who don't skip meals are physiologically younger.
3. *Maintain desirable weight.* People who maintain their body weight close to the average for their height and sex are physiologically younger.
4. *Do not smoke.* People who never take up the habit are physiologically younger.
5. *Drink alcohol moderately or not at all.* People who abstain or who imbibe modest amounts are physiologically younger.
6. *Exercise regularly.* People who work out on a habitual basis are physiologically younger.

These findings illustrate that although you cannot alter the year of your birth, you can change the probable length and quality of your life. Nutrition is involved in at least half of the lifestyle recommendations above, leaving no doubt that it plays a key role in maintaining good health. The Longevity Game Scorecard further demonstrates the point.

Recognizing diet's vital influence on health, in 1988 the Surgeon General released a landmark statement called *The Surgeon General's Report on Nutrition and Health,* which outlines ways to improve health with sound nutrition practices. A year later, a committee of scientists gathered by the National

The Longevity Game Scorecard

You can't look into a crystal ball to find out how long you will live. But you can get a rough idea of the number of years you're likely to survive based largely on your lifestyle today as well as certain "givens," such as your family history. To do so, play the Longevity Game.

Start at the top line—age 74, the average life expectancy for adults in the United States today. For each of the 11 lifestyle areas add or subtract years as instructed. If an area doesn't apply, go on to the next one. If you are not sure of the exact number to add or subtract, make a guess. Don't take the score too seriously, but do pay attention to those areas where you lose years; they could point to habits you might want to change.

Start with:	74
1. Exercise	______
2. Relaxation	______
3. Driving	______
4. Blood pressure	______
5. 65 and working	______
6. Family history	______
7. Smoking	______
8. Drinking	______
9. Gender	______
10. Weight	______
11. Age	______
Your final score	______

1. Exercise. If your job requires regular, vigorous activity or if you work out each day, add three years. If you don't get much exercise at home, on the job, or at play, subtract three years.
2. Relaxation. If you have a "laid back" approach to life (you roll with the punches), add three years. If you're aggressive, hard driving, or anxious (you suffer from sleepless nights or bite your nails), subtract three years. If you consider yourself unhappy, subtract another year.
3. Driving. Drivers under 30 who have received traffic tickets in the past year or who have been involved in an accident should subtract four years. Other violations, minus one. If you always wear seatbelts, add a year.
4. Blood pressure. While high blood pressure is a major contributor to common killers—heart attacks and strokes—it can be lowered effectively through drugs and changes in lifestyle. The problem is that rises in blood pressure can't be felt, so many victims don't know they have it and therefore never receive lifesaving treatment. If you *know* your blood pressure, add one year.
5. 65 and working. If you are at the traditional retirement age or older and still working, add three.
6. Family history. If any grandparent has reached age 85, add two; if all grandparents have reached age 80, add six. If a parent died of a stroke or heart attack before age 50, minus four. If a parent or brother or sister has (or had) diabetes since childhood, minus three.
7. Smoking. Cigarette smokers who finish more than two packs a day, minus eight; one or two packs a day, minus six; one-half to one pack, minus three.
8. Drinking. If you drink two cocktails (or beers or glasses of wine) a day, subtract one year. For each additional daily libation, subtract two.
9. Gender. Women live longer than men. Females add three years; males subtract three years.
10. Weight. If you avoid eating fatty foods and don't add salt to your meals, your heart will probably remain healthy longer, entitling you to add two years.

    Now, weigh in: overweight by 50 pounds or more, minus eight; 30 to 40 pounds, minus four; 10 to 29 pounds, minus two.
11. Age. How long you have already lived can help predict how much longer you'll survive. If you're under 30, the jury is still out. But if your age is 30 to 39, plus two; 40 to 49, plus three; 50 to 69, plus four; 70 or over, plus five.

Source: From "The Longevity Game," by Northwestern Mutual Life Insurance Company, with permission.

Research Council published an equally important document titled *Diet and Health,* which provides similar guidelines for reducing disease risk through diet.[9]

Table 1–2 summarizes the dietary recommendations of the two preceding sources. As you read it, keep in mind that while everyone can benefit from

Table 1–2

Eating to Beat the Odds

Dietary Recommendation	To Help Reduce the Risk of
Fat: Reduce total fat intake to 30% or less of calories. Reduce saturated fat intake to less than 10% of calories and the intake of cholesterol to less than 300 milligrams daily.[a]	Some types of cancer, obesity, heart disease, and possibly gallbladder disease.
Weight: Achieve and maintain a desirable weight.[a]	Diabetes, high blood pressure, stroke, cancers (especially breast and uterine), and gallbladder disease.
Carbohydrates and fiber: Increase consumption of fruits, vegetables, legumes, and whole grains.[a]	Diabetes, heart disease, and some types of cancer.
Sodium: Limit daily intake of salt (sodium chloride).[b]	High blood pressure and stroke.
Alcohol: Avoid completely or drink only in moderation.[a]	Heart disease, high blood pressure, liver disease, stroke, some forms of cancer, and malformations in babies born to mothers who drink alcohol during pregnancy.
Sugar: Limit consumption and frequency of use.	Cavities.
Calcium: Maintain adequate intake.	Osteoporosis and bone fractures.
Fluoride: Maintain optimal intake.	Cavities.

[a]Pay particular attention to this guideline if you have glucose intolerance, high blood cholesterol or high triglyceride levels, or high blood pressure.
[b]Pay particular attention to this guideline if you have high blood pressure.

Source: Adapted from *Surgeon General's Report on Nutrition and Health: Summary and Recommendations* (Washington, D.C.: U.S. Government Printing Office, 1988), pp. 8–17; and *Diet and Health: Implications for Reducing Chronic Disease Risk—Executive Summary* (Washington, D.C.: National Academy Press, 1989), pp. 10–15.

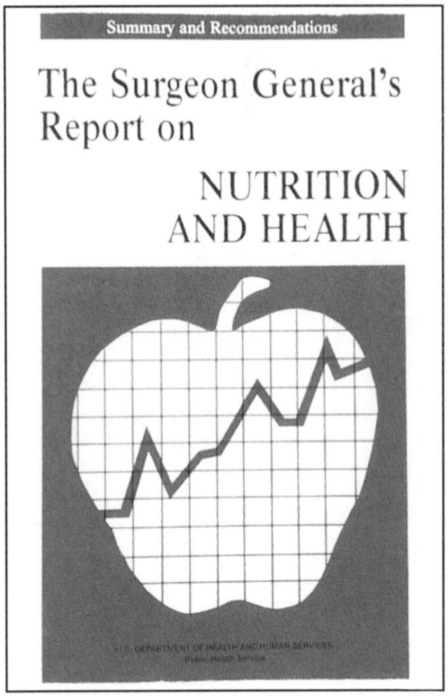

eating a healthful diet that complies with the guidelines, some stand to gain more than others. Those who have high blood cholesterol levels, for instance, are already at risk for heart disease, thereby making it especially important for them to eat a low-fat diet and maintain a healthful weight. By the same token, those who have close relatives with, say, diabetes, would do well to keep their weight down along with paying particular attention to the other nutrition guidelines that help stave off the condition. (The chapters that follow explain the link between diet and chronic diseases in more detail as well as offer advice on how to follow each dietary recommendation.)

The exact proportion dietary factors contribute to each problem can only be estimated, but some experts believe they account for a third or more of all cases of both cancer and heart disease.[10] Moreover, some elements appear to play a more integral role in determining disease risk than others. A high-fat diet, for instance, raises the risk of suffering from some types of cancer, heart disease, and obesity, which in turn contributes to a number of other problems, including diabetes and high blood pressure.

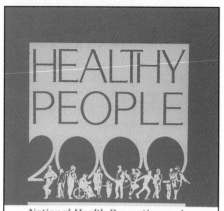

The relative importance of certain dietary recommendations is underscored by their appearance in the U.S. Department of Health and Human Services' official strategy for improving the nation's health during this decade. Dubbed *Healthy People 2000: National Health Promotion and Disease Prevention Objectives,* the plan of action includes a number of nutritional goals geared toward increasing the span of healthy life for Americans:[11]

- Reduce dietary fat consumption among people aged two and older from 36 percent of total calories to an average of 30 percent of calories or less.*
- Increase the amount of fruits and vegetables eaten from two and a half servings a day to five or more, and increase daily servings of grain products (bread and cereals) from three to at least six.
- Decrease salt consumption by increasing from 68 percent to 80 percent the proportion of people who avoid using salt at the table as well as increasing the number of cooks who season dishes without added salt.
- Reduce the prevalence of overweight among adults from 26 percent to 20 percent.

These are just a few of the goals for nutrition spelled out in *Healthy People 2000*. But they represent some of the chief priorities for maintaining health. Much of the practical information presented later in the chapter and in the chapters that follow is aimed at guiding you toward developing eating and lifestyle habits that will help you achieve the goals.

The ABCs of Eating for Health

Given all the statistics and government mandates presented so far, it may seem as if healthful eating is a complicated matter requiring adherence to a rigid regimen in which certain foods must be eliminated from the diet altogether. Fortunately, that's not the case. One of the biggest misconceptions about planning a healthful diet is that some foods, such as carrot and celery sticks, are "good," while others, say cookies and candy, are "bad." Those who think of eating this way often end up feeling guilty every time they "splurge" on a so-called bad food. Individual foods themselves are not bad, however. With a bit of planning, even the most "decadent" high-fat, sugary, high-calorie item can be fit into a healthful pattern. The trick is choosing an overall diet made up mostly of foods that supply adequate nutrients, fiber, and calories without going overboard on fat and sodium.

When you plan a diet for yourself, try to make sure it has certain characteristics: **adequacy** (it will provide enough of the essential nutrients, fiber, and energy—in the form of calories), **balance** (it will not overemphasize any food type or nutrient at the expense of another), **calorie control** (it will supply the amount of energy you need to maintain desirable weight—not more, not less), **moderation** (it will not contain excess amounts of unwanted constituents, such as fat, salt, or sugar), and **variety** (it will be made up of

Adequacy characterizes a diet that provides all of the essential nutrients, fiber, and energy (calories) in amounts sufficient to maintain health.
Balance a feature of a diet that provides a number of types of foods in balance with one another, such that foods rich in one nutrient do not crowd out of the diet foods that are rich in another nutrient.
Calorie control control of energy intake (calories), a feature of a sound diet plan.
Moderation the attribute of a diet that provides no unwanted constituent in excess.
Variety a feature of a diet in which different foods are used for the same purposes on different occasions—the opposite of *monotony*.

*The comparison figures are based on survey results gathered in the 1970s and 1980s and serve as rough estimates of the way Americans are currently eating (and the prevalence of overweight).

Fast Guide to Eating on the Run

Chances are you've stood in line for a burger and fries, slice of pizza, taco, or even just a muffin and coffee at least once this week. You're not alone. Every day an estimated one out of five Americans orders takeout fare from one of the country's 140,000-plus fast-food outlets.[12]

McDonald's golden arches, Domino's Pizza deliveries, and Burger King's "Have It Your Way" slogan are as much a part of our culture as baseball and apple pie. But while a meal eaten on the run fits easily into a busy schedule, it's not necessarily so simple to work it into the dietary guidelines recommended by major health organizations. Two all-beef patties with special sauce and other requisite trimmings, an order of fries, and a milkshake, for example, can chalk up anywhere from 1,000 to 1,500 calories, more than 1,000 milligrams of sodium, and 65 or more grams of fat—more than the amount contained in a half a stick of butter.

The good news is that in the past several years McDonald's and other fast-food giants have begun offering items such as low-fat dairy products and salads that can fit more easily into the high-carbohydrate, low-fat diet experts recommend for good health. With just a little bit of nutrition know-how, you can combine new alternatives with old favorites to place orders more in keeping with the dietary guidelines than the traditional order described above. A regular burger, tossed salad, and cup of low-fat milk, for instance, supply only a third of the calories and a quarter of the fat of a standard double-burger-with-fries-and-a-shake order. (Table 1–3 gives the nutritional breakdown of other fast-food meals.)

The following tips are a guide to help you trim fat and calories from fast-food meals:

- Select an English muffin, bagel, or toast with margarine for breakfast rather than a danish, doughnut, or muffin. You'll save upwards of 150 calories as well as take in about three times less fat. Consider that while a bagel topped with a teaspoon of margarine contains about 200 calories and 5 grams of fat, many takeout muffins contain in the neighborhood of 350 calories and 13 grams of fat.
- Buy breakfast sandwiches or entrees with Canadian bacon or ham instead of sausage. Whereas a three-inch sausage patty provides 200 calories and 17 grams of fat, two slices of Canadian bacon contribute only 85 calories and 4 grams of fat. Three slices of cured bacon supply about 110 calories and 9 grams of fat.
- Sweeten your pancakes with syrup or spread your toast with jelly, but hold the butter. Each tablespoon of butter you spread on your pancakes con-

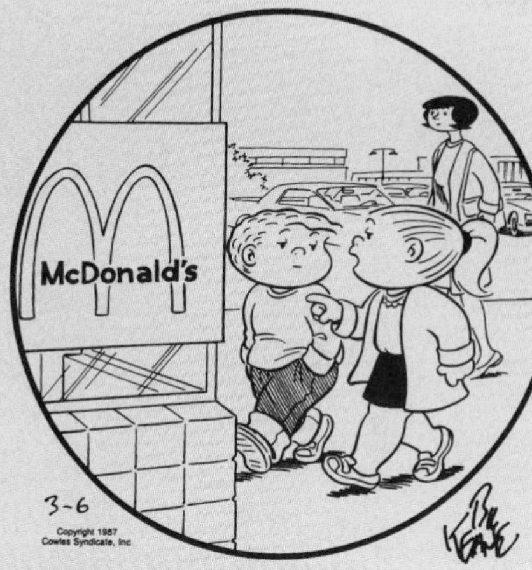

"Before he opened this he had a farm."
Reprinted with special permission of King Features Syndicate, Inc.

tributes 100 calories, virtually all of which come from fat. A tablespoon of syrup or jelly, on the other hand, adds only 50 calories and not a trace of fat.

- Hold the mayo. Each dollop of that condiment adds to a dish about 100 calories, nearly all of which are fat. Most fast-food sandwiches include more than just one spoonful of mayo in their toppings and special sauces. The same goes for tartar sauce. Order a fish sandwich without it, and you'll trim at least 70 fat-laden calories (the amount in just one tablespoon) from your meal.
- Opt for a side salad moistened with reduced-calorie dressing with your burger instead of French fries and ketchup. You'll trim at least 150 calories and a good deal of fat from your meal.
- Wash your meal down with two-percent-fat milk instead of a milkshake, thereby cutting the fat and calorie count at least in half.

Table 1–3

What's in an Order?[a]

	Calories	Grams of Fat	Milligrams of Sodium
Fat and Calories To Go			
Double burger with sauce	625	40	880
Milkshake	410	10	190
French fries (regular size)	240	15	120
Total	1,275	65	1,190
Fish sandwich with cheese and tartar sauce	495	25	676
Soda (12 ounces)	150	0	15
French fries (regular size)	240	15	120
Total	885	40	811
Chicken nuggets (6)	310	20	700
Apple pie	280	15	400
Coffee with cream	65	5	15
Total	655	40	1,115
Slim Pickin's			
Single burger	290	13	435
Tossed salad with low-calorie dressing	50	1	445
Low-fat milk (8 ounces)	105	2	125
Total	445	16	1,005
Baked potato (plain)	150	trace	5
Margarine (1 pat)	35	4	45
Tossed salad with low-calorie dressing	50	1	445
Low-fat milk (8 ounces)	105	2	125
Total	340	7	620
Cheese pizza (1 slice)	155	5	455
Tossed salad with low-calorie dressing	50	1	445
Orange juice (8 ounces)	110	0	0
Total	315	6	900

[a]Figures represent the average nutrient values for similar items from three or more fast-food chains.

Source: Adapted from C. Roberts, Fast-food fare: Consumer guidelines, *New England Journal of Medicine* 321 (1989): 754.

Table 1–4

Topping It Off

	Calories per Tablespoon	Grams of Fat per Tablespoon
Creamy Italian dressing	70	8
Reduced-calorie Italian dressing	15	2
Imitation bacon bits	30	2
Sunflower seeds	50	4
Chopped egg	15	1
Grated process cheese	25	2
Seasoned croutons	5	trace
Raisins	28	trace

Source: U.S. Department of Agriculture, Human Nutrition Information Service, Home and Garden Bulletin No. 232–11, *Eating Better When Eating Out Using the Dietary Guidelines,* p. 9.

- Satisfy your sweet tooth with a cup of hot chocolate. Whereas the hot chocolate contains about 100 to 200 calories per cup, sundaes, pies, milkshakes, and other sweets contribute 300 or more calories per serving (and little else in the way of nutrients).
- Don't let the word *chicken* or *fish* fool you. Granted, many health-conscious consumers have heard the advice to choose skinless poultry and fish instead of relatively high-fat red meat. But when it comes to chicken nuggets and fish patties coated with batter and deep fried, it is a different story. Six chicken nuggets, for example, typically contain as many calories (about 300) as an entire burger. What's more, many chicken- and fish-patty sandwiches chalk up as much fat as a pint and a half of ice cream.
- When ordering a pizza, hold the sausage and pepperoni and ask for mushrooms, green pepper, and onions instead. Pizza is an excellent source of calcium—that bone-building mineral many Americans don't get enough of—as well as protein, carbohydrate and a number of other vitamins and minerals. Two slices of *pepperoni* pizza, however, can easily contain 100 more calories and twice as much fat as the same amount topped with onions, green pepper, and/or mushrooms.
- Cover your plate with fresh greens, fruits, and vegetables at the salad bar, but go easy on some of the toppings. A tablespoon here and a tablespoon there of "fixings," such as bacon bits or rich dressing, can turn a low-fat, low-calorie meal into a high-fat, high-calorie extravaganza (see Table 1–4).
- Ask for lots of lettuce and tomatoes and less sour cream and guacamole on your nachos and tacos. A tablespoon of either sour cream or guacamole adds about 25 calories to Mexican fare. A few extra chunks of tomato, on the other hand, supply a negligible number of calories, no fat, and a good deal of vitamin C.
- Order a plain baked potato with a pat of margarine. While a potato with margarine has under 200 calories, spuds covered with bacon and cheese, sour cream, or chili and cheese can contain as many calories and as much fat as a double burger.

different foods rather than the same meals day after day). Equally important, it will suit you; that is, it will consist of foods that fit your personality, family and cultural traditions, lifestyle, and budget. At best, it will be a source of both pleasure and good health.

Any nutrient could be used to demonstrate the importance of dietary *adequacy*. Iron provides a familiar example. It is an essential nutrient, meaning that you must continually replace daily losses of it by eating iron-rich foods. If your diet is not adequate as far as iron goes—that is, it lacks food sources of the mineral—you can develop a condition known as iron-deficiency anemia. The result: You will feel weak, tired, and unenthusiastic; you may suffer from frequent headaches; and you will be able to do little muscular work without experiencing disabling fatigue. If you add iron-rich foods such as meat, fish, poultry, and legumes to your diet, your symptoms will soon disappear. (More information about iron appears in Chapter 7.)

To appreciate the importance of dietary *balance*, consider a second essential nutrient, calcium. Calcium plays a vital role in building a strong frame that can withstand the gradual loss of bone that occurs with age. Thus, adults are advised to consume daily at least two, and preferably more, servings of milk or milk products—the best sources of the bone-building mineral—to meet their calcium needs. Foods that are rich in iron lack calcium, however, and vice versa, so you have to balance the two in your diet.

Balancing the whole diet is a juggling act that, if successful, provides enough, but not too much, of every one of the 40-odd nutrients the body needs for good health. As you will see in the next chapter, food group plans can help you design a diet that is both adequate and balanced by recommending specific amounts of foods from the different groups that should be eaten each day.

Because not all foods that supply essential nutrients such as calcium and iron contain the same number of calories, diets must be planned with *calorie control* in mind. A cup and a half of ice cream, for example, has about the same amount of calcium as a cup of milk, but the ice cream may contain more than 500 calories, while the milk may have only 90. When it comes to iron, a three-ounce serving of beef pot roast provides the same amount of iron as a three-ounce serving of canned water-packed tuna. But whereas the beef contains 325 calories, the tuna adds only 175 to the diet. The choice of which one to eat depends on personal preference as well as the calorie content of the other foods in the diet.

Nutrient dense refers to a food that supplies large amounts of nutrients relative to the number of calories it contains. The higher the level of nutrients and the fewer the number of calories, the more nutrient dense the food is.

Those who are trying to limit the number of calories they take in each day should be sure to include foods that are rich in nutrients but relatively low in calories. Such foods are referred to as **nutrient dense.** Low-fat milk, for example, contains more calcium, protein, vitamin D, and vitamin A for its calories than ice cream. Hence, it is more nutrient dense. Figure 1–1 compares the nutrient density of ice cream and plain yogurt.

Diet Planning Principles

- Adequacy—enough of each type of food.
- Balance—not too much of any type of food.
- Calorie control—not too many or too few calories.
- Moderation—not too much fat, salt, or sugar.
- Variety—as many different foods as possible.

Another principle of planning a healthful diet is doing everything in *moderation*. In other words, try to eat meals that do not contain excessive amounts of any one nutrient, particularly dietary fat—the culprit linked to a number of chronic diseases. That's not to say that you should choose only foods that supply little or no fat. Such an approach is unrealistic and will only lead to frustration. A more moderate philosophy to adopt is the "80/20 rule": Try to eat low-fat, nutrient-dense foods (and exercise) at least 80 percent of

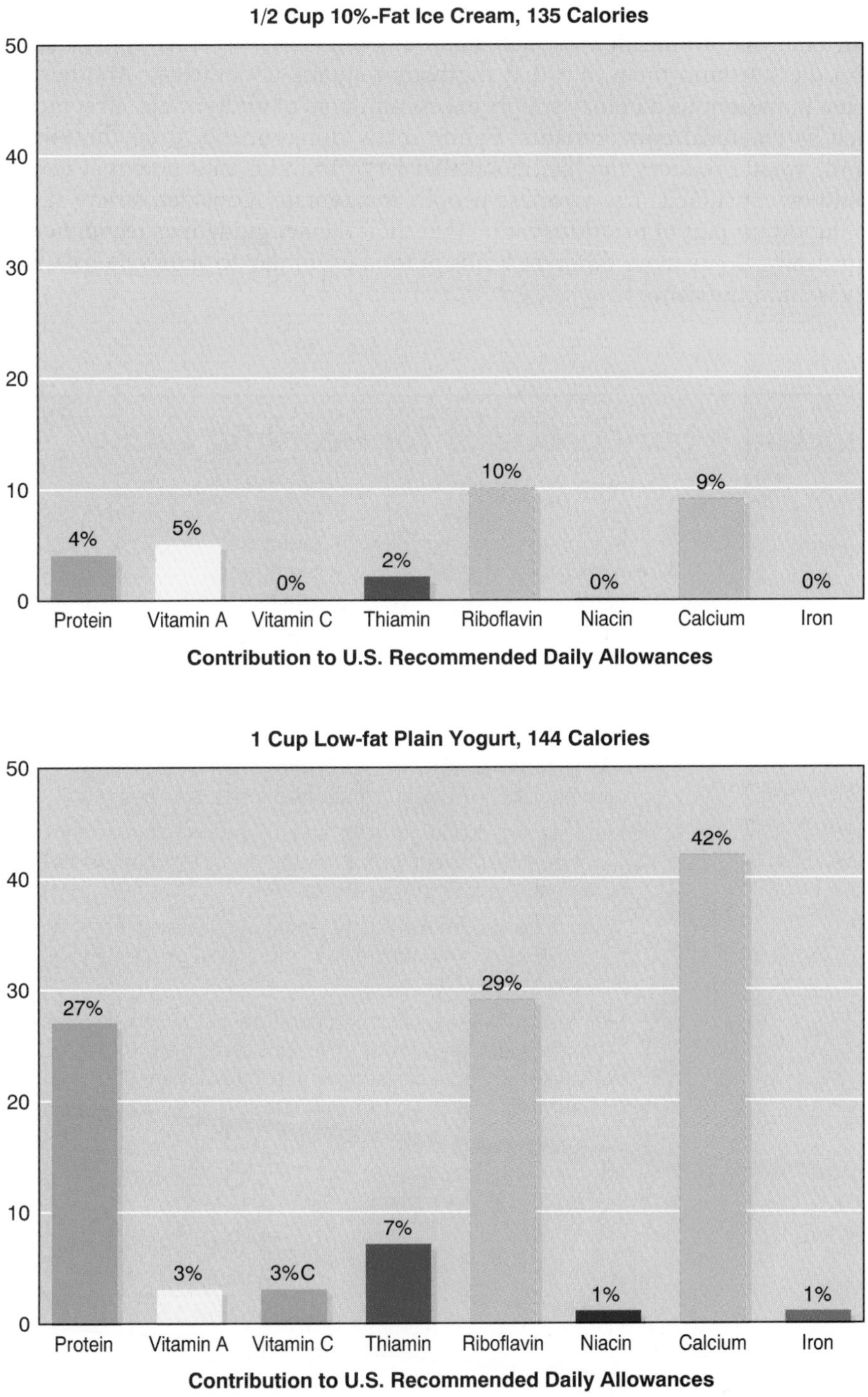

● *Figure 1–1*

Nutrient Density of Ice Cream and Plain Yogurt

The figures show the contribution that ½ cup of ice cream and 1 cup of yogurt make to the U.S. Recommended Daily Allowances for protein, vitamin A, vitamin C, thiamin, riboflavin, niacin, calcium, and iron. While both contain about the same number of calories, compared with the ice cream, the yogurt provides nearly seven times as much protein, three times the riboflavin, and almost five times as much calcium. Thus, the yogurt has a higher nutrient density.

Source: Courtesy of National Dairy Council®. *Comparison Cards*, 1990.

the time, and you're not likely to reverse their benefits to your health if you splurge here and there the remaining 20 percent of the time.

Finally, it is generally held that *variety* is an important characteristic of a healthful diet for two reasons, aside from the sheer monotony of eating the

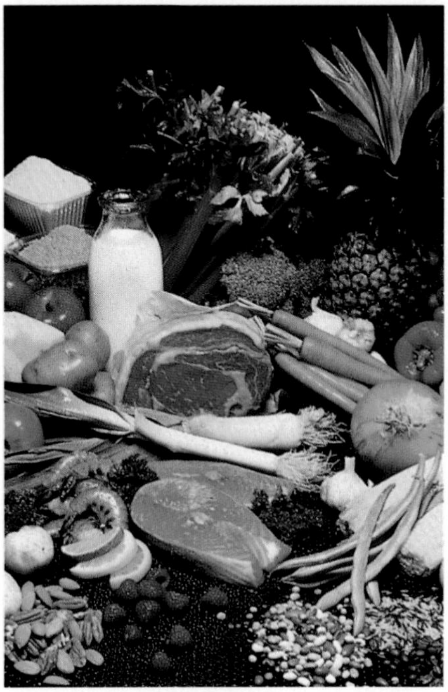

Variety fosters good nutrition.

same foods day after day. One is that some foods may be better sources of nutrients that are needed in such small amounts that we don't consciously plan diets around them, but that the body requires nonetheless. Another is that a monotonous diet may supply excess amounts of undesirable substances such as chemical contaminants. Eating many different foods, on the other hand, greatly reduces the likelihood that large amounts of a potential toxin could be consumed. The Japanese people, incidentally, consider variety such an important part of healthful eating that their dietary guidelines recommend consuming 30 or more different kinds of food every day to achieve a balance of essential nutrients.[13]

Consumer Tips

Stocking Your Cupboards for Healthful Eating

To prepare healthful meals, you need to have the proper ingredients. It helps to keep staples on hand to save time and last-minute trips to the grocery store. Keeping a well-stocked larder containing the following items will make it easier to put to practice the dietary advice and guidelines that appear in later chapters.

Flour, Cereal, and Other Grains

- bran flakes (and other cold cereals)
- bread
- brown and white rice
- corn meal
- graham crackers
- regular or quick-cooking oats
- spaghetti and macaroni
- whole all-purpose flour
- whole-wheat flour

Leavening and Thickening Agents

- baking powder
- baking soda
- cornstarch

Sweeteners

- brown sugar
- honey
- molasses
- white sugar

Seasonings

- basil
- bay leaves
- black pepper
- chili powder
- cinnamon
- dillweed
- garlic cloves and powder
- ginger
- ketchup
- lemon juice
- mustard
- nutmeg
- onion powder
- oregano
- paprika
- salt
- vanilla extract
- vinegar

Other Basics

- beans and peas (dry and/or canned)
- plain low-fat or nonfat yogurt
- carrots
- cheese
- evaporated skim milk
- nonfat milk powder
- nuts
- onions
- peanut butter
- popcorn
- potatoes
- raisins
- tomato paste
- tomato sauce
- vegetable oil

When it comes to storing your staple goods, keep a few tips in mind:[14]

- Rotate foods already in your cupboard or refrigerator with new items to ensure that the older foods are used first.
- Keep staples, including flour, sugar, and cereal, in airtight containers to prevent bug infestation; store whole-wheat flour in the refrigerator or freezer.
- Store frozen foods in airtight containers, freezer bags, or heavy duty freezer wrap or foil in a freezer kept at 0 degrees Fahrenheit or colder.
- Maintain the refrigerator temperature below 40 degrees Fahrenheit and keep foods in airtight containers to prevent the spread of odors or flavors. Keep items far enough from one another to allow air to circulate.
- Place dry foods in clean, cool, dark, and dry shelves above the floor and away from water pipes and air ducts.

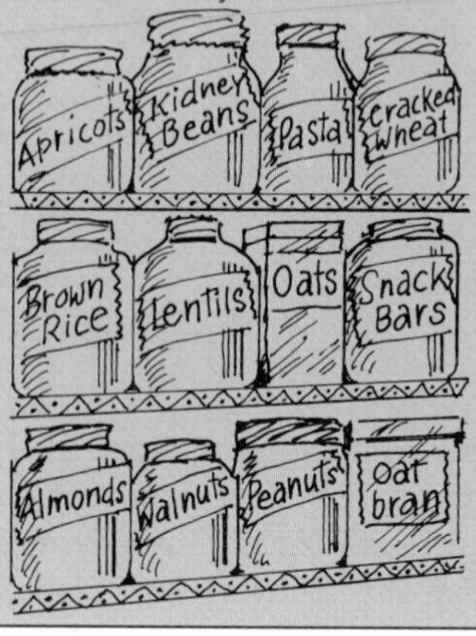

Arrange staple goods attractively and let them inspire you to add variety to your menus.

Spotlight

Separating Nutrition Fact from Fiction

You've just read a headline in a newspaper saying that oat bran does *not* help lower blood cholesterol after all. So you ask yourself whether you should just quit eating it altogether. Or you've heard an advertisement on television for a vitamin supplement guaranteed to produce a laundry list of benefits including fewer colds and a better complexion. Should you buy it? Or maybe your doctor has told you that your blood pressure is too high, so you'd be wise to lose a few pounds. Who do you turn to for help?

We all find ourselves faced with these kinds of dilemmas at one time or another. Knowing how to handle them is essential to protecting yourself from nutrition misinformation. As we pointed out earlier, blatant health fraud costs consumers some $25 billion each year. At the same time, the sale of weight-loss programs and products—not all of them sound—has become a 32-billion-dollar industry.[15] Media attention to "hot" foods generally causes spending on those items to soar. During oat bran's heyday, sales of the grain nearly quadrupled during one year alone.[16]

Money down the drain is just one of the problems stemming from misleading dietary information. While some fraudulent claims about nutrition are harmless and make for a good laugh, others can lead to tragic consequences. Swallowing false claims about nutritional products has been known to bring about malnutrition, birth defects, mental retardation, and even death in extreme cases. Negative effects can happen in two ways. One is that the product in question causes direct harm. Even a seemingly innocuous substance such as vitamin A, for instance, can cause severe liver damage over time if taken in large enough doses. The other problem with using spurious nutritional remedies is that they build false hope and may keep a consumer from obtaining sound, scientifically tested medical treatment. A person who relies on a so-called anti-cancer diet as a cure for the disease, for example, might forego possible lifesaving interventions such as surgery or chemotherapy.

The following questions and answers should answer your questions about the nutrition information you see in the newspapers or on labels. In addition, it should help you develop the skills with which to evaluate nutrition claims with a skeptic's eye or, at the very least, find a qualified professional who can.

• Judging by what I've read in newspapers, it seems as if nutritionists are always changing their minds. One week the headlines say oat bran lowers cholesterol, and the next week they say it doesn't. Why is there so much controversy?

Part of the confusion stems from the way the media chooses to interpret the findings of scientific research. The oat bran story is a good case in point. In the late 1980s, a nutritional "star" was born. Shortly after publication of a study showing that including oat bran as part of a low-fat diet could reduce blood cholesterol levels, spending on the once lowly grain had reached $100 million. Unlikely foods such as potato chips, pretzels, and beer made with oat bran showed up on supermarket shelves.[17] Consumer surveys reportedly indicated that people would buy Life Savers with oat bran added.[18]

In 1990, however, a flurry of headlines including "Is It Still the Right Thing to Do?" and "The Rise and Fallacies of Oat Bran," threatened to pull the bottom out from under the grain's pedestal.[19] A study published in *The New England Journal of Medicine,* one of the most prestigious medical journals, found that Cream of Wheat was just as effective as oat bran at reducing blood cholesterol levels.[20] In other words, it implied that the oat-bran brouhaha had been for naught.

But the oat bran story illustrates how news stories based on one study alone can leave the public with the impression that scientists can't make up their minds. First, oat bran is hailed as the "magic bullet" that will lower Americans' blood cholesterol. One study and several news reports later, oat bran is virtually dismissed as just another fad. However, the truth of the matter is that even those experts who believe that oat bran does have an effect on blood cholesterol levels never suggest that oat bran will do so when it's included in a high-fat diet or put in high-fat muffins or potato chips. Most health professionals advise eating oatmeal or oat bran in place of a high-fat food such as eggs or bacon as part of a low-fat diet.

Contrary to what some headlines imply, reputable scientists do not base dietary recommendations for the public on the findings of just one or two studies. In the case of oat bran, scientists are still conducting experiments to determine if and when the substance does, in fact, help lower blood cholesterol. Researchers design experiments to test theories, such as the notion that adding oat bran to the diet is associated with a drop in blood cholesterol. Other factors, however, sometimes confound the matter at hand. In the case of the oat bran study referred to previously, some critics charged that among other things, the scientists who conducted it did not carefully control the amount of fat in the oat eaters' diets, a factor that may have considerably altered the outcome of the experiment; other research shows that a high-fat diet raises blood cholesterol levels.[21]

Moreover, even if an experiment is carefully designed and carried out, its findings cannot be considered definitive until they have been confirmed by other research. Testing and retesting reduces the possibility that the outcome was simply the result of chance or an error or oversight on the part of the experimenter. When making dietary recommendations for the public, experts pool the results of different types of studies, such as analyses of food patterns of groups of people and carefully controlled studies on people in hospitals or clinics, and then consider all of them before coming to any conclusions. The dietary guidelines spelled out in the 1,300 page *Diet and Health* report, in fact, are based on the results of hundreds of studies. The point is that if you read a report in the paper or hear one on television that advises making a dramatic change in your diet based on just one study, don't believe it. It may make for a good story, but it's not worth taking too seriously.

• What about animal studies? If I hear on the news that a substance in food makes rats sick, should I stop eating it?

Not necessarily. It's wise to be leary of media stories based solely on animal experiments. Admittedly, animal research is an obvious step in gathering information about how chemicals, drugs, or devices may affect living things. It's not practical or ethical to gather this knowledge by allowing humans to use untested products. Translating the findings of animal studies to humans, however, can be just as dangerous and unethical. While different species may respond in some way, for better or for worse, to a treatment, the same response will not necessarily occur in people.

For example, suppose rats became sick when injected with the amount of substance X that a person would normally consume in a year's time. A researcher might conclude correctly that substance X could cause illness. But in a case like this, remember that a rat is a tiny animal compared to a person, and the rodent received a huge dose of substance X all at once. Thus, the experiment does not indicate whether small amounts of substance X taken by a human over the course of a year would produce the same harmful effect. A news story that implies otherwise clearly does not warrant banning the substance from the diet.

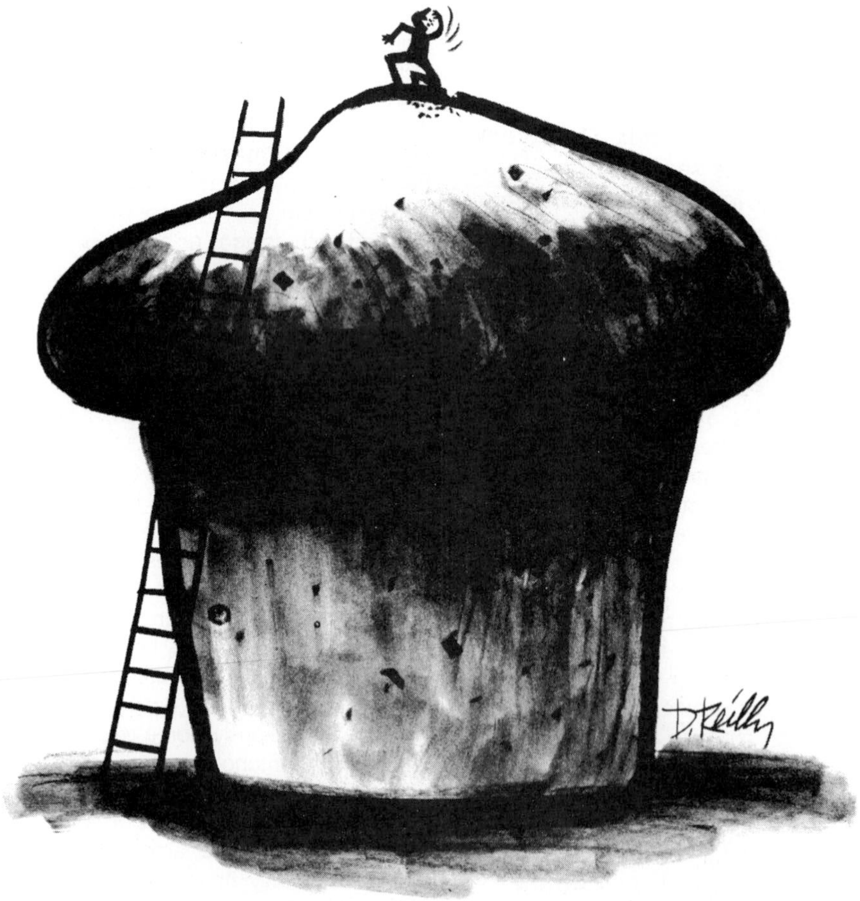

Wellness Update: Thirty-year-old man starting on the twenty-five-thousand-pound oat-bran muffin he must consume over forty years in order to reduce significantly his risk of death from high cholesterol.

Drawing by D. Reilly; © 1989 *The New Yorker* Magazine, Inc.

• Why doesn't the government do something to prevent the media from delivering misleading nutrition information?

The government lacks the power to do so because the **First Amendment** guarantees freedom of the press. Thus, it is possible for people to express whatever views they like in the media, whether sound, unsound, or even dangerous. This freedom is a cornerstone of the U.S. Constitution, and to deny it would be to deny democracy. Writers cannot be punished by law for publishing misinformation unless it can be proved in court that the information has caused a reader bodily harm.

Fortunately, most professional health groups maintain committees to combat the spread of health and nutrition misinformation. A list of organizations that provide reliable scientific information appears in Appendix A, and any of them can serve as sources for your own inquiries about the authenticity of scientific information in their areas.*

●Does the First Amendment also make it legal for companies to say whatever they want about the products they sell?

No. Unlike journalists, purveyors of products are bound by law to make only true statements about their wares. The Food and Drug Administration (FDA) holds the authority to prosecute companies that display false nutrition information on product labels or in advertising materials. Combating health fraud, however, is an overwhelming task requiring enormous amounts of time and money. As one FDA official has put it, ''Quack promoters have learned to stay one step ahead of the laws either by moving from state to state or by changing their corporate names.'' Indeed, the FDA estimates that 38 million consumers have used a fraudulent health product during the past year.[22]

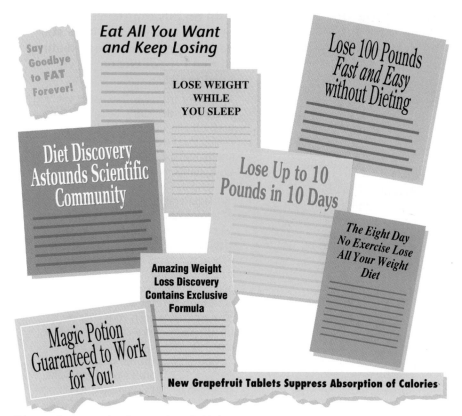

If it sounds too good to be true, it probably is.

●How can I tell whether a product is bogus?

It's not always easy, given that many misleading claims are supposedly backed by scientific-sounding statements, making it difficult even for informed consumers to separate fact from fiction. But the following red flags can help you spot a quack:

- *The promotor claims that the medical establishment is against him or her, and that the government won't accept this new ''alternative'' treatment.*

If the government or medical community can't accept a treatment, it's because the treatment hasn't been proven to work. Reputable professionals don't suppress knowledge about fighting disease. On the contrary, they welcome new remedies for illness, provided the treatments have been carefully tested.

- *The promoter uses testimonials and anecdotes from satisfied customers to support claims.*

Valid nutrition information comes from careful experimental research, not from random tales. A few persons' reports that the product in question ''works every time'' are never acceptable as sound scientific evidence.

- *The promoter uses a computer-scored questionnaire for diagnosing ''nutrient deficiencies.''*

Those computers are programmed to suggest that just about everyone has a deficiency that can be reversed with the supplements the promoter just happens to be selling, regardless of the consumer's symptoms or health.

- *The promoter claims the product will make weight loss easy.*

Unfortunately, there is no simple way to lose weight. In other words, if a claim sounds too good to be true, it probably is.

- *The promoter promises that the product is made with a ''secret formula'' available only from this one company.*

Legitimate health professionals share their knowledge of proven treatments so that others can benefit from it.

---

*If you have questions about a medical book, product, or service, write to the American Medical Association; about an anti-cancer book, product, or service, to the American Cancer Society; about a heart disease preventive, to the American Heart Association; about a diet or nutrient supplement, to the American Dietetic Association; and so forth. Many of the professional organizations have also banded together to form the National Council Against Health Fraud (NCAHF), which has branches in many states. The NCAHF monitors radio, television, and other advertising; investigates complaints; and publishes a bimonthly newsletter to keep consumers informed on the latest health misinformation. You can write to the NCAHF at P.O. Box 1276, Loma Linda, CA 92354.

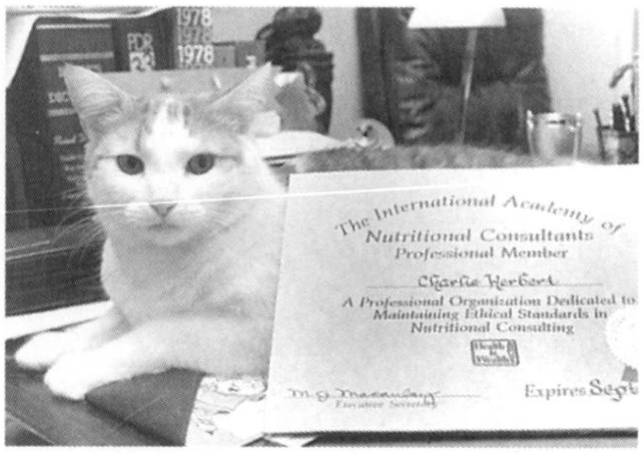

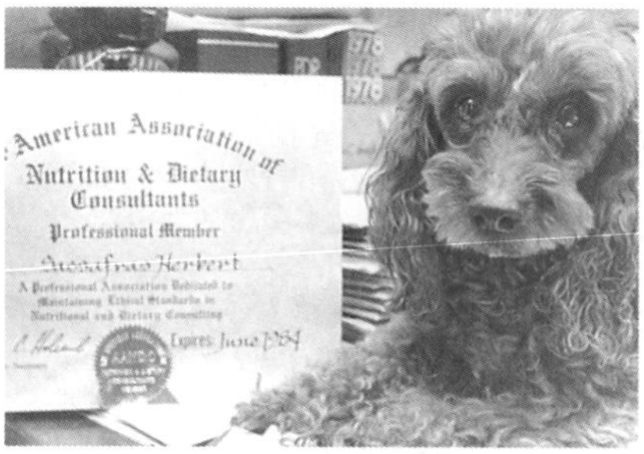

Charlie and Sassafras display their professional credentials.

- *The treatment is provided only in the back pages of magazines, over the phone, or by mail-order ads in the form of news stories or 30-minute commercials (known as infomercials) in talk-show format.*

Results of studies on credible treatments are reported first in medical journals and administered through a doctor or other health professional. If information about a treatment only appears elsewhere, it probably can't withstand scientific scrutiny.*

● If I do buy a product, say, to help me lose weight, but I still need some advice about dieting, should I check with a nutritionist?

To answer that question, we'd like you to consider this story. Several years back Charlie Herbert became a professional member of the International Academy of Nutrition Consultants. Another member of the household, Sassafras Herbert, met all the requirements for membership in the American Association of Nutrition and Dietary Consultants, "a professional association dedicated to maintaining ethical standards in nutritional and dietary consulting." The only qualification for membership, however, is a $50 fee, regardless of your background or even your species. Charlie Herbert is a cat, and Sassafras, a poodle. The two obtained their "credentials" with the help of Victor Herbert, M.D., professor of medicine, chairman of the Committee to Strengthen Nutrition at Mount Sinai School of Medicine, New York City, and a leader in combating nutrition fraud. Dr. Herbert had his pets added to the membership rosters of those organizations to demonstrate how easy it is for anyone to get fake nutrition credentials. That's because, in most states, the term **nutritionist** is not legally defined at present.

Before you pay a fee or follow a nutritionist's advice, inquire about the person's credentials. Some nutritionists obtain their diplomas and titles without undergoing the rigorous training required to obtain a legitimate degree in nutrition. Lax state laws make it possible for irresponsible **correspondence schools**—also called **diploma mills**—to pass out degrees to unqualified individuals for nothing more than a fee.

● How can I check a nutritionist's credentials?

For one, you can call the institution where the person claims to have gotten a degree. To find out about the existence or reputation of an institution of higher learning, you can go to any library and ask for a directory of colleges and universities. Be suspicious

● *Table 1–5*

Contacts for Reliable Nutrition Information

City, county, or state public health department	Nutritionist[a]
Local hospital	Registered Dietitian[a]
Local college or university	Nutrition and food science department or public health/nutrition department
Land grant university and county	Cooperative Extension Service
Local or state Department of Education	Nutrition Education and Training Program (NET)
Family physician (depending on training)	
Community resources	Home economist with utility company, high school, or supermarket; nutrition or dietetic consultant,[a] yellow pages of telephone book (check credentials)

[a]Nutrition professionals who have a degree in nutrition, food science, or public health/nutrition or who are licensed by the American Dietetic Association as registered dietitians are qualified to offer sound food and nutrition information.

Source: Adapted from J. A. Rubey, *Nutrition for Everybody,* (Oakland Calif.: Society for Nutrition Education, 1981), p. 21.

*If you think you've been duped by a quack, write the FDA, Consumer Affairs and Information, 5600 Fishers Lane, HFC-110, Rockville, MD 20857; your state Attorney General's office; the Federal Trade Commission, Correspondence Branch, Room 692, Sixth and Pennsylvania Avenues, N.W., Washington, DC 20580; and/or the newspaper, magazine, TV or radio station running the ad. If you ordered the product by mail, alert the U.S. Postal Service, Chief Postal Inspector, 475 L'Enfant Plaza, Washington, DC 20260. If you want to take legal action and need help finding an experienced lawyer, write or call the National Council Against Health Fraud's Task Force on Victim Redress at P.O. Box 33008, Kansas City, MO 64114; (816)444–8615.

Miniglossary

Accreditation approval; in the case of hospitals or university departments approval by a professional organization of the educational program offered. There are phony accrediting agencies; the genuine ones are listed with the U.S. Department of Education.

Correspondence school a school from which courses can be taken and degrees granted by mail. Those that are accredited offer respectable courses and degrees.

Diploma mill a correspondence school that grinds out degrees the way a grain mill grinds out flour—degrees sometimes worth no more than the cost of the paper they are printed on.

First Amendment The amendment to the U.S. Constitution that guarantees freedom of the press.

Nutritionist a person who claims to be capable of advising people about their diets. Some nutritionists are registered dietitians, whereas others are self-described experts whose training is questionable.

Registered dietitian (R.D.) a professional who has graduated from a program of dietetics approved by the American Dietetic Association (ADA), has passed the ADA's registration examination, has served an internship program or the equivalent to gain practical skills, and maintains competencies through continuing education. Some states require licensing for dietitians; that is, they have legislation in place obligating anyone who wants to use the title "dietitian" to receive permission by passing a state examination. Other states do not require dietitians to be licensed. R.D. (the abbreviation for registered dietitian) is often used to refer to such a professional in the same way M.D. designates a medical doctor.

of diplomas or degrees issued by institutions that cannot prove that they have **accreditation** from the U.S. Department of Education.

Another option is to find out if the person is a special type of nutritionist known as a **registered dietitian** (R.D.). The R.D. is an especially meaningful credential and has a standard definition. An R.D. is a professional who has not only passed coursework required by the American Dietetic Association (ADA) (which are college courses in chemistry, anatomy, physiology, beginning through advanced nutrition, diet therapy, food science, and food service administration) but also completed an internship including on-the-job training for counseling people about the relationship between diet and health. In addition, the R.D. has passed a national registration examination administered by the ADA. All registered dietitians must keep their credentials current by completing regular continuing education requirements.

You can check on any R.D. by asking for that person's registration number and calling the ADA's Commission on Dietetic Registration (312-899-0040) to confirm the credentials. If you'd like to contact an R.D. but don't know where to find one in your area, send a self-addressed, stamped envelope to the Nutrition Resources Department, American Dietetic Association, 216 W. Jackson Boulevard, Suite 800, Chicago, IL 60606-6995, and ask for the State List of Consulting Nutritionists in your particular area, which is a free list of R.D.'s in private practice in your state. Table 1–5 lists other sources of reliable nutrition information.

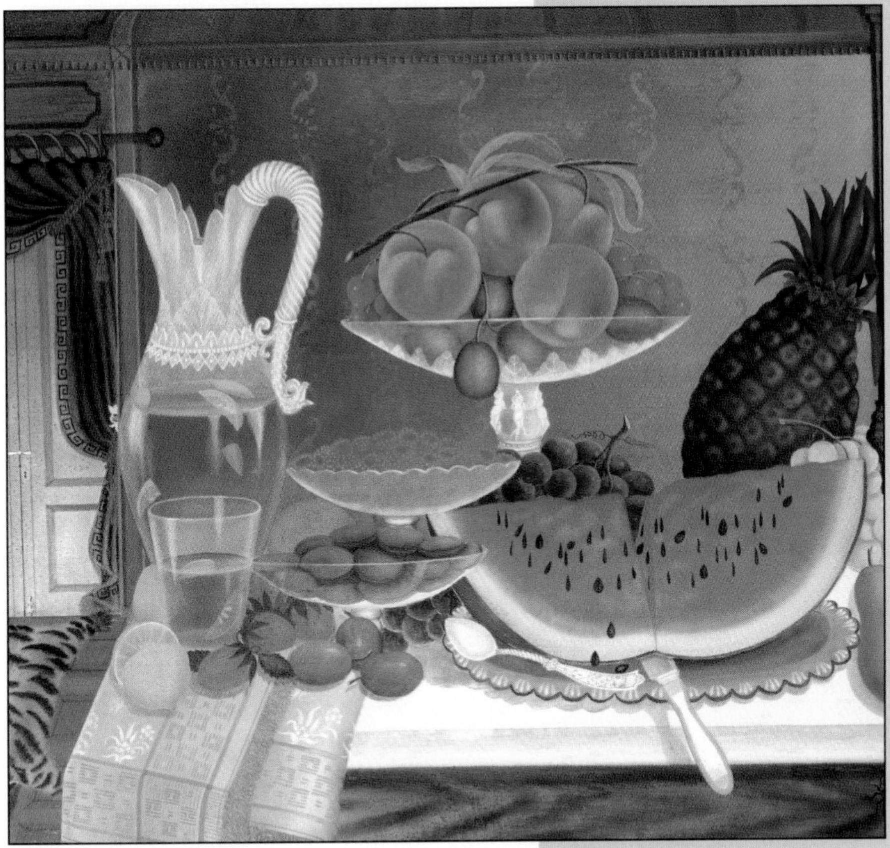

Still Life by *Henry Church. The Collection of Frances O. Stem Babinsky.*

> *Nourishment is a matter of making wise choices in our individual food selection: choosing to eat foods that provide particular nutrients, choosing not to eat foods with no nutrient value at all.*
>
> *—B. Godfrey*

CHAPTER 2
The Pursuit of an Ideal Diet

Contents

Ask Yourself . . . ?

Which of these statements about nutrition are true, and which are false? For the false statements, what *is* true?

1. Malnutrition occurs in people in the United States and Canada.
2. It is possible to have an appetite without being hungry.
3. As far as nutrients are concerned, the more, the better.
4. The vitamins and minerals yield no energy.
5. The closer to the farm the foods you eat, the better nourished you are.
6. If you weigh 150 pounds, your body probably contains about 90 pounds of water.
7. Grazing on snacks all day is okay, at least from the nutrition standpoint, as long as the snacks chosen are nutritious and don't exceed your food energy allowance.
8. Alcohol has the most calories per gram of any substance people ingest; protein has the fewest.
9. If you don't meet your RDA for a nutrient, you will have a deficiency of that nutrient.
10. If a cereal box label states that a serving of the cereal provides 25% of the U.S. RDA for vitamin C, then you can be sure that a serving of the cereal provides at least 25% of *your* vitamin C allowance for a day.

Answers: 1. True. 2. True. 3. False. Too much or too little of a nutrient is equally harmful. 4. True. 5. True. 6. True. 7. True. 8. False. Fat has the most calories per gram—9. Alcohol has 7; carbohydrate and protein each has 4. 9. False. If you don't meet your RDA for a nutrient, you may still have an adequate intake, although you may be approaching deficiency. 10. True.

Nutrition is complex. It nourishes not only the body but also the whole being and outlook of a person. Nutrition is the relationship between food and the body as well as the study of what happens to health, development, and performance when the body receives too few, too many, or the wrong balance of nutrients.

You choose to eat a meal about 1,000 times a year. Each time, you choose particular amounts of the foods you prefer from what is available to you. Eating is so habitual that often people give it hardly any thought, yet it is a voluntary activity. You can choose when to eat, what to eat, and how much to eat— 1,000 times a year, or over 70,000 times in a lifetime.

Not all foods supply the nutrients needed for health. Some people in the United States and Canada, especially those with low incomes, suffer from **undernutrition.** Some pregnant women suffer nutrient deficiencies that retard their infants' growth. Among migratory workers and certain rural populations, more than one in every ten children suffer stunted growth caused by a poor diet.[1] Iron deficiencies occur in all people regardless of income, affecting 1 percent to 5 percent of people severely enough to cause the deficiency disease anemia. Many more are affected in subtly damaging ways. At the same time, **overnutrition** can threaten people's health. About 15 percent of men and 25 percent of women are obese. People's average daily intakes of sodium are substantially higher than is consistent with health of the heart. People are choosing to eat foods higher in fat, cholesterol, and sugar than recommended. High incidences of several **degenerative diseases** are attributed to these habits.[2]

Nutrition affects you both today and in your later years. You will appreciate your knowledge of nutrition when you learn that you can feel better from the moment you wake up until the end of your day by the timing and selection of what you eat. You will thank yourself years from now when you

Undernutrition underconsumption of food energy or nutrients severe enough to cause disease or increased susceptibility to disease; a form of malnutrition.

Overnutrition overconsumption of food energy or nutrients severe enough to cause disease or increased susceptibility to disease; a form of malnutrition.

Degenerative diseases diseases characterized by deterioration of body organs from misuse and neglect; they are often influenced by personal lifestyle choices and are chronic and irreversible. Examples are heart disease, cancer, and diabetes.

receive compliments on your health, appearance, active lifestyle, and vigor. To enjoy the best of health, you must be sure to select foods that contain all the nutrients you need without an excess of calories.

Good nutrition is not the only factor involved in prolonging the body's health into the later years. To remain healthy and energetic involves developing a lifestyle that includes all elements relating to health as discussed in Chapter 1. Good nutrition contributes to the ability to enjoy, in good health, "the best years of life for which the first were made." In effect, you can make yourself younger or older by the way you choose to live. Your accumulated choices profoundly influence your health, and it is worth questioning why you eat when you do, why you choose the foods you do—and, most important, whether they supply the nutrients you need.

Understanding Why We Eat

To the question of what prompts you to eat, you may reply that it is **hunger**. That is often true, but hunger—the physiological need for food—is not the only stimulus that triggers eating behavior. Another cue is **appetite**, the psychological desire for food, which may arise in response to the sight, smell, or thought of food even when you don't need to eat. You may have an appetite when you are not hungry, and conversely, you may be hungry and yet have no appetite. Some people eat more food than they need and more often than they need to, while others eat too little. (Hunger, appetite, obesity, and underweight are the subjects of Chapter 8.)

Hunger the physiological need for food.
Appetite the desire to eat, which normally accompanies hunger.

As for the question of why you choose the particular foods you do, several answers come to mind:

- Temptation (they are delicious).
- Personal preference (you like them).
- Habit or tradition (they are familiar; you always eat them).
- Social pressure (they are offered, and you can't refuse).
- Values or personal beliefs (spiritual or ideological meaning).
- Availability (there are no others to choose from).
- Convenience (you are too rushed to prepare anything else).
- Economy (you can afford them).
- Psychological benefits (as a reward or as consolation).
- Nutritional value (you think they are good for you).

Of all these reasons, only one—the last one—involves making a conscious choice in favor of your health. Yet the foods you eat profoundly influence not only how you feel right now, today, but also how well you will withstand the onslaught of the years. The well-nourished person resists disease and other stresses better, enjoys greater energy, and can be physiologically years younger than the poorly nourished person. Your body derives its energy from the foods you eat and is itself made entirely of materials you have obtained from those foods. You are, as the old saying goes, what you eat.

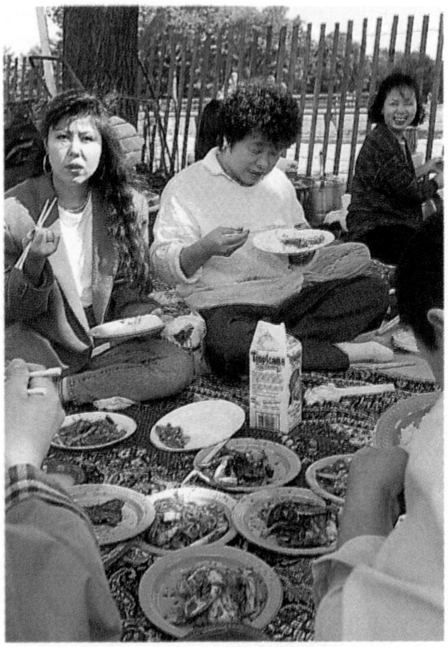
There are many factors that influence our food choices, including advertising, early experiences, economics, habit, health, and social factors.

Why do you like certain foods? One reason, of course, is your preferences for certain tastes, and two of these preferences are widely shared: the tastes

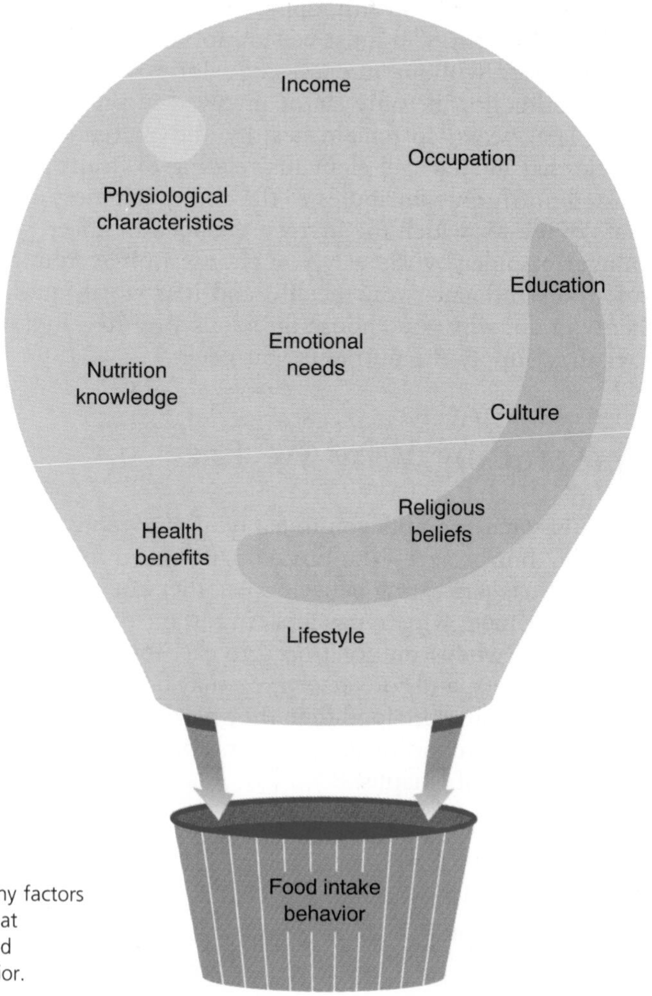

Note the many factors listed here that influence food intake behavior.

for sugar and for salt. You also like foods with which you have happy associations—those you eat in the midst of a warm family gathering at traditional holiday times, those someone who loved you gave you as a child, or those eaten by people you admire. By the same token, intense dislike—strong enough to be unalterable—can be attached to foods that you ate when you were sick, that were forced on you when you weren't hungry, that were served too frequently, or that are eaten by people you don't respect. Your parents may have taught you to like and dislike certain foods for similar reasons of their own, without even being aware that they did so.

Social pressure is another powerful influence on food behavior. How can you refuse when your friends are going out for frozen yogurt or pizza? Such pressure operates in all circles and across cultural lines. It may be considered rude to refuse food or drink; you are not fully a member of the social gathering until you partake with the others.

The influence of availability, convenience, and economy on food selections is clear. You cannot eat foods if they are not available, if you cannot prepare them, or if you cannot afford them.

Food behavior is also intimately related to deep psychological needs such as the infant's association of food with a parent's love. For some people, yearnings, cravings, and addictions with profound meaning and significance reveal themselves in food behavior. Some people respond to stress—positive or negative—by eating; others use eating to ward off loneliness, boredom, or anxiety.

Given the variety of reasons why people eat as they do, you may wonder how good a job they are doing in selecting foods on the basis of the last reason listed: to meet their nutrient needs. Many consumers have become aware that they must select foods that will enable them to achieve optimal health. To do so successfully requires learning what nutrients the body needs and what foods supply them.

Eating well is easy, in principle. All you need to do is choose foods that supply appropriate amounts of the essential nutrients, fiber, and energy. This is a simple enough assignment, but to master it and put it into practice requires that you know the answers to several questions. What are the essential nutrients? How much of each do you need? Which types of foods supply which nutrients and fiber? How much of each type of food do you need to eat to get enough? And how can you eat all these foods without getting fat or getting excess intakes of unwanted substances, such as fat or salt?

Keep the diet-planning principles in mind:

Adequacy—enough of each type of food.

Balance—not too much of any type of food.

Calorie control—not too many or too few calories.

Moderation—not too much fat, salt, or sugar.

Variety—as many different foods as possible.

The Nutrients

Almost any food you eat is composed mostly of water (up to 99 percent). The bulk of the solid materials consists of carbohydrate, fat, and protein. If you could remove these materials, you would detect a tiny residue of minerals, vitamins, and other materials. Water, carbohydrate, fat, protein, vitamins, and some of the minerals are **nutrients.** Some of the other materials are not.

A complete chemical analysis of your body would show that it is made of similar materials in roughly the same order of predominance. If you weigh 150 pounds, your body contains about 90 pounds of water and (if 150 pounds is the proper weight for you) about 30 pounds of fat. The other 30 pounds are mostly protein, carbohydrate, and the major minerals of your bones—calcium and phosphorus. Vitamins, other minerals, and incidental extras constitute a fraction of a pound.

Nutrients substances obtained from food and used in the body to promote growth, maintenance, and repair.

Essential nutrients nutrients that the body cannot make for itself in sufficient quantity but has to obtain from food.

The six classes of nutrients are:

carbohydrate
fat
protein
vitamins
minerals
water

The Essential Nutrients

In nutrition, the words *essential* and *nonessential* are used to distinguish between the nutrients that the body must obtain from food and those that the body can manufacture from its own resources. The body can convert some of the amino acids (parts of protein) into carbohydrate if need be. It can make some of its fats and oils from any of several different raw materials. These are nonessential nutrients. In contrast, certain compounds that the body cannot make for itself are absolutely indispensable to life processes; these are termed the **essential nutrients.** When used this way, the term *essential* means more than just "necessary." Many compounds the body makes for itself are necessary for good health, but an essential nutrient means a necessary nutrient that can be obtained only from the diet.

Organic carbon containing; the organic nutrients are carbohydrate, fat (lipid), protein, and vitamins. The **inorganic** nutrients are minerals and water.
Energy the capacity to do work, such as moving things or heating things.

The energy-yielding nutrients are:

Carbohydrate—provides energy as glucose.

Lipid—provides energy as fatty acids.

Protein—provides structural material but can be transformed into glucose or fatty acids under some conditions.

Calorie the unit used to measure energy. The calories in a food are usually determined by measurement of the heat the food releases when burned; they are familiar to everyone as a reflection of the extent to which a food's energy can be stored in body fat. Technically, a calorie is the amount of heat necessary to raise the temperature of a gram of water 1 degree centigrade. Food energy is measured in thousands of calories (1 kilocalorie = 1,000 calories).
calor = heat

Keep in mind that 1 gram of carbohydrate equals 4 calories, 1 gram of fat equals 9 calories, and 1 gram of protein equals 4 calories.

Alcohol is a nonnutrient that provides energy (more about alcohol appears in Chapter 10).

1 gram alcohol = 7 calories.

About 40 nutrients are now known to be essential for human beings. How can you obtain all these nutrients, and which foods contain which? This chapter shows you how to design a diet that meets all your nutrient needs.

The Energy-yielding Nutrients

Materials from food account both for your body's structure and for its activities. You are made of materials from food—the nutrients—some of which also provide energy to permit you to go about your various pursuits. Four of the six classes of nutrients—carbohydrate, fat, protein, and vitamins—are **organic**, while the other two (minerals and water) are not. On being broken down or metabolized, three of the four organic nutrients (carbohydrate, fat, and protein) can provide **energy** for the body to use. A common misconception people have is that vitamins can yield energy for human use. They cannot, although taking vitamin pills for energy is a common mistake. The only significance to us of vitamins' being organic is that they are easily destroyed by chemical and physical agents such as heat and light. We therefore need to be careful in cooking foods that contain vitamins. In contrast, minerals and water are **inorganic**. They are not broken down in the human body to yield energy but perform other functions, such as maintenance and repair.

The energy from these nutrients is used by the body to do work or generate heat. The units of measure of energy are **calories**, familiar to everyone as a reflection of how "fattening" a food is. The energy content of a food thus depends on how much carbohydrate, fat, or protein the food contains. If you don't use these nutrients soon after you eat them, your body rearranges them (and the energy they contain) into storage compounds, such as body fat, and puts them away for later. Thus, an excess intake of any of the three energy nutrients can lead to overweight. Too much lean meat (a protein-rich food) is just as fattening as too many potatoes (a carbohydrate-rich food) or too many peanuts (a fat-rich food).

Calorie Values of Carbohydrate, Fat, and Protein

If you know the number of grams of carbohydrate, fat, and protein in a food, you can derive the number of calories in it. Simply multiply the carbohydrate grams times 4, the fat grams times 9, and the protein grams times 4, and add them all together.
A note about grams—most people don't think of foods in terms of grams. It's easy to learn to do so, though, and a good idea for those who plan to work with foods in the future. A standard portion (a half cup) of most vegetables or a half cup of milk or juice has a volume of about 100 milliliters and weighs roughly 100 grams. A teaspoon of any dry powder such as sugar or salt weighs (very roughly) 5 grams. For accurate conversion factors, see the inside back cover.

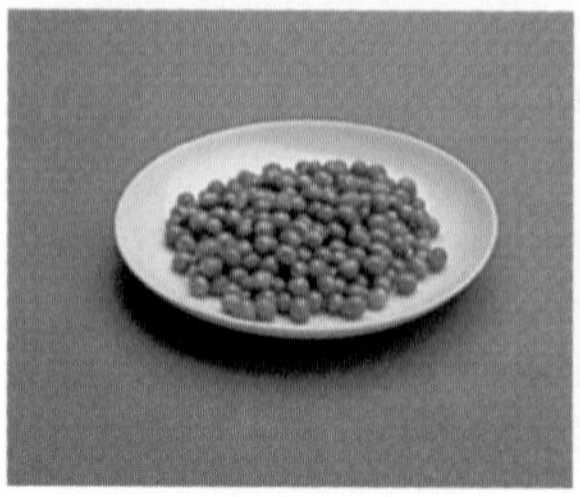

100 g peas

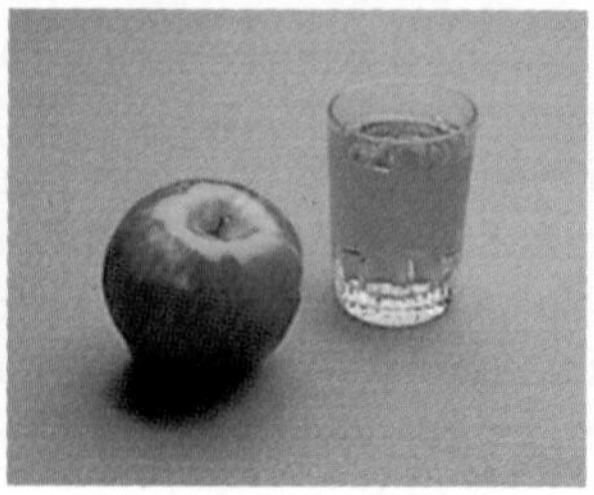

100 g juice

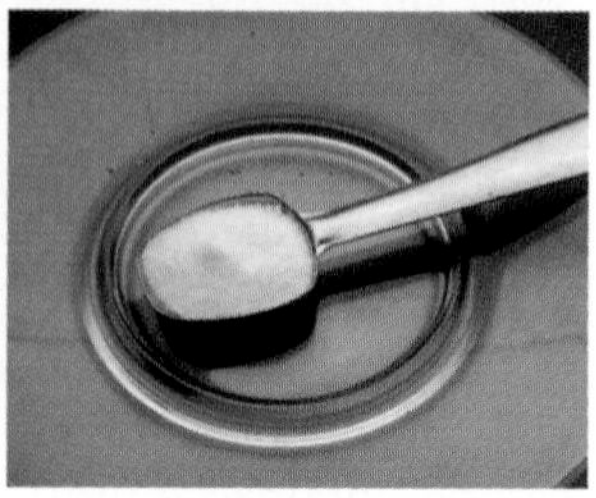

5 g salt

Table 2–1 The Vitamins and Minerals

THE VITAMINS			THE MINERALS			
The water-soluble vitamins		The fat-soluble vitamins	The major minerals		The trace minerals	
B vitamins		Vitamin A	Calcium	Potassium	Chromium	Molybdenum
Thiamin	Vitamin B_{12}	Vitamin D	Chloride	Sodium	Cobalt	Nickel
Riboflavin	Folate	Vitamin E	Magnesium	Sulfur	Copper	Selenium
Niacin	Biotin	Vitamin K	Phosphorus		Fluoride	Silicon
Vitamin B_6	Pantothenic acid				Iodine	Tin
Vitamin C					Iron	Vanadium
					Manganese	Zinc

Only one other compound that people ingest provides energy, and that is the alcohol of alcoholic beverages. Alcohol is not considered a nutrient, because it does not help to maintain or repair body tissues as nutrients do, but it has to be counted as an energy source.

The Other Nutrients: Vitamins, Minerals, and Water

The nutrients known as **vitamins** and **minerals** do not offer energy for the body's use but regulate both the release of energy and the synthesis and breakdown of body tissues. There are 13 vitamins, each with its special roles to play (see Table 2–1). Vitamins are divided into two classes: water-soluble (the B vitamins and vitamin C) and fat-soluble (vitamins A, D, E, and K). This distinction has many implications for the kinds of foods they are found in and the ways the body absorbs, transports, stores, and excretes them. The vitamins and minerals are the subject of Chapters 6 and 7.

Minerals are inorganic compounds, smaller than vitamins and found in even simpler forms in foods. Some minerals are put together into orderly arrays in such structures as bones and teeth. Others float about in the fluids of the body, helping to regulate fluid balance and acidity. You consume small amounts of minerals daily. There are 21 minerals important in nutrition (see Table 2–1).

Water is the forgotten nutrient. It is the medium in which all the body's processes take place. Probably about 60 percent of your body's weight is water. It is the fluid part of the blood and the interior spaces in the cells. Water transports materials to and from cells and provides the warm, nutrient-rich bath in which cells thrive; it also conducts hormonal messages from place to place. When fuel nutrients break down to release energy, they break down to water and other simple compounds. Since you lose water from your

Vitamins organic compounds vital to life, needed in minute amounts; a class of essential nutrients.
vita = life
amine = containing nitrogen
Minerals inorganic elements. Some minerals are essential nutrients.

Vitamins—play regulatory roles.
Minerals—play regulatory roles.
Water—provides the medium for life processes.

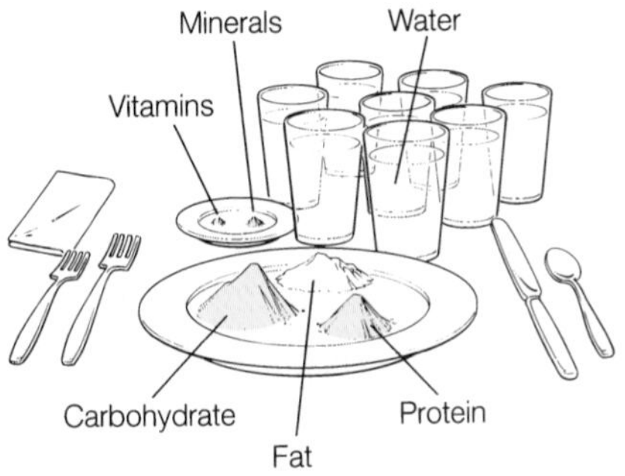

Amounts of nutrients eaten daily. If you could extract and purify the carbohydrate, fat, and protein from your daily diet, they would fill 2 or 3 measuring cups, even though the foods they come in weigh much more and occupy much more volume. A hundred grams of food may contain only 10 or so grams of energy-yielding nutrients, the rest being water, fiber, and other non-caloric materials.

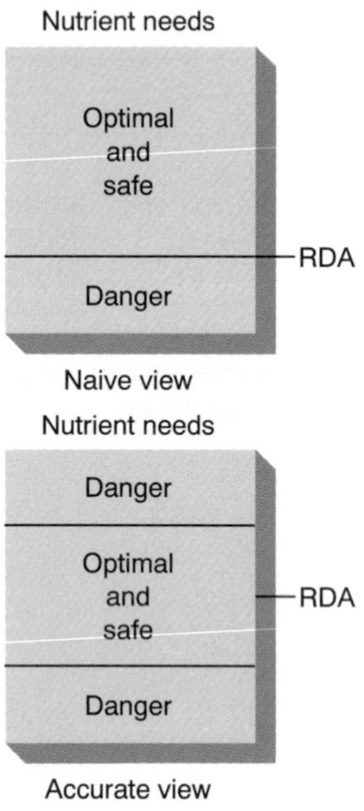

Figure 2–1

The Correct View of the RDA

People used to think that more of an essential nutrient would be better (top figure). Now we know that too much may be dangerous, and the RDA are expressed as optimal amounts with upper and lower limits.

body daily, you must replace it daily. The amounts you must consume relative to the other nutrients are enormous—about 2 or 3 quarts a day. Of course, you need not always drink water as such in these quantities since it comes abundantly in foods and beverages. Second only to oxygen, water is the most vital substance you require; you could live only a few days without it.

Foods are made up of differing combinations of nutrients. How do you know if you are eating the right amount of each nutrient? The following sections explain how.

Recommended Nutrient Intakes

Assuming you are a normal, healthy human adult of average size who engages in average physical activity, you need to consume the following amounts of nutrients daily to remain in optimal health:

- Protein—approximately 50 grams.
- Carbohydrate—at least 100 to 125 grams.
- Fat—perhaps 30 grams or more, including about 5 grams of linoleic acid.
- Vitamins—specific amounts of each of the 13 vitamins (for example, about 1 milligram of thiamin).
- Minerals—specific amounts of each of the 21 minerals (for example, about 1 gram of calcium).
- Water—2 to 3 quarts per day.

The reasons for—and, in fact, the urgency behind—each of these recommendations will become clear through the discussions that follow.

A first, obvious reason is that for any of the essential nutrients, deficiencies can arise. A second reason is that even if you don't develop full-blown deficiency diseases, you may suffer marginal deficiencies. People who are less than optimally nourished may tire more easily, get sick more readily, recover more slowly, and age faster—in short, fail to meet their full health potential. You live only once: why settle for less than you can easily have by choosing foods wisely?

The following section introduces the Recommended Dietary Allowances (RDA) used in the United States as an example of recommended intakes. The Canadian equivalent is the Recommended Nutrient Intakes for Canadians (RNI), presented in Appendix C. The U.S. RDA used on food labels is different from the RDA and is discussed in the Spotlight feature at the end of this chapter.

RDA Recommended Dietary Allowances. The RDA, the recommended daily intakes of nutrients, are intended to provide for individual variations among most normal, healthy people in the United States under usual environmental stresses.

The RDA

The **RDA** are recommendations for nutrient intakes published by a committee of scientists funded by the U.S. government. The RDA are used and referred to so often that they are presented on the inside front cover of this book. Periodically, the committee on the RDA meets to reexamine and revise these recommendations on the basis of new evidence regarding the nutrient needs of Americans. It then publishes an updated set of RDA. The most recent edition was published in 1989. The following facts offer a perspective on the RDA.

- The committee that makes the recommendations is funded by the government but is composed of scientists representing a variety of specialties.
- The RDA are based on reviews of available scientific research to the greatest extent possible.
- The RDA are recommendations, not requirements, and certainly not minimum requirements. They include a substantial margin of safety.
- The RDA take into account differences among individuals and define a range within which most healthy people's intakes of nutrients probably should fall. (See Figure 2–1.) Individuals whose needs are higher than the average are included within this range.
- The RDA are for healthy people only. Medical problems alter nutrient needs.

Separate recommendations are made for different sets of people. Children aged 4 to 6 are distinguished from men and women aged 19 to 24, for example. Each individual can look up the recommendations for his or her own age and sex group.

The RDA are tools best suited for evaluating the nutrient intakes of populations or groups. They are less useful—but still often used—for guessing at an individual's nutrition status. The following discussion is based on the way the committee on the RDA made its recommendation for protein, but it illustrates the limitations and qualifications that apply to all the RDA.

Suppose we were the committee members and we had the task of setting an RDA for nutrient X (any nutrient). Our first step would be to try to find out how much of that nutrient each person needs. We could review studies of such relevant factors as deficiency states and the body's nutrient stores and their depletion. We could also measure the body's intake and excretion of nutrient X (in the case of nutrients that aren't used up or changed in the body) to find out how much of an intake is required to achieve balance (this is called a **balance study**). For each individual, we could determine a **requirement** for nutrient X. Below the requirement, that individual would slip into negative balance, experience declining stores, and develop deficiency symptoms. We would find that different individuals have different requirements. Mr. A might need 40 units of the nutrient each day; Ms. B might need 35; Mr. C, 65. If we looked at enough individuals, we might find that their requirements were distributed as shown in Figure 2–2 with most near the midpoint and only a few at the extremes.

We would then have to decide what intake to recommend for everybody; that is, we would have to set the RDA. Should we set it at the mean (shown in Figure 2–2 at 45 units)? This is the average requirement for nutrient X; it is the closest to everyone's need. But if people took us literally and consumed exactly this amount of nutrient X each day, half of the population would develop deficiencies, Mr. C among them.

Perhaps we should set the RDA for nutrient X at or above the extreme—say, at 70 units a day—so that everyone would be covered. This might be a good idea in theory, but what if nutrient X is expensive or scarce? A person like Ms. B, who needs only 35 units a day, would then try to consume twice that amount, an unnecessary strain on her budget. Or she might overeat as a consequence or overemphasize foods containing nutrient X to the exclusion of foods containing other valuable nutrients.

RDA are set for:

- Energy.
- Protein.
- Vitamins: A, C, D, E, K, thiamin, riboflavin, niacin, B_6, B_{12}, folate.
- Minerals: calcium, phosphorus, magnesium, iron, zinc, iodine, selenium.

Estimated safe and adequate intakes are given in ranges for:

- Vitamins: biotin, pantothenic acid.
- Minerals: copper, manganese, fluoride, chromium, molybdenum.

Estimated minimum requirements of healthy persons are given for:

- Sodium, potassium, chloride.

Balance study a laboratory study in which a person is fed a controlled diet and the intake and excretion of a nutrient are measured.

Requirement the amount of a nutrient that will just prevent the development of specific deficiency signs; distinguished from the RDA, which is a recommended allowance that includes a safety factor to provide for individual variability.

● *Figure 2–2*

Individuality of Nutrient Requirements

Each square represents a person: A, B, and C are Mr. A, Ms. B, and Mr. C.

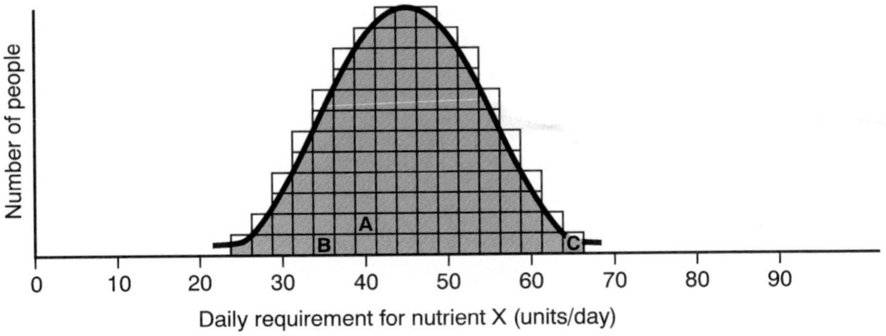

The choice we would finally make, with some reservations, would be to set the RDA at a reasonably high point so that the bulk of the population would be covered. In this example, a reasonable choice might be to set it at 63 units a day. (The committee uses a mathematical formula to find this point, which is intended to cover about 98 percent of the population.) By moving the RDA closer to the extreme, we would pick up few additional people but inflate the recommendation for most people (including Mr. A and Ms. B).

The committee members thus set the RDA for a nutrient well above the mean requirement as best they can determine it from the available information. In theory, relatively few healthy people's requirements, then, are not covered by the RDA.

The RDA cannot be taken literally by any individual; that is, you cannot know exactly what your own personal requirements may be. The committee on the RDA makes several assumptions that may not apply to you at all. It assumes, among other things, that you are eating a generally adequate diet that includes protein of good quality and that you are consuming adequate food energy and nutrients. It assumes that you store and cook your foods with reasonable care and that large amounts of nutrients aren't lost in these processes. In making a recommendation for any one nutrient, the committee assumes that your intakes of all the other nutrients are adequate. When you use the RDA for yourself and compare your nutrient intakes with them, you should keep these qualifications in mind.

The RDA for Energy (Calories)

In setting allowances for energy intakes, the committee took a different approach than it did for the nutrients. Its members set generous allowances for protein, vitamins, and minerals because they felt that small excesses would be less harmful than small deficits. However, *energy* intakes either above or below need are equally undesirable. Underweight is as much to be avoided as is obesity. The committee therefore set the energy RDA as a wide range surrounding the mean for each age-sex group. Figure 2–3 illustrates the difference between the nutrient and the energy RDA set by the committee. As the figure shows, most people's energy needs fall close to the mean, but few fit the mean exactly. The best way to ensure that your energy intake actually fits your own particular requirement is to monitor your food intake over a period of time during which your weight does not change.

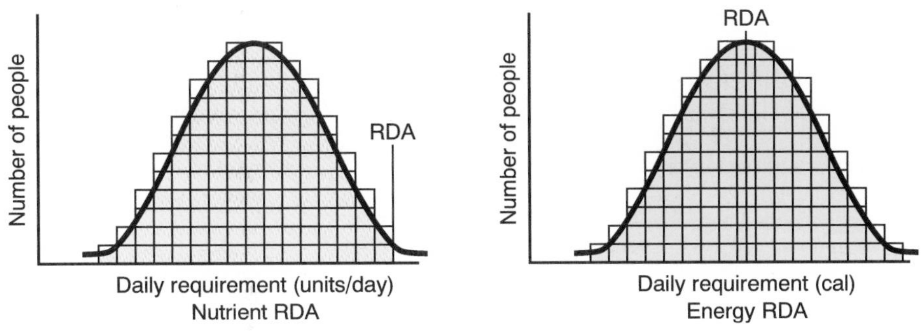

Figure 2–3

The Differences between the Nutrient RDA and the Energy RDA

The nutrient RDA are set so that nearly all people's requirements will be met by them. The energy RDA are set so that half the population's requirements will fall below and half will fall above them.

No RDA is set for carbohydrate or fat. The assumption is that you will first use a certain minimum number of calories for the protein you specifically need and then will use the rest of your energy allowance for carbohydrate, fat, and, possibly, alcohol (according to your personal preference) to balance your energy budget.

Other Recommendations

Different nations and international groups have published different sets of standards similar to the RDA. The Canadian recommendations—the **RNI**—differ from the RDA in some respects, partly because of differences in interpretation of the data they were derived from and partly because people's food intakes and daily lives in Canada differ somewhat from those in the United States.

RNI Recommended Nutrient Intakes for Canadians. (See Appendix C.)

Among the most widely used sets of recommendations are those of two international groups: the Food and Agriculture Organization (FAO) and the World Health Organization (WHO). The FAO/WHO recommendations are considered sufficient for the maintenance of health in nearly all people. They differ from the RDA because they are based on slightly different judgment factors and serve different purposes. The FAO/WHO recommendations, for example, assume a protein quality lower than that commonly consumed in the United States and so recommend a higher intake (see Chapter 5). They also take into consideration that worldwide, people are generally smaller and more physically active than the population of the United States. The United States sets its calcium recommendation higher to keep it in balance with the higher protein intakes of its people. Nevertheless, the recommendations of different nations all fall within the same general range.

The Challenge of Nutrition Guidelines

The RDA make specific recommendations for protein, vitamins, and mineral intakes, but they only make general statements about energy intakes, and they do little to protect people from excess intakes of fat, salt, sugar, cholesterol, and alcohol. Authorities are now as much concerned about achieving moderation in the diet for these substances as they once were about people's consuming too few nutrients.

Table 2–2 Current Dietary Recommendations

Dietary Guidelines for Americans	American Heart Association	American Institute for Cancer Research	Suggestions for Food Choices
Maintain healthy weight.	Consume sufficient calories to maintain recommended body weight.	Avoid obesity.	Control overeating. Take smaller portions. Avoid seconds. Eat fewer fatty foods and sweets. Eat more foods low in calories and high in nutrients.
Eat a variety of foods.	Consume a wide variety of foods.		Include these foods every day: fruits and vegetables; whole-grain and enriched breads and cereals and other products made from grains; milk and milk products; meats, fish, poultry, and eggs; and dried peas and beans.
Choose a diet low in fat, saturated fat, and cholesterol.	Limit total fat intake to less than 30% of calories. Limit saturated fat intake to less than 10% of calories. Limit cholesterol intake to 300 milligrams per day.	Reduce the intake of total dietary fat from the current average of about 37% to a level of no more than 30% of total calories and, in particular, reduce the intake of saturated fat.	Choose low-fat protein sources such as lean meats, fish, poultry, and dried peas and beans. Use eggs and organ meats in moderation. Limit intake of fats on and in foods. Trim fats from meats. Broil, bake, or boil—don't fry. Limit breaded and deep-fried foods. Read food labels for fat contents.
Choose a diet with plenty of vegetables, fruits, and grains.	Consume at least 50 to 55% of calories from carbohydrate sources, especially complex-carbohydrate sources.	Increase the consumption of fruits, vegetables, and whole grains.	Substitute starchy foods for foods high in fats and sugars. Select whole-grain breads and cereals, fruits and vegetables, and dried peas and beans to increase fiber and starch intake.
Use sugars only in moderation.			Use less sugar, syrup, and honey. Reduce concentrated sweets like candy, soft drinks, and cookies. Read food labels for sugar content.
Use salt and sodium only in moderation.	Sodium intake should be no more than 3,000 milligrams (3 grams) per day.		Learn to enjoy the flavors of unsalted foods. Flavor foods with herbs, spices, and lemon juice. Reduce salt in cooking. Add little or no salt at the table. Limit salty foods. Read food labels for salt or sodium contents.

Table 2–2—continued

Dietary Guidelines for Americans	American Heart Association	American Institute for Cancer Research	Suggestions for Food Choices
If you drink alcoholic beverages, do so in moderation.	If alcoholic beverages are consumed, limit intake to 1 to 2 oz of ethanol per day.	Drink alcoholic beverages only in moderation, if at all.	For individuals who drink, limit alcoholic beverages to one or two drinks per day. "One drink" means 12 oz of beer, 3 oz of wine, or 1 ½ oz of distilled spirits. (Pregnant women should not use alcohol. If you drink, do not drive.)
	Consume approximately 15% of calories from protein sources.		
		Eat foods rich in vitamins A and C.	*For Vitamin A:* use dark-green and deep yellow vegetables, cabbage, spinach, carrots, broccoli, tomatoes, and Brussels sprouts.
		Consume salt-cured, salt-pickled, and smoked foods only in moderation.	*For Vitamin C:* use citrus fruits, berries, peaches, melons, green and leafy vegetables, tomatoes, cauliflower, green peppers, and sweet potatoes.

Source: U.S. Department of Agriculture, U.S. Department of Health and Human Services, *Nutrition and Your Health: Dietary Guidelines for Americans.* 3rd ed. (Washington, D.C.: U.S. Government Printing Office, 1990); Nutrition Committee; *Dietary Guidelines for Healthy American Adults: A Statement for Physicians and Health Professionals* (Dallas: American Heart Association, 1991); American Institute for Cancer Research. *Dietary Guidelines to Lower Cancer Risk* (Washington, D.C.: AICR, 1990).

Among the suggestions intended to deal with these issues have been the *Dietary Goals for the United States* (see Figure 2–4). More recent recommendations include the *Surgeon General's Report* (1988) and the National Research Council's *Diet and Health* report (1989)—as discussed in Chapter 1. Others include the *Dietary Guidelines for Americans* (1990) and the American Heart Association's and the Institute for Cancer Research's guidelines for healthy Americans which are revised periodically (these are listed in Table 2–2). These recommendations represent attempts to create broad, noncontroversial recommendations for dietary habits in the United States. The *Nutrition Recommendations for Canadians* are presented in Appendix C.

The ten leading causes of death in the United States, as shown in Chapter 1, are heart disease, cancer, stroke, accidents, lung disease, pneumonia and flu, diabetes, suicide, liver disease, and atherosclerosis. Five of them have been linked to our diet. The various sets of guidelines are proposed to reduce the risks associated with diet. All age groups are expected to benefit from adherence to them. A sedentary lifestyle and overconsumption of foods high in calories, salt, sugar, fat, cholesterol, and alcohol have been associated with obesity, high blood pressure, heart attacks, strokes, diabetes, dental cavities,

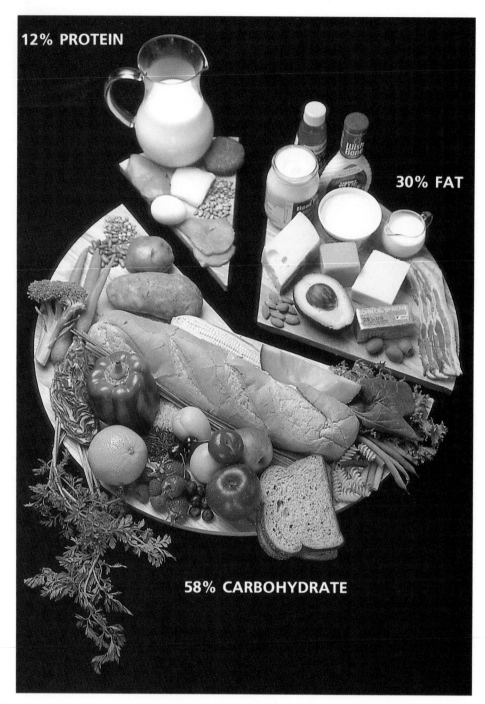

● *Figure 2–4*

The Dietary Goals

A balanced diet is composed of 12 to 15% protein from animal and vegetable sources, 55 to 58% carbohydrate and no more than 30% fat calories, including the fat from meats, whole milk, eggs, cheese, vegetable oils, and nuts.

liver disease, and some forms of cancer—the so-called **lifestyle diseases.** To alter these trends, the recommendations suggest a general increase in the consumption of complex carbohydrates, such as fruits, vegetables, and whole grains; a decrease in the consumption of meats and foods high in fat, sugar, and salt; an increase in the consumption of fish and poultry; and the substitution of polyunsaturated and monounsaturated fats (vegetable oils) for saturated fats such as butter, lard, and shortening (see Figure 2–5).

Lifestyle diseases conditions that may be aggravated by modern lifestyles that include too much eating, drinking, and smoking and too little exercise.

Should you change your diet to meet these guidelines? Two major arguments favor your changing your diet: (1) the risks are not great and the health benefits may be considerable, and (2) the older way of eating—a diet high in plant foods—is better for the earth. The introduction to the *Dietary Goals* took a strong stand in favor of making changes to the effect that the changes do not entail significant risks:

> The diet we eat today was not planned or developed for any particular purpose. It is a happenstance related to our affluence, the productivity of our farmers and the activities of our food industry. The risks associated with eating this diet are large. The question to be asked, therefore, is not why should we change our diet but why not?[3]

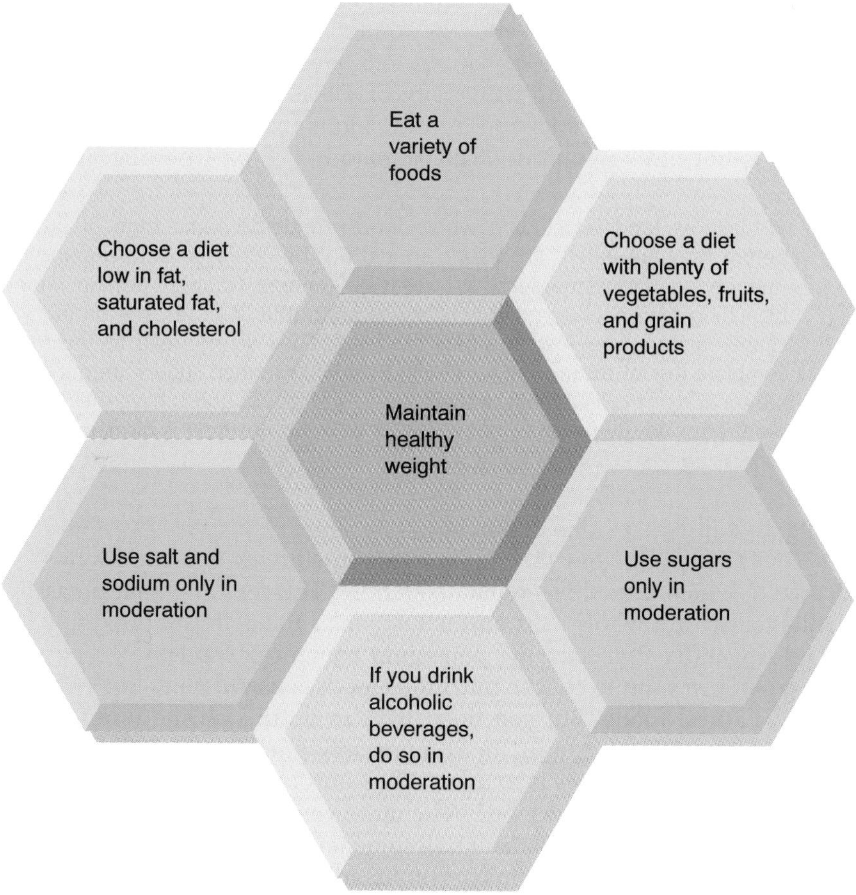

Figure 2–5

Dietary Guidelines

Use the seven guidelines together as you choose a healthful and enjoyable diet.

Whole food has the nutritional advantage

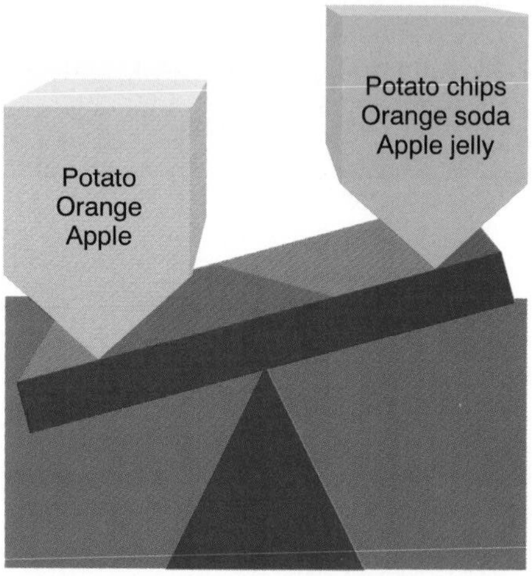

The nutrients supplied by the potato, orange, and apple far outweigh those from their empty-calorie processed forms.

Choosing Whole Foods

A change in our dietary habits would also be good for the earth. As it happens, most of the goals and guidelines offered to date have had one point in common. They tend to favor a return toward a more whole-food, plant-based diet. The Worldwatch Institute (a private organization) has taken the position that the only known risk of such a trend would be to the food industry, whereas important benefits to the economy would counterbalance this effect. An increase in the consumption of fruits, vegetables, and whole grains and a decrease in the consumption of empty-calorie fats, oils, alcohol, and sugar would increase the nutrient density of our diet, thereby reducing malnutrition, including overnutrition.

Generally speaking, the more a food resembles the original, farm-grown product, the more nutritious it is likely to be. During processing, nutrients are lost, and often nutrient-poor additions such as sugar, salt, and fat are made. A potato contains 20 milligrams of vitamin C; the same number of calories in French fries contains only about 7 milligrams; and the same number of calories in potato chips contains only 2 milligrams of vitamin C. An apple contains 12 RE of vitamin A, applesauce with the same number of calories contains about 5, and apple jelly contains less than 1. And so forth. Regardless of where these products are purchased, there is something to be said for buying the potato and the apple. They don't have to be *labeled* natural—they only have to *be* natural—to have a nutritional advantage.

Donald R. Davis of the University of Texas provides a meaningful distinction between nutritious and nonnutritious foods, emphasizing that processing is not, itself, a culprit. "Dismembering," or **partitioning**, *is* a culprit:

> Virtually all foods—including whole foods—undergo some form of processing before they are eaten. *Processing* should not be confused with *refining* or *dismembering*. Processes such as freezing, canning, drying, peeling, grinding, blanching, and cooking all may cause some [nutrient] losses, but ordinarily they cause only a partial loss of a few nutrients. They do not lead to the major or complete loss of most or all nutrients [that] occurs when sugars are purified, fats are separated from whole foods, alcohol is distilled, or grains have their germ and bran removed. By far our biggest enemy of good nutrition is dismembering, not processing.[4]

Table 2–3 illustrates this distinction.

Dr. Davis points out that the potassium content is a good index of the degree to which a food has remained whole. The reason is that potassium is contained within whole cells and is lost when the cells are broken. Chapter 7 and Appendix F present the potassium content of foods.

When you want to choose nutritious foods, a useful guideline is to choose **whole, natural foods.** But you don't have to do this all the time. Not every potato product you use must be recognizably potato. A principle that helps with making food choices is to ask, "What am I using this food for?" or "How big a part of my diet is this food?" The more you depend on a food as a **staple food**, the more important is its wholesomeness. If, for example, bread is one of your staple foods, then whole-grain bread is certainly a better choice than refined, white bread (see Chapter 3).

Natural food one that has been altered as little as possible from the original farm-grown state. As used on labels, this term may misleadingly imply unusual power to promote health; it has no legal definition.

Partitioned food a food that consists of only one or a few components of the original plant or animal tissue from which it was taken—such as sugar (from beets), butter (from milk), or refined flour (from whole grain).

Staple food a food used frequently or daily in the diet—for example, potatoes (in Ireland) or rice (in the Far East).

Whole food a food that is altered as little as possible from the plant or animal tissue from which it was taken—such as beets, milk, or oats.

Table 2–3

Whole Versus Dismembered Foods

Dismembered foods together supply two-thirds of the calories consumed in the United States and other "advanced" nations.

PURIFIED SUGARS	SEPARATED FATS	ALCOHOL	MILLED GRAINS
Dismembered Foods			
Corn sweetener Corn syrup Fructose Fruit "drinks" Gatorade Glucose (dextrose) Honey Lactose Lemonade Raw sugar Syrups Sucrose (table sugar)	Butter Cream Cream cheese Lard Margarine Mayonnaise Salad dressings (most) Shortening Vegetable oils, including "unrefined" and "cold pressed"	Gin Vodka Whiskey All other distilled spirits	Barley (pearled) Cornmeal (degermed) Refined flour Rice (white) Unbleached flour Wheat flour
Partially Dismembered Foods			
Maple syrup (pure) Molasses	Cheese (hard)	Beer Wine	
Whole-food Substitutes for Dismembered Foods			
Date sugar Fruits Raisins Sweet potatoes	Avocados Milk Nuts Peanut butter and other nut butters		Brown rice Whole barley Whole cornmeal Whole-wheat flour

Source: Copyright Donald R. Davis, Clayton Foundation Biochemical Institute, University of Texas, Austin. Used with permission.

Conversely, the less often or heavily you use a food, the less its quality matters. An example is candy bars. If you eat them only on picnics and you picnic only once a year, they'll hardly detract from your nutrition on a year-round basis. But if you are eating nothing but candy bars for breakfast and lunch every day, then they are a staple item in your diet and a very poor choice indeed.

The shift away from animal and toward plant foods would also reduce the amount of land used to feed meat animals, especially if they are grain fed, as most grocery store meat is. Some experts believe that to continue raising meat animals at today's rate is to threaten the world's agricultural future.[5] It takes many tens of thousands of calories in grain to produce a few hundred calories of beef. Thus, it is more economical in terms of resources for people to eat the grain directly and benefit from its calories and nutrients. The Nutrition Action feature in Chapter 11 explores further the relationships between people, what they eat, and the well-being of the earth.

Whether you choose to adopt these recommendations as your own goals is, of course, up to you. In case you are curious to see how your eating style compares with current recommendations, the Diet Variety Scorecard is provided to let you see how your diet measures up to the dietary guidelines. The Spotlight feature at the end of Chapter 3 discusses what is known about the relationship of nutrition to cancer—links that led to the recommendations given in Table 2–2. The Nutrition Action feature in this chapter offers our own guidelines for choosing snacks that meet these guidelines.

Diet Variety Scorecard

How Does Your Diet Rate?

Check one box in each row which best describes how you eat and then total each column.

	Column A	Column B	Column C
Meat			
Red Meat*	☐ I usually eat hot dogs, sausage, bacon, lunch meats such as salami or bologna, prime beef.	☐ I vary my use of high-fat and lean red meat.	☐ I eat only well-trimmed lean red meat: Choice or select grades; flank & round steak, tenderloin, loin chops, wild game, etc.
Fish & Shellfish*	☐ I rarely eat fish of any kind or I eat only fried fish.	☐ I eat fish several times a month.	☐ I eat fish prepared with minimal fat at least once a week.
Poultry*	☐ I rarely eat poultry or I eat only fried poultry.	☐ I always eat poultry with the skin.	☐ I eat poultry at least 2 times a week and remove the skin before eating.
*If you are a vegetarian check box in column C	☐ I eat 12 oz or more of meat, poultry, or fish each day.	☐ I eat 6-12 oz meat, poultry or fish daily.	☐ I eat 6 oz or less meat, poultry, or fish daily.
Dairy Products	☐ I drink whole milk.	☐ I drink 2%-fat milk.	☐ I drink nonfat and 1%-fat milk.
	☐ I eat high-fat cheeses such as cheddar, Swiss, colby, jack, and cream cheese more than 3 times a week.	☐ I eat both high- and low-fat cheeses.	☐ I rarely eat cheese or I use low-fat cheeses such as farmers, cottage, skim-milk mozzarella, and reduced-fat cheese products.
	☐ I eat ice cream more than twice a week.	☐ I eat ice milk or low-fat frozen yogurt instead of ice cream.	☐ I rarely eat frozen desserts or I eat only sherbet, sorbet, or nonfat frozen dessert.

Continued

	Column A	Column B	Column C
Complex Carbohydrates			
Whole grain and starchy products such as oatmeal, bread, rice and pasta.	☐ I eat 2 servings or less a day.	☐ I eat 3–5 servings a day.	☐ I eat 6 or more servings a day.
Fruits & Vegetables	☐ I eat 2 servings or less a day.	☐ I eat 3–4 servings a day.	☐ I eat 5 or more servings a day.
Dried peas & beans such as lima, kidney, pinto, lentil, etc.	☐ I rarely or never eat these foods.	☐ I eat these foods once a week.	☐ I eat these foods 2 or more times a week.
Fats & Oils	☐ I almost always add butter or margarine to my foods.	☐ I add butter or margarine to some, not all, foods.	☐ I rarely add butter or margarine to foods.
	☐ I use regular salad dressings, mayonnaise, and sauces.	☐ I eat both regular and low-fat dressings and sauces.	☐ I use low-fat salad dressings and avoid sauces.
Egg Yolks			
(Include those used in food preparation.)	☐ I eat 8 or more egg yolks a week.	☐ I eat 5–7 egg yolks a week.	☐ I eat no more than 4 egg yolks a week or use egg whites or egg substitutes.
Sweet Baked Goods			
Products such as pies, pastries, cakes, doughnuts.	☐ I eat sweet baked goods at least 4–6 times a week.	☐ I eat these foods 2–4 times a week.	☐ I seldom eat these foods or only eat them on special occasions.
Salt	☐ I usually use salt in cooking and at the table.	☐ I only use salt in cooking.	☐ I prefer to use herbs and spices to flavor my food, and rarely use salt.
Salty Foods			
(Such as snacks, pickles, canned soup, etc.)	☐ I eat some of these foods almost daily.	☐ I eat these foods 2–4 times a week.	☐ I usually avoid these foods.
Totals: Add up how many checks you have in each column.	Total Column A: ________	Total Column B: ________	Total Column C: ________
Scoring:	6 or more checks in column A mean you need help. Choose more from columns B & C.	6 or more checks in column B mean you are making some good food choices. Try more from column C.	10 or more checks mean you are eating smart. Keep up the good work.

Source: Adapted from Heart Smart Nutrition Quiz, American Heart Association, Minnesota Affiliate, Inc.

NUTRITION ACTION

Grazer's Guide to Smart Snacking

Government surveys show that just about everyone reaches for a little something between meals. These findings are supported by the $12 billion Americans spend each year on snack foods such as popcorn and potato chips.[6] But while gobbling is out and **grazing** is in, many people feel a twinge of guilt now and then about between-meal munching. Perhaps the parental warnings of childhood that snacks can spoil a meal linger in the back of many minds. Nevertheless, nutritious nibbling can make it easier for many people to eat healthfully.

Grazing eating small amounts of food at intervals throughout the day, rather than—or in addition to—eating regular meals.

Snacks can supply essential vitamins, minerals, and calories to the diets of small children, whose small stomachs and appetites often cannot handle larger meals. As for teenagers, who typically don't seem to have the time (or the inclination) to eat regularly between going to school, baseball practice, music lessons, or other activities, snacks account for upwards of a third of the calories they eat and as much as 20 percent of their vitamin and mineral consumption.[7] Snacks also contribute to the nutritional needs of adults, who may find fitting meals into a busy schedule difficult. Even senior citizens, whose lifestyles tend to be less hectic, can benefit from grazing. That's because lack of activity, certain medications, and isolation can blunt a formerly hearty appetite, making frequent and small meals more desirable than large breakfasts, lunches, and dinners.

At any age, the key to healthful snacking is choosing foods rich in vitamins, minerals, and fiber as well as low in fat, such as fruits, low-fat cheese and yogurt, whole-grain crackers, and plain popcorn. Cakes, cookies, candy, and potato chips are harder to fit into a healthful eating plan because they add fat and calories to the diet and little else in the way of nutrients.

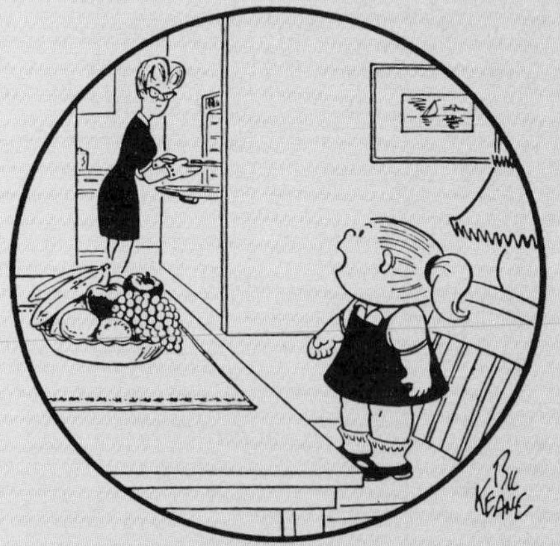

"Grandma, is this fruit the kind for looking at or the kind for eating?"

Source: Reprinted with special permission of King Features Syndicate, Inc.

Some snacks that appear nutritious may be deceiving. For example, fruit drinks, mixes, and punches are loaded with sugar and are more like soft drinks than fruit juice. Fruit rolls and bars are nutritionally similar to jams and jelly, not fresh fruit. Most of the nutrients in the fruit are lost when the fruit is processed with heat, and of course, when sugar and fat are added. Granola bars are often the nutritional equivalent of chocolate candy bars (see Figure 2–6). Many typical granola bars are sweetened with up to fourteen kinds of sugar and are high in fat and salt. Even some varieties of microwave popcorn don't rate well as snacks, since lots of oil and salt are usually added. (You can make your own microwave popcorn without all the extras.) When you feel like snacking, try some of the alternatives offered in Table 2–4. Use Table 2–5 as a guide to see how some of your favorite snacks rate according to number of calories and amount of fat and sodium. In addition, consider the following tips next time you're in the mood to grab a snack.

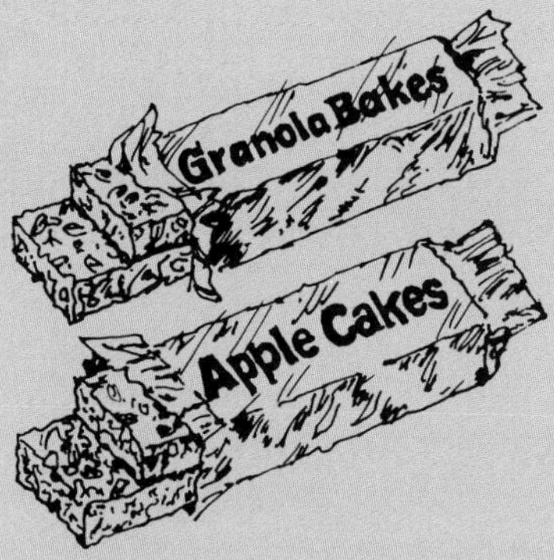

Ingredients: Rolled oats, sugar, coconut oil and/or palm oil, brown sugar syrup, honey, salt, soy lecithin.

Ingredients: 100% whole-wheat flour, applesauce, honey, dates, raisins, soy oil, unsulfured molasses, rolled oats, almonds, amaranth, soy lecithin, wheat germ, baking soda.

Figure 2–6

If You Snack, Do It Well.

Here, both snack items start with a wholesome first ingredient—rolled oats or 100 percent whole-wheat flour. (The majority of available snack items do not.) However, note that one snack includes three sources of sugar on its label (sugar, brown sugar syrup, and honey), whereas the other snack uses only two (honey and molasses). You would have to check the labels and compare total grams of sugar to determine which snack contained more sugar. Also note that the first snack lists saturated fat (coconut and/or palm oil) as an ingredient. The other snack uses polyunsaturated fat (soy oil).

- Stock your refrigerator and kitchen cupboards with nutritious foods such as fruit juices, low-fat yogurt, fresh fruits and vegetables, plain popcorn, pretzels, whole-grain crackers, and low-fat cheeses so that they are close at hand. Nibblers often reach for a snack just to have something to munch on rather than because of a desire for the food itself. If nutritious choices are easy to get to, chances are that's what you'll eat.
- Put fresh fruit and crackers and cheese, or even a half sandwich, in your backpack or briefcase so you won't have to resort to buying candy from a vending machine when you get the urge to munch.
- Create your own snacks. Mix one cup each pretzels, peanuts, raisins, and sunflower seeds together to take with you on your next bicycle trip or hike. Or, instead of cream cheese, blend ½ cup each drained low-fat yogurt and low-fat cottage cheese; add a bit of chopped drained pineapple, strawberries, or any other fruit that suits your taste and spread it on crackers, bagels, English muffins, or rice cakes.
- Make new versions of old favorites, such as **Chili Popcorn**[8] and **Frozen Bananas.**[9]
- Try to brush your teeth—or at least rinse your mouth thoroughly—after snacking to prevent tooth decay. (See Nutrition Action feature in Chapter 10 for a detailed explanation of the role of diet in dental health.)
- Snack with a friend. If you're craving a candy bar or chips and nothing else will do, try splitting a bar or bag with a friend. That way you'll satisfy your craving without going too far overboard on calories and fat or salt.

Chili Popcorn

Mix 1 quart popped popcorn with 1 tablespoon melted margarine. In a separate bowl, mix 1 ¼ teaspoons chili powder, ¼ teaspoon ground cumin, and a dash of garlic powder. Sprinkle seasonings over popcorn and mix well. Makes about 4 1-cup servings.

Frozen Bananas

Mix 1 tablespoon of peanut butter with ¼ cup evaporated milk. Roll 1 banana, cut in half, in the peanut butter mixture. Then roll the coated banana halves in chopped nuts or bran cereal. Place in the freezer until frozen.

Table 2–4 **Snacking Smarter**

INSTEAD OF:	TRY:
Fruit drinks	Fruit juice
Soda pop	Fruit juice concentrate and sparkling water
Milk shake	Shakes made with nonfat milk and fresh fruit
Potato chips	Pretzels (try low salt)
Chips and sour cream dip	Vegetables with buttermilk dip
Granola bars	Homemade oatmeal cookies (reduce the fat and sugar)
Frosted cake	Angel food cake and fruit
Pie	Fruit cobblers
Cookies	Vanilla wafers, gingersnaps, graham crackers

Table 2–5

What's in a Muncher's Menu?

FOOD	GRAMS OF FAT	CALORIES
½ cup corn chips	4	70
1 cup plain popcorn	trace	30
1 cup buttered and salted popcorn	2	50
2 graham cracker squares	1	60
4 saltine crackers	1	50
2 bread sticks	1	75
1 3½"-round bagel	2	200
1 2½"-round bran muffin	6	125
10 thin pretzel sticks	trace	10
2 carrot and 2 celery sticks	trace	5
6 fluid ounces tomato juice	trace	30
10 potato chips	7	105
10 French fries	8	160
Small apple	trace	60
Banana	1	105
1 small box raisins (about 1 ½ tbsp)	trace	40
1 ounce process American cheese	9	105
1 cup nonfat milk	1	90
8-ounce carton lowfat yogurt with fruit	2	230
¼ cup roasted peanuts	18	210
2 tablespoons peanut butter	16	190
½ cup frozen yogurt	2	105
½ cup ice cream	7	135
2 2⅓"-round chocolate chip cookies	6	90
2 chocolate or vanilla sandwich-type cookies	4	100
2 fig bars	2	105
Frosted cream-filled cupcake	4	160
Cake-type doughnut	12	210
1 ½-ounce chocolate candy bar	14	220
12 fluid ounces regular cola soft drink	0	160

Source: Adapted from Muncher's Guide in *Making Bag Lunches, Snacks, & Desserts Using the Dietary Guidelines* (U.S. Department of Agriculture Human Nutrition Information Service, Home and Garden Bulletin No. 232–9): pp. 7–8.

Tools Used in Diet Planning

Given a set of recommendations like the RDA, which tell us about how much of each nutrient we should consume each day, how can we translate those recommendations into a plan of daily menus? After all, we eat foods—not nutrients—and very few people want to know so much about foods that they can mentally add up the zinc, iron, vitamin C, and some 40 other nutrients they are obtaining from each bite of a meal. Fortunately, some guidelines are available for selecting foods, and they are based on the concept of dietary balance, discussed in Chapter 1.

Food group plan a diet-planning tool that sorts foods of similar origin and nutrient content into groups and then specifies that a person eat a certain number of foods from each group.
Fortified food a food to which nutrients have been added.

Food Group Plans

A familiar guideline for diet planning fits the major foods into four groups using a **food group plan.** Table 2–6 shows the Four Food Group Plan. The minimum daily number of servings recommended for an adult from the four food groups (milk/milk products, meats/meat alternates, fruits/vegetables, and grains) is two, two, four, and four from each food group, respectively. Table 2–6 shows some of the major nutrients each food group supplies and offers many specific examples of foods in each group. This helps the planner design an adequate and balanced diet.

The Four Food Group Plan is flexible. For example, it permits you to substitute cheese for milk because both supply similar arrays of nutrients in about the same amounts. You can choose legumes and nuts as alternatives for meats. You can also adapt the plan to casseroles and other mixed dishes and to different national and cultural cuisines.

Legumes are rich in protein and B vitamins, as is meat, but unlike meat, legumes are low in fat and high in healthful complex carbohydrates (both starch and fiber). Long scorned by the middle class as "beans" or "the poor man's meat," legumes are now coming into their own as an inexpensive, health-promoting, land-sparing, nutritious food. From them are made food products that are used in many kinds of cooking: bean curd (tofu) and soy sauce, peanut butter, baked beans, bean sprouts, and refried beans, among others.

Each of the four groups consists of foods that are similar in nutrient content. The nutrients named in the table are representative of all the nutrients; if you have enough of them, it is assumed you will have enough of the others, too. This is true in theory, but in practice people using this plan must be careful to choose mostly *nutrient-dense* foods in each group in order to provide a reasonable foundation for diet planning. A **fortified food** is often an exception because relatively nonnutritious foods are often selected for fortification. In such cases, some eight or ten nutrients may be listed on the label because they were added to the food. This makes the food appear nutritious, but a truly nutritious food has 30 or 40 nutrients. Those on the label of a fortified food may be the only nutrients present. Still, with the precaution that primarily whole foods be used, the Four Food Group Plan provides a suitable foundation for diet planning.

Since the Four Food Group Plan first appeared, many more nutrients have been studied. A person can follow all its rules and still fail to meet the day's needs for some nutrients—especially vitamin B_6, iron, magnesium, zinc, and vitamin E. Two servings of legumes added to the Four Food Group Plan would help to bring these nutrient intakes up to RDA levels.[10] This may increase your food energy intake beyond what you think you can afford, so many nutrition authorities recommend that you increase your activity levels and earn those calories.

Other food grouping systems are available for planning diets. For example, the U.S. Department of Agriculture (USDA) has developed the Food Guide Pyramid (see Figure 2–7), a guide to daily food choices comprising five food groups. Foods grouped together are similar in calories and nutrients. The number of servings called for by the pyramid are 6 to 11 servings a day of grains, 2 to 4 of fruit, 3 to 5 of vegetables, and 2 to 3 each of meat and dairy products—similar to other recommendations. The difference is in the way the information is presented (see Figure 2–7).

The **vegetarian** faces a special challenge in diet planning—that of obtaining the needed nutrients from fewer food groups. There are two major classes

Vegetarian a person who consumes a diet that omits meat, or all animal flesh, or all animal products.
Lacto-ovo vegetarian a vegetarian who eats animal products such as milk and eggs, but no animal flesh.
Vegan (VAY-gun or VEDGE-un) a vegetarian who eats nothing but plant foods; also called a **strict vegetarian.**

Table 2–6 The Four Food Groups

Key: □ Foods generally lowest in calories and highest in nutrient density. △ Foods moderate in calories and nutrient density. ○ Foods generally highest in calories and lowest in nutrient density.

	MINIMUM NUMBER OF SERVINGS	SERVING SIZE	
Milk Group 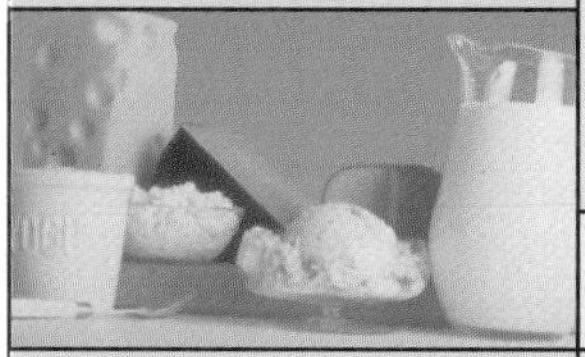	2 servings for adults 3 servings for children 4 servings for teenagers, young adults, and pregnant or breastfeeding women.	1 cup Milk 1 cup Yogurt 1 oz Cheese ½ cup Cottage cheese* ½ cup Ice cream, ice milk, frozen yogurt*	□ Nonfat milk, buttermilk, low-fat milk, plain yogurt. △ Whole milk, cheese, fruit-flavored yogurt, cottage cheese. ○ Custard, milk shakes, pudding, ice cream.
	Good source of: • calcium • riboflavin • protein • vitamin B_{12} • vitamins A and D (when fortified)		
Meat Group 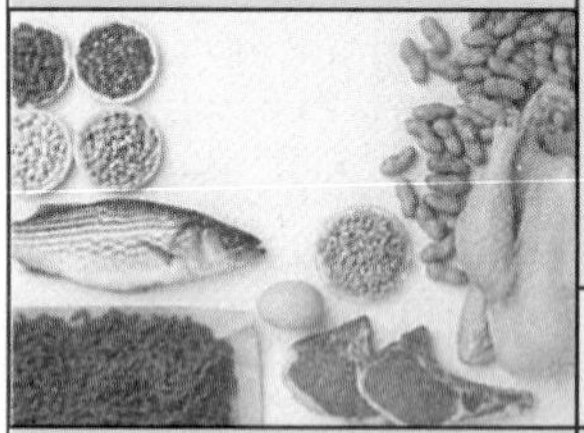	2 servings for all ages 3 servings for all pregnant and lactating women	2–3 oz Cooked lean meat, fish, poultry 1 Egg ½ cup Cooked dried peas, dried beans 2 tbsp Peanut butter ¼ cup Nuts, seeds	□ Poultry, fish, lean meat (beef, lamb, pork), dried peas and beans, eggs. △ Beef, lamb, pork, refried beans. ○ Hot dogs, luncheon meats, peanut butter, nuts.
	Good source of: • protein • phosphorus • vitamin B_6 • vitamin B_{12} • zinc • iron • magnesium • niacin • thiamin		
Fruit-Vegetable Group 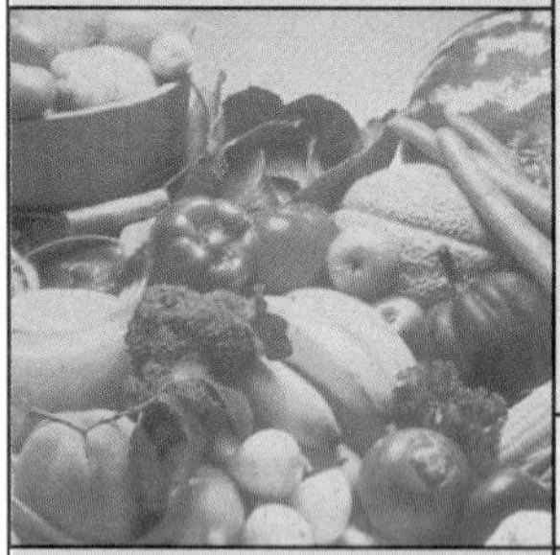	4 servings for all ages	½ cup Juice ½ cup Vegetable, fruit 1 medium Apple, banana, orange ½ Grapefruit ¼ Cantaloupe ¼ cup Dried fruit	□ Apricots, bean sprouts, broccoli, Brussels sprouts, cabbage, cantaloupe, carrots, cauliflower, cucumbers, grapefruit, green beans, green peas, leafy greens (spinach, mustard, and collard greens), lettuce, mushrooms, oranges, orange juice, peaches, strawberries, tomatoes, winter squash. △ Apples, bananas, canned fruit, corn, pears, potatoes. ○ Avocados, dried fruit, sweet potatoes.
	Good source of: • vitamin A • vitamin C • riboflavin • folate • iron • potassium • fiber • magnesium		
Grain Group 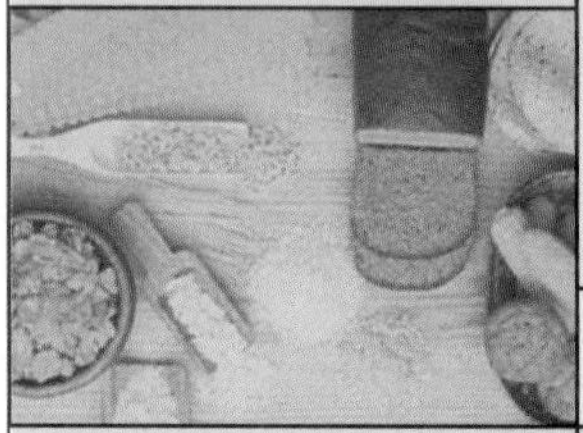	4 servings for all ages	1 slice Bread ½ English muffin, hamburger bun 1 oz Ready-to-eat cereal ½ cup Pasta, rice, grits, cooked cereal 1 Tortilla, roll, muffin	□ Whole grains (wheat, oats, barley, millet, rye, bulgur) enriched breads, rolls, tortillas. △ Rice, cereals, pastas (macaroni, spaghetti), bagels. ○ Pancakes, muffins, cornbread, biscuits, presweetened cereals.
	Good source of: • riboflavin • thiamin • iron • niacin • protein • magnesium • folate • carbohydrate • fiber		

"Others" Category	*Condiments*	*Chips and Related Products*	*Fats and Oils*	*Sweets*	*Alcohol*	*Other*
Foods in the "Others" category are often high in calories and/or low in nutrients. They don't take the place of foods from the Four Food Groups in supplying nutrients.	Barbecue sauce Catsup, mustard Olives, pickles Salt Soy sauce	Corn chips Popcorn Potato chips Pretzels Tortilla chips	Coffee whitener Cream, sour cream Gravy, cream sauce Margarine, butter Mayonnaise Oil, lard, shortening Salad dressing	Brownies, cookies Cakes, pies Candy Jelly, jam Sugar, honey, syrup Sweet rolls, doughnuts	Beer Gin Vodka Whiskey Rum Wine	Coffee, tea Fruit-flavored drinks Soft drinks

These servings provide the nutrients your body needs. They also supply about 1,200 calories. However, most people need more than 1,200 calories. If you do, add more servings.

*Cottage cheese, ice cream, ice milk, and frozen yogurt have about ¼ to ⅓ the amount of calcium per serving as milk, yogurt, and cheese.

Source: Adapted from National Dairy Council, Guide to Good Eating, 1990.

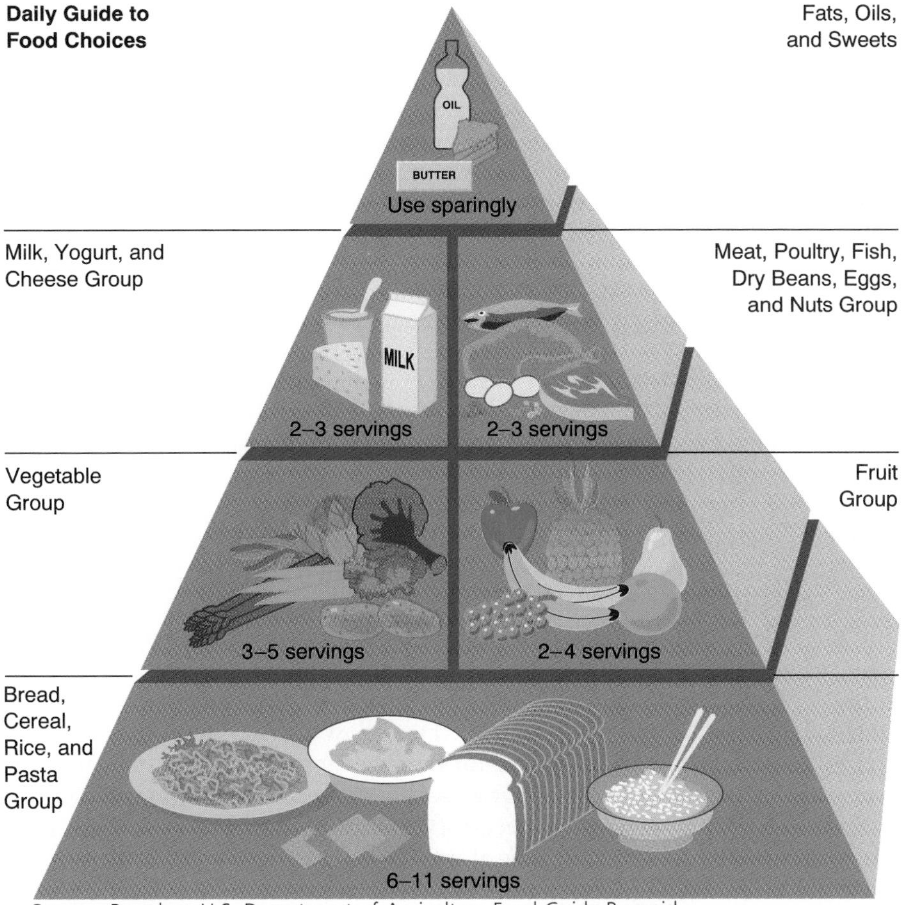

Source: Based on U.S. Department of Agriculture Food Guide Pyramid

Figure 2–7

Start at the Bottom and Eat Up.

"The Food Guide Pyramid emphasizes foods from the five food groups shown in the three lower sections of the pyramid. Each of these food groups provides some, but not all, of the nutrients you need. Foods in one group can't replace those in another. No one food group is more important than another; for good health, you need them all."

The USDA Food Pyramid was created as a food guide intended to provide practical information to the consumer on how to use the Dietary Guidelines. Whereas the traditional Four Food Groups are frequently displayed as a chart or wheel with each group carrying equal weight, the food pyramid assigns the grains group to the base and largest section of the triangle. Fruits and vegetables fill the next highest but slightly smaller section, followed by the meats and dairy groups in a still smaller section. Fats, oils, and sweets—the miscellaneous group—are placed at the tiny tip.*

Source: Adapted from USDA.

* Due to the design of the pyramid, there has been criticism from both meat and dairy producers' groups, with complaints that their products were stigmatized by their location in the triangle—right below the fats and sugars.

of vegetarians (with many variations). The **lacto-ovo vegetarian** uses milk and eggs (animal products) but excludes meat, fish, and poultry (animal flesh), while the **strict vegetarian**, or **vegan**, excludes all these foods and uses only plant foods. For these foodways, it is necessary to know how to choose foods to obtain the nutrients nonvegetarians get from the missing food groups.

The lacto-ovo vegetarian can adapt the Four Food Group Plan by making a change in the meat group (see Table 2–7). The vegan, who doesn't use dairy products, should take a vitamin B_{12} supplement or use soy milk fortified with vitamin B_{12} and calcium. There is more the vegetarian needs to learn, and additional guidelines are offered in the Spotlight feature in Chapter 5.

Portion Sizes

A set of lists is useful along with a food group plan. The plan may tell you to use a **serving** of food from a certain group at each meal. You can then turn to the list to find out exactly what foods are in each group, and what size **portion** will offer the intended amounts of nutrients and calories. Figure 2–8 provides some help with recognizing portion sizes.

The lists most often used with food group plans are called **exchange lists**, because their members are interchangeable. Finding an apple and a peach on the same list, for example, you can trade one for the other without signifi-

Serving an informal term that describes the amount of food a person might eat, similar to a helping.
Portion a defined serving, such as a half cup or a cup.
Exchange lists lists of foods with portion sizes specified; the foods on a single list are similar with respect to nutrient contents and calorie amounts and so can be used interchangeably.

Table 2–7

Vegetarian Food Groups

- 2 servings milk or milk products (or soy milk fortified with calcium and vitamin B_{12}).
- 4 servings fruits and vegetables (women include 1 c dark greens to help meet iron requirements).
- 4 servings whole-grain foods.
- 2 servings protein-rich foods (women include 2 c legumes daily to help meet iron requirements; count 4 tbsp peanut butter as 1 serving).

Table 2–8

The Six Exchange Lists

Milks
- Nonfat
- Low fat
- Whole

Vegetables[a]
Fruits
Starches/grains[b]
Meats
- Lean
- Medium fat
- High fat

Fats

[a]This list includes low-calorie vegetables only.
[b]This list includes starchy vegetables such as lima beans and corn as well as cereal, bread, pasta, and other grain products.

Other food group plans are available. Canada has one of its own—Canada's Food Guide, shown in Appendix C.

cantly altering the nutrient content or calorie count of your meal. Exchange lists help with calorie control and permit you to vary your diet by making different choices on different days. Table 2–8 gives the six common exchange lists.

A person who is serious about controlling calories as well as obtaining the needed nutrients needs to pay attention not only to food types but also to portion sizes. Typical food portions used as the basis for diet planning are as follows:

Milk: 1 cup nonfat milk—90 calories
Vegetable: ½ cup green beans—25 calories
Fruit: 1 small orange—60 calories
Starches/grain: 1 small potato/1 slice bread—80 calories
Meat: 1 ounce lean meat or low-fat cheese—55 calories
Fat: 1 teaspoon butter—45 calories

Figure 2–8 shows food portions that can be substituted without changing calories or the energy-nutrient balance. Cheese can be used as a milk alternate for its calcium or as a meat alternate because its protein and fat contents are similar to those of meat. If you replace meat with cheese, though, you need some other good iron source.

If you are a diet planner who wants to choose foods that contain all the nutrients you need, you are well advised to follow a food group plan because it promotes adequacy and provides for balance among the different kinds of foods to help you avoid overemphasis on any one food. If you want to control calories as well, you will find it necessary to monitor your portion sizes, too. This means that you need to think of nonfat milk as milk and of whole milk as milk with added fat, and of lean meat as meat and of fatty meat as meat with extra fat. Corn and lima beans, nutritious as they are, resemble bread in their nutrient contributions, and olives, bacon, and nuts resemble butter. Think in terms of the portion sizes shown in Figure 2–8.

Food Composition Tables

You now know about how much of each nutrient you need (from the RDA), and you have a rough guideline for setting up a diet plan that will deliver the nutrients. It is useful to have yet another tool—a listing of most of the possible foods you might eat that shows exactly how much iron, calcium, zinc, and so forth, that each food contains.

Such tables do exist. Appendix F provides a food composition table that includes the nutrient contents of over 1,500 different food items. Many people—and you may be one of them—find it worth their while to make careful records of all the foods they eat for several days, look up all these foods in the table or in a computer program that automates the process, add up all the nutrients they have consumed, and compare their intakes with the RDA or RNI.

Such tables have their limitations, of course. Foods vary somewhat in nutrient contents. For example, apricots do not all contain exactly the same amount of vitamin A. People's ways of preparing foods differ, and some cooking methods cause greater nutrient losses than others. Also, not all foods are listed. Nor are all nutrients listed. For example, of the 40 nutrients we have named as essential, only 16 are in this book's table. Still, food composition tables are useful if interpreted with the appropriate judgment.

The last problem is particularly easy to overcome. The more nutrients a diet provides in adequate quantities, the more likely the diet is to provide *other* nutrients in adequate quantities. By the time you have assured yourself that your diet provides ample protein, niacin, and zinc, for example, you probably need not worry about biotin, which is not listed in the table. Your diet is likely to provide enough of that vitamin, too.

As for the other problems, they, too, can be solved. Allow a little leeway: in case your apricot happens to be vitamin A poor, eat two apricots, or better yet, eat many other vitamin A-rich foods. Vary your cooking methods. And, most importantly, select a wide variety of foods so that you will not be depending too heavily on any one food for a given nutrient.

Another objection to food composition tables is that they are terribly cumbersome and time consuming to use. This problem, too, can be solved. In this case, the computer comes to the rescue. Dozens of computer programs are available that can perform the repetitive operations of adding up nutrient amounts in foods. All you have to do is pay, of course, and supply the needed information on the foods you eat in a form the computer can use. Programs differ, with some being easier to use, some more accurate, and some more reasonable in cost than others. The ideal program is one that permits easy and inexpensive use without sacrificing accuracy.

Consumer Tips

Ten Tips for Supermarketing

The first step in preparing a nutritious meal often begins at the supermarket. It takes both preparation and some label reading skills to leave the grocery store with the necessary items for a well-balanced diet. Next time you're shopping for groceries, keep in mind these smart-shopping tips.

1. Use the weekly food section of your local newspaper to give you ideas for the best seasonal buys and special sale items.
2. Make eating healthfully a fun experience. For example, buy at least one new nutritious item and try one new recipe each week.
3. Check to see what foods you already have on hand. Plan to use items that are close to their expiration date or peak freshness.
4. Shop from a list to limit extra trips to the store and to help avoid buying unnecessary items. Keep a running list in your kitchen for noting items you need to replace.
5. Read the nutrition and ingredient labels to compare different brands and types of foods. Ingredients are listed in order of quantity.
6. When available, use unit pricing to determine the best buy per serving.
7. Redeem coupons for items you normally buy to save money.
8. Avoid shopping when you are hungry, since everything looks good on an empty stomach.
9. Use product dating information to assure quality and freshness.
10. Learn to shop using the perimeter of the grocery store. Many of the low-fat, high-carbohydrate foods on your list will be located around the edges of the store—fresh produce, dairy products, whole-grain breads, and meat, poultry, or fish.

Figure 2–8 Exchange List Portion Sizes

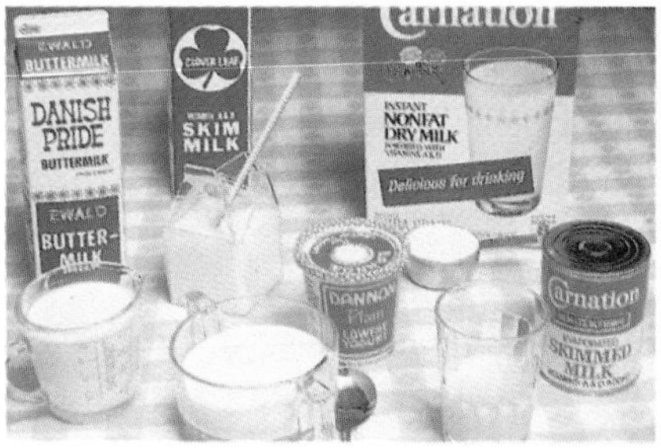

1. Milk
1 c nonfat milk
1 c nonfat yogurt, plain
1 c nonfat buttermilk
½ c evaporated nonfat milk
(1 milk = 12 g carbohydrate, 8 g protein, trace of fat, and 90 cal.)

2. Vegetables
½ c carrots
½ c greens
½ c Brussels sprouts
½ c beets
(1 vegetable = 5 g carbohydrate, 2 g protein, and 25 cal.)

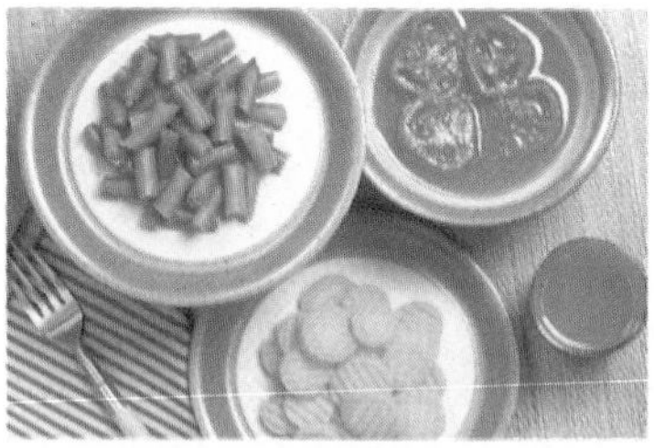

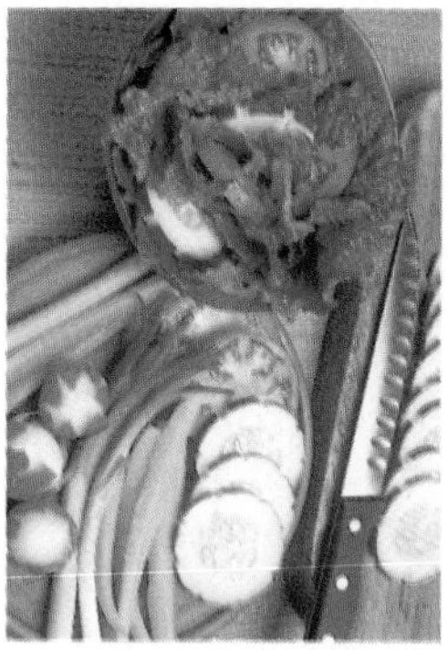

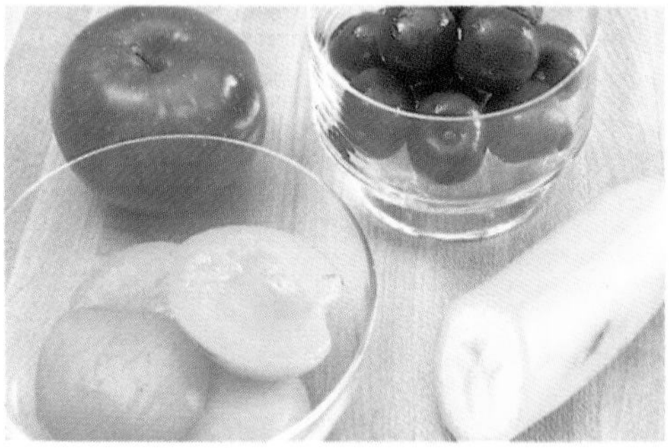

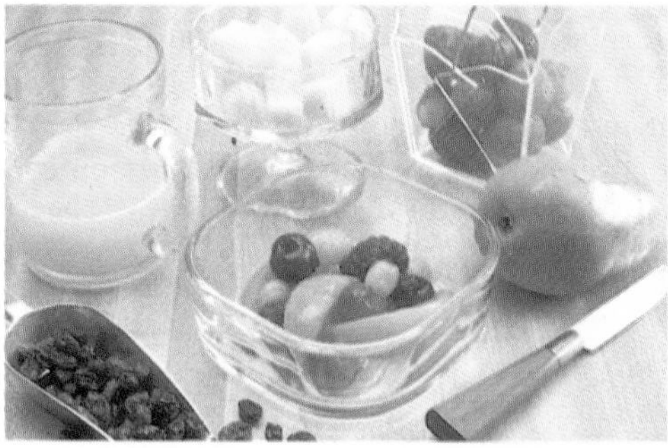

3. Fruits
½ small banana
1 small apple
½ grapefruit
½ c orange juice
(1 fruit = 15 g carbohydrate and 60 cal.)

4. Starches/grains
1 slice bread
¾ c ready-to-eat cereal
⅓ c cooked beans
½ c corn
1 small (3-oz) potato
(1 bread = 15 g carbohydrate, 3 g protein, trace of fat, and 80 cal.)

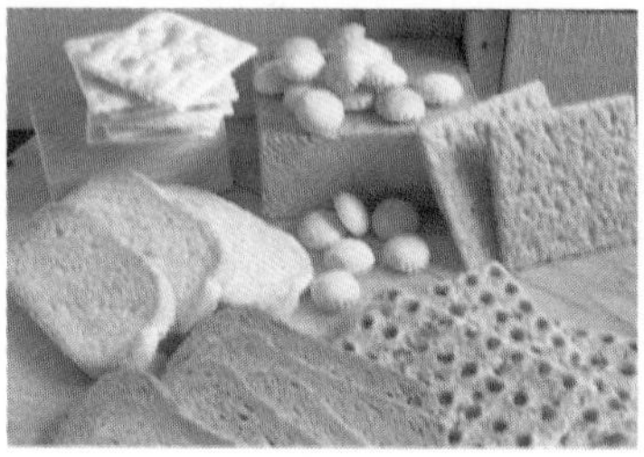

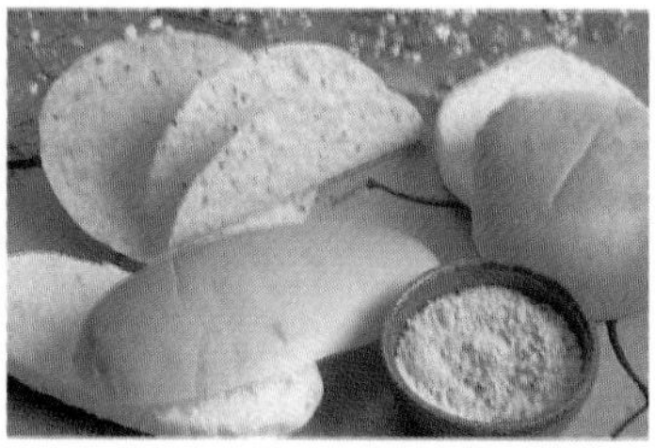

5A. Meats (lean)
1 oz lean meat
1 oz chicken meat without the skin
1 oz any fish
¼ c canned tuna
1 oz low-fat cheese[a]
(1 lean meat = 7 g protein, 3 g fat, and 55 cal.) (One 3-oz portion of meat, such as a hamburger patty = 3 meat exchanges. One meat exchange = ⅓ of a 3-oz hamburger patty.)

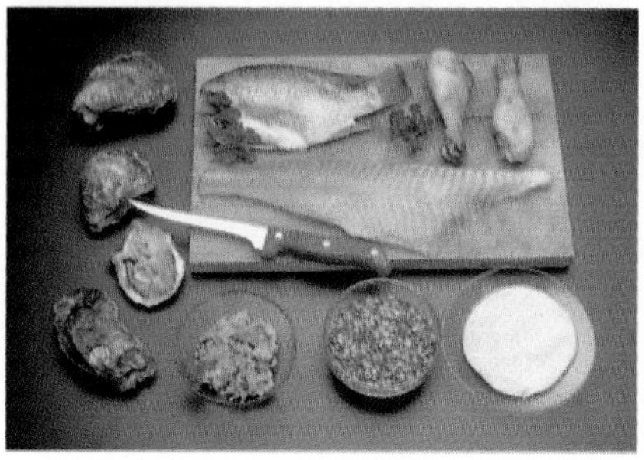

[a]Cheeses are grouped with milk in food group plans because of their calcium content but with meats in this system because, like meat, they contribute calories from protein and fat and have negligible carbohydrate content.

Figure 2–8 continued

5B. Meats (medium fat)
1 oz medium-fat meat is like 1 oz lean meat in protein content but has 5 g fat (2 g more fat than lean meat).
Examples:
1 oz pork loin
1 egg
¼ c creamed cottage cheese[a]
(1 medium-fat meat = 7 g protein, 5 g fat, and about 75 cal.)

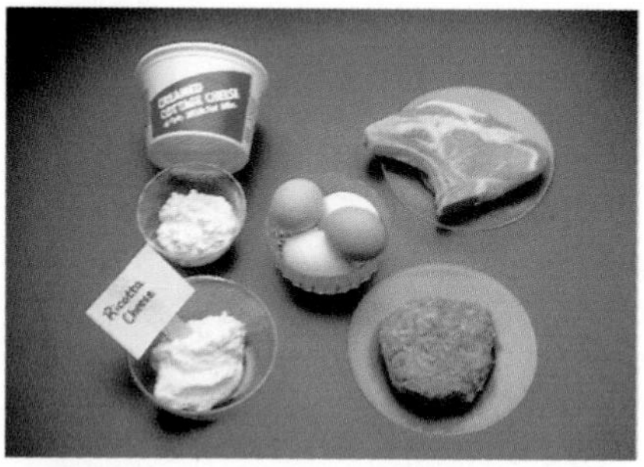

5C. Meats (high fat)
1 oz high-fat meat is like 1 oz lean meat in protein content but is estimated to have an **extra "1 fat"**—that is, to have the 3 g fat of a lean meat and 5 g additional fat.
Examples:
1 oz country-style ham
1 oz cheddar cheese[a]
1 small hotdog (frankfurter)[b]
(1 high-fat meat = 7 g protein, 8 g fat, and 100 cal.)

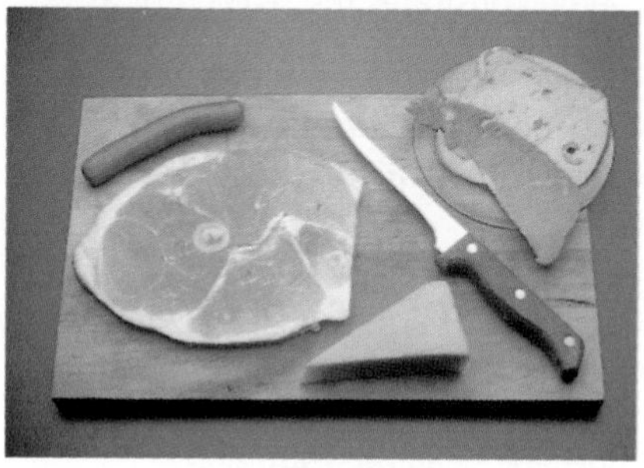

[b]The hotdog counts as 1 high-fat meat exchange plus 1 fat exchange.

5D. Legumes
Legumes are like meats because they are rich in protein and iron, but many are lower in fat than meat. They contain a lot of starch. They can be treated as:
1 c legumes = 1 lean meat + 2 starch.
(1 c legumes = 30 g carbohydrate, 13 g protein, 3 + g fat, and 215 cal.)

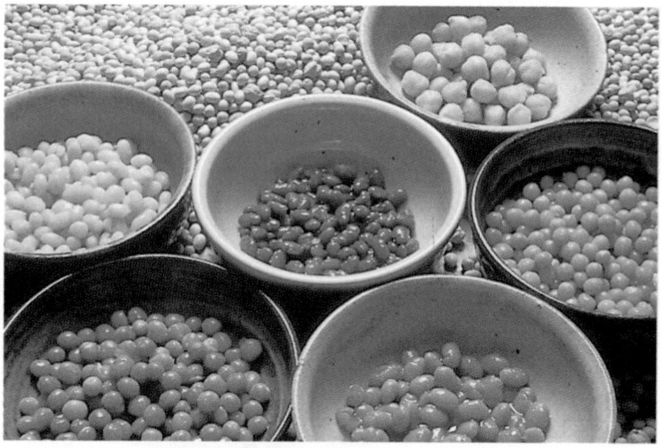

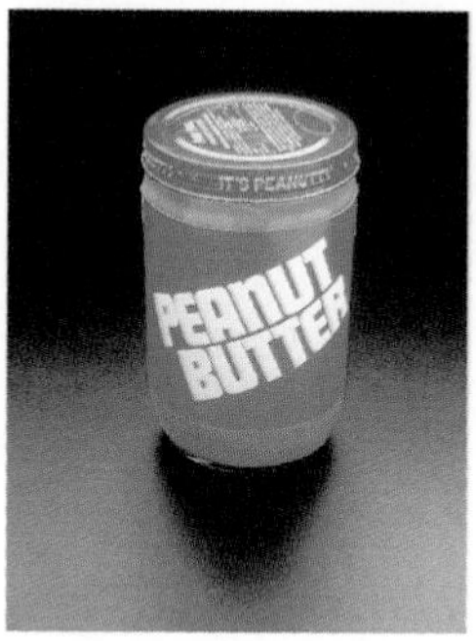

5E. Peanut butter
Peanut butter is like a meat in terms of its protein content. It is estimated as:
1 tbsp peanut butter = 1 high-fat meat (1 tbsp peanut butter = 7 g protein, 8 g fat, and 100 cal.)
Don't swear off peanut butter, necessarily. You'll need to appreciate the unsaturated character of its fat (see Chapter 4) and the B vitamin contributions it makes (see Chapter 6) before deciding how much of a place it should have in your diet.

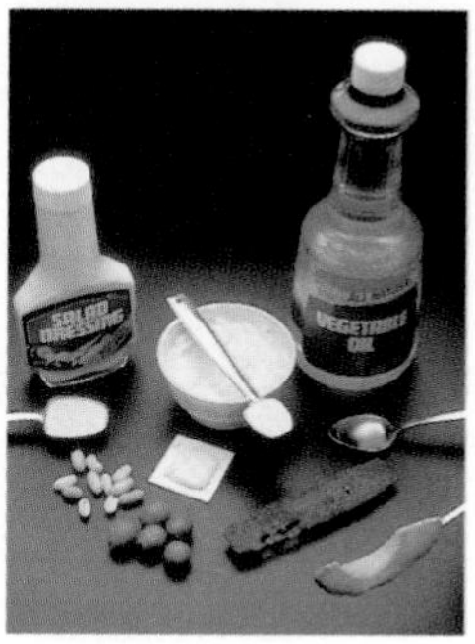

6. Fats
1 tsp butter
1 tsp margarine
1 tsp any oil
1 tbsp salad dressing
1 strip crisp bacon
5 large olives
10 whole Virginia peanuts
(1 fat = 5 g fat and 45 cal.)

Spotlight

Foods and their Labels

Some 25,000 foods line the shelves of the average grocery store. And thousands more are available from fast food operations and restaurants. Yet, as different as each one is, all of these are prepared by people other than ourselves. Reliance on prepared foods, which are easy to store or carry along and quick to cook, is greater than it has ever been before. It's important for people who use these foods daily to understand what sort of nutrient contributions they make and what they lack. A miniglossary of terms explains the various types of foods available in today's market. No matter what a food is called, though, learning how to read its nutrition label can be a big help.

What will the label tell me?

First of all, according to the law all labels must state:

- The common name of the product.
- The name and address of the manufacturer, packer, or distributor.
- The net contents in terms of weight, measure, or count.
- The ingredients listed in descending order of predominance by weight.

If you know how to read the front and side of a package, you're already a step ahead of the naive buyer. This is particularly true in regard to the ingredients list. The ingredient listed first has the largest amount of all the ingredients in the package. Consider the following ingredients lists:

- An orange powder that contains "sugar, citric acid, orange flavor . . ." versus a canned juice that contains "water, tomato concentrate, concentrated juices of carrots, celery . . ."
- A cereal that contains "puffed milled corn, sugar, corn syrup, molasses, salt . . ." versus one that contains "100 percent rolled oats."

Each of these examples contrasts a food that is loaded with nutrient-empty sugar with another that is made of nutrient-rich ingredients. If you read the label, you know what you're getting, and what the main ingredient is. Figure 2–9 demonstrates the reading of a label.

Sometimes labels provide more information than that. Why?

The nutrition-labeling section of the law states that if any nutrition claim is made on the label of a food package, it must conform to the following format under the heading "Nutrition Information":

- Serving or portion size.
- Servings or portions per container.
- Calorie content per serving.
- Carbohydrate grams per serving.
- Fat grams per serving.
- Protein grams per serving.
- Sodium milligrams per serving.
- Protein, vitamins, and minerals as percentages of the U.S. RDA. No claim may be made that a food is a significant source of a nutrient unless it provides at least 10 percent of the U.S. RDA of that nutrient in a serving.

If a nutrient is added to a food (for example, vitamin D added to a breakfast drink) or if an advertising claim is made (for example, that orange juice is a good source of vitamin C), then the package must provide an information panel that complies fully with the nutrition-labeling requirement. Without a complete information panel, nutrition claims could deceive the consumer about the true nutritional value of a food.

Miniglossary of Food Types

Convenience food a food that is cooked or otherwise processed before it is put on the market, then prepared at home.

Engineered food, fabricated food a food made from pure ingredients mixed in laboratories.

Enriched food a food to which nutrients have been added; or specifically in the case of grains, a refined grain food to which four specific nutrients lost in processing (iron, thiamin, riboflavin, and niacin) have been restored, as described in Chapter 3.

Fast food a food prepared in a quick-order restaurant.

Fortified food a food to which nutrients have been added.

Imitation food a food nutritionally inferior to the food it imitates. This term, by law, must appear on the label of a food if it contains 10 percent less of the U.S. RDA of an essential nutrient than the food it imitates.

Nutritious food a food that contains more nutrients than calories relative to a person's need. Enriched and fortified foods are excluded from this definition, because the added nutrients may be the only ones they contain.

Processed food a food that is cooked, frozen, freeze-dried, or otherwise treated before it is put on the market.

Figure 2–9 How to Read a Food Label

The ingredients list on the front or side panel names the ingredients in order of predominance by weight. Significance to you, the consumer: what appears first is present in the largest quantity. Only products with standards of identity (recipes defined by law) have no ingredients list.

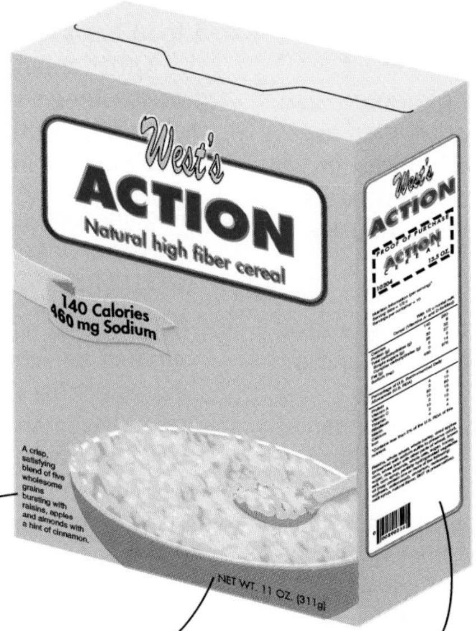

The front of the package must always tell you the product name, the name and address of the company, and the weight or measure; and it may list the ingredients.

The label may also state information about sodium and calories: see the Miniglossary of Terms for Food Labels.

Nutrition Information (per serving) 1
Serving Size = 1 c
Servings per Container = 24 } 2

	Cereal	Cereal + Butter, Milk, Water, Salt*	
Calories	140	280	
Protein (g)	4	6	3
Total carbohydrates (g)	30	32	3
Simple sugars (g)	25	27	4
Complex carbohydrates (g)	5	5	4
Fat (g)	0	14	3
Sodium (mg) 5	460	975	

Percentage of U.S. Recommended Daily Allowances (U.S. RDA)

	Cereal	Cereal + Butter, Milk, Water, Salt*	
Protein	4	8	6
Vitamin A	2	10	6
Vitamin C	80	80	6
Thiamin	10	15	6
Riboflavin	2	8	6
Niacin	10	10	6
Calcium	2	4	6
Iron	4	4	6

*Prepared according to recipe on back of package.

1 The nutrition information panel tells you the nutrients in a serving.

2 The serving size may or may not be the same as the amount you eat. Check the servings per container to get an idea of whether it is.

3 The energy-yielding nutrients are given in grams (units of weight). This is especially meaningful with respect to protein, because you need 40 to 80 g/day, depending on your size and other factors. Protein is also given in percentage of U.S. RDA in the list below.

4 The carbohydrate breakdown tells you how much simple sugar, starch, and fiber are in the product. A fat breakdown may also be listed, including saturated fat, unsaturated fat, and cholesterol.

5 Sodium is listed in milligrams. About 1,000 to 3,000 mg/day is considered a safe intake, but the average U.S. citizen consumes 5,000 to 7,000 mg/day. A teaspoon of salt contains 2,300 mg sodium.

6 Protein, vitamins, and minerals are given in percentages of U.S. RDA (see inside front cover). Significance to you, the consumer: if it meets 10% of the U.S. RDA, it undoubtedly meets at least 10% of your daily needs.

What is the U.S. RDA?

When you read a food label, it would help if it told you how much of your nutrient needs were met by eating one serving of that food. For example, it would be useful to see on the label of a cereal box that one serving of the cereal provides you with 25 percent of the iron you need for the day. Your RDA could be used to give you this information, but the trouble is, the makers of the label don't know who you are: a 20-year-old male or 27-year-old pregnant woman.

To provide useful nutrition information for most of the adult population (people over the age of 2), the U.S. RDA were designed. They provide one recommended amount for each nutrient for use on food labels. You may recall that the RDA table lists different recommendations for each sex and age group. Typically, the U.S. RDA is the highest of all the RDAs. For most nutrients, the U.S. RDA are the same as the RDA for an adult man. But for iron—because a woman's need is greater than a man's—the women's RDA is used. The table on the inside front cover shows the U.S. RDA that are used on the labels that make nutrition claims.

The U.S. RDA table includes two values for protein. If the protein is of high quality, the U.S. RDA is 45 grams. If it's of lower quality, the U.S. RDA is 65 grams (see Chapter 5 for more about protein quality). This rule enables the consumer to use protein of widely different qualities and still meet protein needs efficiently.

• I have to watch my weight, so I look for foods labeled low in calories. Are these foods really low in calories?

Foods labeled "low in calories" must state the absolute number of calories they contain on the label and must contain no more than 40 calories per serving. Any food called a reduced-calorie item must be at least a third lower in calories than the food it most closely resembles and must carry a nutrition label. See the miniglossary that defines terms found on food labels.

• Many of the convenience foods I use are either enriched or fortified. Does this mean they are more nutritious than ordinary foods?

Not necessarily. A fortified breakfast cereal may have such large quantities of nutrients added that one serving provides 100 percent of the U.S. RDA for all of them, yet your body can't absorb that many nutrients all at once. Or a fruit drink may be fortified with vitamin C and so provide more vitamin C than an equal amount of real fruit juice. But the smart consumer will realize that the juice also provides other vitamins and minerals that the drink doesn't. Try your skill at detecting misleading claims on the Nutrition Savvy Scorecard.

• Food Labeling Reform

Today's food shopper, presented with more nutrition information than ever before, faces confusing choices. In competing for the nutrition-conscious shoppers' food dollars, the industry tries to give consumers what the consumers perceive to be more healthful choices. For example, a salad oil is labeled "no cholesterol," and a "lite" fried chicken is labeled as containing "one third less fat" than regular fried chicken. Most of these labels are accurate, but misleading. Labeling a vegetable oil as "cholesterol free" seduces the consumer into ignoring the fact that the oil is rich in potentially heart-clogging fats. And the "lite" fried chicken may be one third leaner than other fried fowl, but it still provides more than one fourth of the suggested daily fat limit.

In 1989, the Food and Drug Administration responded to the need for more useful information on food labels and called for changes on food labels. In 1990, the Nutrition Labeling and Education Act of 1990 became law. This legislation gives the FDA's labeling initiative a solid legal base and an accelerated timetable. Because of the number of changes necessary to bring food labels in line with the new law, the FDA is changing the labels in three phases.

Phase One: Ingredients, Juices, Produce, and Fish

Unlike our grandparents, most people today aren't familiar with the makings of mayonnaise or bread. So the 1990 Act provides for a listing of all ingredients in standardized foods, such as ice cream, peanut butter, mayonnaise, bread, and others. During the 1930s, when the government set standards or recipes for these foods, people were familiar with the ingredients because many of these products were made in the home. The new law also removes the exemption of certified color additives from the labeling requirement. Under the new law each certified color additive used in a food has to be declared by its name.

Other amendments proposed to give consumers more complete information about the components of the foods they eat include the following:

- Require food labels to explain that the list of ingredients is in descending order of predominance by weight.
- Require that all sweeteners used in a product be listed together in the ingredient list under the collective term "sweeteners." Following the collective term, each sweetener will be listed in parentheses in descending order of predominance by weight of the sweetener in the food.
- Require that protein hydrolysates, used in many foods as flavors and flavor enhancers, be declared. For example, if hydrolyzed soy protein is added to a product, it must be declared by that name in the ingredient statement and not by the generalized designation "hydrolyzed protein."
- Require label declaration of sulfiting agents present in standardized foods. Some people are allergic to these preservatives.
- Require the label to identify caseinate as a milk derivative when used in foods that claim to be nondairy, such as coffee whiteners, because some people with milk allergies use nondairy products.

The remaining revisions affect labels on fruit and vegetable juices and nutrition information for the 20 most popular raw fruits, raw vegetables, and seafood.

- Require the percentage of actual fruit or vegetable juice to appear on the label of all juices, whether full strength or diluted.
- Require that multiple juice beverages that name or otherwise identify individual juices on the labels declare

Miniglossary of Terms for Food Labels

Cholesterol terms*

Cholesterol free less than 2 milligrams cholesterol and no more than 5 grams of fat per serving.

Low cholesterol no more than 20 milligrams cholesterol and no more than 5 grams of fat per serving.

Reduced cholesterol 75% lower in cholesterol than the food it most closely resembles.

Sodium terms

Sodium free less than 5 milligrams per serving.

Very low sodium 35 milligrams or less per serving.

Low sodium 140 milligrams or less per serving.

Reduced sodium processed to reduce the usual level of sodium by 75 percent.

Unsalted, no added salt, salt-free processed without the normally used salt.

Sugar terms

Sugar free, sugarless, no added sugar no table sugar (sucrose), but may contain other caloric sweeteners; must meet criteria of low-calorie or reduced-calorie food, or state otherwise.

Energy/calorie terms

Diet, dietetic terms used to indicate that a food is either low in calories or a reduced-calorie food.

Low calorie no more than 40 calories per serving.

Reduced calorie a food with at least a third fewer calories than the food it most closely resembles.

Weight terms

Gram a unit of weight. A teaspoon of any dry powder (such as salt) weighs about 5 grams. A half cup of food (such as vegetables) or liquid (such as juice) weighs about 100 grams. Many food servings are 100-gram servings.

Milligram 1/1000 of a gram.

U.S. RDA the United States Recommended Daily Allowance, used as a standard for the daily intake of nutrients for any normal, healthy adult, and designed for use on food labels. Individual RDA figures specifically for women, children, men, pregnant women, and other groups also exist (see inside front cover).

the percentage of each of the identified juices.

- Require that retail outlets make available to consumers nutrition information close to where raw fruits, vegetables, and fish are displayed for sale.

Phase Two: Nutrition Content

Under the old law only those foods that made an advertising claim (for example, that orange juice is a good source of vitamin C) or that added a nutrient to a food (for example, vitamin A added to milk), had to provide complete nutrition information that complied fully with the nutrition labeling requirements. In 1990, nutrition labeling appeared on about 60 percent of foods. Under the new law, about 90 percent of foods will be labeled. Foods exempted from nutrition labeling include those from small businesses (under $500,000 per year), those from restaurants, bulk foods, institutional foods, foods in bite-size packages, individual foods in multipacks, and foods of no nutritional significance (for example, spices). However, public demand for information may force these to be labeled as well.

Additions and deletions in the 18-year-old label format will reflect advances in nutrition science and provide useful information to consumers. The newest additions are fiber, cholesterol, saturated fat, sodium, and total calories from fat. Other listings of thiamin, niacin, and riboflavin that appeared on the old label format will be optional. Because the U.S. RDA was often confused with the National Research Council's RDAs, the FDA is proposing two groups of nutrient guidelines be used instead: the RDI (Reference Daily Intakes) and the DRV (Daily Reference Values.)

The RDIs reflect average allowances for all persons based on the 1989 RDA (10th revision). RDIs have been established for protein and 26 vitamins and minerals. The DRVs are established for nutrients that have no RDA: fat, fiber, saturated fat, cholesterol, carbohydrate, sodium, and potassium. Some DRVs are nutrient levels to achieve (fiber, carbohydrate) while others reflect limitations on intake (fat, saturated fat, cholesterol, sodium). Many of the DRVs are based on a calorie intake of 2,350 calories per day and so may overestimate amounts of the nutrients, especially for infants, young children, some women, and sedentary individuals whose calorie needs are not as great.

Phase Three: Nutrient Claims, Health Claims, Serving Size

FDA is concerned that nutrient claims made on products, such as "cholesterol-free" or "*X*-percent fat free," mislead and confuse consumers. The new laws

*These cholesterol definitions have been proposed by the FDA.

Nutrition Savvy Scorecard

All four of the label claims below are true. But which claims are misleading?

1. A label says one serving of a food provides 35 times as much iron as an 8-oz glass of whole milk.
2. A label says the lunchmeat is ''92 percent fat free''.
3. A label says a brand of instant nonfat dry milk has ''all the calcium, protein, and B vitamins of whole milk.''
4. A breakfast bar label says that the product has the same amount of protein, fat, carbohydrate, and certain vitamins and minerals as a breakfast of milk, egg, toast, and orange juice.

Scoring:
Labels 1, 2, and 4 are all misleading—label 1, because milk is a poor source of iron; label 2, because 75% of the lunchmeat's calories come from fat (see Chapter 4, Figure 4–10, part B); and label 4 for many reasons: the carbohydrate is sugar, versus the complex carbohydrate in toast; the fat is saturated fat, versus the corn oil the egg might have been fried in; and there may also be considerable salt in the bar. Furthermore, there are other nutrients in the regular breakfast that the breakfast bar does not contain. Label 3 is true and responsible. Give yourself 1 point for each of the four labels that you assessed correctly. If you got 1 point, you did about as well as most consumers would do—average. If 2 points—above average. If 3 points—superior. If all 4 points—outstanding: you are a savvy consumer.

define the use of nutrient labeling claims regarding fiber, vitamins, minerals, sodium, and calories as well as terms such as ''light'' and ''fresh.''

Health claims will be allowed on food labels only if a valid relationship between the nutrient and disease exists. If available scientific data support the health claims and experts agree that the claims are supported, the FDA will publish separate proposals for each health claim.

All of the nutrition information and nutrition claims made about a product hinge on its serving size. In order to fairly compare products, consumers need a consistent and reasonable serving size. For the first time, the FDA is attempting to define serving and portion sizes for 152 foods.

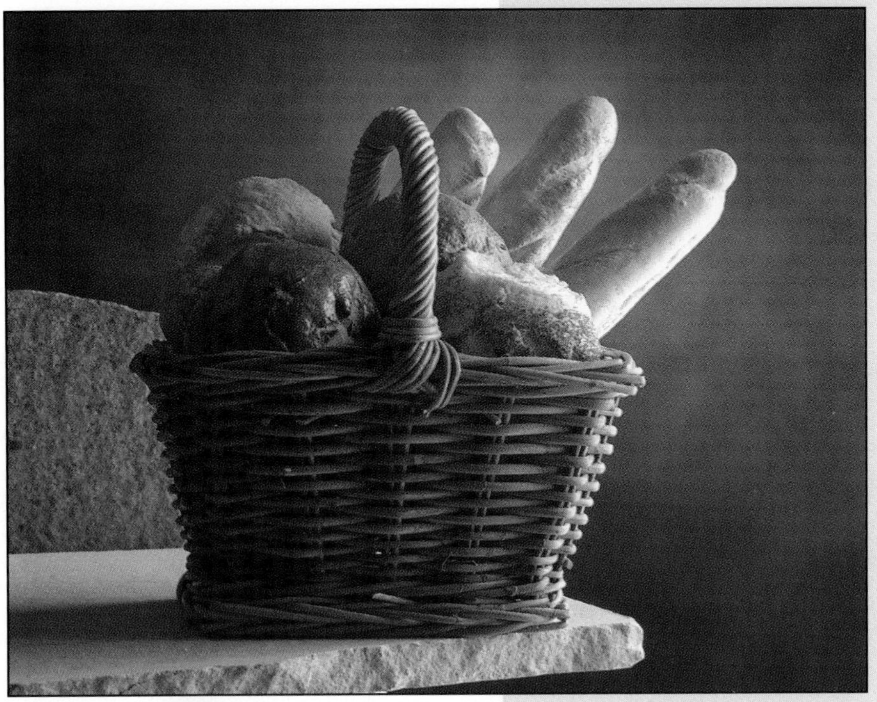

© Peter Wong

> *Rabbit said, "Honey or condensed milk with your bread?" [Pooh] was so excited that he said, "Both," and then, so as not to seem greedy, he added, "But don't bother about the bread, please."*
> *—A. A. Milne, Winnie the Pooh*

CHAPTER 3
The Carbohydrates: Sugar, Starch, and Fiber

Contents

Ask Yourself . . . ?

Which of these statements about nutrition are true, and which are false? For the false statements, what *is* true?

1. Depending on the food it comes in, sugar can make a positive or negative contribution to health.
2. Fruit sugar (fructose) is less fattening than table sugar (sucrose).
3. Foods high in complex carbohydrate (starch and fiber) are good choices when you are trying to lose weight.
4. People with diabetes shouldn't eat carbohydrate.
5. The primary role of dietary fiber is to supply energy.
6. Breads to which nutrients have been added are more nutritious than breads in their original forms.
7. To restore a low blood glucose level to normal, it is best to eat a food that contains a lot of sugar.
8. The Surgeon General recommends that people eat more starch than they did in the past.
9. Some foods labeled "sugar-free" actually contain calorie-bearing sugars.
10. Artificial sweeteners are safe to use in moderation.

Answers: 1. True. 2. False. Fructose and sucrose are equally fattening because they have the same number of calories per gram. 3. True. Foods high in fiber tend to be low in fat and calories. 4. False. People with diabetes need carbohydrate in their diets, just as other people do. 5. False. Although certain fibers may provide negligible calories to the diet, fiber's primary role is in providing bulk for the digestive tract. 6. False. Breads to which nutrients have been added are *less* nutritious than breads in their original forms because more nutrients have been lost than are added. 7. False. To restore a low blood glucose level to normal, it is best to eat a balanced meal. 8. True. 9. True. 10. True.

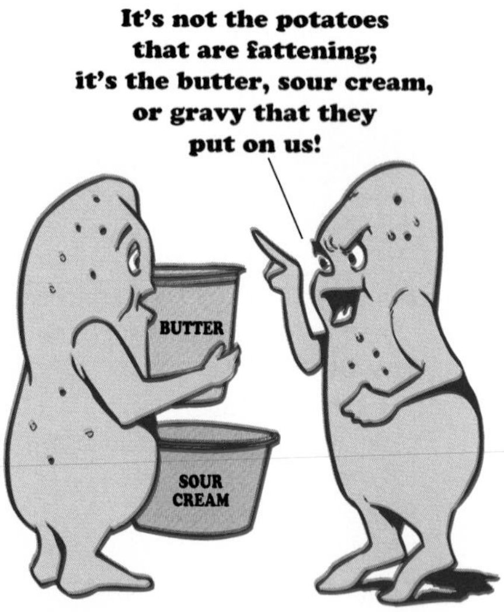
It's not the potatoes that are fattening; it's the butter, sour cream, or gravy that they put on us!
BUTTER
SOUR CREAM

Glycogen is another type of complex carbohydrate composed of glucose, but one that is not a major source of energy; glycogen is made and stored by liver and muscle tissues of human beings and animals as a storage form of glucose.

Once upon a time, bread, potatoes, pasta, and other starchy foods were placed on the dieter's list of most-fattening or "illegal" foods. This unattractive image doubtless comes from the practice of serving many carbohydrate-rich foods laden with fat—potatoes with sour cream and butter, vegetables with rich cream sauces, toast with butter, and salads with fat-rich dressings. People who need to lose weight must limit high-calorie foods, but they are ill-advised to try to avoid all **carbohydrate.** It is the fat, not the carbohydrate, that raises the calorie count the most.

This chapter invites you to learn to distinguish between carbohydrates, such as starch and fiber, and others, such as concentrated sugars. You will learn to choose your calories by the company they keep.

Carbohydrate Basics

The primary role of carbohydrates is to provide the body with energy (calories), and for certain body systems (for example, the brain and the nervous system), carbohydrates are the preferred energy source. Of the three energy nutrients, carbohydrates are the one we are told to increase in our diet. A balanced diet would ideally contain about 58 percent carbohydrate.

The carbohydrates are divided into two categories: complex carbohydrates and simple carbohydrates. **Complex carbohydrates** include starch and fiber. Starches make up a large part of the world's food supply—mostly as grains (breads and pastas). Consider such staples as wheat, rice, and corn, which are rich sources of starch. Fiber is found abundantly in plants, especially in the outer portions of cereal grains, and in fruits, legumes, and most vegetables. **Simple carbohydrates** include naturally occurring sugars in fresh fruits and some vegetables and in milk and milk products and added sugars in concentrated form, as in honey, corn syrup, or sugar in the sugar bowl.

All of these carbohydrates have characteristics in common, but they are of different merit nutritionally. The only carbohydrate we are told to limit is the concentrated form of sugar, not the dilute sugars in fruits, other plant foods, or milk. All of the carbohydrates are made partly or completely of the simple sugar **glucose**, and all carbohydrates but fiber can quickly be converted to glucose in the body, as the following section shows. Table 3–1 introduces the different types of carbohydrates.

The Sugars

All carbohydrates are composed of single sugars, alone or in various combinations. All contain the simple sugar glucose and other sugars much like it in composition and structure. Carbohydrate-rich foods are obtained almost exclusively from plants. Milk is the only animal-derived food that contains significant amounts of carbohydrate. Glucose is not a very sweet sugar, but plants can rearrange its atoms to form another sugar, **fructose**, which is sweet to the taste. Fructose occurs mostly in fruits, in honey, and as part of another sugar—table sugar—to be described in a moment. Glucose and fructose are the most common single sugars in nature.

Some sugars are double sugars, made by bonding two single sugars together. When fructose and glucose are bonded together, they form **sucrose**, or table sugar, the product most people refer to when they use the term *sugar*. The sweet taste of sucrose comes primarily from the fructose in its structure. It occurs naturally in many fruits and vegetables. Sugar cane and sugar beets

Carbohydrate compounds made of single sugars or multiples of them and composed of carbon, hydrogen, and oxygen atoms.
carbo = carbon (C)
hydrate = water (H_2O)

Complex carbohydrates long chains of sugars (glucose) arranged as starch or fiber. Also called polysaccharides.
poly = many
saccharides = sugar unit

Simple carbohydrates (sugars) the single sugars (monosaccharides) and the pairs of sugars (disaccharides) linked together.

Glucose (GLOO-koce) the building block of carbohydrate; a single sugar used in both plant and animal tissues as quick-energy currency. A single sugar is known as a **monosaccharide.**
mono = one

Fructose (FROOK-toce) the sweetest of the single sugars.

Another single sugar, **galactose** (ga-LACK-toce), occurs bonded to glucose in the sugar of milk. A double sugar is known as a **disaccharide.**
di = two

Sucrose (SOO-crose) a double sugar composed of glucose and fructose.

Table 3–1 Categories and Sources of Carbohydrates

CARBOHYDRATE TYPE	OTHER COMMON NAMES	FOOD SOURCES
Monosaccharides		
Glucose	Dextrose, blood sugar	Fruits, sweeteners
Fructose	Fruit sugar, levulose	Fruits, honey, high-fructose corn syrup
Galactose	------	Part of lactose, found in milk
Disaccharides		
Sucrose (glucose + fructose)	Table sugar	Beet and cane sugar, fruit
Lactose (glucose + galactose)	Milk sugar	Milk and milk products
Maltose (glucose + glucose)	Malt sugar	Germinating grains
Polysaccharides	Complex Carbohydrates	
Starches	Dextrins	Potatoes, legumes, corn, wheat, rye, and other grains
Dietary fiber	Roughage, Bulk: Hemicellulose, Pectins, Cellulose, Gums, Mucilages, Psyllium	Whole grains, legumes, fruits, vegetables

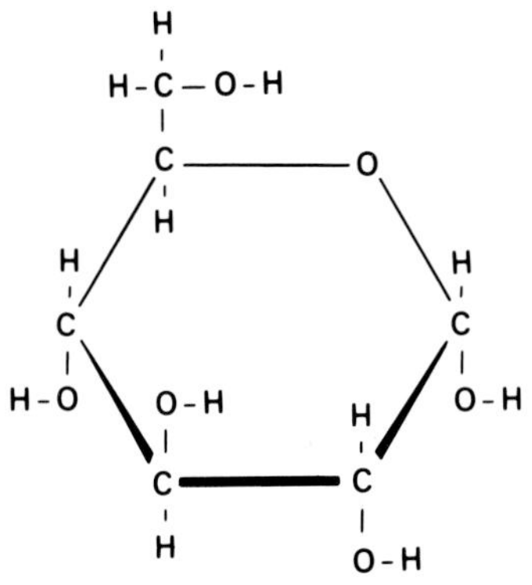
The chemical structure of glucose.

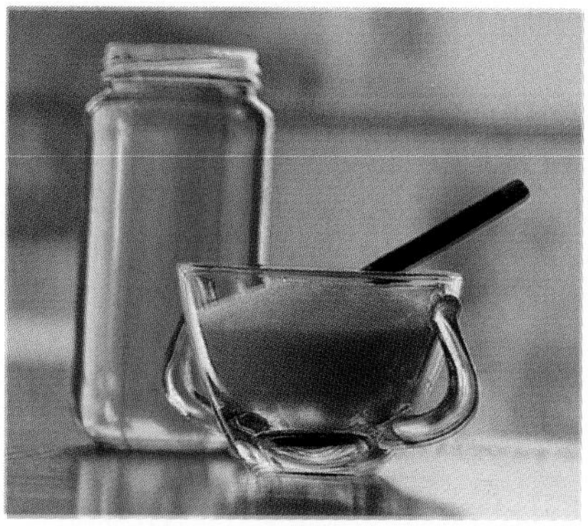

1 tsp honey = 22 cal.
1 tsp sugar = 16 cal.

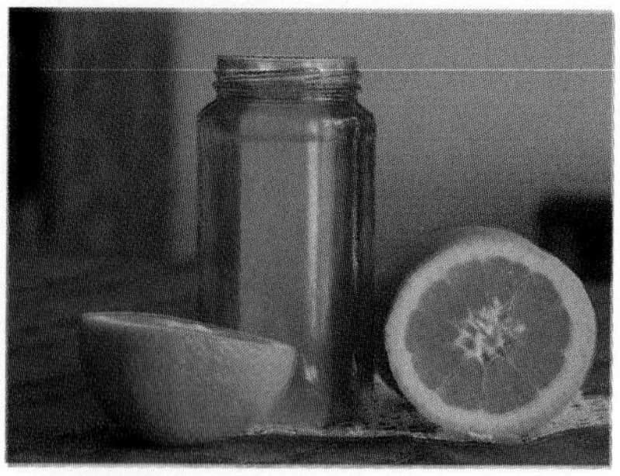

1 tsp honey = 22 cal.
1 tsp fruit = 2 cal with vitamins, minerals, and fiber.

Honey and sucrose contain the same monosaccharides, but in sucrose they are linked together. Compared with honey or sugar, fruit is truly nutritious.

are two sources from which sucrose is purified and granulated to various extents to provide the brown, white, and powdered sugars available in the supermarket. Sucrose is one of the two most calorie-contributing ingredients of candy, cakes, pastries, frostings, cookies, ready-to-eat cereals, and other concentrated sweets. (The other major calorie contributor is fat, described in the next chapter.)

Another double sugar, **maltose**, appears wherever starch is being broken down. It occurs in sprouting seeds and arises during the digestion of starch in the human body. Maltose consists of two glucose units. The malt found in beer contains maltose. Enzymes used in the brewing process break down the long chains of starch in barley and wheat into maltose units. Dry heat can also be used to break down long glucose chains to form maltose. Bread tastes sweeter after toasting for this reason.

Finally, there is **lactose**, the major sugar in milk, a double sugar made by mammals from galactose and glucose units. A human baby is born with the digestive enzymes necessary to split lactose into its two simple sugars—glucose and galactose—so that they can be absorbed. Lactose facilitates the absorption of calcium and promotes the growth of beneficial bacteria in the intestines. Breastmilk or formula, which contain lactose, are ideal foods for babies because they provide a simple, easily digested carbohydrate to meet the infants' energy needs.

When you eat a food containing sugars, **enzymes** in your small intestine first split the double sugars into single sugars so that they can enter your bloodstream. Your liver then quickly converts fructose or galactose to glucose or to smaller pieces that can serve as building blocks of either glucose or fat.

Many people can lose the ability to digest lactose during or after childhood. Thereafter, the person may experience nausea, abdominal pain, diarrhea, or excessive gas after drinking milk or eating lactose-containing products, because the intestinal bacteria will use the lactose for energy, producing gas and other products that irritate the intestine. This condition—**lactose intolerance**—is inherited by about 80 percent of the world's people—including most Africans, Greeks, and Asians. It also can develop temporarily in anyone who is malnourished or sick, making the avoidance of milk and milk products temporarily necessary. Because milk is an almost indispensable source of calcium for growth, a milk substitute must be found whenever children are lactose intolerant. Chapter 7 describes ways to find substitutes for milk when necessary.

Maltose a double sugar composed of two glucose units.
Lactose a double sugar composed of glucose and galactose; commonly known as milk sugar.
Enzymes protein catalysts. A catalyst facilitates a chemical reaction without itself being altered in the process. (Proteins are described in Chapter 5; digestive enzymes, in Appendix B).
Lactose intolerance inability to digest milk sugar due to a lack of the necessary enzyme; a genetic flaw that can occur at any age. Symptoms include nausea, abdominal pain, diarrhea, or excessive gas after consuming milk or milk products.

How the Sugars Rate

The single sugar fructose is sold in purified, crystalline form and advertised as a "natural" sugar that—unlike the "unnatural" sugar sucrose—won't cause weight gain. This is just a sales pitch. What's natural about *any* purified, concentrated sugar? The calories in fructose are used for energy just as those in ordinary table sugar are, and too much of either can cause weight gain if calories are excessive.

Fructose was thought for a while to be a desirable sugar substitute for people with **diabetes.** Diabetics need to avoid most sugars because they cannot produce enough effective **insulin**, the hormone that regulates the body's management of sugar. The idea of giving fructose to people with diabetes was based on a dual rationale. Fructose is sweeter than sucrose, so people with diabetes might use less, and fructose does not raise the blood glucose level as much as glucose does or require such an insulin response. As it turns out, fructose is not really that much sweeter than sucrose, and some of it is converted to glucose after it enters the body, requiring insulin to be used. In any case, most people with diabetes need to control their weight, and fructose does not help with that. It not only supplies nutrient-empty calories but also requires less energy for its metabolism than does glucose, so it is even more fattening.[1]

Diabetes (dye-uh-BEET-eez) a disorder (technically termed *diabetes mellitus*) characterized by insufficiency or relative ineffectiveness of insulin, which renders a person unable to regulate the blood glucose level normally.

Insulin a hormone secreted by the pancreas in response to high blood glucose levels; it assists cells in drawing glucose from the blood.

Empty-calorie foods a phrase used to indicate that a food supplies calories but negligible nutrients. When many empty-calorie foods are eaten regularly, they displace nutrient-dense foods from the diet and contribute to both poor nutritional health and obesity.

Starch a plant polysaccharide composed of glucose, digestible by human beings.

Some people believe that honey is more nutritious than white table sugar because it is "natural." As a matter of fact, chemically, honey and table sugar are almost indistinguishable. Honey contains the two monosaccharides glucose and fructose in approximately equal amounts. Table sugar contains the same monosaccharides, but joined together to form the double sugar sucrose. In the body, after digestion, table sugar and honey are identical. Spoon for spoon, however, table sugar contains *fewer* calories than honey, because its dry crystals take up more space than the crystals of honey dissolved as a liquid.

When people learn that fruit's energy comes from sugars, they may think that eating fruit is the same as consuming concentrated sweets such as candy or soft drinks. However, fruits differ from concentrated sweets in important ways. Their sugars are diluted in large volumes of water, packaged in fiber, and mixed with many vitamins and minerals needed by the body. In contrast, concentrated sweets such as honey and table sugar are merely—as the popular phrase calls them—**empty-calorie foods.**

From the preceding examples, you may see that the most significant difference between sugar sources is not between "natural" and "purified" sugar but between concentrated sweets and the dilute sugars of fruits and vegetables. When you are advised to decrease sugar consumption, it is primarily concentrated sugars like sucrose and corn syrup that you are supposed to limit. How much sugar *do* you eat? Try the Carbohydrate Consumption Scorecard, which checks your diet for sugar, starch, and fiber, to find out.

Complex Carbohydrates: Starch

Starch is made up of many glucose units bonded together—3,000 or so in each molecule of starch. Cooking facilitates the digestive process by spreading out the tightly packaged chains of glucose so that during digestion, the digestive enzymes can break the chains down into glucose units for absorp-

Starch can be broken down during food processing to shorter chains of glucose units known as dextrins. The word *dextrins* sometimes appears on food labels, because dextrins can be used as thickening agents in foods.

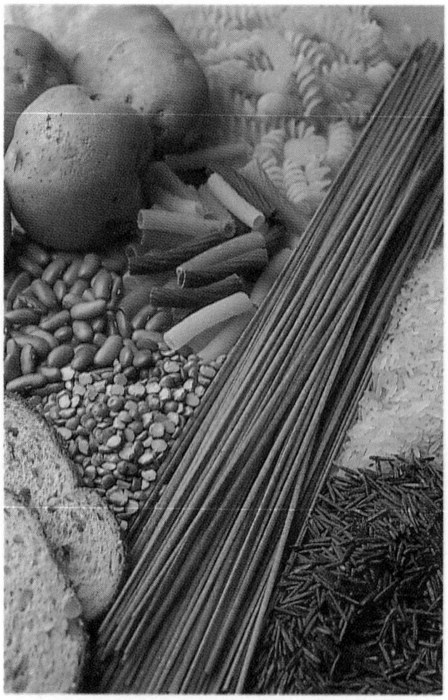

Foods like potatoes, dried beans and peas, rice and whole-grain breads, cereals, and pastas are especially nutritious due to their starch, fiber, vitamin, and mineral content—and because they are virtually fat and cholesterol free.

tion. The first digestive enzymes to work on starch are those in the saliva; they begin taking the starch apart, and enzymes in the intestines continue digestive action. The enzymes release the individual glucose units, which are absorbed across the intestinal wall into the blood (see Appendix B). One to four hours after a meal, all the starch has usually been digested and absorbed and is circulating to the cells as glucose.

All starchy foods are plant foods. Seeds such as grains, peas, and beans are the richest starch source. Most societies have a primary or staple grain that provides most of the people's food energy. In many Asian nations, the staple grain is rice. In Canada, the United States, and Europe, the staple grain is wheat. If you consider all the food products made from wheat—bread (and other baked goods made from wheat flour), cereals, and pasta—you will realize how all-pervasive this grain is in the food supply. The staple grains of other peoples include corn, millet, rye, barley, and oats.

A second important source of starch is the legume family, including such dried beans and peas as butter beans, kidney beans, pinto beans, navy beans, black-eyed peas (cowpeas), chickpeas (garbanzo beans), and soybeans. These vegetables are about 40 percent starch by weight and contain abundant protein. Root vegetables (such as yams) and tubers (such as potatoes) are other sources of starch that are important in many societies.

Complex Carbohydrates: Fiber

The **fibers** of a plant form the supporting structures of the plant's leaves, stems, and seeds. Most fibers are polysaccharides, just as starch is, but with different bonds between the glucose units—bonds that cannot be broken by human digestive enzymes. Thus fibers are "the nonstarch polysaccharides in foods."[2] The term *fiber* is used by almost everyone as if it represented a single entity. It was known generations ago as **roughage.** However, there are many compounds, mostly carbohydrates, that make up fiber.* Such compounds are familiar as the strings of celery, the skins of corn kernels, and the membranes separating the segments in citrus fruits. Isolated from plants, they may be used to thicken jelly (citrus pectin), to keep salad dressing from separating (guar gum), to provide roughage (wheat, oat, and other brans), and to exert other effects on texture and consistency.

The bonds that hold the units of fiber together cannot be broken by human digestive enzymes, but some can be broken by the bacteria that reside in the human digestive tract. Therefore, we obtain a little glucose, some related products, and some energy from fiber molecules. Fibers exert important effects on people's health, as described later in the chapter.

Fibers the indigestible residues of food composed mostly of polysaccharides.

The term *dietary fiber* refers to nutritionally significant fiber in food—that is, the fiber that resists human digestive enzymes. (A chemist might digest food in a test tube by a harsher procedure than the human intestine does and so might find only one third or one half as much undigested material remaining; this fiber is termed crude fiber.)

Roughage (RUFF-edge) the rough parts of food, an imprecise term that has been largely replaced by the term *fiber.*

The best-known of the fibrous polysaccharides are **cellulose, hemicellulose, pectin,** and **gums.**

The Carbohydrates and Health

Carbohydrate is the ideal fuel for the body. There are only two alternative energy-nutrient sources—protein and fat. Protein-rich foods are usually expensive and provide no advantage over carbohydrates when used to provide fuel for the body. Fat-rich foods might be less expensive, but fat cannot be used efficiently as fuel by the brain and nerves, and diets high in fat are

*The woody material of heavy stems and bark is the noncarbohydrate lignin, classed by some as a fiber.

Carbohydrate Consumption Scorecard

Rating Your Diet: How Sweet Is It?

Now that you are aware of some of the sources of added sugars, let's take a look at *your* diet. Check the box that most closely describes your eating habits to see how the foods you choose affect the amount of added sugars in your diet.

How often do you—	SELDOM OR NEVER	1 OR 2 TIMES A WEEK	3 TO 5 TIMES A WEEK	ALMOST DAILY
1. Drink soft drinks, sweetened fruit drinks, or punches?	☐	☐	☐	☐
2. Choose sweet desserts and snacks, such as cakes, pies, cookies, and ice cream?	☐	☐	☐	☐
3. Use canned or frozen fruits packed in heavy syrup or add sugar to fresh fruit?	☐	☐	☐	☐
4. Eat candy?	☐	☐	☐	☐
5. Add sugar to coffee or tea?	☐	☐	☐	☐
6. Use jam, jelly, or honey on bread or rolls?	☐	☐	☐	☐

How Did You Do?

The more often you choose the items listed above, the higher your diet is likely to be in sugars. You may need to cut back on sugar-containing foods, especially those you checked as "3 to 5 times a week" or more. This does not mean eliminating these foods from your diet. You can moderate your intake of sugars by choosing foods that are high in sugar less often and by eating smaller portions.

Check Your Diet for Starch and Fiber

How often do you eat:	SELDOM OR NEVER	1 OR 2 TIMES A WEEK	3 TO 4 TIMES A WEEK	ALMOST DAILY
1. Several servings of breads, cereals, pasta, or rice?	☐	☐	☐	☐
2. Starchy vegetables like potatoes, corn, peas, or dishes made with dried beans or peas?	☐	☐	☐	☐
3. Whole-grain breads or cereals?	☐	☐	☐	☐
4. Several servings of vegetables?	☐	☐	☐	☐
5. Whole fruit with skins and/or seeds (berries, apples, pears, etc.)?	☐	☐	☐	☐

How Did You Do?

The best answer for all of the above is ALMOST DAILY. Breads, cereals, and other grain products and starchy vegetables provide starch. Whole-grain products, legumes, fruits, and vegetables, especially those with edible skins and seeds, are good sources of fiber.

Source: USDA Home & Garden Bulletin, April 1986.

associated with many diseases. Thus, of all alternative food-energy sources, carbohydrate is preferred; it provides most of the day's energy for most of the world's people.

Alcohol can provide calories, but has the same disadvantages as fat as well as others; it is not a nutrient in any sense (see the Chapter 10 Spotlight).

Sweet Alternatives to Sugar

Artificial sweeteners nonnutritive replacements for sugar such as acesulfame K, aspartame, and saccharin.

Saccharin a 0-calorie sweetener discovered in 1879 and used in the United States since the turn of the century. A possible link to bladder cancer has led to its being banned as a food additive in Canada, although it is available there as a sweetener; it is used with a warning label in the United States.

Aspartame a dipeptide (see Chapter 5) containing the amino acids aspartic acid and phenylalanine. While it is digested as protein and supplies calories, it is so sweet that only small amounts, which contribute negligible calories, are needed to sweeten foods. Thus, it is classified as a nonnutritive sweetener. Marketed under the trade name NutraSweet, aspartame is blended with lactose and an anticaking agent and sold commercially as Equal.

Acesulfame K (AY-see-sul-fame) a derivative of acetoacetic acid approved for use in foods in 1988. Since it is not metabolized by the body, acesulfame K does not contribute calories and is excreted from the body unchanged. It is currently approved for use in 20 countries, in more than 100 international products, including chewing gum, gelatins, nondairy creamers, powdered drink mixes, and puddings.[6]

It all started back in 1879. That was the year a substance called saccharin was first discovered and found to be able to sweeten foods without adding calories. Since that time, the sale of **artificial sweeteners** has become a 256-million-dollar-a-year business projected to reach $358 million by 1995.[3] Despite the ever-growing popularity of such sweeteners, doubts about their safety have stirred a good deal of controversy over the years. In addition, confusion about the characteristics of the various available alternatives to sugar (see Table 3–2) and their role in fighting problems such as obesity and tooth decay prevail among the millions of Americans who use them. The following assumptions about sugar substitutes and the facts behind them should help put matters into perspective.

Saccharin Causes Cancer

This assumption has never been proven. It's true that some studies of **saccharin**, the sweetener in Sweet 'n Low, have found that it can cause bladder cancer in laboratory rats. A human, however, would have to drink 850 cans of soda pop a day to take in a dose equivalent to what the rats in those studies were being fed. What's more, investigations of large groups of people have yet to establish any clear-cut link between saccharin consumption and the risk of cancer. One study of more than 9,000 men and women by the National Cancer Institute, for instance, found no association between saccharin use and bladder cancer.[4] Thus, it appears that the health risks, if any, posed by saccharin are miniscule at most. Those fearful of getting cancer would be better off quitting smoking or reducing the amount of fat in their diets than worrying about putting Sweet 'n Low in their coffee now and then. As the American Medical Association's Council on Scientific Affairs has stated, "In humans, available evidence indicates that the use of artificial sweeteners, including saccharin, is not associated with an increased risk of bladder cancer."[5]

Aspartame Can Be Used to Sweeten Baked Goods

Not so. **Aspartame**, the artificial sweetening agent marketed under the trade name NutraSweet, cannot be used in products that require cooking or baking because it breaks down upon heating and releases tiny amounts of methyl alcohol, which imparts a sour flavor. It can only be used to sweeten warm and cold foods and liquids or added to foods once they have already been cooked.

Saccharin, on the other hand, can withstand the high temperatures needed for cooking and baking. The same goes for **acesulfame potassium** (or acesulfame K, the chemical symbol for potassium), marketed as Sunette. The

Table 3–2
How Sweet It Is

NAME (TRADE NAME)	SWEETNESS	CHARACTERISTICS[a]
Sweeteners that have been approved for use in the United States.		
Acesulfame K (Sunette)	200 times sweeter than sucrose.	Stable in high temperatures; soluble in water.
Aspartame (NutraSweet)	180 times sweeter than sucrose.	Loses sweetness at high temperatures and may lose sweetness over time; cannot be used in baking or cooking but can be added to cooked products after heating.
Saccharin	300 times sweeter than sucrose.	Stable at high temperatures.
Sweeteners for which approval in the United States is pending.		
Alitame (Novasweet)	2,000 times sweeter than sucrose.	Stable at high temperatures and in both acidic and nonacidic foods; highly soluble in water.
Cyclamate[b]	30 times sweeter than sucrose.	Stable at high temperatures; long shelf life.
Sucralose	600 times sweeter than sucrose.	Stable at various temperatures.

[a]In addition to the characteristics listed, all of the sweeteners have a synergistic effect when combined with other sweeteners. In other words, together they enhance the sweetness of one another, yielding a combined sweetness greater than the sum of each individual substance's sweetness.
[b]Cyclamate was banned in the United States in 1970 because of studies suggesting that it may cause cancer. The validity of the studies has been questioned, however. Currently there is a petition before the FDA to reapprove cyclamate for use in the United States.

Source: Calorie Control Council Sweetener Fact Sheets: acesulfame K, alitame, aspartame, cyclamate, saccharin, and sucralose.

latest sweetener to be approved for use by the Food and Drug Administration, acesulfame K won't break down upon heating.

Aspartame Causes Headaches

Not in most people. While the Food and Drug Administration has received numerous complaints from consumers who claim to suffer headaches, nausea, anxiety, and other symptoms after consuming aspartame-containing foods or beverages, it has never been confirmed by scientific studies that the sweetener is truly the culprit. Consider that scientists at Duke University who conducted carefully controlled research into the matter concluded that tablets containing the amount of aspartame in about four liters of diet soft drink were no more likely to prompt headaches in people than **placebo** pills administered for the sake of comparison.[7] Furthermore, numerous careful scientific investigations carried out both before and after aspartame first appeared on the market have indicated that the product brings about adverse health effects only in a small group of people with a rare metabolic disorder known as **phenylketonuria**, or PKU. People born with PKU must carefully control their intake of phenylalanine—one of the two amino acids that make up aspartame—to prevent health problems as severe as mental retardation. The American Medical Association's Council on Scientific Affairs, the Centers for Disease Control, and the Food and Drug Administration all consider the sweetener to be safe for use except by people with PKU.[8]

Placebo (plah-SEE-bo) a sham treatment given to a control group; an inert, harmless "treatment" that the group's members cannot recognize as different from the real thing. This will minimize the chance that an effect of the treatment will appear to have occurred due to the **placebo effect**—the healing effect that the *act* of treatment, rather than the treatment itself, often has.

Phenylketonuria an inborn error of metabolism, detectable at birth, in which the body lacks the enzyme needed to convert the amino acid phenylalanine to the amino acid tyrosine. As a result, derivatives of phenylalanine accumulate in the blood and tissues, where they can cause severe damage, including mental retardation.

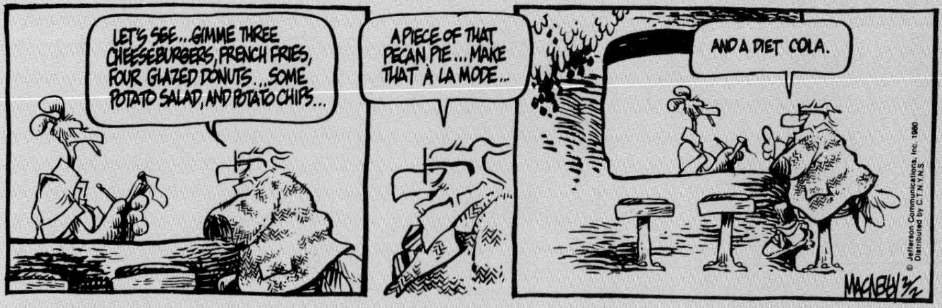
LET'S SEE...GIMME THREE CHEESEBURGERS, FRENCH FRIES, FOUR GLAZED DONUTS...SOME POTATO SALAD, AND POTATO CHIPS...
A PIECE OF THAT PECAN PIE...MAKE THAT A LA MODE...
AND A DIET COLA.

Use of Artificial Sweeteners Will Bring About Weight Loss

If only it were that simple. Obviously, because artificially sweetened foods typically contain fewer calories than their sugar-sweetened counterparts, substituting a low-calorie alternative for a sugar-laden one can help a person who is trying to lose weight enjoy sweet-tasting foods and save calories. But simply *adding* foods sweetened with sugar substitutes to the diet will not do the trick. Moreover, eating artificially sweetened foods to have an excuse to splurge on a high-calorie food defeats the purpose. A person who drinks diet soda pop to justify eating an ice cream sundae later is reaping little, if any, benefit. In other words, it's the way in which you fit artificial sweeteners into the rest of your diet that counts.

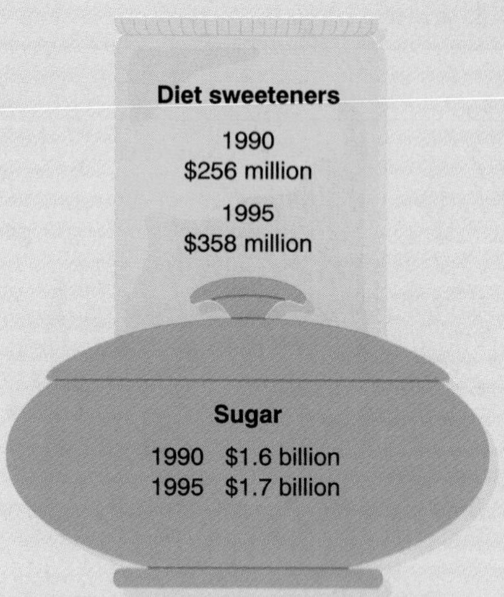

While sugar sales may be leveling off, artificial sweetener sales appear to be rising at a relatively fast rate.

On the flip side, some consumers may be under the impression that artificial sweeteners bolster the appetite. Back in 1986, a report that aspartame sends mixed signals to the brain and thereby increases appetite as well as eating spawned the notion that artificial sweeteners can interfere with weight loss. That report was based on comparisons of the effects of drinking plain water and aspartame- and sugar-sweetened water, however, rather than consuming actual foods or beverages that are typically sweetened with aspartame. Moreover, the researchers did not measure how much food people ate after drinking the liquids. Thus, the study did not show how consuming aspartame-sweetened foods influences appetite and eating behavior in the "real world."

Since that time, about a dozen investigations into the relationship between appetite and foods and beverages sweetened with the substance have indicated that aspartame either lessens, or doesn't affect, feelings of hunger or the amount of food ultimately eaten. So for now, at least, it appears that aspartame's impact on appetite need not be of concern to those trying to lose weight.[9]

Foods Sweetened with Sugar Substitutes Do Not Contribute to Tooth Decay

Not necessarily. Any carbohydrate-containing food, be it sugar-sweetened or otherwise, can promote tooth decay. When you eat a sugary food, the millions of bacteria lurking on the surfaces of and between your teeth feast on the sugar and, in the process, release an acid that eats away at tooth enamel. Once inside the mouth, any carbohydrate can be devoured by cavity-causing bacteria because enzymes in the saliva break the complex carbohydrates into simple sugars, which bacteria thrive on. (See Chapter 10 for a more detailed explanation of food's role in dental health.)

Diabetics Should Only Eat Foods Sweetened with Sugar Substitutes Instead of Sugar

That depends. It is often assumed that because the body absorbs sucrose into the bloodstream quickly, which in turn contributes to a rise in the blood glucose level, diabetics should only eat foods sweetened with alternatives to sugar. But it's not that simple. Many factors, including the amount and type of fat, sugar, and fiber in a food, play a role in the body's blood glucose response to the food. That's one reason the American Diabetes Association recommends that "the use of any sweetener should be individualized with consideration to overall diet and nutritional adequacy."[10]

Another reason that blanket statements about use of sugar substitutes are not made for diabetics is that the various types behave differently in the body. A group of sugar substitutes known as **alternative sweeteners** (fructose, sorbitol, mannitol, and xylitol), for instance, contain calories but are sometimes recommended for diabetics because the body generally absorbs them more slowly than sucrose, and thus minimizes blood glucose fluctuations. Some have side effects that detract from their desirability for certain diabetics, however. Some research suggests that fructose, for example, may contribute to rises in blood triglyceride levels, making it a poor choice for some people. And some people may suffer diarrhea after taking in large amounts of sorbitol, mannitol, or xylitol. Thus, the role sugar substitutes play in the overall diet is a decision that should be made individually with the help of a dietitian or physician.[11]

Alternative sweeteners nutritive (calorie-containing) sugars such as fructose, sorbitol, mannitol, and xylitol, that may be used in place of sucrose because of their different effects in the body.

Sugar-free Chewing Gum Doesn't Contain Any Calories

Not so. Sugar-free chewing gum is sweetened with certain alternative sweeteners, such as xylitol and sorbitol, also known as sugar alcohols. While sugar alcohols impart a sweet taste and supply calories (about eight per stick), unlike sucrose, they do not promote tooth decay.

Sugar and Health

Sugar is often in the headlines and has been accused of contributing to a host of human ills such as tooth decay, obesity, diabetes, heart disease, hyperactive behavior in children, and even criminal behavior. Nevertheless, research studies have not shown a direct link between sugar and any of these conditions, except tooth decay (see the Nutrition Action feature in Chapter 10).

However, if eating a lot of sugar means that you eat a lot fewer foods containing essential nutrients, inadequate consumption of other important nutrients can result. Conversely, if you eat a lot of sugar without eating less of something else, you might get too many calories. Excess calories from any energy nutrient—even protein—are stored as body fat. Evidence from population studies in many countries shows that obesity rates rise as sugar consumption increases. One reason may be that many sugary foods, such as candy bars, are also high in fat.

There is no reason to believe that moderate consumption of sugar (5 percent to 10 percent of calories) is dangerous to a healthy human being. The guideline to limit sugar to less than 10 percent of total calories does not apply to *all* sugars in the diet. The diluted sugars found in milk and fruits should not be confused with concentrated refined sugars, like table sugar, honey, and corn syrups. These concentrated sweets should be avoided if they displace needed nutrients.

After digestion, purified, refined white sugar—sucrose—yields a 50-50 mixture of glucose and fructose. In the body, the mixture becomes equivalent to pure glucose (because fructose is converted to glucose). As such, it differs in no way from the glucose that comes from starch. Starch usually comes in foods with other nutrients, while sugar itself contains no other nutrients—no protein, vitamins, or minerals—and so can be termed an empty-calorie food. If you have 200 calories to "spend" on something and you spend them on sugar, you get very little of value in terms of nutrients for your outlay. If 200 calories equal 10 percent of your total energy allowance, they ought to bring 10 percent of your total needed nutrients with them. If you spend your 200 calories on three slices of whole-wheat bread instead, you get 14 percent of the protein, 18 percent of the thiamin, and 12 percent of the niacin recommended for a day, as well as comparable amounts of many other nutrients (see Table 3–3). Whether you can afford to eat sugar, then, depends on the overall nutrient density of your diet and the number of calories you have to spend altogether.

It is theoretically possible, with careful food selection, to obtain all the needed nutrients within an allowance of about 1,500 calories—but this is not easy for most people. For example, a teenage boy needs as many as 4,000 calories to get all the energy he needs. If he eats some very nutritious foods, then perhaps the empty calories of soft drinks are an acceptable part of his diet. On the other hand, many teenage girls eat 1,200 calories or even less, so they can afford to take in only the most nutrient-dense foods. They should

Table 3–3

Sample Nutrients in Sugars and Other Foods

The indicated portion of any of these foods would provide approximately 100 calories. Notice what nutrients the eater receives along with the energy.

			PERCENTAGE OF U.S. RDA[a]				
Food	Size of 100-cal Portion	Grams of Carbohydrate	Protein	Calcium	Iron	Vitamin A	Thiamin
Lowfat milk	¾ c	9	17	26	—	3	5
Kidney beans	½ c	21	12	4	13	< 1	9
Watermelon	4-by-8" wedge	23	3	3	12	50	9
Whole-wheat bread	1½ slices	19	7	4	7	—	9
Sugar, white	2 tbsp	24	0	0	0	0	0
Molasses, blackstrap	2 tbsp	22	0	27	35	0	3
Cola beverage	1 c	26	0	0	0	0	0
Honey	1½ tbsp	26	—	< 1	1	0	—

[a]Percentages are rounded to the nearest whole number. A dash means the percentage has not been determined and is not significant. The U.S. RDA are recommended adult intakes (see inside front cover).

avoid empty-calorie foods. Overconsumption of sugar can clearly cause malnutrition, then, not by any positive action of its own, but by displacing nutrients that prevent malnutrition. Nutritious foods must come first.

You may wonder whether using artificial sweeteners to reduce some of the total sugar in your diet is a safe and recommended strategy. The Nutrition Action feature beginning on page 62 will help you decide.

Complex Carbohydrates and Health

Complex carbohydrate is thought to be our most valuable energy nutrient. The *Dietary Guidelines for Americans* include the following suggestions:

- Choose a diet with plenty of vegetables, fruits, legumes, and grain products.
- Use sugars only in moderation.

If you have been exposed to as much anticarbohydrate propaganda as most people have been, the statement that we need to consume more complex carbohydrates, rather than less, may be startling. Yet much evidence supports it. It may prompt you to think creatively about your own diet and to make space in your diet for your favorite foods rich in complex carbohydrates. (See Figure 3–1 for a comparison of levels of carbohydrate Americans consume with recommended levels.)

The health benefits to be expected from such a change would be many. A diet lower in pure sugars and higher in foods containing complex carbohydrates would almost necessarily be lower in fat and calories and higher in fiber. Working together, these factors might be expected to bring about, or to contribute to, lower rates of obesity, heart disease, diabetes, cancer, and tooth decay.

Most health recommendations tell us to make reductions in four areas: fats and cholesterol, sodium, alcohol, and body weight. In contrast, complex carbohydrates are the nutrient most promoted by these health recommendations.

All carbohydrates, with the exception of fiber, provide the same number of calories as protein— 4 per gram—as compared with the 9 calories per gram of fats or the 7 per gram of alcohol. Figure 3–2 asks you to add up the calories that various carbohydrate sources provide in a popular breakfast cereal. Foods containing complex carbohydrates are usually lower in calories

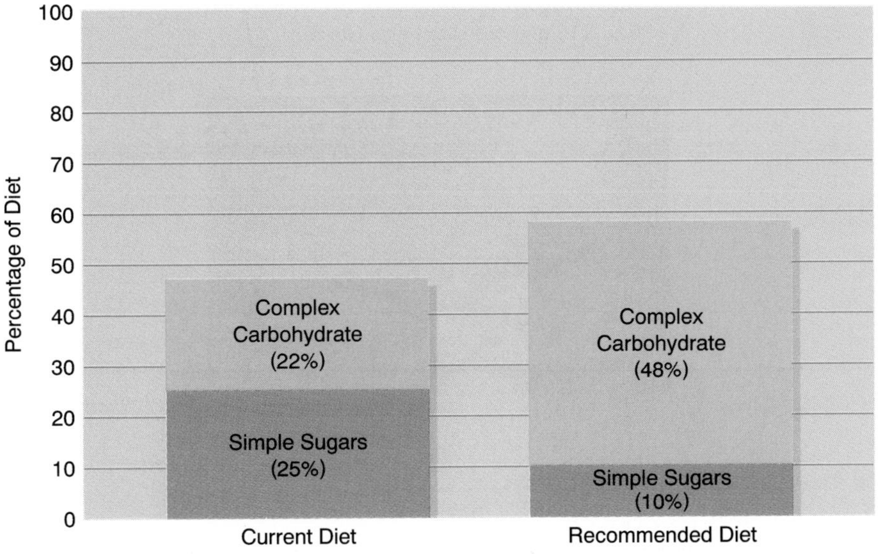

Figure 3–1

Current Versus Recommended Levels of Carbohydrate in the U.S. Diet

While total carbohydrate in the diet is supposed to increase, sugar as a percentage of the carbohydrate and as a percentage of the total diet is supposed to decrease, making a major increase in the amount of complex carbohydrate—starch and fiber—in the diet. The figure shows the percentage of total calories derived from sugar versus complex carbohydrate in the diet.

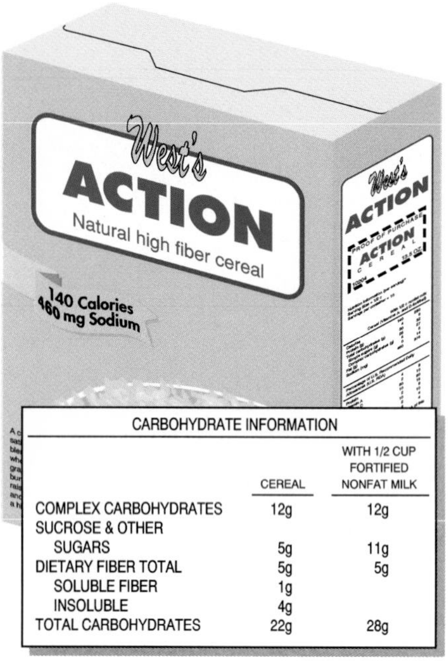

CARBOHYDRATE INFORMATION

	CEREAL	WITH 1/2 CUP FORTIFIED NONFAT MILK
COMPLEX CARBOHYDRATES	12g	12g
SUCROSE & OTHER SUGARS	5g	11g
DIETARY FIBER TOTAL	5g	5g
SOLUBLE FIBER	1g	
INSOLUBLE	4g	
TOTAL CARBOHYDRATES	22g	28g

The feeling of satisfaction and fullness after a meal is known as **satiety** (sat-EYE-uh-tee). The two constituents of food that convey satiety are fiber and fat.

Figure 3–2 Carbohydrate on the Label: Fiber Math

Do you think foods high in fiber (whole-grain breads and cereals) are also high in calories? If a food product is high in fiber and low in fat, it may be lower in calories than you think. For example, the food label shown here gives some interesting nutrition information about its fiber content. Fill in this chart to find out how many calories are provided by fiber, sucrose, and other carbohydrate sources.

Grams of Carbohydrate per Serving (without milk)		Calories per Gram		Total Calories
______ Grams of complex carbohydrate	×	4	=	______
______ Grams of sucrose and other sugars	×	4	=	______
______ Grams of total dietary fiber	×	0	=	______
______ Grams of total carbohydrate			=	______

Source: Adapted from ConAgra Inc., *What's in a label?,* 1990, p. 44

per portion than protein-rich foods because the latter often include considerable fat. A diet high in complex carbohydrates might be more beneficial for weight loss than a diet of comparable calories that is high in fat. A preliminary report states that "altering the composition of the diet in favor of a higher carbohydrate-to-fat ratio may decrease the incidence of obesity."[12] One reason is that switching to a high complex-carbohydrate (high-fiber) diet tends to make you feel full faster, which may reduce caloric intake. Table 3–4 compares foods from the major food classes by carbohydrate, protein, fat, and calorie content, and Figure 3–3 illustrates the amounts of carbohydrate in typical representative foods from the food groups.

Figure 3–3

Carbohydrate in Foods

Four of the six exchange lists contain carbohydrate, so you need only know four values and learn a value for concentrated sugar (which is not on the exchange lists). All whole-plant foods are valuable fiber contributors if you eat enough of them.

ONE EXCHANGE	GRAMS OF CARBOHYDRATE
Starches/grains	15
Vegetables	5
Fruits	15
Milks	12
Sugar	5
Meats	0
Fats	0

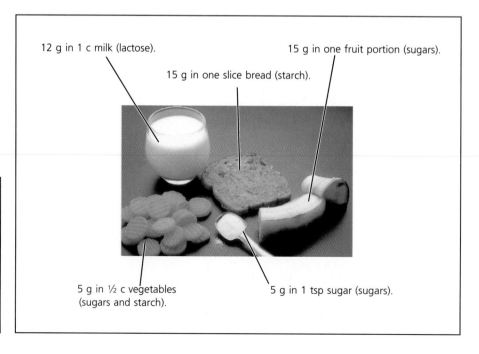

Table 3–4 Food Classes and Calories

FOOD CATEGORY (AND PORTION SIZE)	GRAMS OF CARBOHYDRATE	GRAMS OF PROTEIN	GRAMS OF FAT	CALORIES
Meat (1 oz)				
Lean	—	7	3	55
Medium fat	—	7	5	75
High fat	—	7	8	100
Milk (1 c)				
Nonfat	12	8	trace	90
Low fat	12	8	5	120
Whole	12	8	8	150
Vegetable (½ c)[a]	5	2	—	25
Fruit (1 piece)	15	—	—	60
Starch/bread (1 portion or slice)[b]	15	3	trace	80
Fat (margarine, butter, or oil, 1 tsp)	—	—	5	45

Note: A dash means negligible grams—almost the same as 0 grams.
[a]This includes low-calorie vegetables only.
[b]This includes starchy vegetables, such as lima beans, peas, and corn, as well as cereal, bread, pasta, rice, and other grain products.

The Health Effects of Fiber

Many health experts are encouraging consumers to eat more fiber. According to recent evidence, inadequate levels of fiber in the diet are associated with several diseases (see miniglossary on page 73), while consumption of recommended levels of fiber offers many health benefits. Recall that dietary fiber is found only in plant foods, such as fruits, vegetables, legumes, and grains, and it is the part of plant foods that human enzymes cannot digest.

Fiber has two forms: **insoluble** and **soluble.** Table 3–5 shows the health benefits from the different types of fiber. Since insoluble and soluble fibers have different effects in the body, it is important to eat a variety of high-fiber foods in order to get both types.

Both types of fiber—soluble and insoluble—may help with weight control. In the stomach, they convey a feeling of fullness, because they absorb water, and some of them delay the emptying of the stomach so that you feel fuller longer. If you eat many high-fiber foods, you are likely to eat fewer empty-calorie foods such as concentrated fats and sweets. Indeed, producers of some diet aids base the success of their products on the ability of certain fibers in the products to provide bulk and make you feel full.

Insoluble fibers—the type in wheat bran—hold water in the colon, thus increasing bulk which stimulates the muscles of the digestive tract so that they retain their health and tone. The toned muscles can more easily move waste products through the colon for excretion. This prevents **constipation**, **hemorrhoids** (in which veins in the rectum swell, bulge out, become weak, and bleed), and **diverticulosis** (in which the intestinal walls become weak and bulge out in places in response to pressure needed to excrete waste when bulk is inadequate). These fibers may also speed up the passage of food through the digestive tract, thus shortening the time of exposure of the tissue to agents in food that might cause certain cancers, such as **colon cancer.**

Soluble fibers, the type in beans and oats, are credited with reducing the risks of heart and artery disease—**atherosclerosis**—by lowering the level of

Soluble fiber includes the fiber types called gums, mucilages, and pectin; soluble fibers dissolve in water. Psyllium seed husk is an ingredient in certain bulk-forming laxatives and contains soluble fiber.

Insoluble fiber includes the fiber types called cellulose, hemicellulose, and lignin; insoluble fibers don't dissolve in water.

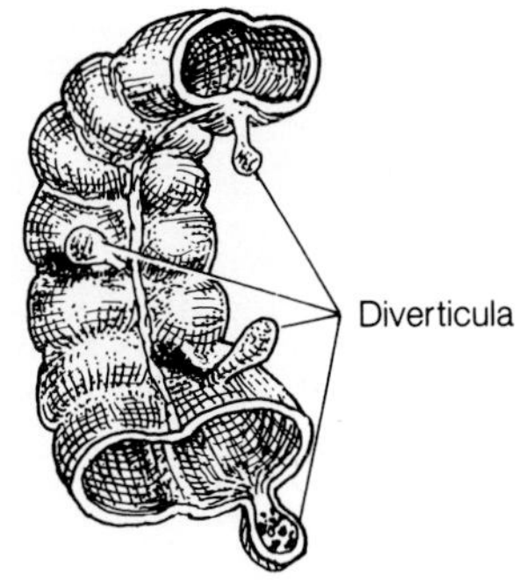

Diverticulosis. The outpocketings of intestinal linings that balloon through the weakened intestinal wall muscles are known as **diverticula.**

Table 3–5

Health Benefits and Sources of Various Types of Fibers

HEALTH PROBLEMS	FIBER TYPE	POSSIBLE HEALTH BENEFITS
Obesity	Soluble Insoluble	Replaces calories from fat, provides satiety, and prolongs eating time due to "chewiness" of food.
Digestive tract disorders: Constipation Diverticulosis Hemorrhoids	Insoluble	Provides bulk and promotes regularity.
Colon cancer	Insoluble	Speeds transit time through intestines and may protect against colon cancer.[1]
Diabetes	Soluble	May improve blood sugar tolerance by delaying glucose absorption.
Heart disease	Soluble	May lower blood cholesterol.[2]

[1]This effect is based on epidemiologic studies and is usually observed along with a reduced-fat intake.
[2]This protective effect is based on epidemiologic evidence that associate a low-fiber diet, typically high in fat, with an increased incidence of disease.

Foods rich in insoluble fiber:

apples	rice bran
bananas	root vegetables
brown rice	pears
cabbage family	peaches
cauliflower	plums
corn bran	seeds
green beans	strawberries
green peas	tomatoes
legumes	wheat bran
mature vegetables	whole-grain breads
nuts	and cereals

Foods rich in soluble fiber:

apples	oat bran
bananas	oatmeal
barley	pears
black-eyed peas	potatoes
broccoli	prunes
carrots	rye
citrus fruits	seeds
corn	sweet potatoes
green peas	zucchini
legumes	

cholesterol in the blood. The products of bacterial digestion of soluble fiber in the colon are absorbed into the body and may inhibit the body's production of cholesterol as well as enhance the clearance of cholesterol from the blood.[13] Cholesterol levels may also decrease if high-fiber foods are used to replace fattier foods in the diet. Certain insoluble fibers also bind cholesterol compounds and carry them out of the body with the feces so that the whole body content of cholesterol is lowered.

Adding one or two servings of oats, beans, or other form of soluble fiber helps lower fasting blood sugar levels in persons with diabetes.

Soluble fibers also improve the body's handling of glucose, even in people with diabetes, perhaps by slowing the digestion or absorption rate of carbohydrate.[14] Blood glucose levels therefore stay moderate, helping to prevent symptoms of diabetes or hypoglycemia. A high-fiber breakfast still exerts regulatory effects on people's blood glucose and insulin responses to lunch. The list of fiber's contributions to human health, therefore, is impressive.

When people choose high-fiber foods in hopes of receiving some of these benefits, they must choose with care. Wheat bran, which is composed mostly of cellulose, has no cholesterol-lowering effect, whereas oat bran and the fibers of legumes, carrots, apples, and grapefruit do lower blood cholesterol. On the other hand, the fiber of wheat bran in whole-wheat bread is one of the most effective stool-softening fibers which help prevent constipation and hemorrhoids. If a single practical conclusion were to be drawn from what is known about fiber, it would have to be that all whole plant foods seem to contain many kinds of fibers and so can be expected to have the whole range of effects previously mentioned. To obtain the greatest benefits from fiber, therefore, you have to eat a variety of foods that contain it rather than take doses of purified fiber such as bran from a single source.

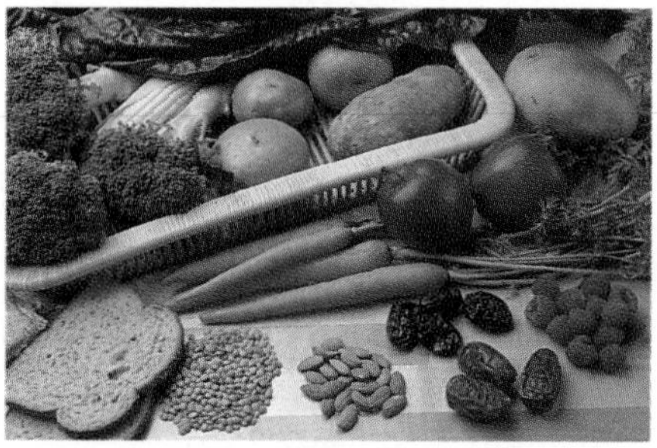

We are advised to increase our intakes of complex carbohydrates and fiber. The best way to get enough fiber in your diet is to eat plenty of fruits, vegetables, legumes, and whole grains rather than use supplements.

The wholesale addition of purified fiber to foods is probably ill advised, because it can be taken so easily to extremes. Taking only one isolated type deprives the taker of the benefits the other types of fiber provide. On the other hand, if you add a variety of whole grains, legumes, nuts, fruits, and vegetables to your diet, you get the various types of fiber you need, together with a package of benefits—water, minerals, vitamins, and the energy nutrients. Fiber out of context is similar to sugar out of context: it can be viewed as nutrient-empty fiber, just as concentrated sugar is sometimes seen as nutrient-empty calories.

Undoubtedly, including fiber in a daily meal plan has benefits—but how much is enough? Even fiber has potential to cause harm if taken in excess. Fiber carries water out of the body and can cause dehydration and intestinal discomfort. Iron is mainly absorbed early during digestion, and because fiber speeds the movement of foods through the digestive system, it may limit the opportunity for the absorption of iron and other nutrients. Binders in some fibers link chemically with minerals such as calcium and zinc, making them unavailable for absorption by carrying them out of the body (more about this in Chapter 7). Too much bulk from the diet could reduce the total amount of food consumed and cause deficiencies of both nutrients and energy. The malnourished, the elderly, and children, because they eat small amounts of food anyway, are especially vulnerable to these concerns.

There is no RDA for fiber, and not everyone agrees on just how to measure a food's fiber content. Still, with all the uncertainties, it is probably true to say that about 20 to 35 grams of dietary fiber daily is a desirable intake. The diet can supply that amount, given ample choices of whole foods, as Table 3–6 and the Consumer Tips feature in this chapter demonstrate. The diet does have to be high in fruits, vegetables, legumes, and grains and moderate in meats, fats, and concentrated sugars—the same recommendations made in the *Surgeon General's Report* and in the *Dietary Guidelines*.

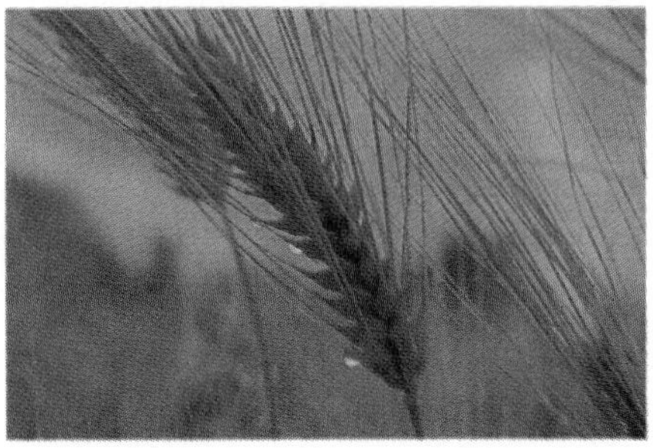

The nutrients present in the wheat plant at harvest are not always present in the wheat products you eat.

The Bread Box: Refined, Enriched, and Whole-grain Breads

For many people, grains supply much of the carbohydrate, or at least most of the starch, in a day's meals. Because they have such a primary place in the diet, be sure that the grains you choose—wheat, rice, oat, or corn—contribute the nutrients you need. Learn the meanings of the words associated with the flours that make up the grain products you use—**refined**, **enriched**, and **whole grain.** This discussion of the nutritional differences between different breads provides an example of an important principle of nutrition: foods far removed from the original state of wholeness may be lacking in significant nutrients.

The part of the wheat plant that is made into flour and then into bread and other baked goods is the kernel. About 50 kernels cluster in the grain head, where they stick tightly until fully ripe. These kernels are first separated from the stem and then further broken apart by the milling process.

The wheat kernel (a whole grain) has four main parts (see Figure 3–4). The **germ** is the part that grows into a wheat plant, and so it contains concentrated food to support the new life. It is especially rich in protein, vitamins, and minerals. The **endosperm** is the soft, white inside portion of the kernel containing starch and protein. The **bran**, a protective coating around

Refined refers to the process by which the coarse parts of food products are removed. For example, the refining of wheat into flour involves removing three of the four parts of the kernel—the chaff, the bran, and the germ—leaving only the endosperm (starch, with only a little protein).

Enriched refers to a process by which the B vitamins thiamin, riboflavin, and niacin and the mineral iron are added to refined grains and grain products at levels specified by law. After enrichment, a grain product has approximately the same amount of thiamin, niacin, and iron, and about twice as much riboflavin, as the original whole-grain product had.

Enriched foods wheat flour, cornmeal, polished rice, and grits.

Whole grain refers to a grain (for example, wheat, oat, corn, or rice) milled in its entirety (all but the husk), not refined.

Table 3–6 Foods that Provide 25 Grams of Dietary Fiber per Day

Fruits (with skins): about 2 grams of fiber per portion; eat four or more per day.	
apple, 1 small	peach, 1
banana, 1 small	pear, ½ small
cantaloupe, ½ melon	prunes, 2
cherries, 16 large	strawberries, ¾ c
Grains and cereals: about 2 grams of fiber per portion; eat four or more per day.	
All Bran, 1 tbsp	popped popcorn, 1½ c
barley, ½ c	Puffed Wheat, 1½ c
cooked oatmeal, 1 c	Rye Crisp, 2 crackers
corn bran, ¼ c	Shredded Wheat, ½ biscuit
cracked-wheat bread, 2 slices	wheat bran, 1 tsp
Grape-Nuts, ⅓ c	whole-wheat bread, 1 slice
oat bran, 2 tsp	
Vegetables: about 2 grams of fiber per portion; eat four or more per day. These values are for cooked portions.	
broccoli, ½ c	green beans, ⅔ c
Brussels sprouts, ½ c	lettuce, raw, 2 c
carrots, ½ c	potato, 1 small
celery, 1 c	tomato, 1 large
corn, ⅓ c	
Legumes (cooked): about 8 grams of fiber per portion.	
baked beans, canned, ½ c	kidney beans, ½ c
dried peas, 1 c	lentils, 1 c
garbanzo beans, ½ c	lima beans, 1 c
Miscellaneous: about 1 gram of fiber per portion.	
peanut butter, 2½ tsp	strawberry jam, 5 tbsp
peanuts, 7 nuts	walnuts, ¼ c
pickle, 1 large	

Source: Values for barley, Puffed Wheat, celery, lettuce, garbanzo beans, walnuts, pickles, and jam from Recommendations for a high-fiber diet, *Nutrition and the MD,* July 1981, in turn adapted from D. A T. Southgate and coauthors, A guide to calculating intakes of dietary fiber, *Journal of Human Nutrition* 30 (1976): 303–313; value for popcorn from Appendix F; all others from E. Lanza and R. R. Burtrum, A critical review of food fiber analysis and data, *Journal of the American Dietetic Association* 86, (1986): 732–743.

Germ the nutrient-rich and fat-dense inner part of a whole grain (removed during refining).
Endosperm the bulk of the edible part of a grain; contains starch grains embedded in a protein matrix.
Bran the outermost covering of a whole grain and the chief source of fiber in grain (removed during refining).
Husk the outer, inedible part of a grain.

the kernel similar in function to the shell of a nut, is also rich in nutrients and fiber. The **husk**, commonly called chaff, is unusable for most purposes except for animal feed.

In earlier times, people milled wheat by grinding it between two stones, then blowing or sifting out the inedible chaff but retaining the nutrient-rich bran and germ as well as the endosperm. Improved milling machinery made it possible to remove the dark, heavy germ and bran as well, leaving a whiter, smoother-textured flour. People came to look on this flour as more desirable than the crunchy, dark brown, "old-fashioned" flour but were unaware of the nutrition implications at first. Bread eaters suffered a tragic loss of needed nutrients in turning to white bread. A U.S. survey done in 1936 revealed that many people were suffering from deficiencies of the nutrients iron, thiamin, riboflavin, and niacin, which they had formerly received from bread. The Enrichment Act of 1942 standardized the return of these four lost nutrients to commercial flour. This doesn't make a single slice of bread "rich" in these four nutrients, but people who eat several or many slices of bread a day obtain significantly more of them than they would from unenriched white bread.

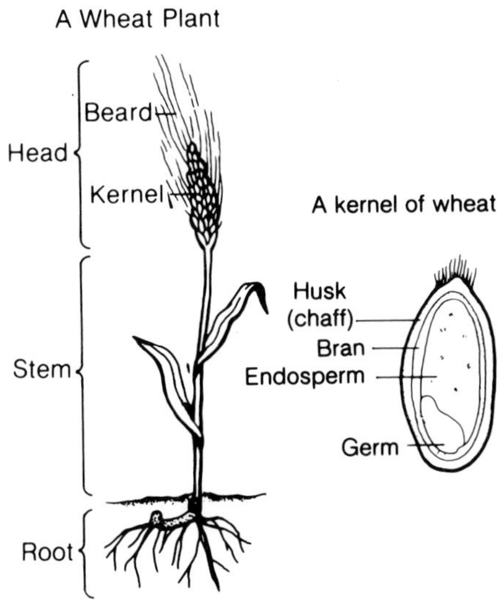

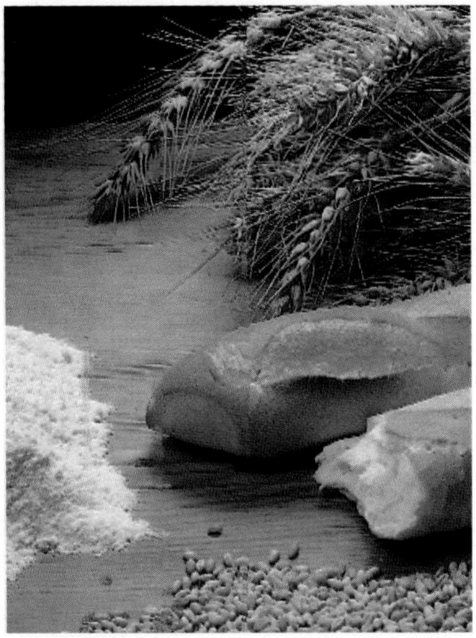

Figure 3–4

A Wheat Plant

To make flour and then bread, kernels are first separated from the stem of the wheat plant and then further broken apart by the milling process. A wheat kernel (a whole grain) has four main parts: the germ, the endosperm, the bran, and the husk.

To a great extent, the enrichment of white flour eliminated the four then-known deficiency problems in the eaters of refined white bread. Today, you can assume that almost all breads, grains like rice, wheat products like macaroni and spaghetti, and cereals, both cooked and ready-to-eat, have been enriched. Figure 3–5 shows that although enrichment makes refined bread comparable to whole-grain bread with respect to the four mentioned nutrients, it does not do so with respect to other important nutrients. Therefore, although the enrichment of flour and other cereal products does improve them, it doesn't improve them enough: whole-grain products are still preferred over enriched products. If bread is a staple food in your diet—that is, if you eat it every day—you would be well advised to learn to like the hearty flavor of whole-grain bread.

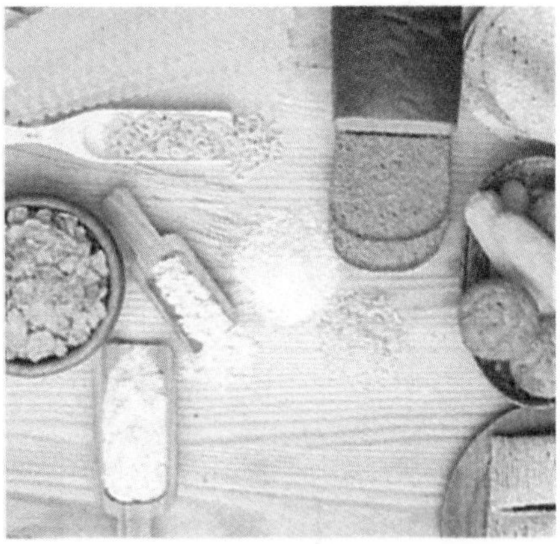

Enjoy the hearty flavor of whole grains.

Miniglossary of Diseases Associated with Fiber Lack

Appendicitis inflammation and/or infection of the appendix, a sac protruding from the large intestine.

Atherosclerosis (ATH-er-oh-scler-OH-sis) the most common kind of hardening of the arteries characterized by the formation of fatty deposits, or plaques, in their inner walls.

Colon cancer cancer of the large intestine (colon), the terminal portion of the digestive tract (see Appendix B).

Constipation hardness and dryness of bowel movements associated with discomfort in passing them.

Diabetes already defined on page 59.

Diverticulosis (dye-ver-tic-you-LOCE-iss) outpocketings of weakened areas of the intestinal wall, like blowouts in a tire, that can rupture, causing dangerous infections.

Hemorrhoids (HEM-or-oids) swollen, hardened (varicose) veins in the rectum, usually caused by the pressure resulting from constipation.

Obesity body weight high enough above normal weight to constitute a health hazard (see also Chapter 8).

Figure 3–5

Nutrients in Whole-grain, Enriched White, and Unenriched White Breads

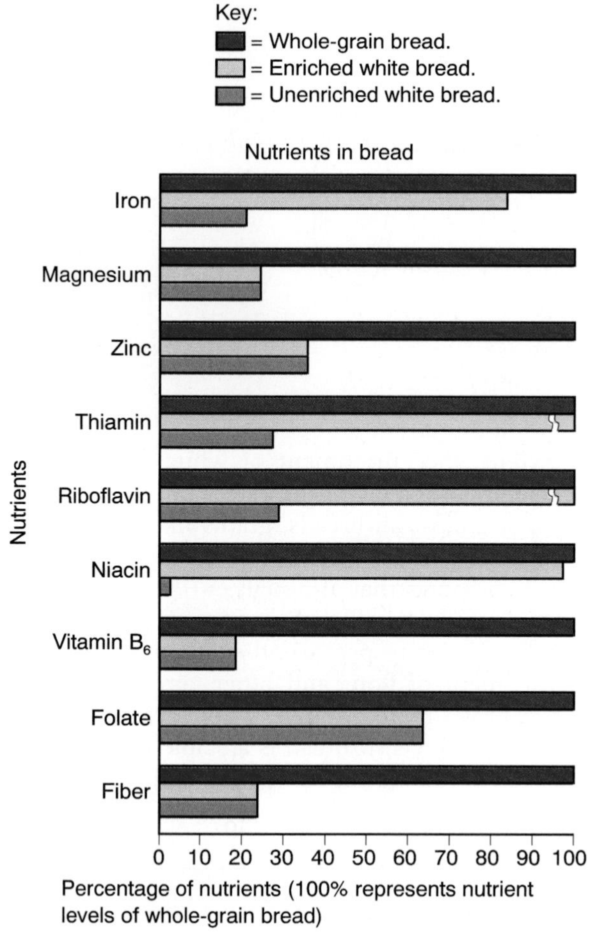

The Body's Use of Carbohydrate

This section refers to many body organs. To review them, turn to Appendix B.

Glycogen (GLY-co-gen) a polysaccharide composed of chains of glucose, manufactured in the body and stored in liver and muscle. As a storage form of glucose, glycogen can be broken down by the liver to maintain a constant blood glucose level when carbohydrate intake is inadequate.

Just as glucose is the original unit from which the variety of carbohydrate foods are made, so is glucose the basic carbohydrate unit that each cell of the body uses. Cells cannot use lactose, sucrose, or starch; they require glucose. The task of the digestive system, then, is to disassemble the double sugars and starch to single sugars and to absorb these monosaccharides into the blood. The liver converts to glucose those carbohydrates that are not already in the form of glucose so that they can be transported to the cells. The cells can then store this glucose, use it for energy, or convert it to fat.

If the blood delivers more glucose than the cells need, the liver and muscles take up the surplus to build the polysaccharide **glycogen.** The muscles hold two-thirds of the body's total store of this carbohydrate and use it during exercise. (Chapter 9 explores this relationship between glycogen and exercise and gives tips on how to make the most of glycogen stores.) The liver stores the other one-third, making it available to maintain the blood glucose level.

After the glycogen stores are full and the cells' immediate energy needs are met, the body takes a third path for using carbohydrate. Say you have eaten a dinner which includes enough carbohydrate to fill your glycogen stores. Now, you watch a movie, eat popcorn, and drink a cola beverage. Your digestive tract is delivering glucose from the popcorn and soda to your liver; your liver breaks these extra energy compounds into small fragments and puts them together into the more permanent energy-storage compound—fat. The fat is then released, carried to the fatty tissues of the body, and deposited there. (Fat cells, too, can utilize excess glucose to make fat for storage.) Unlike the liver cells, though, which can store only about half a day's worth of glucose as glycogen, the fat cells can store unlimited quantities of fat.

Maintaining the Blood Glucose Level

The brain and nervous system are sensitive to the concentration of glucose in the blood. Normal blood glucose levels are important for a feeling of well-being. When your blood glucose level becomes too concentrated, you get sleepy; when the concentration falls too low, you get weak and shaky. Only when blood glucose is within the normal range can you feel energetic and alert. The person who wants to feel energetic and alert all day should make the effort to eat so as to maintain blood glucose levels in the normal range to fuel the critical work of the brain and nervous system.

The maintenance of a normal blood glucose level depends on two safeguards, as shown in Figure 3–6. When the level gets too high—for example, immediately after a meal—it can be corrected by siphoning off the excess into liver and muscle glycogen and into body fat. When it gets too low—for example, following an overnight fast—it can be replenished by drawing on liver glycogen stores.

When the blood glucose level rises, the body adjusts by storing the excess. The first organ to detect the excess glucose is the pancreas, which releases the hormone insulin in response. Most of the body's cells respond to insulin by taking up glucose from the blood to make glycogen or fat. Thus, the blood glucose level is quickly brought back down to normal as the body stores the excess. Insulin's opposing hormone, released by the pancreas when blood glucose is too low, is **glucagon**, which draws forth glucose from storage, making it available to supply energy. Insulin and glucagon both work to maintain the concentration of glucose in the blood within the normal range—neither too high nor too low.

The hormone insulin (previously mentioned on page 59) is secreted in response to high blood glucose levels; it assists cells in drawing glucose from the blood.

Glucagon (GLUE-cuh-gon) insulin's opposing hormone, released by the pancreas when blood glucose is too low; it draws forth glucose and other fuels from storage, making them available to supply energy to cells.

Balanced meal a meal containing sufficient but not excessive amounts of foods from each of the food groups and therefore sufficient but not excessive amounts of carbohydrate, fat, protein, vitamins, and minerals.

Obviously, when the blood glucose level falls and stores are depleted, a meal or a snack can replenish the supply. An appropriate choice is to eat a **balanced meal** containing several different kinds of food that offer carbohydrate, protein, and fat:

- The carbohydrate in the meal provides a quick source of glucose. (Glucose, remember, is quickly put away by insulin.)
- The protein in the meal stimulates glucagon secretion, which opposes insulin and keeps it from putting away glucose too fast.
- The fat in the meal slows down digestion so that you receive a steady stream of nutrients rather than a sudden flood.

By these standards, a doughnut for breakfast (high in sugar and fat, low in protein) is a poor choice. The boost it gives to blood glucose does not last.

Figure 3–6

Blood Glucose Regulation

A. High blood glucose (sugar) stimulates the pancreas to release insulin. Insulin serves as a key for entrance of blood glucose into cells. Liver and muscle cells store the glucose as glycogen. Excess glucose can also be stored as fat.

B. Later, low blood glucose stimulates the pancreas to release glucagon, which serves as the key for the liver to break down stored glycogen to glucose and release it into the blood.

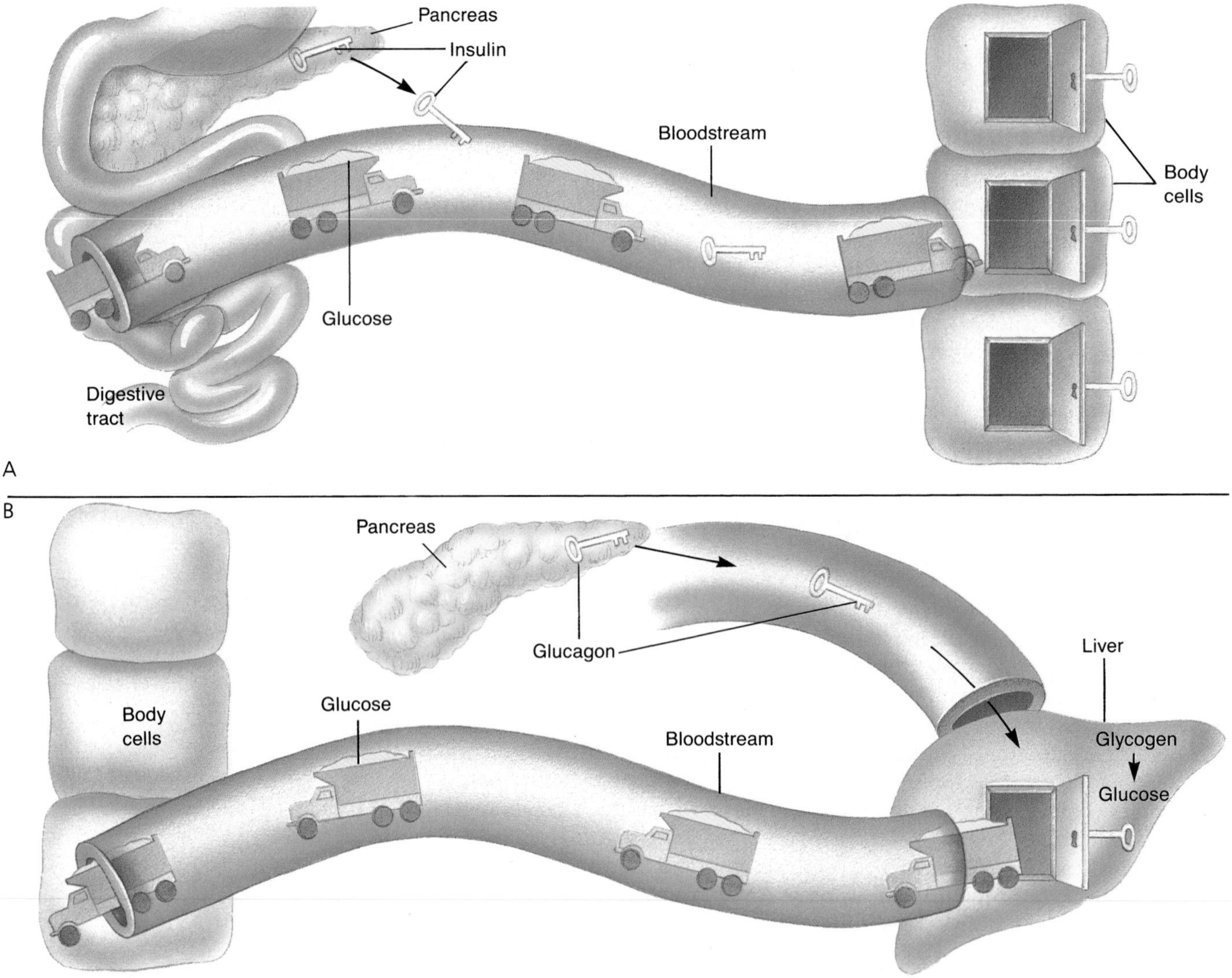

Eating well-spaced, carefully chosen meals that provide the balance of protein, carbohydrate, and fat recommended in the *Dietary Guidelines* can prevent rapid rises and falls in the blood glucose level.

The effect of a food on the blood glucose level is important to people with abnormalities of blood glucose regulation, notably diabetes and **hypoglyce-**

mia.* Rapid swings in blood glucose can affect the performance of both an athlete during an endurance event and an office employee following lunch. People are wise to avoid foods producing too great a rise and too sudden a fall in the blood glucose level. Researchers are attempting to rank foods according to their effects on blood glucose. In general, legumes produce the most even blood glucose response, dairy products next, and fruits and cereals next; pure sugar produces the greatest rise in the blood glucose level.[15]

Hypoglycemia (HIGH-po-gligh-SEEM-ee-uh) an abnormally low blood glucose concentration—below about 60 to 70 mg/100 ml.

Hypoglycemia

Suppose the blood glucose falls, the glycogen reserves are exhausted, and you do *not* eat. Gradually, your body will shift into a fasting state, breaking down its muscle to provide amino acids to the liver. The liver converts some of these into glucose to fuel the brain. The fat released from the muscle cells is used to fuel other cells. (Chapter 8 describes this state—ketosis—in more detail.) Most times, the transition is smooth and is not noticeable. But there may be times when your blood glucose level falls rapidly or below what is normal for you, and you may experience symptoms of glucose deprivation to the brain: anxiety, hunger, and dizziness. Your muscles become weak, shaky, and trembling, and your heart races in an attempt to speed more fuel to your brain. These symptoms of low blood glucose signify that your system is out of balance, but this is usually no cause for concern. All of us, at times, experience the ordinary type of hypoglycemia—low blood glucose levels occurring within six hours of a meal. The treatment consists of learning to eat promptly and properly.

There is another type of hypoglycemia, however, that requires treatment. It is a rare and often serious condition in which abnormal amounts of hormones are secreted, perhaps because of tumors or other abnormalities. As a result, the person's blood glucose is constantly too low—independent of dietary intake. This kind of hypoglycemia causes symptoms (headache, confusion, fatigue, amnesia, seizures, or unconsciousness), even after only 8 to 14 hours without food (for example, overnight). A person with this kind of hypoglycemia urgently needs diagnosis and medical treatment.

Hypoglycemia has been a popular buzzword for many decades. It is not a single entity; it is a symptom, not a disease. It may be simple and easy to avoid, or it may be a serious matter. Diagnosis and treatment are properly left to a qualified professional. But for anyone who has a hard time making it from one meal to the next, there can be no harm in eating balanced, sustaining meals of a kind most likely to blunt the glycemic effect—meals containing adequate protein; a bit of fat; ample fluid; and abundant carbohydrate, including fiber, from vegetables, grains, fruits, and especially legumes.[16]

Diabetes

Knowing how the blood glucose level is maintained, you can appreciate the problem of the person with diabetes whose insulin response is slow or inef-

*The effect of food on a person's blood glucose and insulin response is called the *glycemic effect*—how fast and how high the blood glucose rises and how quickly the body responds by bringing it back to normal. A *glycemic index* ranks foods on the basis of the extent to which the foods raise the blood glucose level as compared with pure glucose.

Table 3–7
Differences Between the Two Main Types of Diabetes

	TYPE I: INSULIN-DEPENDENT DIABETES	TYPE II: NON-INSULIN DEPENDENT DIABETES
Incidence	10% of cases.	90% of cases.
Insulin lack	Yes, pancreas unable to make insulin to meet needs.	No, but there may be insufficient insulin, or cells may be unresponsive to insulin.
Risk factors	Genetic predisposition plus environmental factor (for example, viral infection).	Genetic predisposition plus obesity.
Treatment	Insulin injections. Dietary intervention.	Weight loss. Dietary intervention.

Table 3–8 Sugar in Food

FOOD	TEASPOONS SUGAR PER SERVING
Angel food cake (1/12 of cake)	6
Apple pie (1/6 of pie)	12
Apricots (4–6 halves)	4
Catsup (1 tbsp)	1
Cereal, sweetened (1 c)	8
Chewing gum (2 sticks)	1
Chocolate cake, iced (1/12 of cake)	15
Cola (12 oz)	9
Corn, canned (5 oz)	3
Dairy creamer (1 tbsp)	2
Doughnuts, glazed (1)	6
Doughnuts, plain (1)	4
Fig bars (2)	10
Fruit, canned with syrup (1 c)	9
Fudge (1 oz)	5
Gingersnaps (1 medium)	1
Ice cream (½ c)	3–6
Jam, jelly, syrup (1 tbsp)	3
Jellybeans (10)	6½
Kool-Aid (8 oz)	6
Oatmeal cookies (1 medium)	1½
Peanut butter, commercial (2 tbsp)	½
Raisins (¼ c)	4
Salad dressing, French (1 tbsp)	1
Sherbet (½ c)	4½–8
Yogurt, fruit type (1 c)	6

Source: Adapted from Too much sugar, *Consumer Reports,* March 1978, and data from the U.S. Department of Agriculture.

fective. Most adults with diabetes fall into this category (see Table 3–7).* Even if the blood glucose level rises too high (hyperglycemia), glucose still fails to get into cells and so stays too high for an abnormally long time. The kidneys may respond by shifting some glucose out of the body into the urine so that it can be excreted—hence the notion that people with diabetes should not eat carbohydrate. They should; they need it. But they must be careful to eat balanced meals—providing a constant, steady, moderate flow of glucose to the bloodstream—and avoid concentrated sugar so that the insulin response can keep up. Recent research indicates that people with diabetes actually do best on a diet that is high in complex-carbohydrate-rich foods—as high as is recommended for any healthy person. The starch and protein in these foods help to regulate the blood glucose level, as already described.

People with the common type of diabetes—those who make insulin but resist responding to it—tend to become obese, storing more fat than normal and being constantly hungry. This is because the liver takes up from the blood the glucose that the cells cannot take up, converts the glucose to fat, and then ships it out to the fat cells for storage. The fat cells respond—slowly, to be sure—but ultimately they store all the fat that is sent to them. Being slow to get the message that energy fuels are coming in from food, the person with diabetes is constantly hungry. Being slow to detect the presence of glucose in the blood, the person is hungry for sweets. Unfortunately, the larger the fat cells become, the more resistant they are to insulin, thus making the diabetes worse. People with diabetes in their families are urged not to gain excess weight, for it is likely to precipitate the onset of the disease.

A rarer type of diabetes occurs in about 10 percent of all cases. It involves a total lack of insulin, and it requires insulin shots. The person who secretes no insulin is likely to experience a sudden onset of the disease. Such a person may lose weight rapidly, because without insulin, the cells cannot store glucose or fat. Thus, the two types of diabetes have opposite effects on body weight—one making the person fat; the other, thin.

*Most diabetes is of the type known as type II, or non-insulin-dependent, diabetes. People with this diabetes secrete insulin, but secretion is ineffective or delayed. Often the diet can be adjusted to enable the body's own insulin to do its work so that no shots or drugs need to be taken. The rarer type of diabetes is called type I, or insulin-dependent, diabetes.

Keeping Sweetness in the Diet

The taste of sweetness is a pleasure; the liking for it is innate. However, the *Dietary Guidelines for Americans* recommend that people use concentrated sweets only in moderation. To help with this task while still catering to the sweet tooth, consider the following pointers:

- Use less of all sugars, including white sugar, brown sugar, raw sugar, honey, and syrups.
- Eat less of foods containing sugars, such as soft drinks, candy, ice cream, cakes, and cookies.
- Select fresh fruits or fruits canned without sugar or in light syrup rather than heavy syrup to satisfy your urge for sweets.
- Read food labels for clues on sugar content—if the name sucrose, glucose, maltose, dextrose, fructose, or syrup appears first, the food contains a large amount of sugar (see Figure 3–7). Use sparingly foods in which these sweeteners are among the first three ingredients listed. Table 3–8 shows the amounts of sugar in some common products.
- Remember, for dental health, how frequently you eat sugar is as important as—and perhaps more important than—how much sugar you eat at one time (see the Nutrition Action feature on dental health in Chapter 10).

Alternatives to sweet desserts might be whole-grain crackers, lowfat cheese, and yogurt. Snacks for children need not be sugar-water drinks but

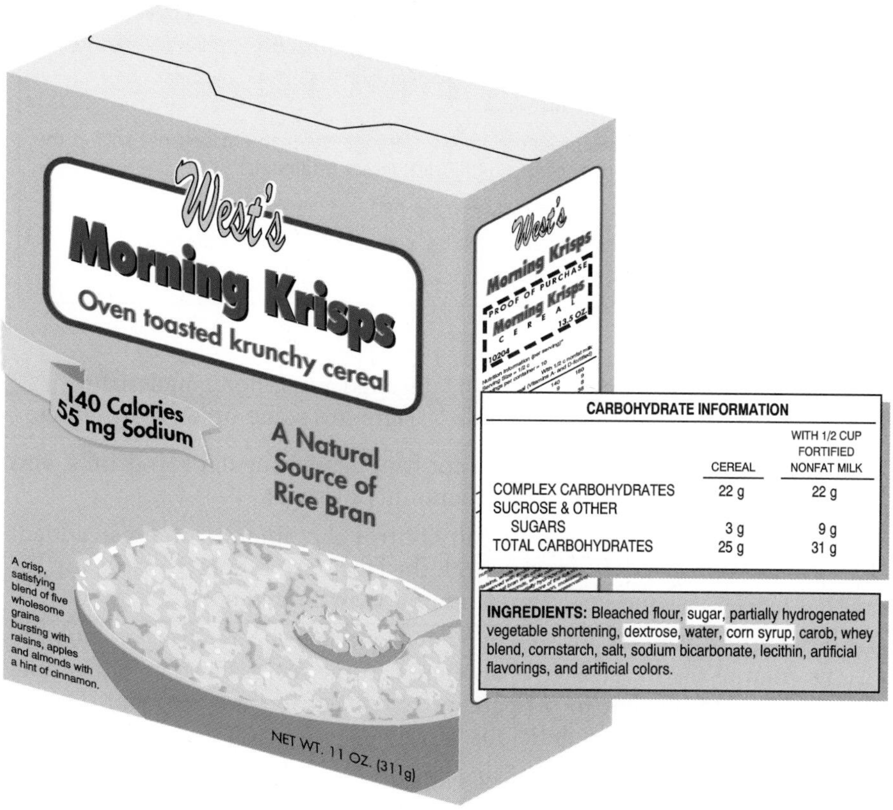
West's
Morning Krisps
Oven toasted krunchy cereal
140 Calories
55 mg Sodium
A Natural Source of Rice Bran
A crisp, satisfying blend of five wholesome grains bursting with raisins, apples and almonds with a hint of cinnamon.
NET WT. 11 OZ. (311g)
PROOF OF PURCHASE
CARBOHYDRATE INFORMATION
CEREAL
WITH 1/2 CUP FORTIFIED NONFAT MILK
COMPLEX CARBOHYDRATES 22 g 22 g
SUCROSE & OTHER SUGARS 3 g 9 g
TOTAL CARBOHYDRATES 25 g 31 g
INGREDIENTS: Bleached flour, sugar, partially hydrogenated vegetable shortening, dextrose, water, corn syrup, carob, whey blend, cornstarch, salt, sodium bicarbonate, lecithin, artificial flavorings, and artificial colors.

Figure 3–7

Using the Food Label

The cereal shown contains sugars. To find out how much, check the carbohydrate information panel for sucrose and other sugars. Many cereals contain considerably more sugar than this cereal contains. Check labels and make your own comparisons. How do you know if sugar has been added to a food if the nutrition information doesn't list sucrose and other sugars by grams? The more processed the food is, the more likely it is to contain sugar. Learn to read labels (see label at left). Labels list ingredients in order of amount, with the greatest amount of an ingredient present in the food listed first. In addition to *sucrose,* check labels for the sugar terms listed in the miniglossary. If one or more of these sweeteners are listed first, second, or third on the label, there is a large proportion of sugar in the food. Use sparingly foods in which these sweeteners are among the first three ingredients listed.

This product contains three different added sugars: sugar, dextrose, and corn syrup. Notice that these sugars are the second, fourth, and sixth ingredients on the label. This indicates that the product is probably high in sugar.

Source: Adapted from ConAgra Inc., *What's in a label?,* 1990, p. 74.

Miniglossary of Sweeteners

Brown rice syrup similar to honey in taste and consistency; also available as a powder.

Brown sugar white sugar with molasses added; about 95% pure sucrose.

Confectioners' sugar finely powdered sucrose; 99.9% pure sucrose.

Corn sweeteners corn syrup and sugars derived from corn.

Corn syrup a syrup produced by the action of enzymes on cornstarch; contains mostly glucose.

Dextrose another name for glucose.

Fructose, galactose, glucose the monosaccharides; see page 57.

Granulated sugar common table sugar; crystalline sucrose—99.9% pure.

High-fructose corn syrup (HFCS) the predominant sweetener used in processed foods and beverages; contains mostly fructose, with some glucose and maltose.

Honey primarily a mixture of glucose and fructose made by bees from the sucrose in nectar.

Invert sugar a mixture of glucose and fructose formed by splitting sucrose in processing; sold in liquid form and used as an additive to prevent crystallization of sucrose in candies and other confections.

Lactose, maltose, sucrose the disaccharides; see page 57.

Levulose another name for fructose.

Maple sugar a concentrated form of sucrose purified from the sap of the sugar maple tree.

Molasses a thick brown syrup; a leftover from the process of refining sucrose from sugar cane; blackstrap molasses contains certain minerals—notably iron—picked up from the machinery used to process it.

Natural sweeteners a term without a legal definition; refers to any sugar or sweetener other than refined table sugar.

Raw sugar the first crystals produced during the sugar refining process; not sold in the United States due to the presence of "filth" (dirt, insect fragments).

Turbinado sugar raw sugar that has been washed to remove the filth.

White sugar pure sugar; made by dissolving, concentrating, and recrystallizing raw sugar.

rather, fruits, raw vegetables, popcorn, unsalted nuts, homemade fruit-juice popsicles, and other wholesome foods.[17] Here are some other suggestions:

- Substitute fruit *juices* or plain water for fruit *drinks,* regular soft drinks, and punches that contain considerable amounts of sugar.
- Buy *unsweetened* cereals so you can control the amount of sugar added. Many cereals are presweetened. Check the label (see Figure 3–7). Many list sugar first—or second and third—among their ingredients.
- Experiment with reducing the sugar in your favorite recipes, or look for recipes that use fruit juices as a sweetener. Some recipes taste just the same even after a 25 percent to 50 percent reduction in sugar content. Others taste different but just as delicious.
- The sweet spices—allspice, anise, cardamom, cinnamon, cloves, fennel, ginger, and nutmeg—can replace substantial sugar in recipes. Use half as much sugar and one and a half times as much spice as the recipe calls for.

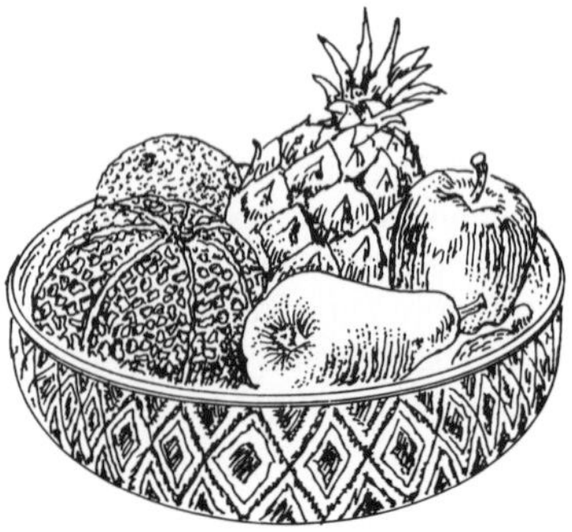

Naturally sweet foods like fruit can satisfy your sweet tooth.

Still another alternative is to use sugary foods that convey nutrients as well as calories. Examples: rather than sugar cookies, serve oatmeal cookies; rather than brownies, eat apricot bars; and rather than table sugar as a topping, add raisins and banana slices, which are really very sweet.

Keep in mind that sugar is delicious and that you can use it with discretion, but use it in moderation. The person with nutrition sense and a taste for sweets can artfully combine the two by using sugar with creative imagination to enhance the flavors of nutritious foods.

Consumer Tips

Adding Fiber to the Diet

Current recommendations advise people to eat 20 to 35 grams of dietary fiber a day. However, most Americans now eat only 11 grams of fiber. This fact is largely due to the number of refined foods, fats, and sweets that have displaced the higher fiber foods our grandparents used to enjoy—the basic, whole foods like fruits, vegetables, legumes, and whole-grain breads and cereals. Adding fiber to your diet can be easier and tastier than you may think. Here are some easy tips for including more fiber-rich foods in your diet.

- Increase consumption of a variety of fiber-rich foods, including fruits, vegetables, legumes, and whole-grain breads, pastas, and cereals (refer to Table 3–6 for the fiber content of various foods).
- Select high-fiber foods when shopping for groceries—whole-grain cereals, breads, and snack foods, for example. Buy products that list a whole-grain, or whole-wheat or other whole-grain flour as the first ingredient. Check the food label for "dietary fiber" content.
- Choose whole fruits instead of juice; leave the peel on fruits and vegetables.
- Add berries to muffin and pancake batters.
- Whenever possible, substitute whole-grain flour for all-purpose flour when baking.
- Use oats in place of flour in crumb-type toppings for fruit crisps; using a blender, grind whole-grain oats into flour, and use it to replace one-third or more of the all-purpose flour called for in recipes; try toasting whole-grain oats as a replacement for bread crumbs on top of casseroles, cooked vegetables, or fish fillets; add cinnamon to the toasted oats and sprinkle over fresh fruit and yogurt.
- Eat whole, baked, or boiled potatoes, including skins, instead of mashed.
- Use unpeeled vegetables in salads, soups, and stews.
- Experiment with legumes: add beans to salads, soups, stews, tacos, or burritos; one-half cup of cooked kidney beans in a bowl of chili adds about 8 grams of dietary fiber.
- Use brown rice instead of white rice for added fiber and nutrients.
- Eat high-fiber snacks—popcorn, fresh fruits, raw vegetables, dried fruits, and nuts (go easy on the nuts, since 1 cup of most nuts has 800 calories).
- Start your day off with a high-fiber selection: a warm bowl of oatmeal with fresh fruit; bran cereals or shredded wheat with sliced fruit; banana bread; oat- or wheat-bran muffins; compote of prunes with citrus fruits; whole-grain English muffin.
- Remember to add high-fiber foods to the diet gradually, with adequate fluids, giving your body time to adjust.

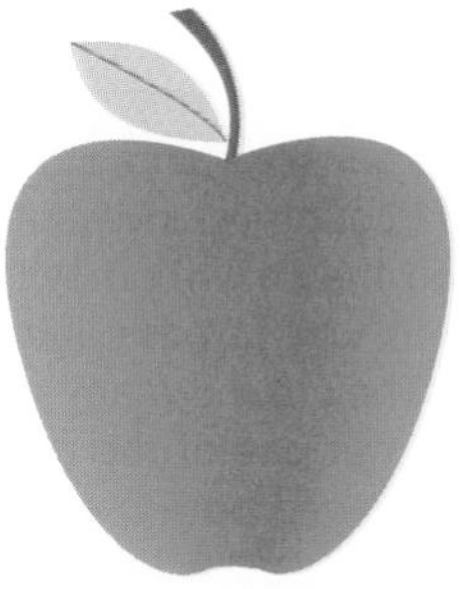

Large whole apple with peel: 5.0 g fiber

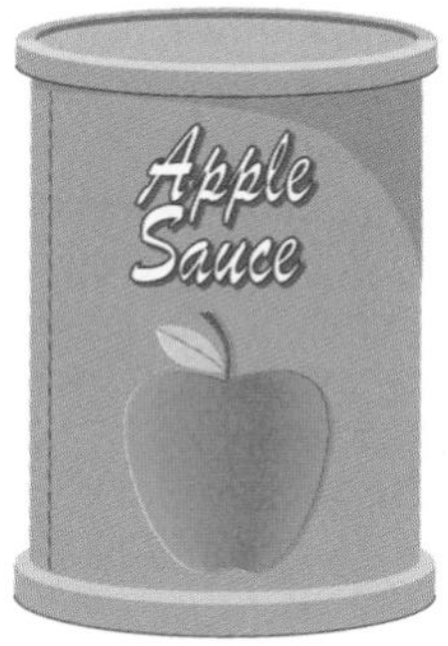

Applesauce, 1/2 cup: 2.0 g fiber

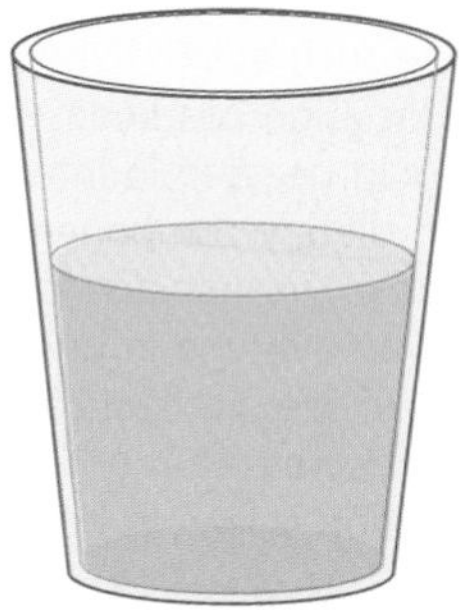

Apple juice, 3/4 cup: 0.2 g fiber

Spotlight

Diet and Disease Prevention—Cancer

You probably know someone who has cancer or who has recovered from it or who has died of it. After heart disease, cancer is our most prevalent disease and can be expected, in one form or another, to affect one out of every four Americans living today. Given what is known now about the link between diet and cancer, you are well advised to learn about this connection. Unlike so many factors in our environment, the food you choose to eat is a factor you can control to a great extent. This discussion attempts to answer questions about the connection between diet and cancer.

• How is diet associated with cancer?

Numerous studies conducted in both laboratory animals and humans over the past two decades have shown that many connections exist between diet and cancer. Constituents in foods may be responsible for starting the cancer (a process called *initiation*) or for speeding its development (a two-step process that includes tumor *promotion* and *progression*), or they may protect against cancer. Also, for the person who has cancer, diet can make a crucial difference to recovery by helping to restore body weight and improve nutritional status.

Not all studies have shown a firm relationship between cancer and food and nutrient intake. In particular, some epidemiologic studies—that is, studies of disease rates and food patterns of groups of people—have failed to demonstrate such a link. Where a positive association has been found, caution should be used in interpreting data linking dietary components with cancer or other chronic diseases. Remember, an increase in one component of the diet can cause increases or decreases in others.[18] If a close correlation is shown between cancer and, say, the consumption of animal protein by a human population, how can we be sure that the critical factor is the animal protein? It may be increased fat consumption, because fat goes with animal protein in foods. Or the cancer may occur because of what is crowded out: vitamins, minerals, or fiber contained in the missing fruits, vegetables, and cereals.

These issues must be considered when examining the results of studies describing a connection between diet and cancer. Our diets are complex and diverse, making it difficult to separate the effect of a single dietary component from the hundreds of other constituents found in foods. In addition, the difficulty of evaluating the diet-cancer link is compounded by the fact that many cancers take up to 20 years to develop. Thus, assessing a cancer patient's diet today is not as helpful as knowing how that patient ate 10, 20, or even 30 years before the cancer was diagnosed. Finally, our eating pattern is only one of many factors that contribute to the development of cancer.

• Is nutrition related to cancer causation the way other environmental factors are—such as smoking or air pollution?

Yes. The National Cancer Institute estimates that 90 percent of all cancers are associated with lifestyle and environmental factors including nutrition. Lifestyle factors can usually be controlled by the individual and include tobacco use, diet, consumption of alcohol, exposure to sunlight, patterns of sexual behavior, and personal hygiene. Individuals typically have little control over environmental factors, such as the exposure to carcinogens in the workplace, radiation during medical and dental procedures, or contaminants (either naturally occurring or artificially-created) present in the soil, air, and water. Of course, we have no control over the genetic factors that contribute to the development of cancer.[19]

Nutrition is a lifestyle factor that may account for as much as a third of all cancer deaths. Thus, researchers have taken the study of nutrition and cancer seriously. They are attempting to discover what dietary differences exist between people who do and do not get cancer. In the process, they are trying to identify the various dietary factors that may contribute to or protect against many different types of cancer, including cancer of the esophagus, stomach, liver, pancreas, colon, rectum, breast, ovary, prostate, and lung.

• What is some of the evidence linking diet and cancer?

Studies of the eating habits of different population groups provide some of the knowledge we have about the diet-cancer connection. Particularly telling is research involving Seventh-Day Adventists, a group of people with a remarkably low death rate from cancers of all kinds. This religious group has rules against smoking and using alcohol, discourages the use of hot condiments and spices, and encourages a meatless diet. After cancers linked to smoking and alcohol are discounted, these people still have a cancer mortality rate about one-half to two-thirds that of the rest of the population. This may be due to a low consumption of meat (and, therefore, *fat*) and to a high consumption of vegetables and cereal grains.

On a larger scale, in a study involving 37 countries, investigators documented the daily food available per person as well as other indicators of lifestyle. They found many correlations, but one of the most interesting showed both breast cancers and cancers of the large intestine (colon) to be strongly associated "with indicators of affluence, such as a high-fat diet rich in animal protein."[20]

When it comes to colon cancer, other studies lend weight to their conclusion. In one study, people with colon cancer were compared with a carefully matched set of people without cancer. Those with cancer were found to have a strikingly higher consumption of meat, especially beef. Another study showed fiber consumption to be lower in colon cancer victims than in comparable people who did not have cancer. Still another showed colon cancer victims to be eating less fiber and more saturated fat than people without cancer. Furthermore, among U.S. women between the ages of 34 and 59, the risk of colon cancer was related to their intake of animal (but not vegetable) fat, according to researchers at Harvard Medical School.[21] These examples are just a few of the many studies that have led researchers to the view that a diet high in total fat, especially animal fat, and low in fiber is associated with cancer of the colon.[22]

So, diet is associated with the development of colon cancer. What about breast cancer?

The case of the connection between diet and breast cancer is a good example of the difficulty of interpreting study results. Laboratory animals, particularly rodents, consistently develop mammary or breast tumors when fed a high-fat diet.[23] Despite the strength of this link in the animal model, similar results have not been seen consistently in human studies.

In one study of more than 88,000 registered nurses in the United States, there was no evidence of a link between the intake of fat, saturated fat, or dietary cholesterol and the risk of breast cancer.[24] A similar finding was reported by a group of researchers in Athens, Greece, who studied 120 women with breast cancer and 120 women without cancer: there was no association between breast cancer and the consumption of fats and oils.[25] By comparison, a research group in Israel reported that Israeli women with a high intake of animal fat and protein and a low intake of dietary fiber had an increased risk of breast cancer.[26] Several studies from Canada and the United States have also supported a link between breast cancer and fat intake. However, despite these apparently conflicting study results, the National Cancer Institute has determined that the bulk of the evidence suggests a link between fat intake and breast cancer.

What should consumers do?

The American Cancer Society and the National Cancer Institute have reviewed the evidence independently and have pointed out to consumers the following specific concerns:

- *Total energy intake.* Studies on animals show that reduced food intakes reduce cancer incidence at any age, but the evidence is less clear for human beings. Obesity, however, does increase risks for some cancers in both animals and people (see Chapter 8).
- *Fat.* Both animal studies and epidemiological studies support the view that high-fat intakes increase the incidence of cancers of the breast, ovaries, colon, and prostate. Evidence on the relationship between cholesterol and cancer is unclear at this point.
- *Protein.* High protein intakes may be associated with increased risks of certain kinds of cancer, but the evidence is not yet firm enough to permit a definitive statement.
- *Carbohydrate.* There is little evidence that carbohydrates as such play a role in cancer development. High intakes of simple carbohydrates (for example, sucrose) may contribute to caloric excess, weight gain, and obesity.
- *Vitamin A.* Inadequate intakes of vitamin A and/or its relatives correlate with a high incidence of cancers of the lung, bladder, and larynx; by inference, adequate intakes may help protect against these cancers.

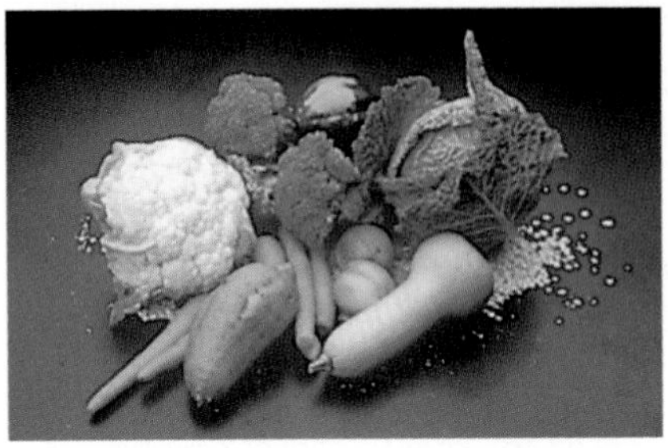

Cruciferous vegetables, such as cauliflower, broccoli, and Brussels sprouts contain nutrients and nonnutrients that protect against cancer.

- *Vitamin C.* Vitamin C may help prevent the formation of cancer-causing agents and thereby protect against cancers of the esophagus and stomach.
- *Other vitamins and minerals.* Bits of evidence suggest that other nutrients may protect against certain types of cancer, but no firm conclusions can yet be made. Selenium, for example, is believed to have a protective effect against cancer of the esophagus, stomach, colon, and rectum.[27] Likewise, vitamin E may protect against cancer, particularly cancer of the gastrointestinal tract.[28]
- *Vitamin A-rich and cruciferous vegetables.* The consumption of vitamin A-rich and cruciferous vegetables is associated with a reduced incidence of cancer at several sites. Cruciferous vegetables are a group of vegetables named for their cross-shaped blossoms. They have been shown to protect against cancer in laboratory animals. Examples of cruciferous vegetables are cauliflower, cabbage, Brussels sprouts, broccoli, turnips, and rutabagas.
- *Calcium.* Low calcium intakes have been associated with increased colon cancer.

What about fiber?

Wherever the diet is high in fat-rich foods it is usually low in vegetable fiber. This raises the question whether the absence of fiber may promote cancer independently of the presence of fat. The answer is difficult to discern, but the association of cancer with fat is stronger than with the lack of fiber. Still, fiber might help protect against some cancers, for example, by speeding up the passage of all materials through the colon so that its walls are not exposed for long to cancer-causing substances.

Evidence from Finland supports fiber's independent protective effect. The Finns eat a high-fat diet, but unlike other such diets, theirs is very high in fiber as well. Their colon cancer rate is low, suggesting that fiber has a protective effect even in the presence of a high-fat diet.[29]

• Fat is linked to certain cancers, and fiber is associated with cancer prevention. Do vegetarians have a lower incidence of those cancers?

Yes, they do. The Seventh-Day Adventists have already been mentioned. Vegetarian women also have less breast cancer than do women who eat meat.

A number of studies have examined the relationship between cancer and vegetable consumption. Many of them have shown that people with colon cancer use vegetables less frequently than do others; one study revealed that colon cancer victims specifically used less cabbage, broccoli, and Brussels sprouts than did people free of cancer. Similarly, comparisons of stomach cancer victims' diets with those of carefully matched people without cancer showed less use of vegetables in the cancer group—in one case, vegetables in general; in another, fresh vegetables; in others, lettuce and other fresh greens or vegetables containing vitamin C.[30] Some of the suspects for the causation of stomach cancer are the chemicals known as nitrosamines, produced in the stomach and intestines from nitrites found in foods. Vegetables may help in cancer prevention by contributing vitamin C, which inhibits the conversion of nitrites to nitrosamines.

• What about alcohol: is it connected with cancer?

Yes. Environmental causes of head and neck cancer have been studied, and the major factor appears to be the combination of alcohol and tobacco use. However, dietary factors have turned up, pointing to a low intake of fruits and raw vegetables, specifically of the fruits and vegetables that contribute the orange pigment carotene (which converts to vitamin A in the body) and the vitamin riboflavin. Carotene—noted for giving carrots, winter squash, sweet potatoes, apricots, cantaloupe, oranges, and other fruits and vegetables their familiar colors—and its relatives (known as the retinoids, which are found in milk, cheese, butter, ice cream, and certain fish) may also be important in reducing the risk of skin cancer.[31]

• What is the association between vitamin A and cancer?

Among the known actions of vitamin A are important roles it plays in maintaining immune function. A strong immune system may be able to prevent cancers from gaining control, even after they have gotten started in the body.

A five-year study has shown lung cancer incidence to be 60 percent to 80 percent lower in men with a high vitamin A intake than in those with a low intake. Another study has shown lung cancer rates to be 20 percent to 30 percent lower in smokers who ate vitamin A-rich yellow or green vegetables daily than in those who did not. In ex-smokers who ingested yellow or green vegetables daily, the reduction was much greater, indicating that the *repair* of damage done by smoking might be enhanced by something in the vegetables.[32]

• Would that "something" in the vegetables be vitamin A?

Not necessarily. Green vegetables appear to have a protective effect beyond those already discussed for vitamin A, vitamin C, and fiber. These vegetables also contain folate, a vitamin, which is involved in cell multiplication and may prove to play an important role in cancer prevention. The effects of the members of the cabbage family may be due to their containing substances known as indoles, which may act by inducing an enzyme in the host that destroys cancer-causing agents.[33]

• Do these findings have any implications for the way a person should eat today?

Although clearly there is still much to learn, many experts believe that enough is known to take the first preventive steps. The following recommendations are commonly offered:

- Reduce total fat and food energy intake if necessary to meet recommended levels.
- Ingest more complex carbohydrates, both starch and fiber.
- Eat plenty of green, orange, and yellow vegetables and fruits, including generous servings from the cabbage family.
- Vary your choices. Don't let your diet become monotonous.

The National Cancer Institute has added three other recommendations: (1) avoid obesity; (2) consume alcoholic beverages in moderation, if at all; and (3) eat salt-cured, salt-pickled, or smoked foods sparingly.[34] Taken together, this advice agrees with most recommendations made to the public for helping prevent heart disease, diabetes, and many other ills, as well as cancer.

• Does it make a difference if I choose to take supplements instead of eating vegetables?

Yes. Fiber, vitamin A, vitamin C, carotene, riboflavin, indoles, and other components found in *foods* rather than pills appear to have preventive effects on cancer development. And because it is obvious that researchers do not have *the* answer—just many partial answers—it is best to stick with foods. Supplements may not contain some as yet unidentified components found in foods that may help protect against cancer. Also, with vitamin/mineral supplementation, there is always the risk of an excessively high intake; recall that vitamin A, selenium, and other vitamins and minerals can be toxic at high doses. *It is best to rely on foods.* Fruits and vegetables will add vitamins, minerals, and fiber to your diet—and color and flavor as well.

● Why should I vary my diet?

The recommendation to eat a varied diet is based on an important cancer-prevention strategy—dilution. The standard advice to eat a variety of foods takes on new meaning in this quote: "The wider the variety of food intake, the greater the number of different chemical substances consumed, and the less is the chance that any one chemical will reach a hazardous level in the diet."[35] In other words, whenever you add new foods to the diet, you are diluting whatever is in one food with what is in another.

The variety principle has traditionally meant to eat foods from each of the four food groups. This principle needs to be applied within each of the food groups as well. Don't alternate just between corn and potatoes. Select different vegetables each time you go to the store—broccoli, peas, green beans, squash, and many others.

Although there are many cancer-causing factors that you cannot control, you can decide which food habits you will keep and which ones you will change. By using these guidelines in making your choices, you will have every reason to feel confident that you are providing your body with the best nutrition at the lowest possible risk. Remember that in the final analysis, your risk of developing cancer can be reduced significantly by not smoking and by adopting healthful eating habits.

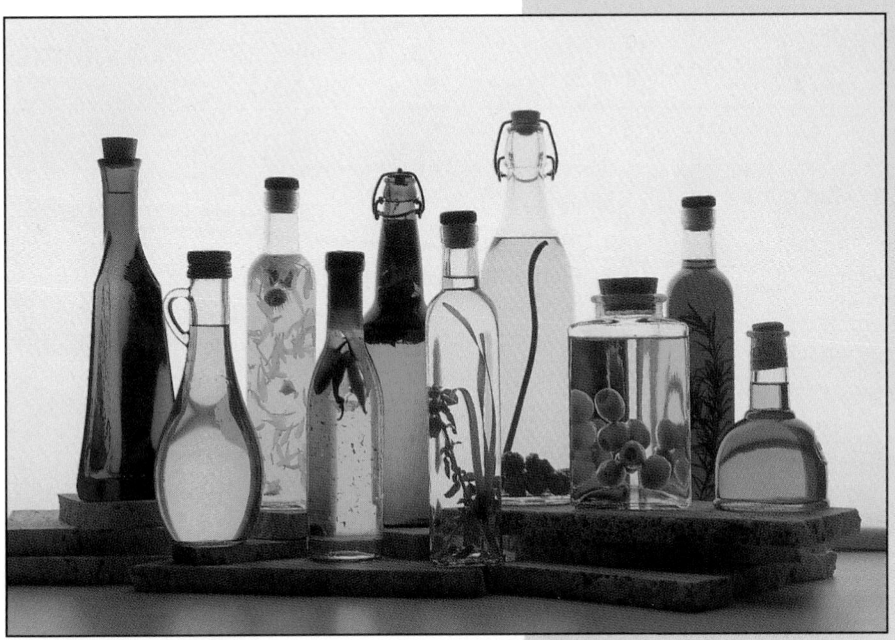

© Peter Wong

> *The ultimate reality of nutrition rests with the chemistry of the food we eat and its effects on the processes of life.*
>
> —R. M. Deutsch

CHAPTER 4
The Lipids: Fats and Oils

Contents

Ask Yourself . . . ?

Which of these statements about nutrition are true, and which are false? For the false statements, what *is* true?

1. The less fat you have in your diet, the better.
2. The body can store fat in virtually unlimited amounts.
3. A person's blood level of cholesterol is a predictor of that person's risk of having a heart attack.
4. For the health of your heart, the fat you should avoid eating most of all is cholesterol.
5. The more omega-3 fatty acids you eat, the better it is for your health.
6. Fruits are essentially fat-free.
7. In general, the softest margarines are the most polyunsaturated.
8. High HDL-cholesterol in the blood is a sign of good health.
9. Nondairy creamers, because they are made from plant fats, do not contribute to heart disease.
10. No one is free of atherosclerosis.

Answers: 1. False. It is important not to cut fat from the diet altogether. 2. True. 3. True. 4. False. For the health of your heart, the fat you should avoid eating most of all is saturated fat. 5. False. Omega-3 fatty acids are good for the health of your heart, but like all fats, they should be eaten in moderation. 6. True. 7. True. 8. True. 9. False. Some nondairy creamers, even though they are made from plant fats, contain saturated fats, which can contribute to heart disease. 10. True.

Lipids a family of compounds that includes triglycerides (fats and oils), phospholipids (for example, lecithin), and sterols (cholesterol).
Fats lipids that are solid at room temperature.
Oils lipids that are liquid at normal room temperature.

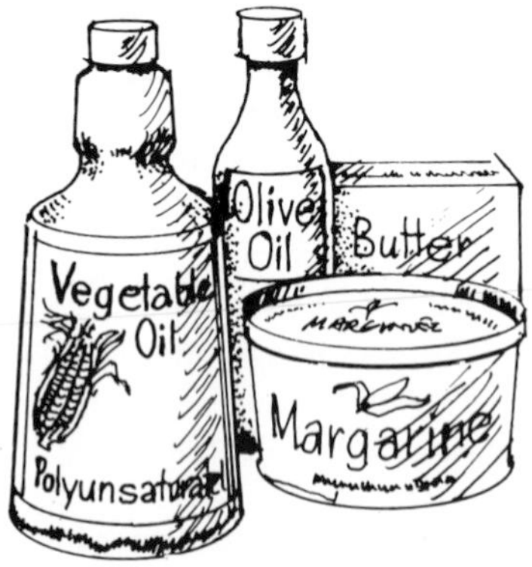

Fats in common use. The vegetable oil is highly polyunsaturated, the olive oil is highly monounsaturated, the butter is largely saturated, and the margarine, no doubt, is partially hydrogenated.

When you and your friend visit a health fair at a local shopping mall you learn that your blood cholesterol level is high. Your friend, a registered dietitian, urges you to see your health care provider to request a blood lipid profile to determine the level of triglycerides and the ratio of "good" to "bad" cholesterol in your blood. On your way out of the mall, you notice a bookstore display for a new diet book that urges you to "cut fat intake to reduce cancer risk." Then you stop at the window of a health-food store. Your friend points to the freshly ground peanut butter, mentioning to you that it is not hydrogenated, while you stare at the bottles of lecithin and fish oil supplements that line the wall. Later during the evening news, your attention is drawn to the television commercials—one features a tub of margarine touted as being better than butter, and another shows a loving couple promising to use heart-healthy spreads on their morning muffins. "What does all of this mean?" you ask.

Actually you may know more than you think you do about the **lipids**, more commonly called **fats** and **oils.** The most obvious common sources of fat are oil, butter, margarine, and shortening. Other sources are meats, nuts, mayonnaise, salad dressings, eggs, bacon, gravy, cheese, ice cream, and whole milk. You may know that egg yolk and liver are high in cholesterol, and you probably know that the cholesterol in the body is in some way related to heart disease. However, you may be confused by the many terms related to the fat in your diet. This chapter explores the terminology of fat and will describe how fats can both contribute to health and detract from it.

A Primer on Fats

Most people have the impression that fat is bad for them, and it might come as a surprise that fats are valuable. More than valuable, some are absolutely necessary, and some fats must be present in the diet for you to maintain good health. Even if you wanted to, it would be impossible to remove all the fat from your diet, because at least a trace of fat is found in almost all foods.

The Functions of Fat

Fat is the body's chief storage form for the energy from food eaten in excess of immediate need. Fats provide most of the energy needed to perform much of the body's work, and especially muscular work.

Fat serves as an energy reserve. Whenever you eat, you store some fat, and within a few hours after a meal, you take the fat out of storage and use it for energy until the next meal. Thus, both glucose and fat are stored after meals, and both are released later when needed as fuel for the cells' work. However, whereas excess carbohydrate and protein can be converted to fat, they cannot be recovered from it; fat can serve only as an energy fuel for cells equipped to use it.

The body has scanty reserves of carbohydrate and virtually no protein to spare, but it can store fat in practically unlimited amounts. A pound of body fat is worth 3,500 calories, and a person's body can easily carry 30 to 50 pounds of fat without looking fat at all. In fact, a man of normal weight might have about 15 percent of the body weight as fat and a woman, about 20 percent.

Fat is a nutrient found in many foods. As the most concentrated source of food energy, fat contains more than twice as many calories, ounce for ounce, as protein or carbohydrate. High-fat foods may therefore deliver many *unneeded* calories in only a few bites to the person who is not expending much energy in physical work. A pound of pure fat contains more than 4,000 calories, while a pound of pure carbohydrate or protein contains about 1,800 calories. It is easy, therefore, to overconsume fat calories long before you feel full. This is the reason you feel hungry again not long after a Chinese meal, which is usually low in fat and high in complex carbohydrate. The complex carbohydrate gives you a feeling of fullness before you have eaten as many calories, because it has more bulk, but the feeling does not last as long as the satiety from a meal rich in fat. Fat provides satiety by slowing the stomach's motility.

Both fats and oils are found in your body, and both help to keep your body healthy. Fat is important to all your body's cells as part of their cell membranes. Natural oils in the skin provide a radiant complexion; in the scalp they help nourish the hair and make it glossy. Fat insulates the body and cushions its vital organs. It serves as a shock absorber. The fat blanket under the skin also provides insulation from extremes of temperature, thus achieving internal climate control.

Fat is important for another reason. Some essential nutrients are soluble in fat and therefore are found mainly in foods that contain it. These nutrients

Normal weight man: 5′ 10″ 160 pounds. 15% of 160 is 24 pounds of body fat.
Normal weight woman: 5′ 5″ 128 pounds. 20% of 128 is 26 pounds of body fat.

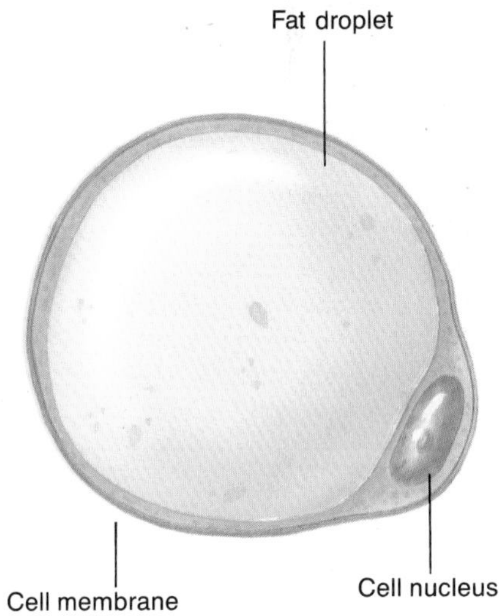

A Fat Cell. Within the fat cell, lipid is stored in a droplet. This droplet can greatly enlarge, and the fat cell membrane will grow to accommodate its swollen contents. More about fat cells and obesity in Chapter 8.

1 gram carbohydrate = 4 calories.
1 gram fat = 9 calories.
1 gram protein = 4 calories.
1 gram alcohol = 7 calories.

Triglycerides (try-GLISS-er-ides) the major class of dietary lipids. A triglyceride is made up of three units known as fatty acids and one unit called glycerol.
Phospholipids (FOSS-foh-LIP-ids) one of the three main classes of lipids; a lipid similar to a triglyceride but containing phosphorus.
Lecithin (LESS-ih-thin) a phospholipid, a major constituent of cell membranes, manufactured by the liver and also found in many foods.
Sterols (STEER-alls) one of the three main classes of lipids; a lipid with a structure similar to that of cholesterol.
Cholesterol (koh-LESS-ter-all) one of the sterols, manufactured in the body for a variety of purposes and also found in animal-derived foods.
Blood lipid profile a test performed by a medical laboratory to determine the amounts and kinds of lipids in the blood, normally as part of a diagnosis for cardiovascular disease risk.
Cardiovascular disease (CVD) disease of the heart and blood vessels—atherosclerosis (see this chapter's Spotlight feature).

are the essential fatty acids (to be described shortly) and the fat-soluble vitamins—A, D, E, and K (Chapter 6 describes these vitamins). Fat also carries many dissolved compounds that give foods their aroma and flavor. This accounts for the aromatic smells associated with foods that are being fried, such as onions or French fries. It also helps explain why a doughnut is more flavorful than a plain roll—it is higher in fat.

The Terminology of Fat

About 95 percent of the lipids in foods and in the human body are **triglycerides.** Other members of the lipid family are the **phospholipids** (of which **lecithin** is one) and the **sterols** (**cholesterol** is the best known of these). The **blood lipid profile** refers to a test conducted by a medical laboratory that reveals the amounts of various lipids (especially triglycerides and cholesterol) found in the blood and the carriers (such as LDL and HDL, described later) in which they are found. The results of this test tell much about a person's risk of heart and artery disease, or **cardiovascular disease (CVD).** The blood cholesterol level is especially telling, and it bears on the question of whether people should avoid foods containing fat, those containing cholesterol, or both.*

Two kinds of lipids in foods are:

- triglycerides (commonly called fat)
- cholesterol

Similarly, two kinds of lipids in the blood are:

- triglycerides
- cholesterol

A person's *blood* level of cholesterol is considered to be a predictor of that person's likelihood of suffering a heart attack or stroke. The fat in *food* that contributes most to a high blood cholesterol level is triglycerides (fat), *not cholesterol.* People often fail to understand this point, and the question arises again and again: "Should I eat cholesterol?" When told "It doesn't matter much," the questioner often jumps to the wrong conclusion—the conclusion that cholesterol doesn't matter. It does matter. High *blood* cholesterol is an indicator of risk for CVD, but the main *food* factor associated with it is a high *fat intake.*† One more distinction must be made clear about fats on the plate: they come in two varieties—saturated and unsaturated. The saturated type is strongly implicated in raising blood cholesterol. The differences between saturated and unsaturated fats are described later.

**Blood, plasma,* and *serum* cholesterol all refer to about the same thing; this book uses the term *blood* cholesterol. Plasma is simply blood with the cells removed; serum has the clotting factors also removed. The concentration of cholesterol is not much altered by these treatments.

†A few individuals have a hereditary inability to clear from their blood the cholesterol they have eaten and absorbed. This condition is rare, but well-known, because the study of it led to the discovery of how cholesterol is transported in the body. People with hereditary high blood cholesterol levels must refrain from eating cholesterol in foods; perhaps this is where the general public's fear of dietary cholesterol has come from. The vast majority of people can eat eggs and other cholesterol-containing foods without fear of incurring high blood cholesterol levels.

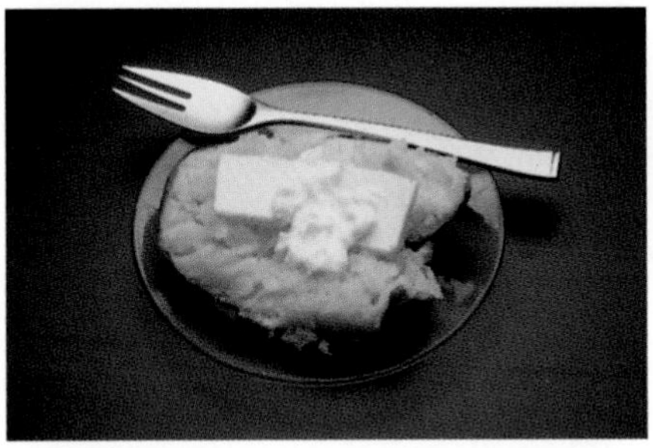

Large potato with 1 tablespoon butter and 1 tablespoon sour cream (14 grams fat, 350 calories).

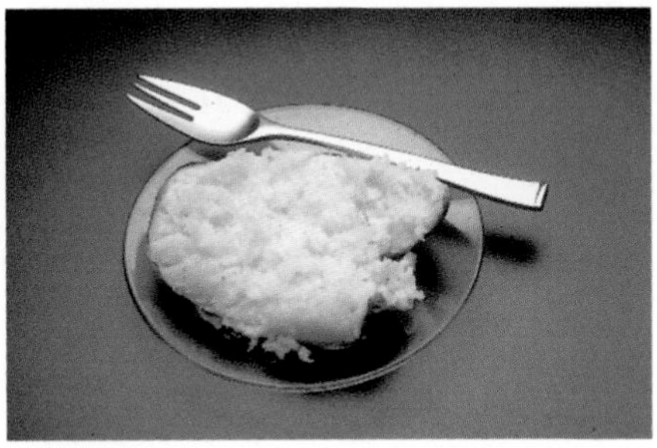

Plain large potato (less than 1 gram fat, 220 calories).

"Fat on the plate" includes visible fats and oils, such as butter, the oil in salad dressing, and the fat you trim from a steak. It also refers to some you cannot see, such as the fat that marbles a steak or that is hidden in foods like nuts, cheese, biscuits, crackers, doughnuts, cookies, muffins, avocados, olives, fried foods, and chocolate. The single most effective step you can take to reduce the energy value of a food is to eat the food without fat. This step is also an effective dietary weapon against high blood cholesterol levels.

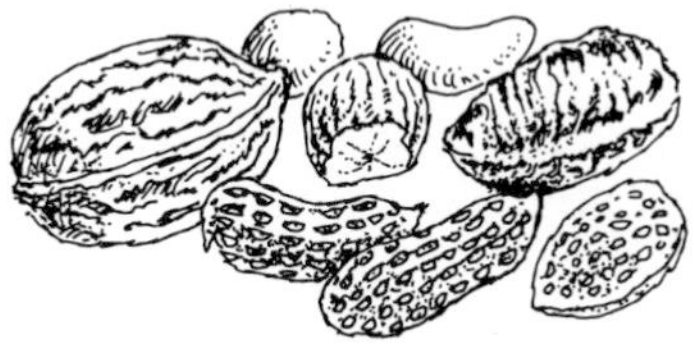

Nuts are rich in many nutrients, but are also high in fat. Two whole walnuts or ten large peanuts contain the same amount of fat as is found in a teaspoon of butter or margarine (5 grams of fat and 45 calories).

A Closer View of Fats

Most of the lipid in our diet comes from animal flesh or animal products. Animal fat, in turn, may have come from the fats and oils in plants; from the carbohydrate in plants, as you learned in the last chapter; or from protein, which will be discussed in Chapter 5. When the energy of carbohydrate or protein is to be stored in fat, it is first broken into fragments—small molecules made of carbon, hydrogen, and oxygen. These fragments are then linked together into chains known as **fatty acids.** Fatty acids are the major building blocks of triglycerides, the chief form of fat.

Fatty acids basic units of fat, composed of chains of carbon atoms with oxygen atoms at one end and hydrogen atoms attached all along their length.

Saturated fatty acid a fatty acid carrying the maximum possible number of hydrogen atoms (having no points of unsaturation). A saturated fat is one that is made up primarily of saturated fatty acids.

Fatty Acids and Triglycerides

Fatty acids may differ from one another in two ways: in chain length and in degree of saturation. Chain length refers to the number of carbons that are hooked together in the fatty acid (see Figure 4–1).* Chain length is significant because it affects solubility of the fat in water—the short-chain fatty acids are somewhat soluble in water. Milk, butter, and cheese are rich in the short-chain fatty acids; vegetable oils and red meat contain triglycerides with long-chain fatty acids.

Of more significance than chain length is the term *saturation,* mentioned earlier in relation to heart disease. Saturation refers to the chemical structure—specifically, to the number of hydrogens the fatty acid chain is holding. If every available bond from the carbons is holding a hydrogen, we say the chain is a **saturated fatty acid**—filled to capacity, or saturated, with hydrogen (see Figure 4–1).

Foods high in saturated fats:

butter
cheese
chocolate
coconut
coconut oil
cream
meat
milk
palm oil

*Short-chain fatty acids contain 4 to 6 carbons; medium-chain fatty acids contain 8 to 10 carbons; long-chain fatty acids contain 12 or more carbons.

Figure 4–1

The Fatty Acids

The types of fatty acids:

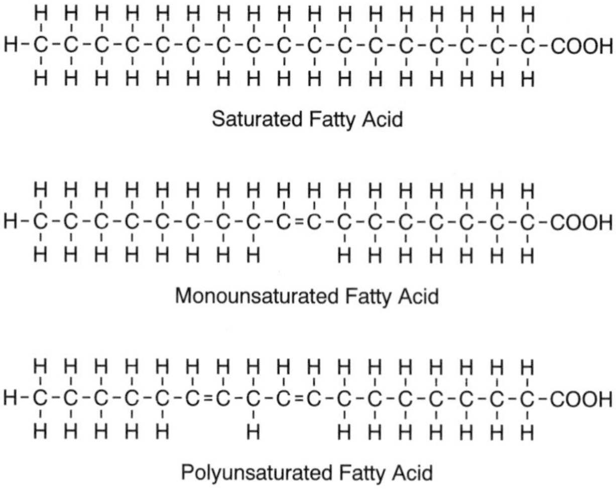

C is a carbon atom.
H is a hydrogen atom.
- is a single bond.
= is a double bond.

Sometimes, especially in the fatty acids in plants and fish, there is a place in the chain where hydrogens are missing—an "empty spot," or **point of unsaturation** (see Figure 4–1). A chain that possesses a point of unsaturation is an **unsaturated fatty acid.** If there is one point of unsaturation, it is a **monounsaturated fatty acid.** If there are two or more points of unsaturation, it is a **polyunsaturated fatty acid.** The higher the percentage of unsaturation a fat or oil has, and the lower the percentage of saturation, the more healthful it is (see the Spotlight feature at the end of this chapter).

Point of unsaturation a site in a molecule where the bonding is such that additional hydrogen atoms can easily be added.
Unsaturated fatty acid a fatty acid in which one or more points of unsaturation occur. An unsaturated fat is a triglyceride in which one or more of the fatty acids is unsaturated.
Monounsaturated fatty acid (sometimes abbreviated MUFA) a fatty acid containing one point of unsaturation.
Polyunsaturated fatty acid (sometimes abbreviated PUFA) a fatty acid in which two or more points of unsaturation occur.

Foods high in monounsaturated fats:

avocados	peanut butter
canola oil	peanut oil
cashews	peanuts
lard	poultry
olive oil	vegetable shortening
olives	

The Essential Fatty Acids

The human body can synthesize all the fatty acids it needs from carbohydrate, fat, or protein, except two—**linoleic acid** and **linolenic acid.** These two cannot be made from other substances in the body or from each other, and they must be supplied by the diet; they are, therefore, **essential fatty acids.** These fatty acids are polyunsaturated fatty acids, widely distributed in the diet, especially in plant and fish oils. To be sure, they are readily stored in the adult body, making deficiencies unlikely. Still, deficiency symptoms can appear in the person deprived of these acids—a characteristic skin rash and, in children, poor growth.

One further classification system for unsaturated fatty acids classifies the fatty acids as either an **omega-6** or an **omega-3** fatty acid. Of the two essential fatty acids, linoleic acid is an omega-6 fatty acid, related to a whole series of others. Linolenic acid is an omega-3 fatty acid, with a similar family of its own.

Of interest in relation to dietary fat are findings on the omega-3 fatty acids found in fish oils, which offer a protective effect beyond merely substituting for saturated fat. Interest in fish oils was first kindled when someone thought to ask why the Eskimos of Greenland, who eat a diet very high in fat, have such a low rate of heart disease.[1] The trail led to the abundance of fish they eat, then to the oils in those fish, and finally to the omega-3 fatty acids in the oils. Now scientists are unraveling the mystery of what those fatty acids do.

The omega-3 fatty acids—primarily found in seafood—have a profound effect on the synthesis of certain hormonelike compounds that play many regulatory roles in the body.[2] They affect a number of body functions, including the formation of blood clots, the raising and lowering of blood pressure and blood lipid levels, the immune response, and the inflammatory response to injury and infection.* The types of these compounds made in the body determine the degree of vulnerability to cardiovascular disease, cancer, and other diseases. For example, one study from the Netherlands reported that one or two fish meals a week in place of meat are all it takes to exert a significant positive effect.[3] The fatty acids in the fish alter the body's blood-clotting balance favorably and provide protection against heart disease, possibly by reducing the synthesis of compounds that raise blood pressure and promote the formation of cholesterol buildup in the arteries.[4] Researchers are currently exploring the possibility that adequate amounts in the diet protect against hypertension.[5]

People who eat large amounts of fish tend to have lower blood cholesterol and triglyceride levels and slower clot-forming rates.[6] More than 70 studies have now documented other connections, too. Diets high in omega-3 fatty acids seem to bring about enhanced defenses against cancer (via the immune response) and reduced inflammation in arthritis and asthma sufferers. The Eskimos apparently did well using fish for food. Perhaps we, too, could benefit from eating fish in abundance.

If our diets need modification, it is not by taking supplements of fish oils. Many hazards may be associated with the taking of such supplements. One reason is that they could unbalance the diet too far; you do need omega-6, too, remember. Too much fish oil might make a person susceptible to stroke or hemorrhage due to its effect of prolonging bleeding and clotting time. Fish oils—made from fish livers—accumulate toxins, not only the fat-soluble vitamins A and D but also pesticides and other contaminants. Excesses of unsaturated oils can precipitate vitamin E deficiency. These and other risks do not accompany the eating of a variety of fish. Furthermore, fish contain other beneficial nutrients. The purified oils contain just oil, and oil is high in calories. If you tried to take enough fish oil to match the Eskimos' intake, you would need 300 to 500 calories a day—enough to gain about 25 pounds a year. Instead, substitute two or three fish meals a week for meals based on other protein-rich foods and you will improve your health more safely.

Characteristics of Fats in Foods

The presence of unsaturated fatty acids in a fat affects the temperature at which the fat melts. The more unsaturated a fat, the more liquid it is at room temperature. In contrast, the more saturated a fat (the more hydrogens it

*The hormonelike compounds referred to here are the **eicosanoids** (eye-COSS-uh-noyds)—compounds that regulate blood pressure, clotting, and other body functions. Names of classes of eicosanoids are prostaglandins, thromboxanes, prostacyclins, and leukotrienes.

Foods high in polyunsaturated fats:

almonds	mayonnaise
corn oil	pecans
cottonseed oil	safflower oil
filberts	soybean oil
fish	sunflower oil
margarine (soft)	walnuts

Linoleic (lin-oh-LAY-ic) **acid, linolenic** (lin-oh-LEN-ic) **acid** polyunsaturated fatty acids, essential for human beings.
Essential fatty acid a fatty acid that cannot be synthesized in the body in amounts sufficient to meet physiological need.
Omega the last letter of the Greek alphabet (ω), used by chemists to refer to the position of the end-most double bond in a fatty acid. The **omega-6** fatty acids have their end-most double bonds after the sixth carbon in the chain; the **omega-3** acids, after the third.

Seafood especially high in omega-3 fatty acids:
Anchovies, herring, mackerel, sablefish, salmon, sardines, sturgeon, tuna (white albacore—canned in water—or bluefin), and whitefish.
Seafood moderately high in omega-3 fatty acids:
Bass, bluefish, catfish, cod, crab, flounder, haddock, hake, halibut, lobster, mullet, ocean perch, oysters, pike, pollack, shrimp, rainbow trout, rockfish, scallops, sea trout, smelt, and swordfish.
Other good sources of omega-3 fatty acids (linolenic acid) besides fish and seafood include: leafy vegetables, canola oil, soybean oil, and walnuts. (Most whole foods add some omega-3 fatty acids to the diet.)

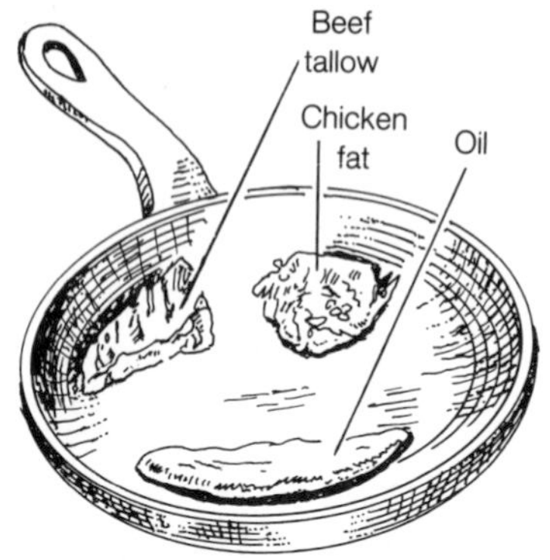

The more unsaturated a fat, the more liquid it is at room temperature. The more polyunsaturated the fat is, the sooner it melts.

has), the firmer it is. Thus, of three fats—beef fat, chicken fat, and corn oil—beef fat is the most saturated and the hardest; chicken fat is less saturated and somewhat soft; and corn oil, which is the most unsaturated, is a liquid at room temperature (and the only one of the three that comes from a plant). If your health care provider tells you to use **monounsaturated fats** or **polyunsaturated fats**, you can usually judge which ones to choose by their hardness at room temperature. Figure 4–2 compares the most common fats and oils with regard to their percentages of the various types of fat.

Because fats differ chemically, they behave differently in foods. To control their characteristics, food manufacturers sometimes alter them—and sometimes the alterations have health consequences, as described next.

Points of unsaturation in fatty acids are like weak spots in that they are vulnerable to attack by oxygen. When the unsaturated points react with oxygen, the oils become rancid. This is why unprocessed oils should be stored in tightly covered containers. If stored for long periods, they need refrigeration to prevent spoilage.

One way to prevent spoilage of oils containing unsaturated fatty acids is to change them chemically by **hydrogenation**, but this causes them to lose their unsaturated character and the health benefits that go with it. When food producers want to use a polyunsaturated oil such as corn oil to make a spreadable margarine, they hydrogenate the oil. Hydrogen is forced into the oil, some of the unsaturated fatty acids accept the hydrogen, and the oil

Monounsaturated fat a triglyceride in which one or more of the fatty acids is monounsaturated.
Polyunsaturated fat a triglyceride in which one or more of the fatty acids is polyunsaturated.
Hydrogenation (high-droh-gen-AY-shun) the process of adding hydrogen to unsaturated fat to make it more solid and more resistant to chemical change.

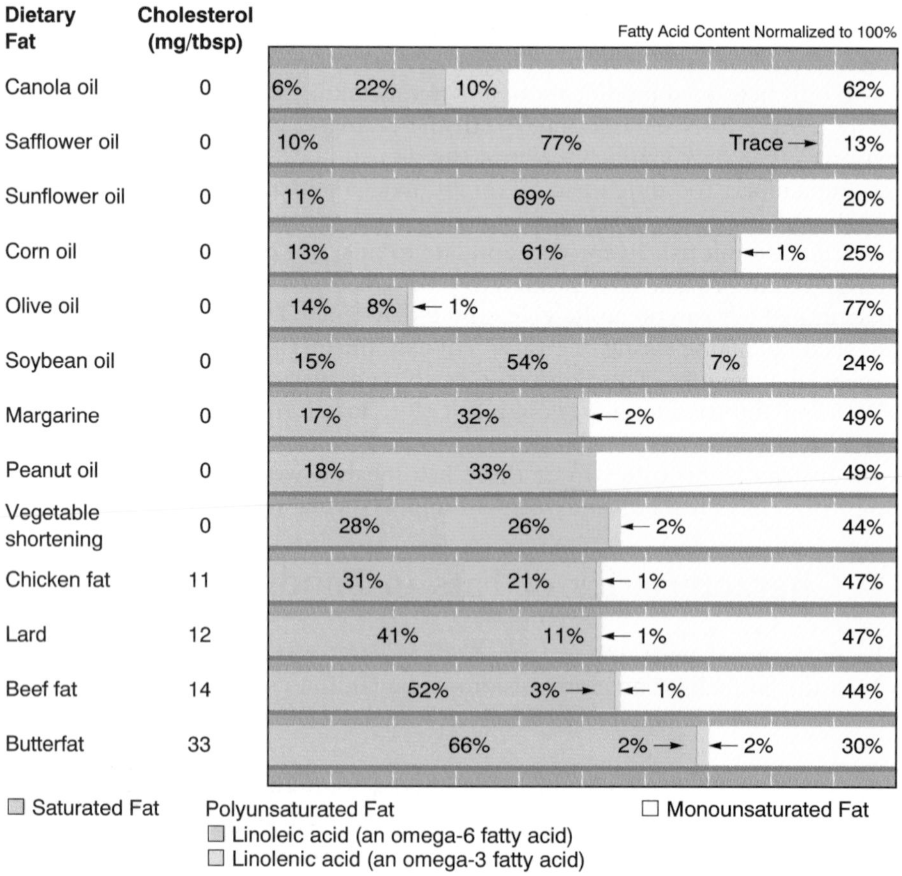

Dietary Fat
Cholesterol (mg/tbsp)
Fatty Acid Content Normalized to 100%
Canola oil 0 6% 22% 10% 62%
Safflower oil 0 10% 77% Trace 13%
Sunflower oil 0 11% 69% 20%
Corn oil 0 13% 61% 1% 25%
Olive oil 0 14% 8% 1% 77%
Soybean oil 0 15% 54% 7% 24%
Margarine 0 17% 32% 2% 49%
Peanut oil 0 18% 33% 49%
Vegetable shortening 0 28% 26% 2% 44%
Chicken fat 11 31% 21% 1% 47%
Lard 12 41% 11% 1% 47%
Beef fat 14 52% 3% 1% 44%
Butterfat 33 66% 2% 2% 30%
Saturated Fat
Polyunsaturated Fat
Linoleic acid (an omega-6 fatty acid)
Linolenic acid (an omega-3 fatty acid)
Monounsaturated Fat

Figure 4–2

Comparison of Dietary Fats

Source: Canola oil, vegetable shortening data on file. Procter & Gamble. All others: J. B. Reeves and J. L. Weihrauch, *Composition of Foods.* Agriculture Handbook No. 8–4 (Washington, D.C.: U.S. Department of Agriculture, 1979). Reprinted with permission from Procter & Gamble.

becomes harder. The spreadable margarine that results is more saturated than the original oil, but not as saturated as butter.

A chemical accident occurs when polyunsaturated oils are hydrogenated. They change in form, creating fatty acids that are not made by the body's cells and that occur only rarely in foods. These unfamiliar fatty acids, or ***trans*-fatty acids**, can be taken up into our cell membranes and may have the potential to alter cell functions. The issue is not clear, but some researchers believe that *trans*-fatty acids may make people prone to develop certain kinds of cancer. However, so many dietary factors are implicated in cancer causation that it is hard to sort them all out and decide which are significant. Undoubtedly, total fat consumption has much more bearing on susceptibility to cancer than does consumption of *trans*-fatty acids.

A second way to prevent spoilage of oils is to add a chemical that will compete for the oxygen and thus protect the oil. Such an additive is called an **antioxidant.** Examples are the well-known additives BHA and BHT, listed on some breakfast cereal and snack food labels, and the natural antioxidants vitamin C and vitamin E. A third alternative, already mentioned, is to keep the product refrigerated.

Another way that the food industry alters natural fats and oils is by adding an **emulsifier** to a food product to allow fats and water to mix and remain mixed in a food product. Mayonnaise, margarines, salad dressings, and cake mixes often list an emulsifier on their labels. Mono- and diglycerides are good emulsifiers, as is the emulsifier found in egg yolk—lecithin.

The question of what kind of fat to use can be puzzling. Research has linked the fat in the diet to several diseases, including breast and colon cancer, heart disease, arthritis, and gallbladder disease. For both cancer and heart disease, the most important strategy is to lower the total fat content of the diet. For heart disease, it is recommended that you replace whatever saturated fats you use, at least partially, with mono- and polyunsaturated fats. That means replacing butter, cream, and beef fat with mono- or polyunsaturated vegetable and fish oils and soft margarine made from corn, sunflower, safflower, or soybean oil with as little hydrogenated oil as possible. More information on fats in the diet is offered later in the chapter.

Trans-fatty acids fatty acids with unusual shapes that can arise when polyunsaturated oils are hydrogenated.

Antioxidant (anti-OX-ih-dant) a compound that protects other compounds from oxygen by itself reacting with oxygen.

Emulsifier a substance that mixes with both fat and water and can break fat globules into small droplets, thereby suspending fat in water.

How the Body Handles Fat

When you eat carbohydrate or protein, some of it can be made into fat in the body, as you have already seen for carbohydrate in Chapter 3. The carbohydrate is first digested to glucose. Some can be stored as glycogen, but some is broken down to fragments. Some of these fragments are used for energy; some are joined together to make fatty acids. The fatty acids are attached to **glycerol** to make triglycerides. Finally, these are transported to the fat depots—muscles, breasts, the insulating fat layer under the skin, the abdominal region, and others.

When you eat animal flesh (meat, fish, or poultry) or animal products (milk, cheese, or eggs), you are eating a combination of fat and protein. Of the fat, 95 percent is triglyceride that has been made in the animal body, mostly from carbohydrate, the same way you make it. Animal fat can end up in fat stores in you own body (as can excess glucose or protein), but first it has to

Glycerol (GLISS-er-all) an organic compound, three carbons long, of interest here because it serves as the backbone for triglycerides.

Let Them Eat Cake (Fat-free, That Is)

Fat-free ice cream, cookies, cakes, and salad dressings have long been the stuff that dieters' dreams are made of. Recently the food industry made such fatless fare a reality. In 1990 alone, manufacturers introduced more than 1,000 low-fat and fat-free items into supermarkets across the country.[7] Sales of nonfat products are expected to soar during the next decade, as more and more fat-conscious consumers discover that they can eat cake, ice cream, and cookies and take in less fat at the same time.

The boom in both low-fat and fat-free products has to do with the country's expanding health consciousness. While most Americans have heard the warnings that fat can contribute to heart disease, cancer, and obesity, many people find low-fat diets particularly unpalatable. Fat adds a desirable flavor and texture, known as "mouth feel," to foods. With innovations in food chemistry, however, the food industry can concoct new recipes or ingredients that yield low-fat or nonfat products that retain the characteristic flavor and mouth feel of fat. Entenmann's, manufacturer of a line of fat-free cakes and cookies, for example, makes such products by substituting egg whites for whole eggs and nonfat milk for whole milk as well as removing the butter from its recipes. The end product: sweets that contain fewer calories and four to five fewer grams of fat per serving than the company's traditional desserts.[8] (See Table 4–1 for a comparison of regular and low-fat and nonfat foods.)

Carrageenan a seaweed derivative used by food manufacturers to add "body" to numerous products including ice cream, frozen yogurt, and salad dressings.

Simplesse® the trade name for a protein-based, low-calorie artificial fat, approved by the FDA for use in foods such as frozen desserts; cannot be used for frying or baking.

Similarly, McDonald's cooks reduced-fat burger patties by adding an ingredient called **carrageenan** to beef. Derived from seaweed, carrageenan helps retain moisture, which in turn makes up for the loss of juiciness that accompanies a reduction in fat. In addition, McDonald's adds extra seasonings to its patties to compensate for any lost flavor brought about by removing fat. Dubbed McLean Deluxe, the low-fat, quarter-pound burger contains 11 fewer grams of fat and 90 fewer calories than the company's Quarter Pounder.[9]

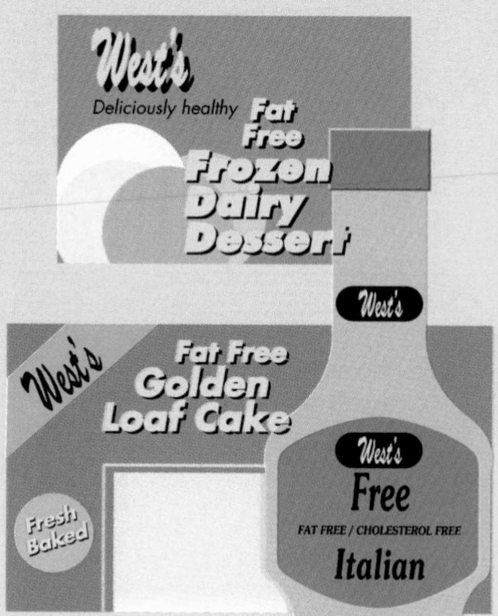

Another technique manufacturers use to replace fat is to add starches, gums, and gels to their products. For example, Kraft uses cellulose gel, a complex carbohydrate, as a filler to make fat-free salad dressings and Sealtest nonfat dairy dessert.[10] Other companies add starches and gums—also complex carbohydrates—to items such as sauces and yogurts to skim fat from those foods. That's because starches and gums hold water and impart a smooth, creamy texture similar to that of fat as well as add form and structure to foods. These substitutes cannot, however, replace the fat used for cooking and frying.[11]

Yet another more innovative approach the food industry has taken to provide fat-free fare is the development of fat substitutes. In 1990, a substance called **Simplesse®** became the first such product to gain the approval of the Food and Drug Administration.

● *Table 4–1*

Fat-Free Fare: Before and After

	GRAMS OF FAT	CALORIES
Entenmann's All Butter Pound Loaf (1-oz slice)	5	110
Entenmann's Golden Loaf Cake (fat-free)	0[a]	70
Ice Cream Sandwich	6	180
Fat Freedom Eskimo Pie Sandwich	0	130
Kraft Zesty Italian Dressing (1 tablespoon)	5	50
Kraft Free Italian Dressing	0	6
McDonald's Quarter Pounder	21	410
McDonald's McLean Deluxe Sandwich	10	320
Sealtest Vanilla Ice Cream (½ cup)	7	140
Sealtest Free Vanilla Nonfat Frozen Dessert	0	100
Cookies 'n' Cream Ice Cream (½ cup)	17	270
Simple Pleasures Cookies 'n' Cream Light Frozen Dairy Dessert	2	150

[a]The Food and Drug Administration allows food companies to round down to the nearest gram of fat per serving. Thus, a product's label can say "0" grams of fat as long as the item contains no more than 0.49 gram of fat per serving.

Source: Manufacturers' information and *Bowes and Church's Food Values of Portions Commonly Used,* 15th ed., (N.Y.: Harper & Row), 1989.

Six years in the making, Simplesse® is a mixture of food proteins such as egg white, whey, and milk protein that are cooked and blended to form tiny round particles that trap water. Inside the mouth the particles roll over one another, and the tongue perceives them as a creamy, smooth liquid similar to fat.

The FDA allows use of Simplesse® in foods including cheese, baked goods, frozen desserts, salad dressings, and sour cream. Foods made with the fat substitute contain considerably less fat and fewer calories than their traditional fat-containing counterparts. The reason is that while fat contains 9 calories per gram, Simplesse® supplies only 1 to 2. Although Simplesse® cannot be used for frying or baking, since heat causes it to gel and lose its creaminess, if approved by the FDA it can be used in other dairy products as well as such foods as salad dressings, margarines, and mayonnaise.[12] Figure 4–3 illustrates the role of Simplesse® in the reduction of fat and calories in the diet.

Another artificial fat on the horizon (pending FDA approval) is a type of **sucrose polyester** called Olestra. The Olestra molecule resembles a triglyceride but is structured in a way that prevents its breakdown by digestive enzymes in the body, thereby allowing it to pass through the digestive tract completely unabsorbed. If approved for use, Olestra can be used anywhere regular fats and oils are used, such as in deep-fat frying for French fries and the like. Some scientists have raised concern that it may interfere with the absorption of fat-soluble vitamins such as vitamin E, however. To get around the problem, Procter & Gamble, Olestra's manufacturer, plans to fortify it with vitamin E if and when it is allowed on the market.[13]

Sucrose polyester (SPE) an artificial fat derived from edible oils such as soybean, corn, and cottonseed as well as sucrose. It can be substituted for oil, butter, margarine, and the like in meals and is indigestible, so it does not contribute calories to food or raise blood cholesterol.

Certainly, the growing number of fat-free foods and fat substitutes provides consumers with viable alternatives to fattier fare. Nevertheless, many experts view the fat-free boom with skepticism. While reduced-fat foods can help lower the overall fat content of the diet, they are not a replacement for

Figure 4–3

The Role of Simplesse® in Fat and Calorie Reduction

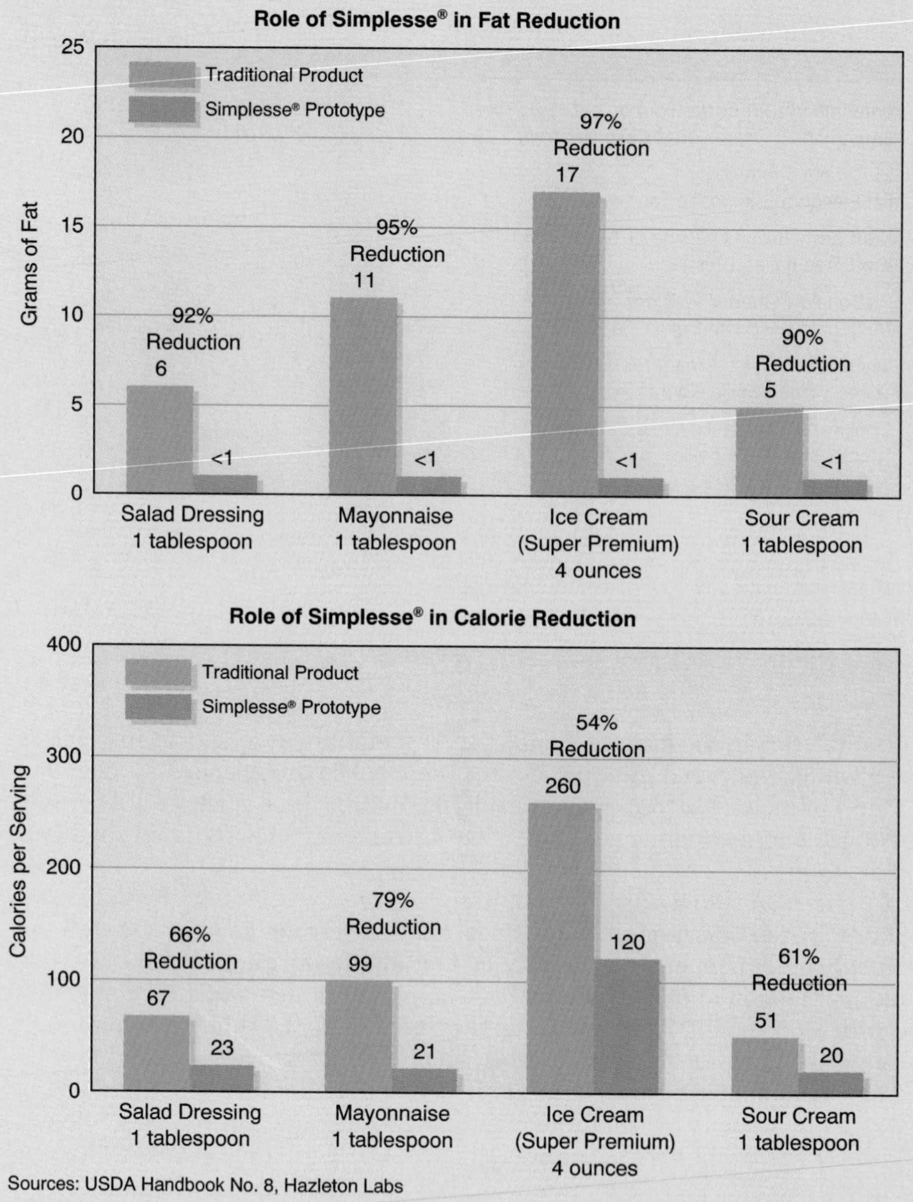

Sources: USDA Handbook No. 8, Hazleton Labs

a healthful diet rich in whole grains and fresh fruits and vegetables. Nor are they likely to become the panacea that will prevent problems such as heart disease and obesity. Fit into a low-fat diet, however, they can help consumers reach and adhere to the goal of taking in no more than 30 percent of total calories as fat. (For ideas on how to choose a low-fat diet, see Table 4–6 and Table 4–9 later in this chapter.)

be digested, absorbed, and transported to its cell destinations. Figure 4–4 shows how the body makes fat ready for absorption.

After digestion in the upper small intestine, the products of fat digestion—fatty acids, glycerol, and monoglycerides—must enter the bloodstream if they are to be of use to the body's cells. If not absorbed, they will be excreted. The shortest free fatty acids pass by simple diffusion into the cells that line the intestine. Because these short-chain fatty acids are somewhat water soluble, they can, without any further processing, enter the body's capillaries. Like the products of carbohydrate digestion, the short-chain fatty acids are transported from these capillaries through collecting veins to the capillaries of the liver. The liver cells pick them up and convert them to other substances the body needs. The glycerol follows the same path as the short-chain fatty acids because it, too, is water soluble.

The larger products of fat digestion (long-chain fatty acids, cholesterol, phospholipids) are insoluble in water, a difficulty that must be overcome. The body's fluids—lymph and blood—are watery and will not accept these larger molecules as they are. The longer-chain fatty acids do pass into the intestinal cells, but there they reconnect with glycerol or with monoglycerides, forming *new* triglycerides. Then the cells package them for transport before releasing them into the lymph system. The cells allow triglycerides and other lipids to form and combine with special proteins to make **chylomicrons**, one of the four types of **lipoproteins** found in the blood. Within the body, the larger fats always travel in lipoproteins. In this ingenious configuration, the water-soluble proteins enable the fats to travel in the watery body fluids. That way, when the tissues of the body need energy from fat, they can extract what they need from lipoproteins. The remnants that remain are picked up by the liver, which dismantles them and reuses their parts.

Bile a mixture of compounds including cholesterol made by the liver, stored in the gallbladder, and secreted into the small intestine. Bile emulsifies lipids to ready them for enzymatic digestion and helps transport them into the intestinal wall cells. Bile works like a detergent (detergents, too, are emulsifiers; they remove grease spots from clothing—molecule by molecule, they dissolve the grease out of the cloth and hold it suspended in the wash water to be rinsed away).

Monoglyceride (mon-oh-GLISS-er-ide) one of the products of digestion of lipids; a glycerol molecule with one fatty acid attached to it.

Figure 4–4 Digestion of Fats

A. In the stomach, fats float to the top of the watery stomach fluid; fat slows digestion, lending satiety to the meal. Little digestion of fats takes place in the stomach.

B. Once in the small intestine, fat encounters **bile,** an emulsifier made in the liver. The gallbladder, a storage organ, squirts bile into the contents of the small intestine to blend the fat with the watery digestive secretions.

C. Enzymes from the pancreas enter the small intestine. The enzymes can attack fat only after emulsification by bile. They break down the triglycerides to fatty acids, glycerol, and **monoglycerides.**

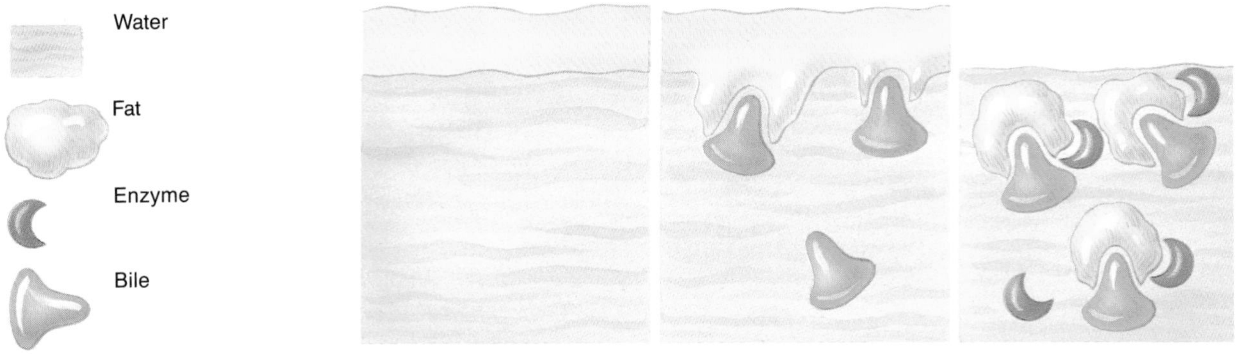

Lipoproteins (LIP-oh-PRO-teens) clusters of lipids associated with protein that serve as transport vehicles for lipids in blood and lymph. The four main types of lipoproteins are **chylomicrons, VLDL, LDL,** and **HDL.**

Lipoproteins are very much in the news these days. In fact, the health-care provider who measures your blood lipid profile is interested not only in the types of fats in your blood (triglycerides and cholesterol) but also in the lipoproteins that carry them. One distinction among types of lipoproteins is of great importance because it has implications for the health of the heart and blood vessels—the distinction between **low-density lipoproteins (LDL)** and **high-density lipoproteins (HDL)**. The more protein in the lipoprotein molecule, the higher the density; a large percentage of lipids characterizes the lower-density molecules. Both LDL and HDL carry similar lipids around in the blood, but there is a functional difference between them. Raised LDL concentrations in the blood are a sign of high heart attack risk because LDL in the blood tend to deposit cholesterol in the arteries. Raised HDL concentrations are associated with a low risk of heart attack because HDL tend to carry cholesterol out of the arteries. (A later section of this chapter clarifies this relationship.) The characteristics of the four types of lipoproteins circulating in the blood are shown in Figure 4–5.

This description of the intestine's processing of fat has omitted the few other dietary fats, such as phospholipids and cholesterol (discussed below), that may have entered the body in food. These fats enter the circulation the same way the triglycerides do and travel packaged in chylomicrons. After transport, they end up in the liver as part of the chylomicron remnants.

Figure 4–5

Characteristics and Functions of Lipoproteins

Chylomicron (KIGH-loh-MY-cron) a type of lipoprotein (very low in density) made by the cells of the intestinal wall; serve as a means of transporting newly digested fat from the intestine through lymph and blood. Chylomicrons donate lipids to all body cells, and the remnants are ultimately cleared from the blood by liver cells.

VLDL (very-low-density lipoprotein)—carries fats made by the liver to various tissues in the body.

LDL (low-density lipoprotein)—carries cholesterol (much of it synthesized in the liver) to body cells. A high blood cholesterol level usually reflects high LDL.

HDL (high-density lipoprotein)—carries cholesterol in the blood back to the liver for recycling or disposal.

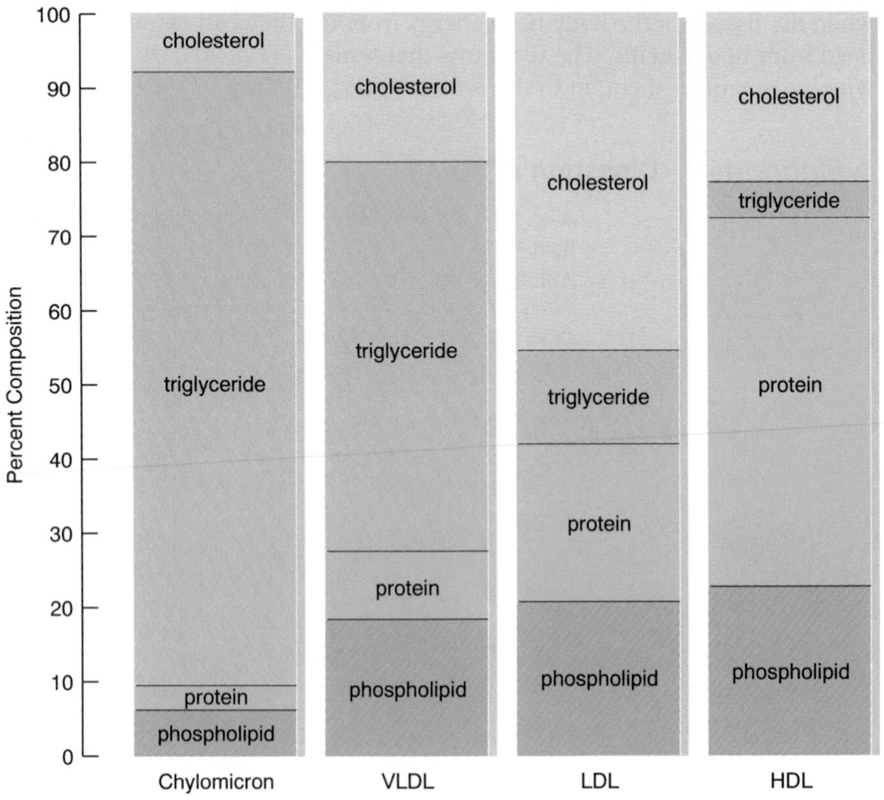

Lecithin

Lecithin and other phospholipids play key roles in the structure of cell membranes. Because of the way the phospholipids are constructed, they can join with both water and fat, so they can help fats back and forth across the lipid-containing membranes of cells into the watery fluids on both sides. Magical properties are sometimes attributed to lecithin, and health-food advertisers try to persuade people to supplement their diets with it. But lecithin is widespread in food and is also made by the body in abundant quantities and therefore is not an essential nutrient.

One of the claims made for lecithin is that it helps to lower blood cholesterol. Actually, among the factors that lower blood cholesterol, lecithin is probably not significant. If it has any effect, it is probably because it has polyunsaturated fatty acids as part of its structure; any other polyunsaturated fat would work equally well.

Another claim made for lecithin is that it helps improve people's memory. If only this were true, we could all benefit by eating lecithin; but if it is true at all, it seems to be so only for people with a specific kind of memory disorder. Even in those people, high doses are needed, suggesting that the effect is like that of a drug, not a nutrient. Lecithin probably works by contributing choline, which helps in several neurological disorders. Memory weakness in general, however, is not a sign of lecithin deficiency.[14]

The Fat in the News: Cholesterol

Cholesterol, as mentioned, is found in animal foods and is also made and destroyed in the body, where it is an important compound with many functions. It is a part of bile, which is necessary in the digestion of fats. It is the starting material from which the sex hormones and many other hormones are made. In the skin, one of its derivatives is made into vitamin D with the help of sunlight. It is an important lipid in the structure of brain and nerve cells. In fact, cholesterol is a part of every cell. But while it is widespread in the body and necessary to its function, it also is the major part of the plaques that narrow the arteries in the killer disease atherosclerosis.

"Good" Versus "Bad" Cholesterol

A silent, symptomless risk factor for heart and artery disease is much talked about but little understood—elevated blood cholesterol levels. Blood cholesterol may be high for a number of reasons. Some people inherit tendencies to make too much cholesterol or to fail to destroy it on schedule. Others have high blood cholesterol for lifestyle reasons: they eat too much fat or too much saturated fat, experience too much stress, exercise too little, carry too much weight, or all of these.[15] The blood lipid profile mentioned earlier can give you an idea of your standing as to this risk factor. Figure 4–6 shows how to interpret your blood cholesterol level.

Acceptable cholesterol levels go up as a person ages. Table 4–2 shows how an elevated blood cholesterol level combines with other risk factors of

● *Figure 4–6*

What Is Your Cholesterol Level and Risk for Heart Disease?

A diet high in fiber and complex carbohydrates and low in fats and cholesterol plus regular exercise can help you achieve heart-healthy cholesterol levels.

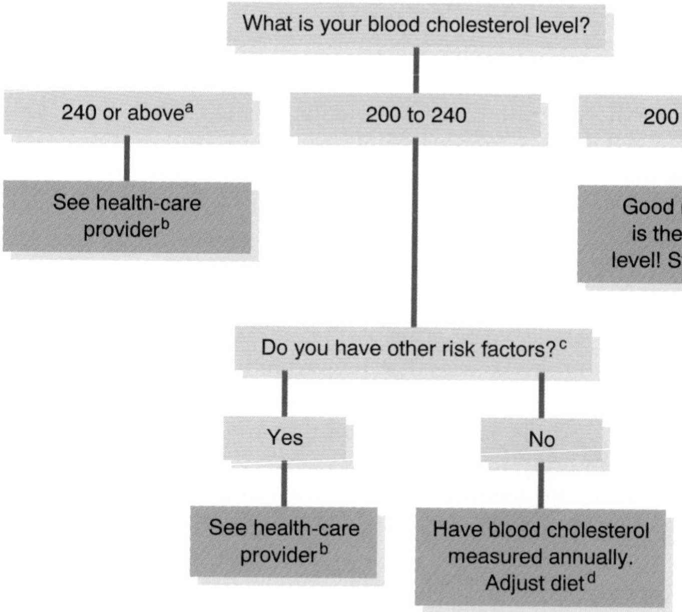

[a]Blood cholesterol is measured in milligrams per deciliter (mg/dL) of blood. 100 ml is sometimes called a dL. Values for blood cholesterol given in mg/100 ml are the same as those given in mg/dL.

[b]Ask to have your low-density-lipoprotein (LDL) level determined. If LDL is high, your health-care provider may suggest diet and/or drug therapy.

[c]Risk factors: being male, family history of premature death from heart disease, hypertension, smoking, diabetes, obesity, history of stroke, low HDL levels.

[d]Restrict total fat, saturated fat, and cholesterol in the diet.

[e]A reading of 200 mg/dL or below is recommended. Stay heart-healthy with a nutritious diet and exercise. Recheck cholesterol every five years or with physical exams.

heart disease to worsen atherosclerosis. As the table indicates, a person with a cholesterol reading of 300 could expect the onset of the critical phase of heart disease 20 years earlier than if it were 200.[16]

Some cases of elevated blood cholesterol do not respond to changes in lifestyle. In these cases, cholesterol-lowering drugs might be prescribed.

● *Table 4–2*

The Effect of Blood Cholesterol Level and Other Risk Factors on Age of Onset[a] of Heart Disease

BLOOD CHOLESTEROL	200 mg/ 100 ml[b]	250 mg/ 100 ml	300 mg/ 100 ml
Age of nonsmoker	70	60	50
Age of smoker	60	50	40
Age of smoker with hypertension	50	40	30

Note: The table shows that a nonsmoker with normal blood pressure and cholesterol of 200 would reach the critical phase at age 70. A smoker with high blood pressure and cholesterol of 300 would reach that phase at age 30.

[a]The age listed is the hypothetical age of onset of the critical phase of heart disease risk (60 percent coverage of artery surfaces by atherosclerosis).

[b]Milligrams cholesterol per 100 milliliters of blood.

Source: Data from S. M. Grundy, Cholesterol and coronary heart disease, *Journal of the American Medical Association* 256 (1986): 2849–2858.

However, for many, a few simple changes in diet can improve cholesterol readings, as discussed next.

Lowering Blood Cholesterol Levels

Among the most influential dietary factors that raise blood cholesterol level are total fat intake, high calories, and saturated fat intake.[17] As it turns out, the changes in diet that reduce blood cholesterol concentrations mostly do so by reducing LDL-cholesterol. Dietary modifications that lower LDL include substituting monounsaturated fats for saturated fats (use of canola, peanut, and olive oils), and substituting for saturated fats polyunsaturated fats, including vegetable oils and fish oils. As for dietary cholesterol, it raises LDL levels slightly for some people, depending on the amount being eaten and on the body's ability to compensate by making less.

The current recommendations for diet, based on these findings, include the following:

- Eat no more than 30 percent of calories as fat.
- Eat no more than 10 percent of calories as saturated fat.
- Eat no more than 10 percent of calories from polyunsaturated fats.
- Eat 10 to 15 percent of calories from monounsaturated fat.
- Limit cholesterol intake to no more than 300 milligrams daily.

The meals listed in the Fat Scorecard that appears later in the chapter meet these guidelines. See Table 4–3 for additional diet tips offered by the American Heart Association.

Most blood cholesterol is carried in LDL and correlates *directly* with heart disease risk, but some is carried in HDL and correlates *inversely* with risk. In fact, for men over 50, the most potent single predictor of heart attack risk may be the HDL level.[18] Raised HDL concentrations relative to LDL represent

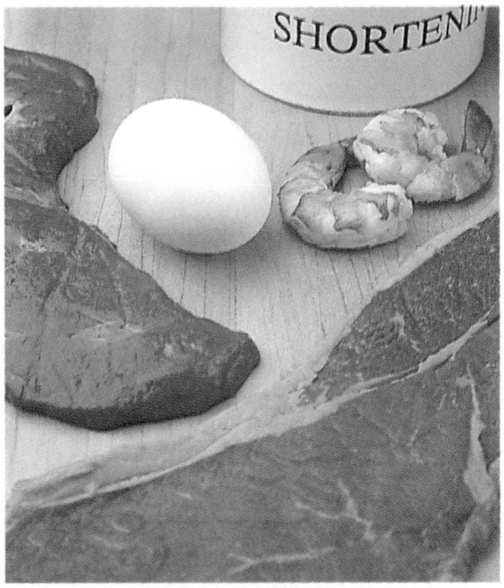

Saturated fats and cholesterol contribute to high blood cholesterol levels.

Table 4–3

The American Heart Association Diet

Control the amount and kind of fat you eat:

- Limit your intake of lean meat, seafood, and poultry to no more than 6 oz/day.
- Use chicken or turkey (without skin) or fish in most of your main meals.
- Choose lean cuts of meat, trim all the fat you can see, and throw away the fat that cooks out of the meat.
- Substitute meatless or low-meat main dishes for regular entrees. Use no more than a total of 5 to 8 tsp of fats and oils per day for cooking, baking, and salads.
- Use low-fat dairy products.

Control your intake of cholesterol-rich foods to take in no more than 300 mg/day:

- Use no more than three to four egg yolks a week, including those used in cooking.
- Limit your use of organ meats such as liver.

Also control:

- Alcohol: have no more than one to two drinks per day.
- Protein: consume no more than 15% of calories as protein.
- Sodium: use no more than 3 g/day.
- Calories: eat just enough to maintain recommended weight.

Source: Adapted from *The American Heart Association Diet, An Eating Plan for Healthy Americans,* a booklet (1991) available from the American Heart Association National Center, 7320 Greenville Ave., Dallas, TX 75231.

Figure 4–7

Fat in Foods

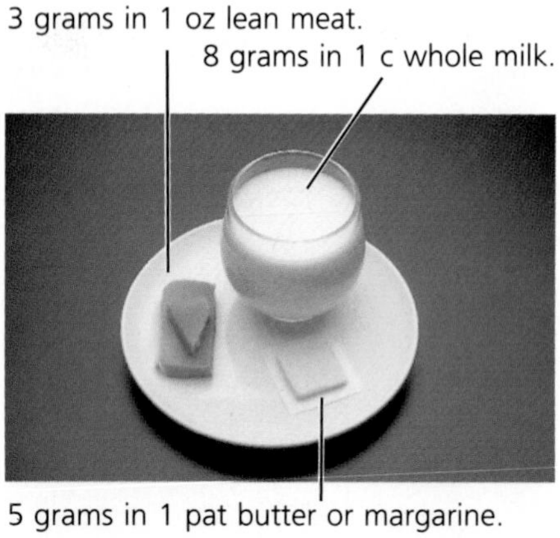
3 grams in 1 oz lean meat.
8 grams in 1 c whole milk.
5 grams in 1 pat butter or margarine.

ONE PORTION	FAT (g)
Milk (1 c)	
Nonfat	Trace
2%	5
Whole	8
Meat (1 oz)	
Lean	3
Medium fat	5
High fat	8
1 tbsp peanut butter	8
Fat (1 tsp)	
Butter, margarine, or oil	5
Vegetables	0
Fruits	0
Breads and starchy vegetables	0
Sugar	0

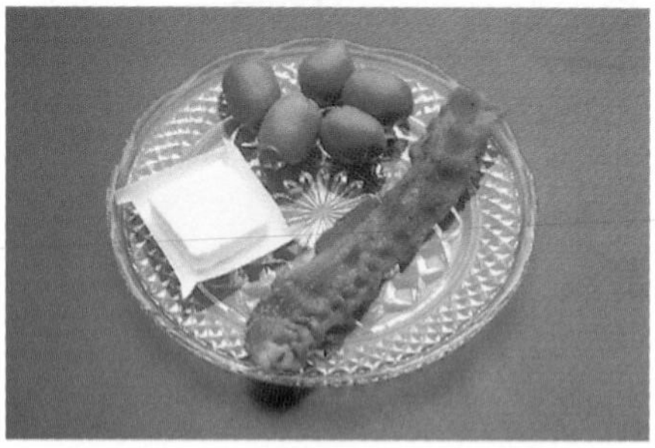

Fat exchanges. Each contributes 5 g fat.

cholesterol on its way out of the arteries back to the liver, and a reduced risk of heart attack. The Spotlight feature at the end of this chapter gives further tips on how to raise your HDL level and lower your LDL level.

Fat in the Diet

The remainder of this chapter will help you to apply what you have learned about fats—that is, how to choose foods that supply enough, but not too much, of the right kinds of fat to support optimal health and provide pleasure in eating.

To start, you must know where the fats are in the food groups. Three food groups—fats and oils; meat, poultry, and fish; and dairy products—have traditionally accounted for about nine-tenths of the fat in the U.S. diet. Recently, however, there has been a shift from animal fats to fats of vegetable origin. The rising consumption of vegetable fats and oils has come about because of three factors: (1) their increased use by some of the fast-food chains serving fried foods such as French fries and chicken, (2) a shift away from the use of lard, and (3) a shift from butter to margarine. A healthful trend is appearing: people are decreasing their total fat intakes and increasing the proportion of unsaturated to saturated fat in their diets.[19]

The listings in Figure 4–7 show exactly where the fats are in foods. Two groups always contain fat (the fats and the meats), and two sometimes contain fat (the milks and the breads). The unprocessed vegetables and fruits are, for the most part, fat-free.

The Fat Group

One fat portion contains about 5 grams of fat, donating 45 calories and negligible protein and carbohydrate. Examples are:

- A teaspoon of butter or margarine.
- One-eighth of an avocado or 5 small olives.
- Two large whole pecans or 1 tablespoon of salad dressing.
- Two tablespoons of sour cream or 1 tablespoon of heavy cream.
- A strip of crisp bacon.

Many people are surprised to find crisp bacon listed with the fat group. They expect to find bacon fat included but think of crisp bacon as meat. It is classified as a fat, however, because its protein content is negligible, even if it is fried crisp and the melted fat is drained away.

The Meat Group

Meats probably conceal most of the fat that people unwittingly consume. Many people, when choosing a serving of meat (or certain meat alternates), don't realize that they are electing to eat a large amount of fat. To help you see the fat in meats, meats are divided into three categories according to their fat content—lean, medium-fat, and high-fat meats (see Table 4–4). The three

Table 4–4

Some Examples of Lean, Medium-Fat, and High-Fat Meats and Meat Alternatives

LEAN MEAT	MEDIUM-FAT MEAT	HIGH-FAT MEAT
Beef tenderloin, round steak	Corned beef, chuck	Hamburger; club or rib steaks
Chicken or turkey without skin	Ground round steak	Fried chicken or fish patties as in fast food
Pork tenderloin	Pork roast, liver, heart, kidney	Breast of lamb
Leg of lamb	Eggs, creamed cottage cheese	Duck, goose
Fish		Cold cuts
Dry cottage cheese		Hot dogs
		Cheddar cheese

categories of meats contain about the same amount of protein per exchange, but the calorie amounts vary significantly among them depending on their fat content.

The meat portion listed in Figure 4–7 is only 1 ounce. This is a very small amount of meat and is not a serving size. A small fast-food hamburger, for example, weighs about 3 ounces, and 3 or 4 ounces of meat is thought of as a normal serving size for meal planning (see Figure 4–8).

People think of meat as protein food, but the calculation of its nutrient content shows a surprising fact. A quarter-pound (4-ounce) hamburger contains 28 grams of protein and 23 grams of fat. Because protein offers 4 calories per gram and fat offers 9, the hamburger provides 112 calories from protein and 207 calories from fat, with a total of more than 300 calories, 65 percent of them from fat. A hot dog is even higher in fat, which contributes 84 percent

Figure 4–8

Compare the Saturated Fat Content of Fish, Poultry, and Beef.[1]

	GRAMS PER 3 OZ SERVING[2]	
	Total fat	Saturated fat
Turkey breast, roasted (without skin)	1	<1
Halibut, baked	2.5	<1
Chicken breast, roasted (without skin)	4	1
T-bone steak, broiled	10	4

[1]To compare the saturated fat and total fat content of other foods, see Table 4–9, later in this chapter's Spotlight feature.
[2]How Much Is Three Ounces? A three-ounce portion of lean beef, chicken, or fish has roughly the dimensions of a deck of playing cards. Three ounces is also the approximate size of the palm of the average woman's hand.

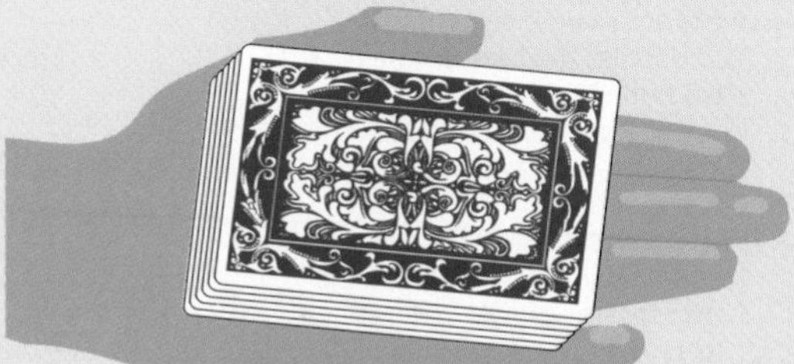

Fat Scorecard

How To Estimate Fat Intake

The values presented in Figure 4–7 provide a way to estimate the amount of fat eaten at a meal or in a day. Two reminders are needed. First, fat is often hidden in cooked vegetables; as a rule of thumb, vegetables served with butter or margarine can be assumed to contain 1 teaspoon of fat per half-cup serving. Second, meats and milks come in low-, medium-, and high-fat categories; be sure not to forget to count the fat in meats and milks.

Let us estimate the amounts of fat in the meals shown below. The cereal and fruit can be assumed to contain no fat, so the only foods to inspect are the meats, grains/starches, vegetables, and milks.

As you can see, the amounts of fat in meats (even low-fat meats, as in this example), and the fat the person adds at the meal (for example, the 2 teaspoons of butter used at dinner) make a considerable difference. These meals are very low in fat and fit the American Heart Association's recommended guidelines.

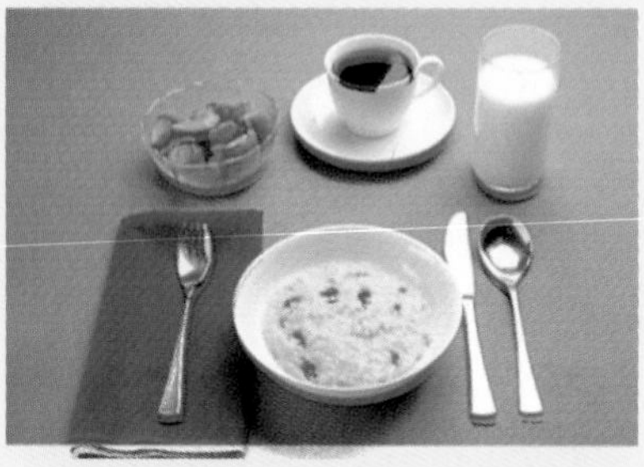

BREAKFAST	GRAMS OF FAT
1 c oatmeal = 2 starch/grains	Trace
¼ c raisins = 2 fruits	—
1 c nonfat milk = 1 milk	Trace
1¼ c strawberries = 1 fruit	—

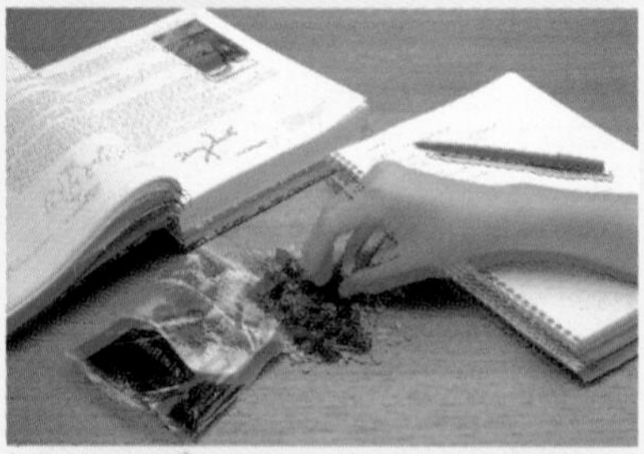

MORNING SNACK	
2 tbsp raisins = 1 fruit	—
2 tbsp sunflower seeds = 2 fats	10

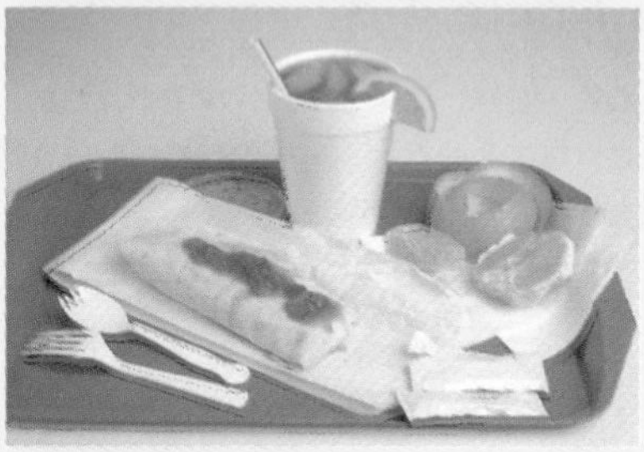

LUNCH	
1 beef and bean burrito	
(1 large tortilla = 2 starch/grains	Trace
⅓ c beans = 1 starch/grain +	Trace
½ high-fat meat)	4
1 orange = 1 fruit	—
1 packet sugar	—

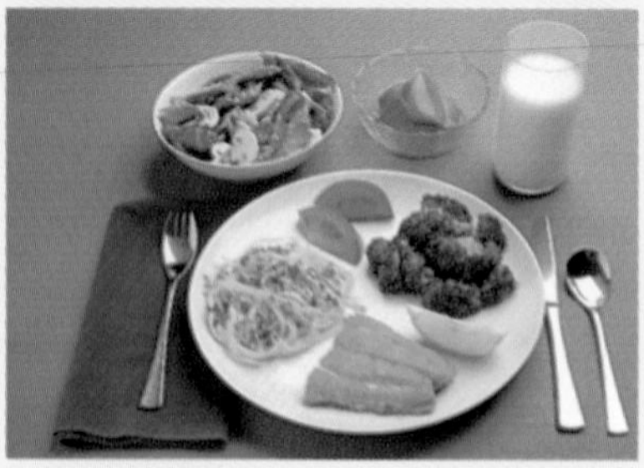

DINNER	
4 oz broiled salmon = 4 lean meats	12
1 c broccoli = 2 vegetables	—
½ c noodles = 1 starch/grain	Trace
2 tsp butter = 2 fats	10
¼ c parsley = ¼ vegetable	—
¼ tomato = ¼ vegetable	—
¼ c mushrooms = ¼ vegetable	—
¼ c water chestnuts = ¼ vegetable	—
1 c fresh spinach = 1 vegetable	—
1 tbsp sesame seeds = 1 fat	5
1 tbsp vinaigrette dressing = 1 fat	5
⅓ c garbanzo beans = 1 starch/grain	Trace
½ c sherbet = 2 starch/grains	Trace
1 c nonfat milk = 1 milk	Trace
Day's total	46 grams[a]

[a]Since there are 9 calories per gram of fat, you can calculate the number of calories derived from fat in this day's meals: 9 calories per gram × 46 grams = 414 calories. This is 24 percent of the total 1,750 calories and well below the recommended 30 percent of calories from fat.

of its calories. From this, you might predict that overeaters of meat would tend to be overweight. This is because so much of the energy in a meat eater's diet is *hidden* fat.

Recently, some animal breeders have begun producing beef and pork that is lower in fat. This is a help to those people who choose lean cuts—they get less fat in the same quantity of meat. When selecting beef or pork, look for the words *loin* or *round* on the label—these words represent lean cuts from which the fat can be trimmed.

Other Food Groups

Figure 4–7 showed that milk can also contain fat. This is because milk processors homogenize or blend the cream (which normally floats and could be removed by skimming) into the milk. As stated in Chapter 2, it is best to view nonfat milk as milk and to view whole milk as milk with added fat. The portion size is 1 cup; a cup of whole milk, then, contains the protein and carbohydrate of nonfat milk but, in addition, contains 8 grams (72 calories) of fat. A cup of low-fat (2 percent) milk is halfway between whole and nonfat, with nearly 5 grams of fat. The fat occupies only a teaspoon of the volume in the milk but adds more than double the calories.

Breads also sometimes contain fat. Notable are biscuits, corn bread, quick breads, snack and party crackers, pancakes, and waffles. People are often surprised to learn of the high fat content of these items. The Fat Scorecard will help you to find the fat in foods.

Shopping for Fats

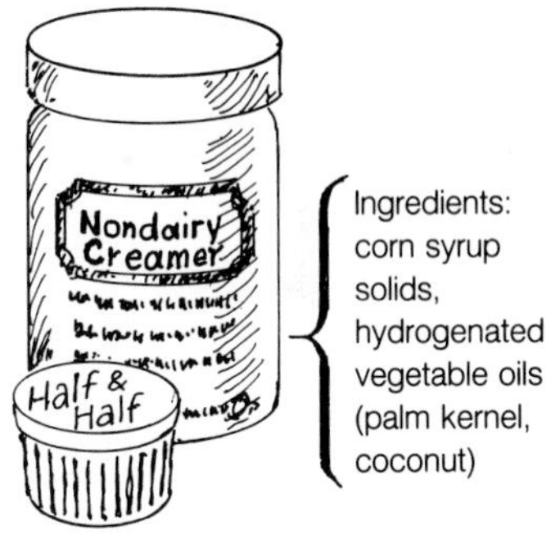
Nondairy Creamer
Half & Half
Ingredients: corn syrup solids, hydrogenated vegetable oils (palm kernel, coconut)

If you were looking for a substitute for cream, you might be inclined to choose a nondairy creamer. However, many nondairy creamers substitute coconut oil or palm kernel oil for the cream, and the product is more saturated than the cream. Notice, too, that sugar (corn syrup) is listed as the first ingredient on the label.

Generally speaking, vegetable and fish oils are rich in polyunsaturates; olive, peanut, and canola oils are rich in monounsaturates; and the harder fats—animal fats—are more saturated. However, not all vegetable oils are polyunsaturated. When you read food labels, don't let words like *vegetable fat* and *unsaturated fat* mislead you. Coconut, palm, and palm-kernel "oils," for example, are often used in nondairy creamers, crackers, and frozen desserts, and these oils are predominantly saturated fats. If you are looking for a substitute for cream, be aware that many nondairy creamers substitute coconut oil (coconut *fat*) for cream (butterfat). Coconut oil is actually more saturated than cream and therefore is no better for you. You have to know your fats; it is not enough simply to use plant oils over animal fats. Remember, too, that some vegetable oils are hydrogenated to make them solid and are not much better than the saturated fats themselves. Thus, to call a lipid product "vegetable" or "oil" is not the same as to say that it is polyunsaturated.

When buying margarine, choose one with the *lowest* amount of saturated fats and hydrogenated oils. There should be at least twice as many polyunsaturated fats as saturated (see Figure 4–9). In general, the softest margarines are the most polyunsaturated.

Some margarine and oil labels state "contains no cholesterol." This is meaningless information, since no vegetable oil contains cholesterol (see Figure 4–9). Butter does because it is an animal product; margarine does only when it is made from beef or other animal oils.

Keep in mind that cholesterol is found only in foods of animal origin.

One strategy for using fats is to use a variety but to keep the amounts as low as possible. Try reducing the fat in recipes by a tablespoon at a time and notice that you can do so and still get a good-tasting product. If you reduce

Figure 4–9

Shopping for Spreads

If you use margarine, choose one that lists liquid vegetable oil as the first ingredient. A spread's P : S ratio (polyunsaturated: saturated fat) should be 2 to 1 or higher. To calculate the P : S ratio for this margarine: Divide 5 grams (P) by 2 grams (S).
P : S ratio = 2.5.

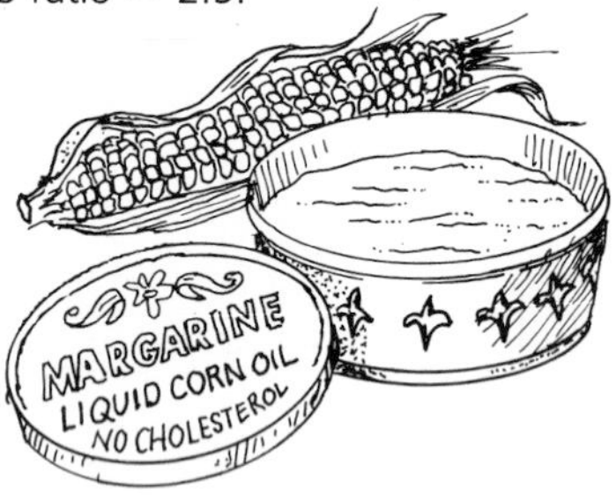

INGREDIENTS: Liquid Corn Oil, Partially Hydrogenated Corn Oil, Water, Salt, Whey, Vegetable Mono- and Diglycerides and Lecithin (emulsifiers), Artificially Flavored and Colored (Carotene), Vitamin A Palmitate and Vitamin D_2 added.

NUTRITION INFORMATION	
PER SERVING	
Serving size: 1 tbsp	14 g
Servings per pound:	32
Calories:	100
Protein:	0 g
Carbohydrate:	0 g
Fat (99% of calories from fat):	11 g
Polyunsaturated:	5 g
Saturated:	2 g
Cholesterol (0 mg per 100 g):	0 mg
Sodium:	95 mg

Diseases associated with high-fat diets:

heart disease, obesity, cancer of the breast and colon, gallbladder disease, and arthritis.

fat by 1 tablespoon of butter or oil, you lower the total fat in the product by about 12 grams and at least 100 calories.

If you use oils often, alternate among them to obtain the benefits different oils offer. Peanut and sunflower oils are especially rich in vitamin E. Olive oil, a monounsaturated oil, may also be beneficial. The people of the Mediterranean areas use large quantities of olive oil and enjoy heart health superior to ours.[20] Canola oil, another oil rich in monounsaturated fatty acids, also offers benefits.[21]

Moderation is a good word to keep in mind when you find yourself wanting to butter foods. Be conscious of where you are adding the fat—often, it isn't necessary. For example, you don't really need to add butter (or mayonnaise) to the bread when making a tuna salad or egg salad sandwich, nor do you need to add that oil to the pasta's cooking water. If you eat your toast with jam and butter, try using the jam without the butter. Most fruit butters and jams contain half the calories per teaspoon that butters contain, and the calories are from sugar, not from fat. Some low-sugar and all-fruit varieties are available—look for them. More tips on cutting the fat out of your diet are offered later in the chapter.

Using the Food Label

As a consumer, you need to remember two important points when reading food labels: the type of fat and the amount of fat. As mentioned earlier, both can affect your blood cholesterol level.

Health professionals recommend that total fat account for no more than 30 percent of total calories. Check Table 4–5 to see the amount of fat (in calories and in grams) you should be eating daily based on your total calorie intake. You can also determine what percentage of a food's calories come from fat by following the steps in Figure 4–10.

Be Fat Wise

Ample evidence exists that people in the developed countries continue to consume a high-fat diet and that this diet is causing an increase in some of the modern diseases. With that in mind, the *Dietary Guidelines* advise us to choose a diet low in fat, saturated fat, and cholesterol.

It is not the food itself but how you prepare it that often determines the total calories in a food. Compare the calories in three ounces of broiled chicken (115) versus three ounces of fried chicken (210). What makes the difference? Fat. The single most effective step you can take to reduce the calorie value of a food is to eat the food without the fat.

Foods you purchase in the grocery store can tell you much about their fat content—if you take the time to read their labels. The margin lists some words that can alert you to the fat foods contain. On a food label, the ingredients are listed in order of predominance in the product; if fat is one of the first ingredients listed, you know you are holding in your hands a high-fat product. Whether or not to choose the food depends on how you intend to use it in your diet: as a staple item, as an occasional treat, or as a garnish for other foods.

Table 4–5

Guide to Determine Total Daily Fat Allowance

We are advised to limit our total daily fat intake to no more than 30% of our total daily calories, and to limit our saturated fat intake to no more than 10% of our total daily calories. Use this table to find your total daily fat and your daily saturated fat allowances. For instance, a 2,000 calorie diet could contain up to 67 grams of total fat (30% of total calories) and 22 grams of saturated fat (10% of total calories).

DAILY CALORIC INTAKE	CALORIES FROM FAT PER DAY	MAXIMUM GRAMS FAT PER DAY	MAXIMUM GRAMS SATURATED FAT PER DAY
1,200	360	40	13
1,400	420	47	16
1,500	450	50	17
1,600	480	53	18
1,800	540	60	20
2,000	600	67	22
2,200	660	73	24
2,400	720	80	27
2,600	780	87	29
2,800	840	93	31
3,000	900	100	33

Example: If you are eating 1,500 calories per day, multiply 1,500 by 30% to determine the maximum number of calories that should come from fat in one day (1,500 × .30 = 450 calories from fat). Since 1 gram of fat provides 9 calories, divide the calories from fat by 9 to see how many grams of fat you should have per day (450 ÷ 9 = 50 grams fat per day):

Total daily calories × .30 = total fat calories

Total fat calories ÷ 9 = total fat grams

To determine your saturated fat goal: Multiply your total daily calories by 10% (1,500 × .10 = 150). Next divide the saturated fat calories by 9 (150 ÷ 9 = 17) to find out how many grams of saturated fat this equals:

Total daily calories × .10 = saturated fat calories

Saturated fat calories ÷ 9 = saturated fat grams

This list suggests a variety of ways to reduce the fat content of your diet significantly:

- Read manufacturers' labels to determine both the amounts and the types of fat contained in foods.
- Check the nutrition information on the packages you buy—it lists the amount of fat in grams per serving. Each gram of fat you eliminate saves you 9 calories.
- Reduce consumption and portion size of animal protein foods, especially meats. Serve 4-ounce portions or less of meats, adding them to stews, soups, stir-fry recipes, or pasta.
- Eat fatty and processed meats (sausages, luncheon meats, bacon, and frankfurters) only occasionally, if at all.
- Choose water-packed canned fish rather than oil-packed varieties.
- Choose lean cuts of meat; remove "visible" fat from meat and skin from poultry.

Use the ingredients list on food labels to identify products containing saturated fat. You can find fat listed on a label as animal fat, butter, cocoa butter, coconut or palm or palm kernel oils, cream, egg yolk solids, hardened fat or oil, vegetable shortening, hydrogenated vegetable oil, and lard.

Figure 4–10 Finding Fat on the Food Label

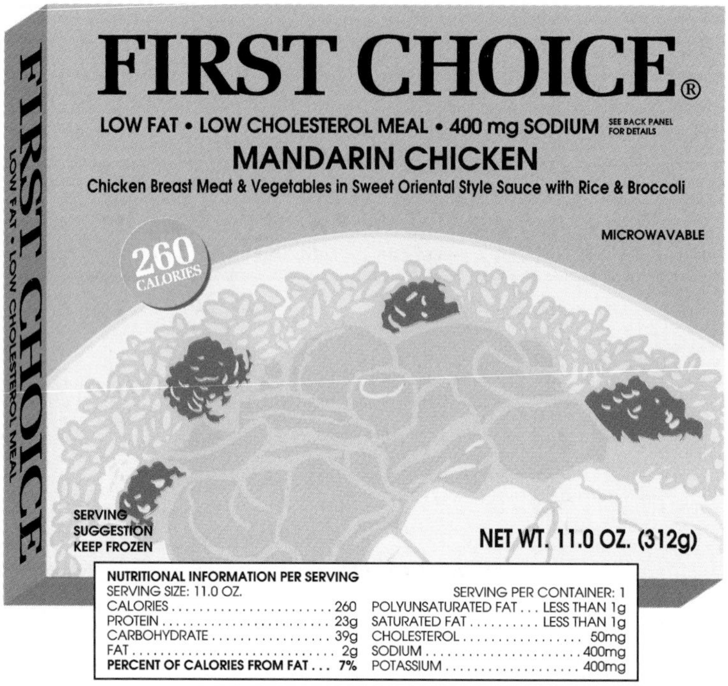

A. First, find out how many calories and how many **grams of fat** are in a serving. As you can see from the nutrition information found on this product's label, there are 260 calories and 2 grams of fat per serving. Then, figure the **percent of calories from fat.** Remember for each gram of fat there are 9 calories. To determine percent of calories from fat:

$$\frac{\text{Grams of fat per serving} \times 9 \text{ (calories per gram of fat)}}{\text{total calories}} \times 100$$

Inserting the number of calories and fat in this product:

$$\frac{2 \text{ grams fat} \times 9}{260 \text{ calories}} \times 100 = 7\% \text{ calories from fat}$$

In many instances, using this criteria helps you identify lower-fat foods. Still, the recommendation itself to limit fat to no more than 30% of our total calories applies to the *total* daily intake of fat, and not to individual foods. Many protein foods (red meat, poultry with skin, dairy products) exceed the 30% level, but contribute to a healthful diet. The key is to choose lower-fat varieties of these foods and prepare them without added fat. If you choose to eat a higher-fat food, you will need to balance it with other foods with a low percentage of calories from fat if you want your diet's average fat content to meet current recommendations to limit fat to 30% of total calories. Table 4–5 can also be used as a guide to help you keep your fat consumption to 30% of calories or less.

B. Examine carefully items which state that they are "___ % fat free." For instance, a package of turkey bologna may state that it is "85% fat free." What this means is that 15% of the product's *weight* is contributed by fat. If you determine percent calories from fat, you might be surprised that the product is not as nutritious as it sounds. For example, if the label reads:

Calories	120	Sodium, mg	428
Protein, g	7	Cholesterol, mg	40
Carbohydrates, g	1	Fiber, g	0
Fat, g	9		

Applying the formula above for percent calories from fat:

$$\frac{9 \text{ grams fat} \times 9}{120 \text{ calories}} \times 100 = 68\% \text{ calories from fat}$$

As you can see, this product is not as heart-healthy as it claims to be. It claims to be 85% fat-free, but 68% of its calories come from fat.

- Include vegetable protein sources in your diet, such as dried peas, beans, and lentils.
- Do not fry; rather, **bake**, **braise**, **broil**, **steam**, **poach**, and **sauté** (see Miniglossary of Cooking Terms). Cook meats on a rack so that the "invisible" fat can drain off.
- Experiment with some new low-fat, low-cholesterol recipes. Your local American Heart Association has many such recipes. Call or write for them.
- Use low-fat dairy products. Learn to substitute: low-fat or nonfat milk for whole milk, low-fat yogurt for sour cream, Neufchatel cheese for cream cheese, and part-skim ricotta and mozzarella cheese for whole-milk varieties.
- Limit your intake of butter, cream, hydrogenated margarine, vegetable shortenings, coconut and palm oils (and nondairy creamers containing them), half-and-half, sour cream, and mayonnaise.
- Use polyunsaturated vegetable oils such as corn, safflower, soybean, and sunflower oils and soft margarine containing these oils; diet margarine; reduced-calorie mayonnaise; and diet salad dressings or salad dressings that contain the polyunsaturated oils.
- When you use margarine, butter, or cream cheese, try the whipped varieties; they contain half the calories of the regular types.
- Use oil-and-vinegar salad dressings instead of creamy ones, which usually have a higher fat content.
- For flavor, experiment with using herbs and spices, onions or garlic, ginger, lemon juice, plain nonfat yogurt with lemon juice, or mustard instead of butter, margarine, or oil.
- Use nonstick sprays rather than fat to coat pans.
- If you are sautéing a vegetable such as onion in butter, margarine, or oil, try reducing the amount used and substituting water or cooking wine in its place.
- Eat fewer high-fat desserts (cheesecake, ice cream, pies, pastries, and butter-and-cream-frosted cakes).
- Prepare broths, soups, and stews ahead of time, refrigerate them, and then skim off hardened fat from the surface. This also gives the flavors time to blend and develop.

Miniglossary of Cooking Terms

Bake to cook in an oven surrounded by heat.

Braise to cook by browning in fat and then simmering in a covered container with a little liquid.

Broil to cook quickly over or under a direct source of intense heat, allowing fats to drip away.

Steam to cook foods suspended over boiling water.

Poach to cook foods (fish, an egg without its shell, etc.) in water near the boiling point.

Sauté (saw-TAY, the French word for stir-fry) to cook in a pan using little fat; foods are stirred frequently to prevent sticking.

Table 4–6

How to Cut Back on Fat in Your Diet

SUBSTITUTE THIS...		WITH THIS...		AND SAVE FAT/CALORIES	
Food	Fat (g)	Food	Fat (g)	Fat (g)	Calories*
Whole milk, 8 oz	8	Nonfat milk, 8 oz	Trace	8	72
Sour cream, 4 oz	24	Yogurt, 4 oz	4	20	180
Ice cream, 1 c	14	Ice milk, 1 c	7	7	63
Hamburger, 3 oz	17	Lean hamburger, 3 oz	10	7	63
Fish sticks, 5	10	Broiled fish, 3 oz	5	5	45
Biscuits, 2 dinner	6	Bread, 2 slices	2	4	36
Butter/margarine, 1 tbsp	12	Parmesan cheese, 1 tbsp	2	10	90
Asparagus, 1 c, with hollandaise sauce	18	Asparagus, 1 c, with lemon	0	18	162
French fries, 15	12	Baked potato with 1 pat butter	4	8	72
Fried egg, 1	9	Boiled or poached egg, 1	6	3	27
Round steak, 8 oz	30	Round steak, 4 oz	15	15	135
Apple pie, 1 slice	18	Apple crisp, 1 portion	8	10	90
Potato chips, 2 oz (1 small bag)	24	Unbuttered popcorn, 3 c	2	22	198
Danish pastry, 1	15	Bran muffin, 1	4	11	99
Yellow cake with icing, 1/12 cake	13	Angel food cake, 1/12 cake	Trace	13	117

*Grams of fat × 9.

Source: Adapted from The Potato Board.

- Use low-fat or nonfat milk when making cream soups.
- Learn to substitute. See Table 4–6 for some ways to reduce both fat and calories. The Consumer Tips feature offers more suggestions to help you lighten your own favorite recipes.

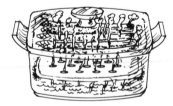

Bake, broil, poach, or steam.

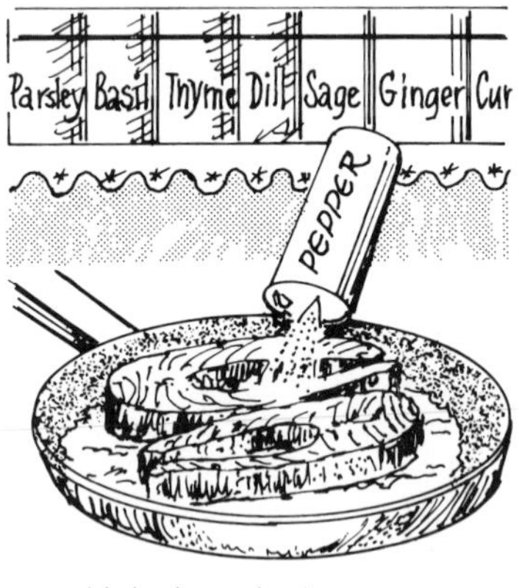

Season with herbs and spices.

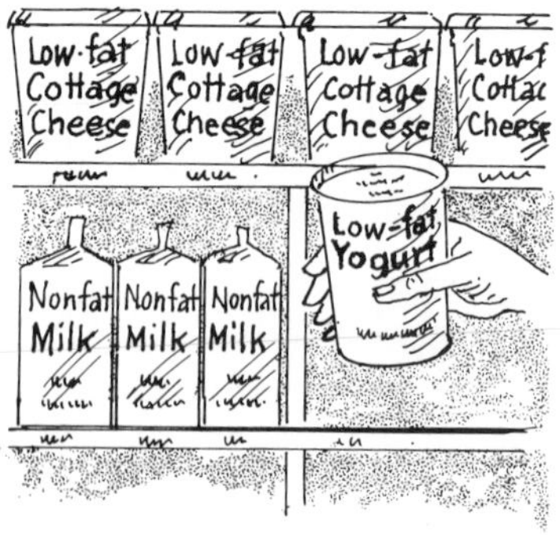

Buy low-fat foods.

Consumer Tips

Recipe Modification

Use this substitution information to modify your own favorite recipes. They'll be more healthful but still look and taste as good as your originals!

INSTEAD OF:	SUBSTITUTE:	RESULT:
1 whole egg	2 whipped egg whites	less fat, less cholesterol, fewer calories
whole milk	nonfat milk	less fat, less cholesterol, fewer calories
evaporated milk	evaporated nonfat or low-fat milk	less fat, less cholesterol, fewer calories
sugar (baking)	use ⅓ less than called for in baking, add a small amount of vanilla, cinnamon or nutmeg	fewer calories
oil	use a vegetable oil spray for preventing foods from sticking	less fat, fewer calories
cake frosting	sprinkled powdered sugar	less sugar, less fat, fewer calories
heavy cream (which does not need to be whipped)	evaporated nonfat or low-fat milk	less fat, less cholesterol, fewer calories
sour cream	plain, low-fat yogurt (add 1½ tbsp cornstarch to each cup yogurt)	less fat, less cholesterol, fewer calories
solid shortening (baking)	vegetable oil, margarine	less saturated fat
solid shortening (stir-frying)	peanut oil	less saturated fat
mayonnaise	plain yogurt (mixed with 1 tbsp mayo per cup yogurt)	less fat, less cholesterol, fewer calories
salt	use ½ the salt called for in recipes (try seasoning with herbs & other spices) except yeast breads	less sodium
cream cheese	reduced-fat cream cheese	less fat, fewer calories
regular cheese	cheese made from part-skim milk (mozzarella, Swiss lace, farmer)	less fat, less cholesterol, fewer calories
salad dressing	reduced-calorie dressing	less fat, less cholesterol, fewer calories
white sauce (made with cream & butter)	use low-fat milk and cornstarch or flour by blending the starch into cold liquid to eliminate the need for fat	less fat, less cholesterol, fewer calories

Spotlight

Diet and Heart Disease

More than half the people who die in the United States each year die of heart and blood vessel disease. The underlying condition that contributes to most of these deaths is atherosclerosis, which leads to closure of the arteries that feed the heart and brain and thus to heart attacks and strokes. In terms of direct health-care costs, lost wages, and lost productivity, heart disease costs the United States more than $60 billion a year.[22] There is little wonder, then, that much effort has been focused on preventing it.

The twin demons that lead to most forms of heart disease are atherosclerosis and hypertension. Atherosclerosis, the subject of this Spotlight, is the common form of hardening of the arteries; hypertension (discussed in the Nutrition Action feature of Chapter 7) is high blood pressure; and each makes the other worse.

• How can I know if I have atherosclerosis?

No one is free of atherosclerosis. The question is not whether you have it but how far advanced it is and what you can do to retard or reverse it. It usually begins with the accumulation of soft mounds of lipid—known as plaques—along the inner walls of the arteries, especially at the branch points (see Figure 4–11). These plaques gradually enlarge, making the artery walls lose their elasticity and narrowing the passage through them. Most people have well-developed plaques by the time they are 30.

Normally, the arteries expand with each heartbeat to accommodate the pulses of blood that flow through them. Arteries hardened and narrowed by plaques cannot expand, so the blood pressure rises. The increased pressure puts a strain on the heart and further damages the artery wall. At damaged points, plaques are especially likely to form; thus, the development of atherosclerosis is a self-accelerating process.

Hypertension makes atherosclerosis worse. A stiffened artery, already strained by each pulse of blood surging through it, is stressed even more if the internal pressure is high. Injured places develop more frequently, and plaques grow faster.

Atherosclerosis also makes hypertension worse. By hardening the arteries, it makes the arteries unable to expand with each beat of the heart, so the pressure rises instead. This leads to further hardening of the arteries, as already explained. Hardened arteries also fail to let blood flow freely through the body's blood pressure-sensing organs—the kidneys—which respond as if the blood pressure were too low and raise it further.

• How can I slow the process down?

Learn your risk factors and control the ones you can control. Among the many factors linked to heart disease are smoking, gender (being male), heredity, high blood pressure, lack of exercise, obesity, stress, high blood cholesterol level, many nutrient excesses and deficiencies, and personality characteristics (see Table 4–7). Some of the risk factors are powerful predictors of heart disease. If you have none of them, the statistical likelihood of your developing heart disease may be only one in 100. If you have three major ones, the chance may rise to over one in 20. The three factors that have emerged as the most powerful predictors of risk are high blood cholesterol, high blood pressure, and smoking.

The accompanying Heart Health Scorecard shows one way of calculating your risk score based on present knowledge. Such a quiz not only helps you look at what your risks may be but also points out areas that you can change to reduce your risk.

• What can I do to improve my risk score?

Obviously, some risk factors cannot be altered. Being born male or inheriting a predisposition to develop high blood cholesterol or high blood pressure are factors beyond your control. Even so, you can make conscious choices that may reduce your risk of developing heart disease. Let's examine one of the two major risk factors related to diet—high blood cholesterol—with an eye toward learning which dietary and lifestyle changes will help reduce your heart disease risk.

• *Table 4–7*

Risk Factors for Heart Disease

- High blood cholesterol
- Cigarette smoking
- High blood pressure
- Obesity
- Diabetes
- Gender (males are at higher risk)
- Family history of heart disease before the age of 55
- Low HDL-cholesterol (less than 35 mg/dL)
- Circulation disorders of blood vessels to the legs, arms, and brain

Source: Adapted from National Cholesterol Education Program, *Report of the Expert Panel on Detection, Evaluation, and Treatment of High Blood Cholesterol in Adults,* Bethesda, MD: U.S. Department of Health and Human Services, Public Health Service, National Institutes of Health, National Heart, Lung, and Blood Institute, NIH Publication No. 88–2925, January 1988.

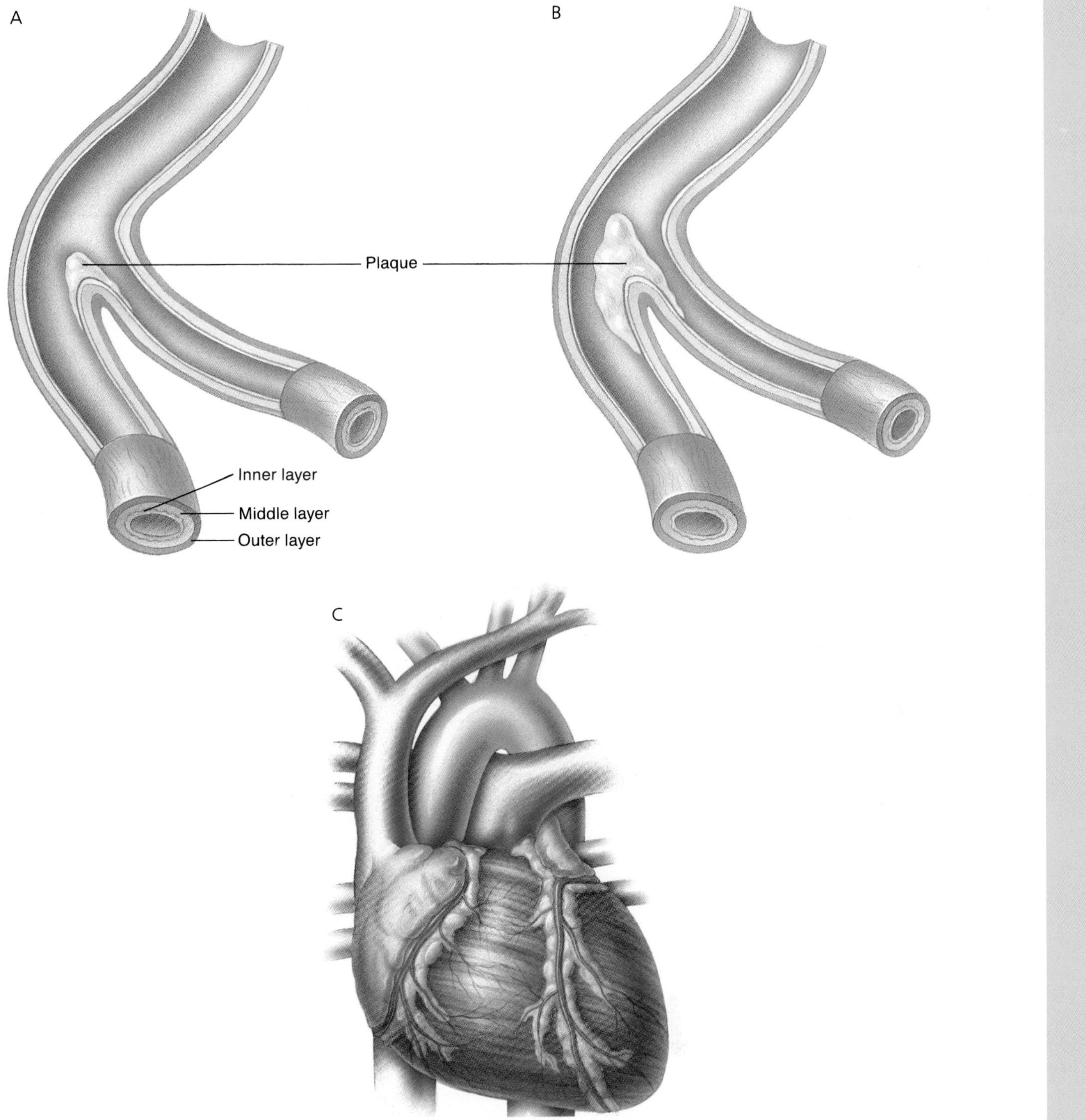

Figure 4–11 Development of Atherosclerosis

A. An artery (section) with plaque just beginning to form. Plaques can easily appear in a person as young as 15. **B.** The same artery, years later, half blocked by plaque. **C.** These are the coronary arteries, which bring nourishment to the heart muscle. If one of these arteries becomes blocked by plaque, the part of the heart muscle that it feeds will die.

Heart Health Scorecard

Every disease has risk factors; those for heart disease are among the best known. The better you know the nature of the risks you face, the better you can decide what prevention measures may be appropriate. To determine your risk of heart disease, add up the numbers in each category that most nearly describe you:

Heredity[a]	1 No known history of heart disease	2 One relative over 60 years old with heart disease	3 Two relatives over 60 years old with heart disease	4 One relative under 60 years old with heart disease	6 Two relatives under 60 years old with heart disease
Exercise	1 Intensive exercise, work, and recreation	2 Moderate exercise, work, and recreation	3 Sedentary work and intensive recreational exercise	5 Sedentary work and moderate recreational exercise	6 Sedentary work and light recreational exercise
Age	1 10 to 20	2 21 to 30	3 31 to 40	4 41 to 50	6 51 to 65
Lb	0 More than 5 lb below standard weight	1 ± 5 lb of standard weight	2 6 to 20 lb overweight	4 21 to 35 lb overweight	6 36 to 50 lb overweight
Tobacco	0 Nonuser	1 Cigar or pipe	2 10 cigarettes or fewer per day	4 20 cigarettes or more per day	6 30 cigarettes or more per day
Habits of eating fat[b]	1 No animal or solid fat	2 Very little animal or solid fat	3 Little animal or solid fat	4 Much animal or solid fat	6 Equal to the typical meat eater's diet
Your risk of heart attack: 4 to 9: Very remote. 10 to 15: Below average.		16 to 20: Average. 21 to 25: Moderate.		26 to 30: Dangerous. 31 to 35: Urgent danger—reduce score!	

Other conditions—such as stress, high blood pressure, and increased blood cholesterol level—detract from heart health and should be evaluated by your physician.

[a]Diabetes and hypertension in the family are also predictors.
[b]If you know your blood cholesterol level, use it instead. Below 180 = 0 points; 181 to 200 = 1; 201 to 235 = 2; 236 to 260 = 4; 261 to 300 = 5; over 300 = 6.

Source: Courtesy of Loma Linda University.

• To what extent does a high blood cholesterol level raise the risk of developing heart disease?

The likelihood of a person developing or dying from heart disease increases as blood cholesterol level rises. Figure 4–12 presents this relationship graphically: the number of deaths from heart disease increases steadily among those with elevated blood cholesterol levels, particularly when it rises above 200 milligrams per deciliter. Individuals with blood cholesterol levels in the neighborhood of 300 milligrams per deciliter run four times the risk of dying from heart disease as those whose cholesterol levels are less than 200 milligrams per deciliter.

Thus, reducing high blood cholesterol levels, particularly the "bad" LDL-cholesterol, is an important strategy toward lowering the risk of heart disease. This is especially true for persons having one or more of the other major heart disease risk factors, such as smoking. Refer to Figure 4–6 and Table 4–8 for information on determining what to do if your blood cholesterol level is high and if you might need to seek treatment.

• What sorts of dietary changes should I make to reduce my total cholesterol and LDL-cholesterol?

Probably the most significant dietary change you can make is to reduce the amount of fat you eat, particularly saturated fat, since high intakes of these dietary constituents are related to high blood levels of LDL-cholesterol. The goals to work toward are to reduce your intake of total fat to 30 percent of total calories or less and your intake of saturated fat to 10 percent of total calories or less. How do these target goals compare to current dietary patterns? A recent analysis of the trend in U.S. fat consumption showed that the average intake of fat in 1984 (the latest year for which population data are available) was about 37 percent of total calories, down from a high of 41 percent in the 1930s; saturated fat intake was about 12 percent on the average in 1984, down from 17 percent in the 1950s.[24]

These figures suggest that many Americans are on the right track toward reducing their intakes of fat and saturated fat and lowering their blood LDL-cholesterol levels. In addition to these strategies, other dietary changes may also help lower LDL-cholesterol.

Dietary fiber, for example, may confer benefits. People on high-fiber diets have been shown to excrete more cholesterol and fat than those on low-fiber diets. One reason is that the high-fiber diet decreases food's transit time through the digestive tract, which allows less time for cholesterol to be absorbed. When cholesterol from the diet is thus reduced, the body must turn to its own supply to use in making necessary body compounds. Diets high in fiber are typically low in fat and cholesterol anyway—another advantage to emphasizing fiber.

The various dietary fibers have varying effects on blood cholesterol. Rolled oats, oat bran, and psyllium have favorable effects on blood cholesterol, whereas wheat bran does not appear effective.[25] Apples, pears, peaches, oranges, and grapes are good sources of pectin, another type of cholesterol-lowering fiber.

• Should I also reduce my cholesterol intake?

The *Dietary Guidelines* recommend that we limit the cholesterol in our diets to 300 milligrams daily. On the average, men consume 400 to 500 milligrams of cholesterol and women consume about 300 milligrams of cholesterol daily. The average for men is above that consumed in countries with little heart disease.

Some experts say all adults should cut their cholesterol intakes; others say only those medically identified as at risk for heart disease should do so. The question remains open, but most people who develop "heart healthy" eating habits such as decreasing saturated fat tend to lower their cholesterol intake along with their fat intake.

• What factors determine my HDL-cholesterol level?

One is gender. Women have higher HDL-cholesterol levels than men. Another, interestingly, seems to be smoking habits. Nonsmokers have uniformly higher HDL levels than smokers. Still another is weight reduction for those who are overweight.

• *Figure 4–12* Relationship Between Blood Cholesterol Level and Death Rate from Heart Disease

Persons with blood cholesterol levels of 300 mg/dL are four times as likely to die from heart disease as those with blood cholesterol levels below 200 mg/dL.

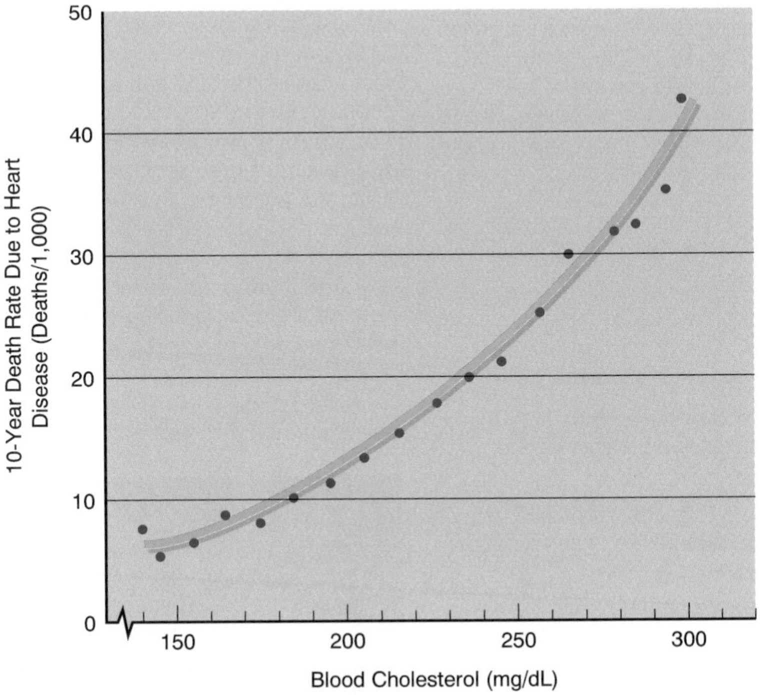

Source: Data from 361,662 men screened for the Multiple Risk Factor Intervention Trial (MRFIT). Adapted from National Cholesterol Education Program, *Report of the Expert Panel on Population Strategies for Blood Cholesterol Reduction,* Bethesda, MD: U.S. Department of Health and Human Services, Public Health Service, National Institutes of Health, National Heart, Lung, and Blood Institute, NIH Publication No. 90–3046, November 1990, p. 7.

Table 4–8

Standards for Blood Cholesterol Levels and Risk of Heart Disease

TOTAL BLOOD CHOLESTEROL CATEGORIES			LDL-CHOLESTEROL CATEGORIES		
Desirable	Borderline-High Risk	High Risk	Desirable	Borderline-High Risk	High Risk
< 200 mg/dL	200–239 mg/dL	≥ 240 mg/dL	< 130 mg/dL	130–159 mg/dL	≥ 160 mg/dL

Note: These categories apply to anyone 20 years of age or older.

Source: Adapted from National Cholesterol Education Program, *Report of the Expert Panel on Detection, Evaluation, and Treatment of High Blood Cholesterol in Adults,* Bethesda, MD: U.S. Department of Health and Human Services, Public Health Service, National Institutes of Health, National Heart, Lung, and Blood Institute, NIH Publication No. 88–2925, January 1988.

If there are dietary factors of any significance, one may be the use of fish rather than meat.[26] Another may be the use of foods containing certain fibers that lower LDL levels selectively and leave HDL levels unchanged.[27] The evidence with regard to alcohol and blood lipids is mixed. A few investigators have reported that the consumption of moderate amounts of alcohol appears to raise HDL levels. However, there is more than one kind of HDL,[28] and the kind of HDL affected by alcohol may not be the "good" kind. In addition, alcohol has profoundly negative effects on the body, and it is associated with many disease states (see the Spotlight feature at the end of Chapter 10).

By far the most powerful influence on HDL levels is not a dietary factor at all—it is regular exercise. The discovery that exercise raises HDL levels has given great impetus to the physical fitness movement—and especially to the popularity of running and walking. The earliest reports were of raised HDL levels in long-distance runners, and the continuing study of this elite group has repeatedly demonstrated that running does indeed elevate HDL.[29] Luckily, however, people do not have to become competitive athletes to raise their HDL—moderate or even light exercise such as walking may both lower LDL levels and raise HDL levels if the activity is consistently pursued.[30] Evidently, then, almost all people are capable of exercising enough to reap this and many other benefits (see Chapter 9).

How do I translate these recommendations into a healthful eating pattern?

Most people have a difficult time translating the dietary recommendations into actual meal patterns. What foods should you eat, for example, to achieve the goal of reducing your fat intake to 30 percent of total calories? It's virtually impossible to know exactly what your fat intake is without having your daily food intake analyzed using a computerized nutrient program. Even so, some general guidelines will help you make the "heart healthy" food choices needed to achieve these goals. If you were to take *all* of the steps suggested, you would:

- Eat skinless poultry and fish often, especially fatty fish, such as mackerel and salmon.
- Choose nonfat or low-fat dairy products, such as nonfat milk and low-fat or nonfat yogurt.
- Consume abundant legumes of many varieties, including soybeans and chickpeas.
- Eat generous quantities of fiber-rich fruits and vegetables, including many raw ones.
- Eat whole grains (especially oat bran, and not especially wheat bran) and sprouts often.
- Limit your use of foods particularly rich in saturated fat, such as fatty red meats. (See Table 4–9.) Trim away all visible fat from meats before cooking.
- Adopt low-fat cooking methods, such as broiling, roasting, steaming, braising, and stir-frying.
- Become a savvy supermarket shopper—learn to read food labels to help you choose low-fat food products.
- Consume alcohol in moderation.

It seems that the factors affecting the health of the heart are all tangled together. The exact relationships among them have not yet been worked out; we don't know which causes what, but all evidence points to the same general recommendations. For good health and to avoid heart disease, stop smoking; reduce blood pressure and weight, if necessary; eat a balanced, adequate, and varied diet; reduce total fat intake, especially saturated fat; and exercise regularly.[31]

Attention to emotional health is also important in reducing the risk of heart disease. People who are normally tense, impatient, and competitive—the so-called Type A personality—tend to have high blood cholesterol levels. Both

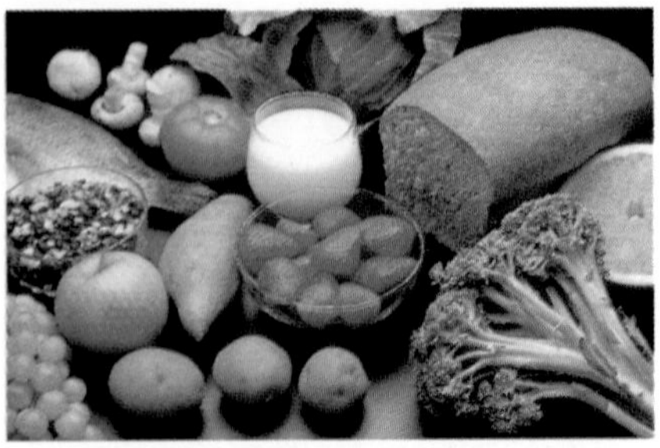

Enjoy a variety of low-fat foods for the health of your heart.

love and affection affect the heart. People with many social ties appear to develop less heart disease than people with few or none. Married men have less heart disease than single men, and pet owners (even owners of pet fish) have lower blood pressure than do people without pets.[32] Clearly, the mystery of heart disease, like all the great human mysteries, involves the mind and spirit as well as the body. So nourish yourself in all ways—not just physically.

The verdict is not yet in as to whether following these suggestions will reverse the process of atherosclerosis. However, the evidence collected to date tends to show that following these suggestions will help prevent the condition from getting any worse and may also begin to clear the arteries.

• Should children, like their parents, eat low-fat diets for heart health?

In 1991 a panel of experts representing 42 major U.S. health and professional organizations recommended that children aged two and older eat diets containing no more than 30 percent of total calories from fat, less than 10 percent of calories from saturated fat, and no more than 300 milligrams of cholesterol daily. The reason is that hardening of the arteries often begins in childhood. However, from birth to two years of age a child's fat consumption should not be restricted because fat is a concentrated source of the calories needed to insure proper physical development.

The panel also advised that youngsters or teens should get their blood cholesterol measured if they have one parent with a high blood cholesterol level. For children and adolescents, a total of 200 milligrams per deciliter or more is considered high; 170 to 199 is borderline high; and less than 170 is acceptable. In addition, youngsters born to families with a history of premature heart disease should have both total blood cholesterol and HDL-cholesterol checked.[33]

Table 4–9

Comparison of Saturated Fat, Total Fat, and Cholesterol in Selected Foods[1]

The following foods within each grouping are ranked from low to high saturated fat.[2] The foods chosen for this chart are meant to be representative of their type. You will want to select most often the low saturated fat and cholesterol foods from the upper portion of each group.

	GRAMS OF SATURATED FAT	GRAMS OF TOTAL FAT	MILLIGRAMS OF CHOLESTEROL	TOTAL CALORIES
Beef (3½ oz)				
Top round	1.7	5.0	90	199
Sirloin	2.6	6.8	89	191
Chuck, arm pot roast	2.8	7.6	101	210
Ground lean	7.2	18.5	87	272
Salami, about 4 slices	8.4	20.1	60	254
Pork (3½ oz)				
Ham steak, extra lean	1.4	4.2	45	122
Fresh tenderloin	1.7	4.8	93	166
Fresh, leg, rump half	3.7	10.7	96	221
Lamb (3½ oz)				
Leg	2.8	7.7	89	191
Loin chop	3.5	9.7	95	216
Arm chop	5.0	14.1	121	279
Poultry (3½ oz)				
Turkey, fryer-roasters:				
Light meat without skin	0.4	1.2	86	140
Light meat with skin	1.3	4.6	95	164

continued

[1]If you want to check whether you are eating 30 percent of your total calories from fat (or 10 percent of your total daily calories from saturated fat), use this table to add up the grams of fat (or saturated fat) you eat each day and refer to Table 4–5 to see the amount of fat and saturated fat you should be eating based on your total caloric intake.

[2]All values for meat, poultry, and fish are for products prepared by broiling, braising, roasting, or moist heat cooking methods rather than frying, unless otherwise indicated.

Table 4–9, Continued

	GRAMS OF SATURATED FAT	GRAMS OF TOTAL FAT	MILLIGRAMS OF CHOLESTEROL	TOTAL CALORIES
Chicken, broilers:				
Light meat without skin	1.3	4.5	85	173
Dark meat without skin	2.7	9.7	93	205
Light meat with skin	3.0	10.9	84	222
Dark meat with skin	4.4	15.8	91	253
Ground turkey	3.8	13.8	69	229
Fish (3½ oz)				
Haddock	0.2	0.9	74	112
Halibut	0.4	2.9	41	140
Tuna	1.6	6.3	49	184
Salmon	1.9	11.0	87	216
Shellfish (3½ oz)				
Lobster	0.1	0.6	72	98
Clam	0.2	2.0	67	148
Shrimp	0.3	1.1	195	99
Oyster	1.3	5.0	109	137
Clam, breaded and fried	2.7	11.2	61	202
Milk (8 oz)				
Nonfat	0.3	0.4	4	86
Buttermilk	1.3	2.2	9	99
Low-fat, 1%	1.6	2.6	10	102
Low-fat, 2%	2.9	4.7	18	121
Whole	5.1	8.2	33	150
Yogurt (4 oz)				
Plain nonfat yogurt	0.1	0.2	2	63
Plain yogurt	2.4	3.7	14	70
Soft cheeses (4 oz)				
Cottage cheese, low-fat	0.7	1.2	5	82
Cottage cheese, creamed	3.2	5.1	17	117
Ricotta, part-skim	5.5	8.9	34	171
Ricotta, whole milk	9.3	14.5	57	216
Hard cheeses (1 oz)				
Mozzarella, part-skim	2.9	4.5	16	72
Mozzarella	3.7	6.1	22	80
Swiss	5.0	7.8	26	107
American processed	5.6	8.9	27	106
Cheddar	6.0	9.4	30	114
Frozen Desserts (1 cup)				
Orange sherbert	2.4	3.8	14	270
Vanilla ice milk	3.5	5.6	18	184
Vanilla ice cream	8.9	14.3	59	269
Eggs (1 large)				
Egg white	0	trace	0	16
Egg yolk	1.6	5.1	213	59

continued

Table 4–9, Continued

	GRAMS OF SATURATED FAT	GRAMS OF TOTAL FAT	MILLIGRAMS OF CHOLESTEROL	TOTAL CALORIES
Fats and Oils (1 tbsp)				
Canola oil	1.0	14.0	0	124
Safflower oil	1.2	13.6	0	120
Peanut butter	1.5	7.9	0	94
Corn oil	1.7	13.6	0	120
Olive oil	1.8	13.5	0	119
Margarine, soft tub	2.1	11.4	0	101
Margarine, stick	2.1	11.4	0	101
Butter	7.1	10.8	31	101
Nuts and Seeds (1 oz)				
Almonds	1.4	14.8	0	167
Pecans	1.5	19.2	0	190
Sunflower seeds	1.5	14.1	0	162
English walnuts	1.6	17.6	0	182
Pistachio	1.7	13.7	0	164
Peanuts	1.9	13.8	0	159
Breads (1 whole item)				
Corn tortilla	0.1	1.0	0	65
English muffin	0.3	1.0	0	140
Bagel	0.3	2.0	0	200
Whole wheat bread	0.4	1.0	0	70
Hamburger bun	0.5	2.0	trace	115
Croissant	3.5	12.0	13	235
Sweets and Snacks				
Air-popped popcorn, 1 cup	trace	0	trace	30
Angel food cake, 1⁄12 cake	trace	trace	0	125
Vanilla wafers, 5	0.9	3.3	12	94
Fig bars, 4	1.0	4.0	27	210
Potato chips, 1 oz	2.6	10.1	0	147
Pound cake, 1⁄17 cake	3.0	5.0	64	110
Chocolate chip cookies, 4	3.9	11.0	18	185

Source: Adapted from *Facts about blood cholesterol,* Bethesda, MD: National Heart, Lung, and Blood Institute, U.S. Department of Health and Human Services, Public Health Service, National Institutes of Health, NIH Publication No. 90–2696, October 1990, pp. 12–16.

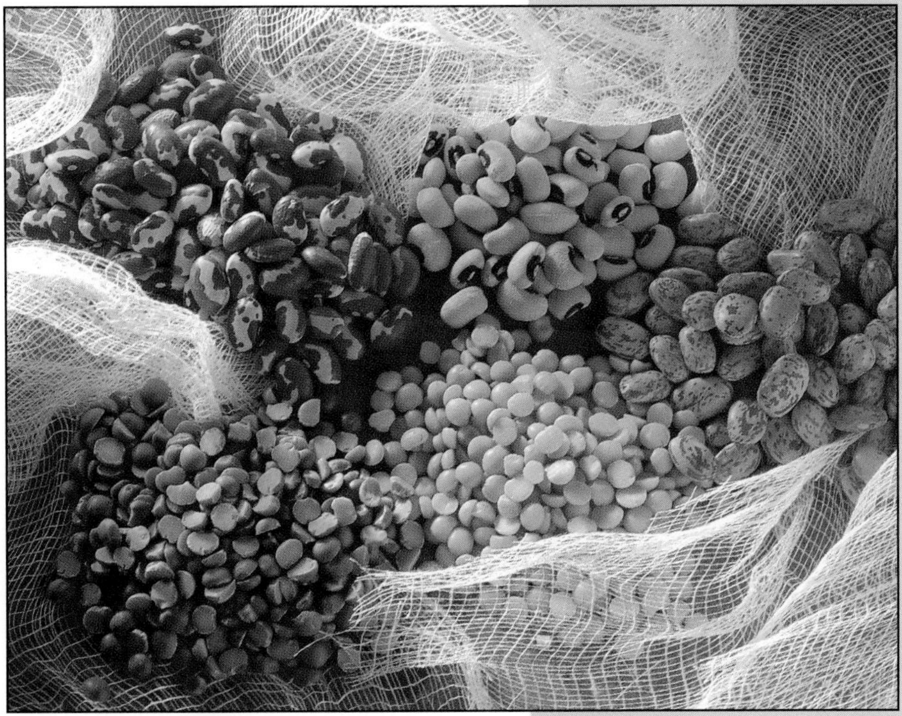

© Peter Wong

> *The amino acids of proteins are the raw materials of heredity, the keys to life chemistry, handed from generation to generation.*
> —*R. M. Deutsch*

CHAPTER 5
The Proteins and Amino Acids

Contents

Ask Yourself . . . ?

Which of these statements about nutrition are true, and which are false? For the false statements, what *is* true?

1. Protein eaten in excess of need is stored intact in the body, as fat is, so that it can be used when a person's diet falls short of supplying the day's need for essential proteins.
2. No new living tissue can be built without protein.
3. Whenever cells are lost, protein is lost.
4. All enzymes and hormones are made of protein.
5. When antibodies enter the body, they produce illness.
6. When a person doesn't eat enough food to meet the body's energy needs, the body devours its own protein tissue.
7. Once the body has assembled its proteins into body structures, it never lets go of them.
8. Milk protein is the standard against which the quality of other proteins is usually measured.
9. It is impossible to consume too much protein.
10. People who eat no meat have to eat a lot of special foods to get enough protein.

Answers: 1. False. Protein eaten in excess of need is not stored in the body, as fat is, so it has to be eaten every day if it is not to become depleted. 2. True. 3. True. 4. False. All enzymes, but not all hormones, are made of protein. 5. False. Antibodies protect the body from illness caused by antigens. 6. True. In an energy deficiency, the body devours its own protein tissue. 7. False. Your body loses protein every day. 8. False. Egg protein, not milk protein, is the standard against which the quality of other proteins is usually measured. 9. False. It is possible to consume too much protein. 10. False. People who eat no meat can easily get enough protein without eating a lot of special foods.

The **proteins** are perhaps the most highly respected of the three energy nutrients, and the roles they play in the body are far more varied than those of carbohydrate or fat. Without them, life would not exist. First named 150 years ago after the Greek word *proteios* ("of prime importance"), proteins have revealed countless secrets about the ways living processes take place, and they account for many nutrition concerns. How do we grow? How do our bodies replace the materials they lose? How does blood clot? What makes us able to become immune to diseases we have been exposed to? The answers to these and many other such questions arise to a great extent from an understanding of the nature of proteins.

Proteins compounds—composed of atoms of carbon, hydrogen, oxygen, and nitrogen—arranged as strands of amino acids. Some amino acids also contain atoms of sulfur.

Amino (a-MEEN-o) acids building blocks of protein; each is a compound with an amine group at one end, an acid group at the other, and a distinctive side chain.

Amine (a-MEEN) group the nitrogen-containing portion of an amino acid.

Essential amino acids amino acids that cannot be synthesized at all by the body or that cannot be synthesized in amounts sufficient to meet physiological need.

What Proteins Are Made Of

To appreciate the many vital functions of proteins, we must understand their structure. One key difference from carbohydrate and fat, which contain only carbon, hydrogen, and oxygen atoms, is that proteins contain nitrogen atoms. These nitrogen atoms give the name *amino* ("nitrogen containing") to the **amino acids** of which protein is made. Another key difference is that in contrast to the carbohydrates—whose repeating units, glucose molecules, are identical—the amino acids in a strand of protein are different from one another.

All amino acids have the same, simple chemical backbone with an **amine group** (the nitrogen-containing part) at one end and an acid group at the other end. The differences between the amino acids depend on a distinctive structure—the chemical side chain—that is attached to the backbone (see Figure 5–1). It is the nature of the side chain that gives identity and chemical nature to each amino acid. Twenty amino acids with twenty different side chains make up most of the proteins of living tissue.

The side chains vary in complexity from a single hydrogen atom like that on glycine to a complex ring structure like that on phenylalanine (see Figure 5–2). Not only do these structures differ in composition, size, and shape, they also differ in electrical charge. Some are negative, some are positive, and some have no charge. These side chains help to determine the shapes and behaviors of the larger protein molecules that the amino acids make up.

Essential and Nonessential Amino Acids

The body can make the majority of the amino acids for itself, given the needed parts: nitrogen to form the amine group, along with backbone fragments derived from carbohydrate or fat. But there are some amino acids that the healthy body cannot make. These are the **essential amino acids.** If the diet does not supply them, the body cannot make the proteins it needs to do its work. The indispensability of the essential amino acids makes it necessary for people to eat protein food sources every day.

The distinction between essential and nonessential amino acids is not quite as clear-cut as the list in the margin makes it appear. Histidine often appears not to be essential, perhaps because the diet supplies it in abundance; now, however, it has been added to the list of essential amino acids.[1] Arginine, under some conditions, may be synthesized too slowly to meet the human need fully.[2] States of illness can interfere with amino acid transformations in the body and so make other amino acids essential for certain individuals.*

Proteins as the Source of Life's Variety

In the first step of **protein synthesis**, each amino acid is hooked to the next. A bond, called a peptide bond, is formed between the amino end of one and the acid end of the next. Proteins are made of many amino acid units, from several dozen to many hundred.

A strand of protein is not a straight, but a tangled, chain. The amino acids at different places along the strand are attracted to one another, and this

*Cysteine and tyrosine normally are not essential, because the body makes them from methionine and phenylalanine—but if there is not enough of these precursors from which to make them, they have to be supplied in the diet. Another amino acid, taurine, is not listed with the standard 20 because it is not used in making protein strands. However, it is used to make materials important in brain and eye function and in the digestion of fat. Its concentration in human milk is high, and under special circumstances, human infants may require an external dietary source.

Figure 5–1

The Structure of an Amino Acid

The "backbone" of an amino acid is the same as that of carbohydrate or fats—two carbon atoms joined together. The structure includes an amino group, an acid group, and a side group of one or more atoms which is different for each amino acid.

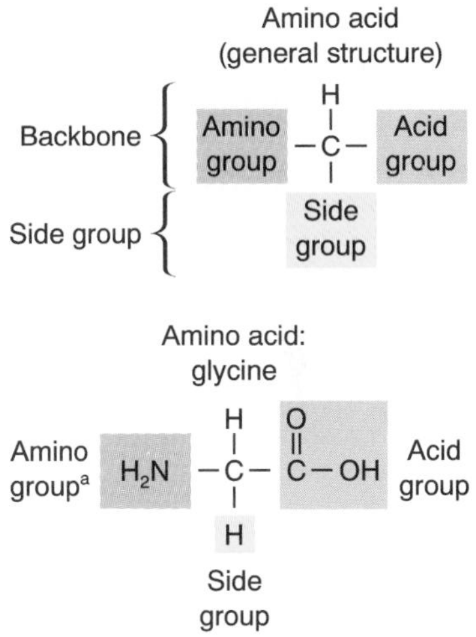

[a]Note that the distinctive element of all amino acids—nitrogen—is in the amino group.

The nine amino acids known to be essential for human adults:

tryptophan	lysine
valine	phenylalanine
threonine	methionine
isoleucine	histidine
leucine	

The nonessential amino acids—also important in nutrition:

alanine	cystine	proline
arginine	glutamic acid	serine
aspartic acid	glutamine	tyrosine
cysteine	glycine	

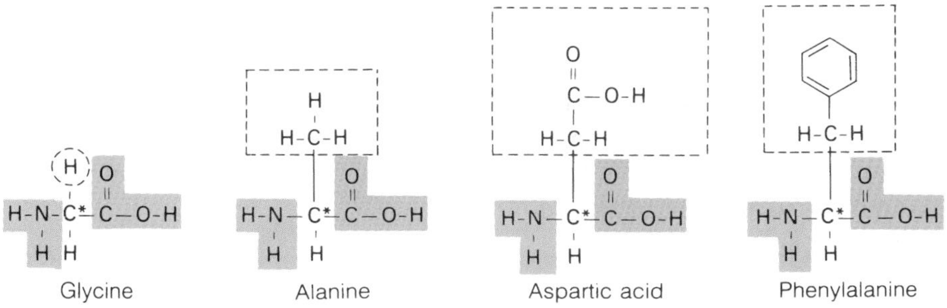

Figure 5–2

Examples of Amino Acids with Different Side Chains

Note that the side chains are different in each. The asterisk denotes the central carbon.

Protein synthesis the process by which cells assemble amino acids into proteins. Each individual is unique because of minute differences in the ways his or her body proteins are made. The instructions for making every protein in a person's body are transmitted in the genetic information the person receives at conception.

Denaturation the change in shape of a protein brought about by heat, acids, bases, alcohol, heavy metals, or other agents.

attraction causes the strand to coil into a shape similar to that of a metal spring. Not only does the strand of amino acids form a long coil, but the coil tangles, forming a globular structure.

The charged amino acids are attracted to water, and in the body fluids they orient themselves on the outside of the globular structure. The neutral amino acids are repelled by water and are attracted to one another; they tuck themselves into the center, away from the body fluid. All these interactions among the amino acids and the surrounding fluid result in the unique architecture of each type of protein. Additional steps may be needed for the protein to become functional. A metal ion (mineral) or a vitamin may be needed to complete the unit and activate it, or several proteins may gather to form a functioning group.

The differing shapes of proteins enable the proteins to perform different tasks in the body. In proteins that give strength and elasticity to body parts, several springs of amino acids coil together and form ropelike fibers. Other proteins, like those in the blood, do not have such structural strength but are water-soluble, with a globular shape like a ball of steel wool. Some are hollow balls that can carry and store minerals in their interiors. Still others provide support to tissues. Some—the enzymes (see page 127)—act on other substances to change them chemically.

Denaturation of Proteins

Proteins can undergo **denaturation**, resulting in distortion of shape by heat, alcohol, acids, or the salts of heavy metals. The denaturation of a protein is the first step in the protein's breakdown. Denaturation is useful to the body in digestion. During the digestion of a food protein, an early step is denaturation by the stomach acid, which opens up the protein's structure, permitting digestive enzymes to get at it.

Many well-known poisons are salts of heavy metals like mercury and silver; these salts alter the structure of proteins wherever they touch them. The common first-aid remedy for swallowing a heavy-metal poison is to drink milk. The poison then acts on the protein of the milk rather than on the protein tissues of the mouth, esophagus, and stomach. Afterwards, vomiting is induced to expel the poison.

The Functions of Body Proteins

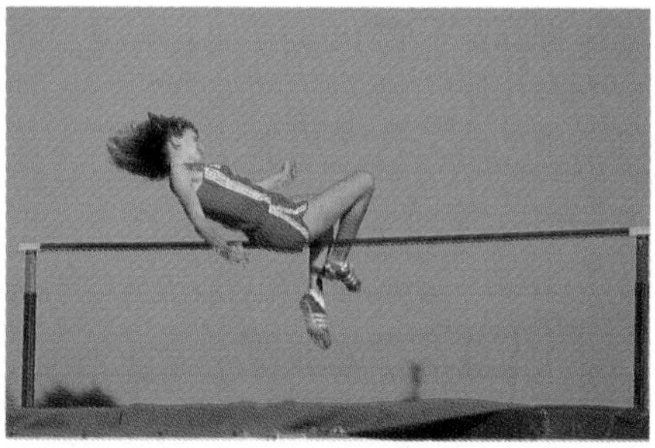

Proteins perform many different tasks in the body—for example, our muscles are made of protein.

No new living tissue can be built without protein, for protein is part of every cell. About 20 percent of our total body weight is protein. Proteins come in many forms: enzymes, antibodies, hormones, transport vehicles, cellular "pumps," oxygen carriers, tendons and ligaments, scars, the cores of bones and teeth, the filaments of hair, the materials of nails, and more. A few of the many vital functions of proteins are described here to show why they have rightfully earned their position of importance in nutrition.

Growth and Maintenance

One function of dietary protein is to ensure the availability of amino acids to build the proteins of new tissue. The new tissue may be in an embryo; in a growing child; in the blood that replaces that which has been lost in burns, hemorrhage, or surgery; in the scar tissue that heals wounds; or in new hair and nails. Not so obvious is the protein that helps replace worn-out cells. The cells that line the digestive tract live for about three days and are constantly being shed and excreted. You have probably observed that the cells of your skin die, rub off, and are replaced from underneath. For this new growth, amino acids must constantly be resupplied from food.

Enzymes

All enzymes are proteins, and they are among the most important proteins formed in living cells. Enzymes are catalysts—biological spark plugs—that help chemical reactions take place. There are thousands of enzymes inside a single cell, each type facilitating a specific chemical reaction. Enzymes are involved in such processes as the digestion of food, the release of energy from the body's stored energy supplies, and tissue growth and repair.

A mystery that has been partially explained in recent years is how an enzyme can be specific for a particular reaction. The surface of the enzyme is contoured so that the enzyme can recognize the substances it works on and ignore others. The surface provides a site that attracts one or more specific chemical compounds and promotes a specific chemical reaction. For example, two substances may become attached to the enzyme and then to each other. The newly formed product is then expelled by the enzyme into the fluid of the cell (see Figure 5–3). For another example, one compound may attach to the enzyme, then split into two products and be released. Enzymes are the hands-on workers in the production and processing of all substances needed by the body.

Hormones and Antibodies

Similar to the enzymes in the profoundness of their effects are the **hormones.** However, these molecules differ from the enzymes. For one thing, not all of them are made of protein. For another, they don't catalyze chemical reactions directly. Rather, they are messengers that elicit the appropriate responses to maintain a normal environment in the body. Hormones regulate overall body conditions, such as the blood glucose level (the hormone insulin) and the metabolic rate (thyroid hormone).

Of all the great variety of proteins in living organisms, the **antibodies** best demonstrate that proteins are specific for one organism. Antibodies are

Hormones chemical messengers. Hormones are secreted by a variety of glands in the body in response to altered conditions. Each affects one or more target tissues or organs and elicits specific responses to restore normal conditions.

Antibodies large proteins of the blood and body fluids, produced by one type of immune cell in response to invasion of the body by unfamiliar molecules (mostly proteins). Antibodies inactivate the invaders and so protect the body. The invaders are called **antigens.**

anti = against

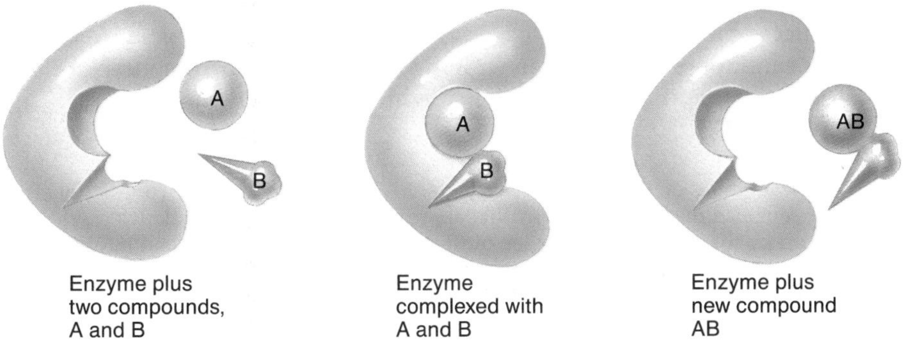

Figure 5–3

Enzyme Action

Each enzyme facilitates a specific chemical reaction.

● *Figure 5–4*

Development of Immunity

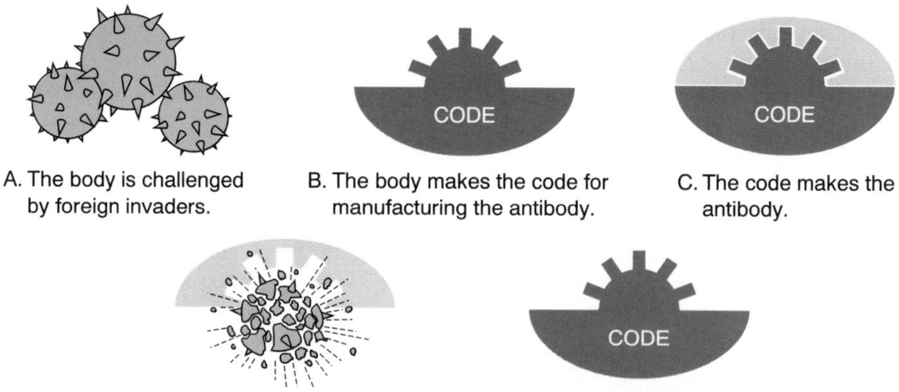

A. The body is challenged by foreign invaders.

B. The body makes the code for manufacturing the antibody.

C. The code makes the antibody.

D. The antibody inactivates the foreign invader.

E. The code remains to make antibodies faster the next time a foreign invader attacks.

formed in response to the presence of foreign proteins (or other large molecules) that invade the body. The foreign protein may be part of a bacterium, a virus, or a toxin, or it may be present in food that causes allergy. The body, after recognizing that it has been invaded, manufactures antibodies, which inactivate the foreign protein. Without sufficient protein to make antibodies, the body cannot maintain its resistance to disease.

One of the most fascinating aspects of this response is that each antibody is designed specifically to destroy one invader. An antibody that has been manufactured to combat one strain of flu virus would be of no help in protecting a person against another strain. Once the body has learned to make a particular antibody, it never forgets; and the next time it encounters that same invader, it will be equipped to destroy it even more rapidly (see Figure 5–4). In other words, it develops an **immunity.** This is the principle underlying the vaccines and antitoxins that have nearly eradicated most childhood diseases in the Western world.

Clearly, malnutrition injures the immune system. Without adequate protein in the diet, the immune system will not be able to make its specialized cells and other tools to function optimally. Often protein deficiency and immune incompetence appear together. For this reason, measles in a malnourished child can be fatal. It also can put the malnourished person at risk for increased incidence of **opportunistic infections**—as is the case with many of those diagnosed with **acquired immune deficiency syndrome** (AIDS). These infections are often the cause of death in the AIDS patient. While nutrition cannot prevent infection with the AIDS virus, nutrition intervention can be important in preventing the weight loss and malnutrition seen in people with AIDS.*

*As of the beginning of 1989, more than 87,000 AIDS cases had been reported; nearly 50,000 persons had died. Some predict that approximately 365,000 cumulative cases will be diagnosed by the end of 1992. For the most part, AIDS is preventable, and information regarding prevention is available. The Centers for Disease Control operates a National AIDS Hotline available 24 hours per day at 1-800-342-AIDS.

Immunity specific disease resistance, derived from the immune system's memory of prior exposure to specific disease agents and its ability to mount a swift defense against them.

Opportunistic infections infections produced by organisms that do not affect people whose immune systems are working normally. An example is the unusual form of pneumonia caused by *Pneumocystis carinii* often seen in individuals with AIDS.

Acquired immune deficiency syndrome (AIDS) an immune system disorder caused by the human immunodeficiency virus (HIV). Its attack on the individual's immune cells (T-cells) results in a decreased ability to fight foreign organisms, thus increasing the individual's susceptibility to a variety of opportunistic infections. AIDS is transmitted to a person from direct contact of the person's body fluids with contaminated body fluids. It is most often transmitted through sexual intercourse, contaminated needles or blood products, or from mother to infant during pregnancy or lactation. Since the early 1980s, AIDS has become a major health problem.

Many other nutrients besides proteins participate in conferring immunity, and many factors besides the antibodies are involved. The immune system is extraordinarily sensitive to nutrition, and almost any nutrient deficit can impair its efficiency and reduce resistance to disease.

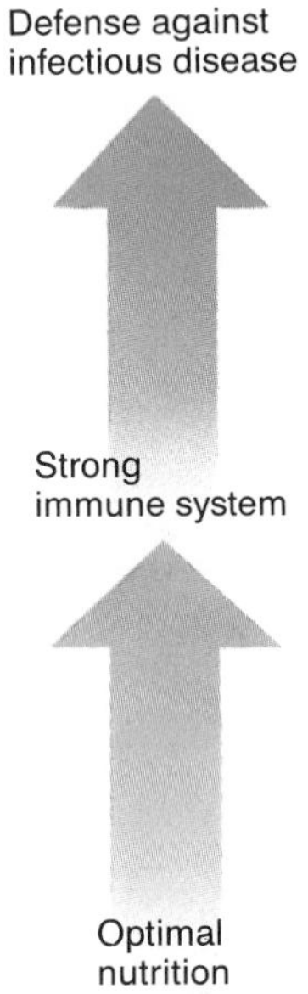

An optimal diet helps provide strength and support to the body's immune system.

Fluid Balance

Proteins help regulate the quantity of fluids in the compartments of the body to maintain the **fluid balance.** To remain alive, a cell must contain a constant amount of fluid. Too much might cause it to rupture, and too little would make it unable to function. Although water can diffuse freely into and out of the cell, proteins cannot—and proteins attract water. By maintaining a store of internal proteins, the cell retains the fluid it needs (it also uses minerals this way). Similarly, the cells secrete proteins (and minerals) into the spaces between them to keep the fluid volume constant in those spaces. The proteins secreted into the blood can't cross the vessel walls, and thus they help maintain the blood volume in the same way.

Acid-Base Balance

Normal processes of the body continually produce **acids** and their opposite, **bases**, which must be carried by the blood to the organs of excretion. The blood must do this without allowing its own **acid-base balance** to be affected. To accomplish this, some proteins act as buffers. They pick up hydrogens when there are too many in the blood (the more hydrogen, the more concentrated the acid). Likewise, protein buffers release hydrogens again when there are too few. The secret is that the negatively charged side chains of the amino acids can accommodate additional hydrogens (which are positively charged) when necessary.

The acid-base balance of the blood is one of the most accurately controlled conditions in the body. If it changes too much, the dangerous condition **acidosis** or the opposite basic condition **alkalosis** can cause coma or death. The hazards of these conditions are a result of their effect on proteins. When the proteins' buffering capacity is exceeded—for example, when proteins have taken on board or released all the acid hydrogens they can—additional acid or base deranges their structure by pulling them out of shape; that is, it denatures them. Knowing how indispensable the structures of proteins are to their functions and how vital their functions are to life, you can imagine how many body processes would be halted by such a disturbance.

Fluid balance distribution of fluid among body compartments.

Acids compounds that release hydrogens in a watery solution.

Bases compounds that accept hydrogens from solutions.

Acid-base balance equilibrium between acid and base concentrations in the body fluids.

Acidosis (a-sih-DOSE-iss) blood acidity above normal, indicating excess acid.

Alkalosis (al-kah-LOH-sis) blood alkalinity above normal.

Transport Proteins

A specific group of the body's proteins specializes in moving nutrients and other molecules into and out of cells. Some of these act as pumps—picking up compounds on one side of the membrane and depositing them on the other—and thereby decide what substances the cell will take up or release. The protein machinery of cell membranes can be switched on or off in response to the body's needs. Often hormones do the switching with a marvelous precision.

Other transport proteins move about in the body fluids, carrying nutrients and other molecules from one organ to another. Those that carry lipids in the lipoproteins are an example. Special proteins also can carry fat-soluble vitamins, water-soluble vitamins, and minerals.

These are but a sampling of the major roles proteins play in the body but should serve to illustrate their versatility, uniqueness, and importance. All the body's tissues and organs—muscles, bones, blood, skin, and nerves—are made largely of proteins. No wonder proteins are said to be the primary material of life.

Protein as Energy

Only protein can perform all the functions described above, but it will be sacrificed to provide needed energy if insufficient fat and carbohydrate are eaten. The body's number one need is for energy. All other needs have a lower priority.

Urea (yoo-REE-uh) the principal nitrogen-excretion product of metabolism, generated mostly by the removal of amine groups from unneeded amino acids or from those being sacrificed to a need for energy.
Protein-sparing a description of the effect of carbohydrate and fat, which, by being available to yield energy, allow amino acids to be used to build body proteins.

When amino acids are degraded for energy, their amine groups are usually incorporated by the liver into **urea** and sent to the kidney for excretion in the urine. The fragments that remain are composed of carbon, hydrogen, and oxygen, as are carbohydrate and fat, and these fragments can be used to build those substances or be metabolized like them.

Only if the **protein-sparing** calories from carbohydrate and fat are sufficient to power the cells will the amino acids be used for their most important function—making proteins. Thus, energy deficiency (starvation) is always accompanied by the symptoms of protein deficiency.

If amino acids are oversupplied, the body has no place to store them. It will remove and excrete their amine groups and then convert the fragments that remain to glucose and glycogen, or to fat, for energy storage. Amino acids are not stored in the body except in the sense that they are present in proteins in all the tissues. In case there is a great shortage of amino acids, tissues like the blood, muscle, and skin have to be broken down so that their amino acids can be used to maintain the heart, lungs, and brain.

How The Body Handles Protein

When a person eats a food protein, whether from cereals, vegetables, meats, or dairy products, the digestive system breaks the protein down and delivers the separated amino acids to the body cells. The cells then put the amino acids together in the order necessary to produce the particular proteins they need.

Dipeptides (dye-PEP-tides) protein fragments two amino acids long. A peptide is a strand of amino acids.
Tripeptides (try-PEP-tides) protein fragments three amino acids long.

If you need to review the digestive and absorptive systems relevant to the body's handling of protein, turn to Appendix B.

The stomach initiates protein digestion (see Appendix B). By the time proteins slip into the small intestine, they are already broken into different-sized pieces—some single amino acids and many strands of two, three, or more amino acids—**dipeptides**, **tripeptides**, and longer chains. Digestion continues until almost all pieces of protein are broken into dipeptides, tripeptides, and more free amino acids. Absorption of amino acids takes place all along the small intestine. As for dipeptides and tripeptides, the cells that line the small intestine capture them on their surfaces, split them into amino acids on the cell surfaces, absorb them, and then release them into the bloodstream.

Once they are circulating in the bloodstream, the amino acids are available to be taken up by any cell of the body. The cells can then make proteins, either for their own use or for secretion into the circulatory system for other uses (see Figure 5–5).

If a *non*essential amino acid (that is, one the body can make for itself) is unavailable for a growing protein strand, the cell will make it and continue attaching amino acids to the strand. If, however, an essential amino acid (one the cell cannot make) is missing, the building of the protein will halt. The cell cannot hold partially completed proteins to complete them later, for example, the next day. Rather, it has to dismantle the partial structures and return surplus amino acids to the circulation, making them available to other cells. If other cells do not soon pick up these amino acids and insert them into protein, the liver will remove their amine groups for the kidney to excrete. Other cells will then use the remaining fragments for other purposes. Whatever need prompted the calling for that particular protein will not be met.

Protein Quality of Foods

The role of protein in food, as already mentioned, is not to provide body proteins directly but to supply the amino acids from which the body can make its own proteins. Since body cells cannot store amino acids for future use, it follows that all the essential amino acids must be eaten as part of a balanced diet.[3] To make body protein, then, a cell must have all the needed amino acids available. Three important characteristics of dietary protein,

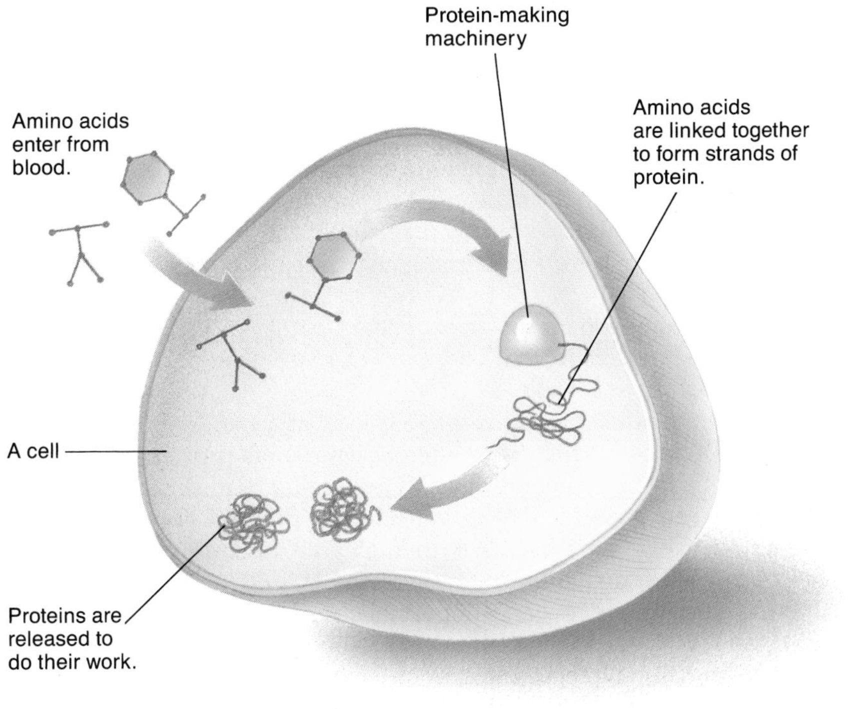
Protein-making machinery
Amino acids enter from blood.
Amino acids are linked together to form strands of protein.
A cell
Proteins are released to do their work.

Figure 5–5

How the Body Handles Protein

Amino acids from the diet or from cell breakdown travel in the blood. These amino acids can be absorbed by cells to build body proteins, as shown here, or used for energy, if needed. Liver cells can also convert part of the amino acid's structure to fat or glucose.

Complete proteins proteins containing all the essential amino acids in the right balance.

Incomplete protein a protein lacking or low in one or more of the essential amino acids.

Biological value (BV) a measure of protein quality, assessed by determining how well a given food or food mixture supports nitrogen retention.

Reference protein egg protein, the standard with which other proteins are compared to determine biological value.

Protein efficiency ratio (PER) a measure of protein quality assessed by determining how well a given protein supports weight gain in laboratory animals.

therefore, are (1) that it should supply at least the nine essential amino acids, (2) that it should supply enough other amino acids to make nitrogen available for the synthesis of whatever nonessential amino acids the cell may need to make, and (3) that it should be accompanied by enough food energy (preferably from carbohydrate and fat) to prevent sacrifice of its amino acids for energy. This presents no problem to people who regularly eat **complete proteins**, such as those of meat, fish, poultry, cheese, eggs, or milk, as part of balanced meals. The proteins of these foods contain ample amounts of all the essential amino acids, and the rest of the diet provides protein-sparing energy and needed vitamins and minerals. An equally sound choice is to eat two or more **incomplete protein** foods from plants, each of which supplies the amino acids missing in the other—also, of course, as part of a balanced meal. This strategy is described later in the chapter.

A person in good health can be expected to use dietary protein efficiently. However, malnutrition or infection can seriously impair digestion (by reducing enzyme secretion), absorption (by causing degeneration of the absorptive surface of the small intestine or losses from diarrhea), and the cells' use of protein (by forcing amino acids to meet other needs). In addition, infections cause the stepped-up production of antibodies made of protein. Malnutrition or infection may greatly increase protein needs while making it hard to meet them.

People usually eat many foods containing protein. Each food has its own characteristic amino acid balance, and together, a mixture of foods almost invariably supplies plenty of each individual amino acid. However, when food energy intake is limited, this is not the case (see "Protein-Energy Malnutrition," later in the chapter). Also, even if food energy intake is abundant, if the selection of foods available is severely limited (where a single food such as potato or rice provides 90 percent of the calories), then protein intake may not be adequate. The primary food source of protein must be checked, for its protein quality is of great importance. Researchers have studied many different individual foods as protein sources and have developed many different methods of evaluating their quality.

When amino acids are wasted, their amine groups (which contain their nitrogen) cannot be stored. Therefore, the efficiency of a protein can be assessed experimentally by measuring the net loss of nitrogen from the body. The higher the amount of nitrogen retained, the higher the quality of the protein. This is the basis for determinations of the **biological value (BV)** of proteins.

A high-quality protein by this standard is egg protein. It has been designated the **reference protein** and given a score of 100; other proteins are compared with it (see Table 5–1).

Table 5–1
Protein Scores

Protein	Chemical Score*
Eggs	100
Milk	93
Rice	86
Beef	75
Fish	75
Corn	72

*Chemical scores are derived by a method that evaluates protein quality by comparing its chemically determined amino acid composition, on paper, with human amino acid requirements.

Source: Adapted from Assessment of proteins, *Nutrition and the M.D.,* June 1985, pp. 3–4.

The **protein efficiency ratio (PER)** is used as a standard for food labeling. The U.S. RDA recommends two different daily intakes of protein, depending on the quality. If the protein is of as high a quality as milk protein (casein) or higher, then 45 grams a day is considered sufficient for an adult; if the protein's quality is lower than that, then 65 grams a day is recommended (see Figure 5–6). (See inside front cover for the U.S. RDA table.)

Protein scores are of great importance in dealing with widespread malnutrition. For the average well-fed North American, however, perhaps the most relevant lesson to be learned from them is that although animal proteins tend to have slightly higher scores than plant proteins, the two overlap con-

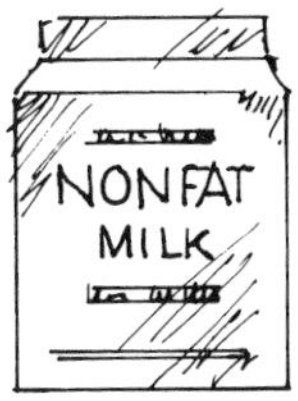

NUTRITION INFORMATION PER SERVING

SERVING SIZE	1 C
SERVINGS PER CONTAINER	2
CALORIES	90
PROTEIN, GRAMS	9
CARBOHYDRATE, GRAMS	12
FAT, GRAMS	1
SODIUM, MILLIGRAMS	135

SERVING SIZE	9½ OZ.
SERVINGS PER CONTAINER	2
CALORIES	170
PROTEIN, GRAMS	11
CARBOHYDRATE, GRAMS	28
FAT, GRAMS	1
SODIUM, MILLIGRAMS	970

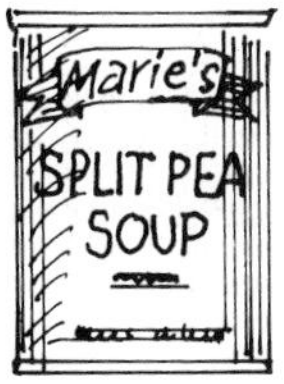

PERCENTAGE OF U.S. RECOMMENDED DAILY ALLOWANCES (U.S. RDA)

PROTEIN	20	NIACIN	0
VITAMIN A	10	CALCIUM	30
VITAMIN C	0	IRON	0
THIAMIN	2	VITAMIN D	25
RIBOFLAVIN	20	PHOSPHORUS	25

PROTEIN	15	RIBOFLAVIN	6
VITAMIN A	45	NIACIN	10
VITAMIN C	4	CALCIUM	2
THIAMIN	15	IRON	15

DIETARY FIBER PER SERVING = 4 GRAMS

INGREDIENTS: SKIMMED MILK, VITAMIN A, AND VITAMIN D.

INGREDIENTS: WATER, GREEN SPLIT PEAS, CARROTS, CELERY, SALT, ONION POWDER, SPICES.

Figure 5–6

Protein Quantity and Quality As Expressed on Nutrition Labels

According to these food labels, a serving of milk contains 9 grams of protein; a serving of split pea soup contains 11 grams. However, the quality of the milk protein is better than that of the split peas. To reflect this difference on food labels, different protein standards exist in the U.S. RDA for higher-quality protein (45 grams a day) and lower-quality protein (65 grams a day). Therefore, the percentage of the U.S. RDA standards that the split pea soup satisfies (15 percent) is lower than that for the milk (20 percent)—even though the soup contains more grams of protein per serving.

siderably. The best guarantee of amino acid adequacy is to eat mixtures of foods containing protein in the presence of adequate amounts of vitamins, minerals, and energy from carbohydrate and fat.

Recommended Protein Intakes

Recommended protein intakes can be stated in one of two ways: as a percentage of total calories or as an absolute number (grams per day). It is recommended that protein provide about 12 percent of total caloric intake.

The committee on the RDA of the Food and Nutrition Board of the National Academy of Sciences states the RDA in grams per day. It considers that a generous protein allowance for a healthy adult would be 0.8 gram per kilogram (or 2.2 pounds) of desirable body weight per day. Protein RDA for people of average heights at all ages are presented in Table 5–2. If your height is not average, you can compute your own individualized RDA for protein. Suppose your desirable weight is 50 kilograms; your protein RDA would then be 0.8 times 50, or 40 grams of protein each day.

The committee uses the desirable, not the actual, weight for a given height, because the desirable weight is proportional to the *lean* body mass of the average person. Lean body mass determines protein need. If you gain weight, your fat tissue increases in mass; but fat tissue is composed largely of fat and, as mentioned, does not require much protein for maintenance.

In setting the RDA, the committee assumes that the protein eaten would be a combination of plant and animal proteins, that it will be consumed with adequate calories from carbohydrate and fat, and that other nutrients in the diet will be adequate. The committee also assumes that the RDA will be applied only to healthy individuals with no unusual metabolic need for protein.

Table 5–2

The Protein RDA (1989)

Age (yr)	RDA (g/kg)[a]
0–½	2.2
½–1	1.6
1–3	1.2
4–6	1.1
7–14	1.0
15–18 (males)	0.9
15–18 (females)	0.8
19 and up	0.8

[a]The RDA is 10 g/day higher during pregnancy, 15 g/day higher during the first six months of lactation, and 12 g/day higher during the remainder of lactation.

Protein and Health

With all the attention that has been paid to the health effects of starch, sugars, fibers, fats, oils, and cholesterol, protein has been slighted. Protein deficiency effects are well-known because together with energy deficiency, they are the world's main form of malnutrition. But the effects of too much protein, and particularly the effects of proteins of different kinds, are far less well-known. The following sections discuss, in turn, protein deficiency, protein excess, and types of protein.

Protein-energy malnutrition (PEM), also called **protein-calorie malnutrition (PCM)** the world's most widespread malnutrition problem, including both kwashiorkor and marasmus as well as the states in which they overlap.

Kwashiorkor (kwash-ee-OR-core) a deficiency disease caused by inadequate protein in the presence of adequate food energy.

Marasmus (ma-RAZ-mus) an energy-deficiency disease; starvation.

Edema (eh-DEEM-uh) swelling of body tissue caused by leakage of fluid from the blood vessels, seen in (among other conditions) protein deficiency.

Dysentery (DISS-en-terry) an infection of the digestive tract that causes diarrhea.

Protein-Energy Malnutrition

Protein deficiency and energy deficiency go hand in hand so often that public health officials have given a nickname to the pair: **protein-energy malnutrition (PEM).** The two diseases and their symptoms overlap all along the spectrum, but the extremes have names of their own. Protein deficiency is **kwashiorkor**, and energy deficiency is **marasmus.**

Kwashiorkor is the Ghanaian name for "the evil spirit that infects the first child when the second child is born." In countries where kwashiorkor is prevalent, parents customarily give their newly weaned children watery cereal rather than the food eaten by the rest of the family. The child has been receiving the mother's breast milk, which contains high-quality protein designed beautifully to support growth. Suddenly the child receives only a weak drink with scant protein of very low quality. It is not surprising that the just-weaned child sickens when the new baby arrives.

The child who has been banished from its mother's breast faces this threat to life by engaging in as little activity as possible. Apathy is one of the earliest signs of protein deprivation. The body is collecting all its forces to meet the crisis and so cuts down on any expenditure of protein not needed for the heart, lungs, and brain. As the apathy increases, the child doesn't even cry for food. All growth ceases; the child is no larger at four than at two. New hair grows without the protein pigment that gave hair its color. The skin also loses its color, and open sores fail to heal. Digestive enzymes are in short supply, the digestive tract lining deteriorates, and absorption fails. The child can't assimilate what little food is eaten. Proteins and hormones that previously kept the fluid correctly distributed among the compartments of the body now are diminished, so that fluid leaks out of the blood (**edema**) and accumulates in the belly and legs. Blood proteins, including hemoglobin, are not synthesized, so the child becomes anemic; this increases the child's weakness and apathy. The kwashiorkor victim often develops a fatty liver, caused by a lack of the protein carriers that transport fat out of the liver. Antibodies to fight off invading bacteria are degraded to provide amino acids for other uses; the child becomes an easy target for any infection. Then **dysentery**, an infection of the digestive tract that causes diarrhea, further depletes the body of nutrients, especially minerals. Measles, which might make a healthy child sick for a week or two, kills the kwashiorkor child within two or three days.

If the child is taken into the hospital, this starved condition may not be obvious. Water in the tissues may cause the body to look almost fat. Only when the fluid balance is restored will it be seen that the child is just a skeleton thinly covered with skin.

If the condition is caught in time, a kwashiorkor child's life may be saved by careful nutrition therapy (see Figure 5–7). The fluid balances are most critical. Diarrhea will have depleted the body's potassium stores and upset other salt balances. Careful remediation of these critical balances will prevent sudden death from heart failure about half the time. Only later can nonfat

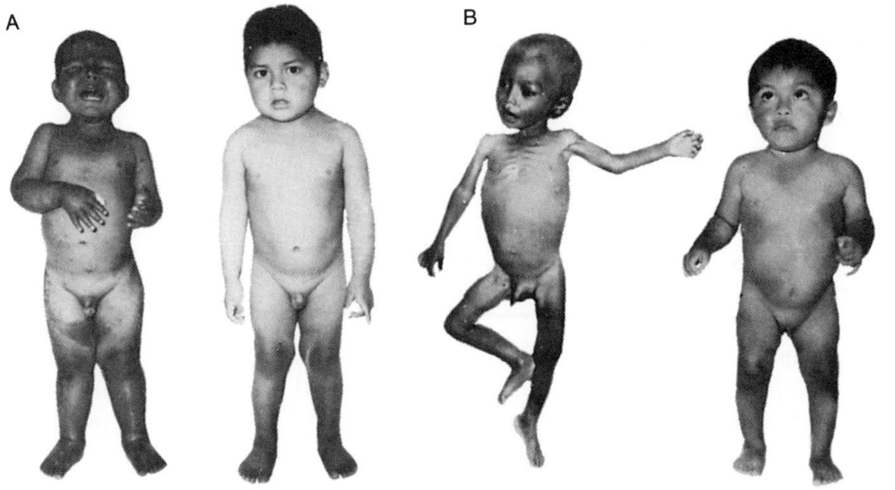

Figure 5–7

Kwashiorkor and Marasmus

A. Kwashiorkor. The child at the left has the characteristic "moon face" (edema), swollen belly, and patchy dermatitis (from zinc deficiency) often seen with kwashiorkor. At the right, the same child after nutritional therapy.
B. Marasmus. The child at the left is suffering from the extreme emaciation of marasmus. At the right is the same child after nutritional therapy.

milk containing protein and carbohydrate be safely given; then comes fat, when body protein is sufficient to provide carriers.

Children with marasmus suffer symptoms similar to those of children with kwashiorkor, since both conditions cause loss of body protein tissue, but there are differences between the two conditions. Kwashiorkor children retain some of their stores of body fat (because they are still consuming calories), accumulate fat in their livers (because they can't make protein to carry it away), and develop edema (from protein lack). Marasmus children experience **ketosis** to conserve body protein, while kwashiorkor children do not, because they are receiving some carbohydrate. Thus, kwashiorkor is actually a less balanced state and a more fatal disease than marasmus for children at any given age.

Ketosis (kee-TOE-sis) an adaptation of the body to prolonged (several days') fasting or carbohydrate restriction: body fat is converted to ketones, which can be used as fuel for some brain cells. (More about ketosis in Chapter 8.)

A marasmic child looks like a wizened little old person—just skin and bones (see Figure 5–7). The child is often sick because his or her resistance to disease is low. All the muscles are wasted, including the heart muscle, and the heart is weak. Metabolism is so slow that body temperature is subnormal. There is little or no fat under the skin to insulate against cold. The experience of hospital workers with victims of this disease is that their primary need is to be wrapped up and kept warm. They also need love, because they have often been deprived of parental attention as well as food.

Unlike the kwashiorkor child, who is fed milk until weaning, the marasmic child may have been neglected from early infancy. The disease occurs most commonly in children from 6 to 18 months of age in all the overpopulated city slums of the world. Since the brain normally grows to almost its full adult size within the first two years of life, marasmus impairs brain development and so may have a permanent effect on learning ability.

Kwashiorkor occurs not only in Ghana but also in other African countries, Central America, South America, the Near East, and the Far East. Cases have also been reported on American Indian reservations and in the inner cities of the United States. Both marasmus and kwashiorkor also occur in adults in countries where PEM is prevalent. In recent years, PEM has also been recognized in many undernourished hospital patients, including those with anorexia nervosa, AIDS, cancer, and other wasting conditions. The ex-

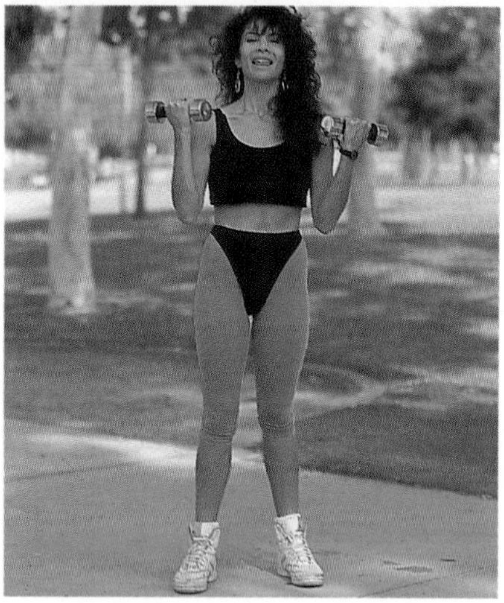

We cannot force extra protein into our muscles just by eating more of it—the way to make muscles grow is to make them work (see chapter 9).

To calculate the percentage of calories you derive from protein:

1. Use your total calories as the denominator (example: 1,900 cal).
2. Multiply your protein *grams* by 4 cal/g to obtain calories from protein as the numerator (example: 70 g protein × 4 cal/g = 280 cal).
3. Divide to obtain a decimal, multiply by 100, and round off (example: 280/1,900 × 100 = 15% cal from protein).

To figure your protein RDA:

1. Look up the desirable weight for a person your height (inside back cover). Assume this weight is appropriate for you.
2. Change pounds to kilograms (one kilogram = 2.2 pounds).
3. Multiply kilograms by 0.8 g/kg.

Example (for a 5′ 8″ medium-frame male):

1. Desirable weight: about 150 lb.
2. 150 lb ÷ 2.2 lb = 68 kg (rounded off).
3. 68 kg × 0.8 g/kg = 54 g protein (rounded off).

tent and severity of malnutrition worldwide is a political and economic problem and is discussed further in the Spotlight feature in Chapter 11.

Too Much Protein

Many of the world's people struggle to obtain enough food and enough protein to keep themselves alive, but in the developed countries, protein is so abundant that the problems of protein excess are seen. Infants and children do not adjust well to diets containing large amounts of protein; their body composition is altered.[5] Animals fed high-protein diets experience a protein overload effect, seen in the enlargement of their livers and kidneys. In human beings, high-protein diets eaten over a lifetime may cause problems in kidney function.[6] Excess protein also creates an increased demand for vitamin B_6 in the diet so that the body can utilize the protein. As a result, a deficiency of this vitamin could result.

Animals experimentally fed high-protein diets similar to those that people typically eat in the United States experience losses of zinc from their tissues as they age.[7] Such zinc excretion is also seen in pregnant women and infants on protein supplements. The use of such supplements during pregnancy may do more harm than good, even to undernourished women.[8] In infants, the use of protein supplements has been linked to deficits in cognitive development.[9]

High dietary protein also increases the tendency to obesity, a finding in direct contrast to the popular belief that such diets cause people to "burn off fat." People who wish to lose weight may lose less rapidly on a high-protein diet than on a moderate-protein diet offering the same food energy amount.[10] Protein-rich foods are often high-fat foods. The higher a person's intake of such protein-rich foods as meat and milk, the more likely it is that fruits, vegetables, and grains will be crowded out of the diet, making it inadequate in other nutrients. Diets high in protein necessitate high intakes of calcium because such diets promote calcium excretion.[11]

There are evidently no benefits to be gained by consuming excessive protein, and the committee on the RDA has suggested an upper limit for protein intake of no more than twice the RDA amount when food energy is adequate. Note the qualification, "when food energy is adequate," in the preceding statement. Remember that protein intakes are stated in two ways—as a percentage of calories and as an absolute number (grams per day). An absolute number, such as 40 grams a day for a 50-kilogram person, offers a reasonable percentage of daily calories but only if the person eats a reasonable number of calories—say, 2,000 a day. In that case, 50 grams of protein, equal to 200 calories, provide 10 percent of the total. But if the person reduces caloric intake drastically—to, say, 800 a day—then 200 calories from protein is suddenly 25 percent of the total, yet it is the same absolute number. It is still a reasonable intake, but it is the food energy intake that is not reasonable. Similarly, if the person eats far too many calories—say, 4,000—the protein intake represents only 5 percent of the total, yet it is *still* a reasonable intake. Again, it is the food energy intake that is unreasonable.

Be careful when judging protein intakes as a percentage of calories. Always ask what the absolute number of grams is, too, and compare it with the RDA or some such standard given in grams. Recommendations stated as a percentage of calories are useful only when food energy intakes are within reason.

Amino Acid Essentials

Back in 1989, Dr. Gerald Gleich had a hunch. After receiving telephone calls from several doctors baffled over the cause of a bizarre set of symptoms, including muscle pain, mouth sores, and abnormally high levels of a certain type of white cell in the blood of a handful of patients, the blood disorder expert at Minnesota's Mayo Clinic identified a suspect: a nutritional supplement called **L-tryptophan.** One of the essential amino acids, L-tryptophan has been sold in supermarkets, drug stores, health food stores, and other retail outlets and has been self-prescribed for everything from sleeping problems to depression to stress to premenstrual syndrome to drug addiction. All of the victims had been taking the supplement before their symptoms appeared.

L-tryptophan an essential amino acid that has been sold in tablets, capsules, and powders as a nutritional supplement.

Eosinophilia-myalgia syndrome a disease characterized primarily by a high level of eosinophils, a type of white blood cell, as well as myalgia—that is, muscle pain and weakness.

Dr. Gleich contacted the Centers for Disease Control, the Atlanta-based health watchdog, sparking a national investigation that confirmed his suspicions within two weeks and prompted the Food and Drug Administration to ban the supplement shortly thereafter.[12] Nevertheless, by February 1990, five months after Dr. Gleich had received the first phone calls, more than 1,200 consumers had reported similar symptoms linked to popping L-tryptophan supplements.[13] The cause of the illness, dubbed **eosinophilia-myalgia syndrome**, was later traced to an impurity that contaminated a particular manufacturer's L-tryptophan supplements.[14]

While the amino acid itself did not cause the epidemic, the case of the contaminated tryptophan underscores one of the potential hazards of self-prescribing large doses of amino acids—or any other nutrient supplement, for that matter. The Food and Drug Administration cautions that swallowing excesses of one or another of those building blocks of protein can, aside from posing the threat of contamination, be toxic and create imbalances of other amino acids in the body. That's why the FDA back in 1974 removed amino acid supplements from its list of substances that are generally recognized as safe. (The only use of amino acids approved by the FDA is their addition to foods to improve the value of an item's protein or in the making of special "medical foods" designed to be used under a physician's supervision by people who require special protein formulations because of health problems such as kidney or liver disease.)[15]

Beyond the health risks amino acid supplements pose, there are other reasons not to take such supplements. One is cost. As Table 5–3 illustrates, while special protein supplements command a high price, foods supply ample amounts of protein at a fraction of the cost. One glass of milk or three ounces of chicken, for example, provides a generous helping of all nine essential amino acids for less than half the price of a dose of most amino acid tablets, liquids, or powders. That's why it's easy for most Americans to take in with food alone more than enough protein to supply the body with all of the amino acids it requires each day.

Table 5–3

The High Cost of Protein Supplements

Food or Supplement	Amount Needed to Obtain about 15 Grams of Protein	Cost[a]
Nonfat milk	2 cups	$ .32
Tuna (canned in water)	2 ounces	.33
Twinlab Amino Fuel Liquid Concentrate	3 tablespoons	1.02
Joe Weider's Amino 2500 Capsules	30 capsules	4.99

[a] Based on 1991 prices at Boston-area stores.

Source: Manufacturers' information; J.A.T. Pennington, *Bowes and Church's Food Values of Portions Commonly Used,* 15th ed., (New York: Harper & Row), 1989.

Another reason not to take amino acids is that they don't do what their manufacturers say they do. L-tryptophan, for instance, has never been shown to relieve depression, insomnia, stress, premenstrual syndrome or any other ills its manufacturers claim it treats. The same goes for arginine, an amino acid that has been touted as "causing weight loss overnight" by stimulating secretion of a substance called human growth hormone, which in turn supposedly promotes weight loss. While it's true that arginine can prompt the release of the hormone, it will do so only when people take in whopping doses of it that are unlikely to be found in supplements. And even if a person were to take enough arginine to bring about a rush of the hormone into the body, he or she wouldn't automatically shed pounds; human growth hormone has not been found to cause weight loss. Thus, claims that arginine "burns fat" are spurious, at best. In fact, in 1978 an FDA advisory panel on over-the-counter weight-loss products investigated arginine along with 11 other amino acids touted as diet aids—namely, cystine, histidine, isoleucine, leucine, L-lysine, methionine, phenylalanine, threonine, tryptophan, tyrosine, and valine—and found no basis for claims about the effectiveness of any of them in controlling weight.

See the Spotlight feature in Chapter 1 for some tips on how to spot fraudulent nutritional products.

Despite the uselessness of amino acid supplements, it's no wonder that consumers swallow fraudulent claims about them. Many supplement manufacturers take evidence from a study or two and use it to "prove" that a particular amino acid has curative powers, a ploy used to lure people eager for simple solutions to a myriad of health problems. Some research with the amino acid lysine, for example, indicated that it could help treat herpes infections, a suggestion that has been used to hawk the substance. That evidence was based on poorly conducted studies, however, which carefully controlled research failed to confirm. Thus, lysine is not recommended by reputable professionals as a treatment for herpes.[16]

In addition to those suffering from certain ailments, athletes rank as prime targets of amino acid manufacturers. Pick up any copy of one of the bodybuilding magazines and you're likely to see ads for all manner of supplements packed with "free-form," "predigested," and "peptide-bond" amino acids touted as optimum sources of protein for athletes. Scientific-sounding names notwithstanding, such products have never been shown to increase muscle size or enhance athletic prowess. Consider that one comparison of Marine officer candidates given protein supplements with another set of trainees who received a placebo indicated that the groups performed equally well overall before, during, and after the program, regardless of supplement use or lack thereof.[17]

Finally, consumers should note that some companies reportedly sell tests costing in the neighborhood of $150 to measure the amino acid content of blood and urine. The tests are then used to help sell concoctions designed to replace the "missing" amino acids. That practice, however, is completely fraudulent; amino acid levels in the blood and urine vary greatly from day to day and have no bearing on the body's supply of or requirement for amino acids.[18]

Choose Your Protein Wisely

Misconceived notions abound regarding protein in the diet; the most obvious of these is that more is better. North Americans, on the average, consume more than 90 grams of protein daily, and about 70 percent of this protein comes from animal flesh and dairy products (see Figure 5–8).[19] As you know, saturated fats supply half or more of the calories in animal protein foods. You could better balance your food choices by selecting one-half or less of your protein from animal sources and the rest from plants.

Foods that supply protein in abundance are milk and milk products, eggs, meats, fish, poultry, and legumes (see Figure 5–9). Other vegetables and

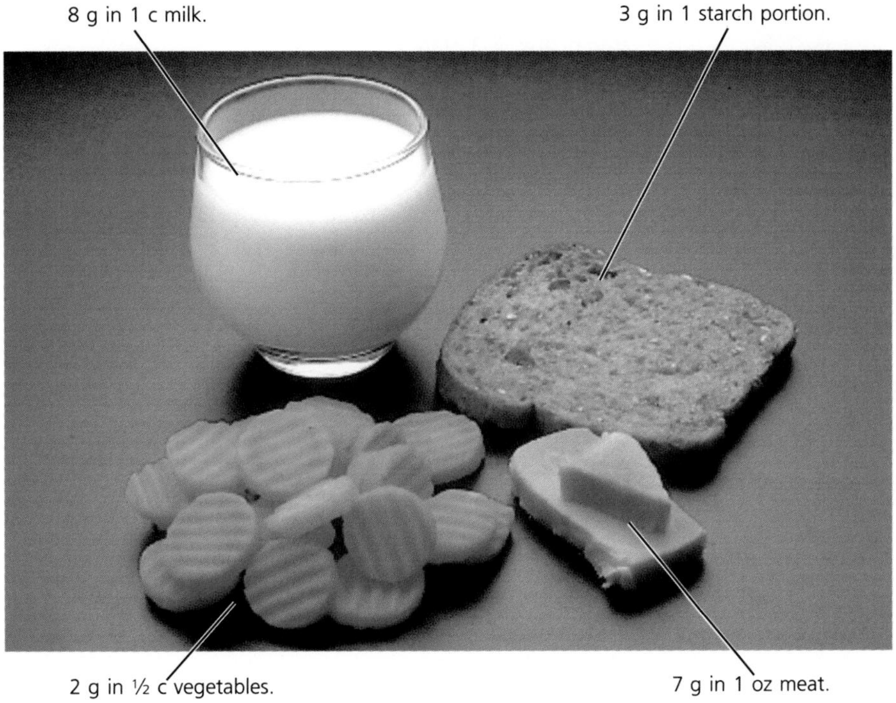
8 g in 1 c milk.
3 g in 1 starch portion.
2 g in ½ c vegetables.
7 g in 1 oz meat.

Figure 5–8

Protein Consumption in the Average American Diet

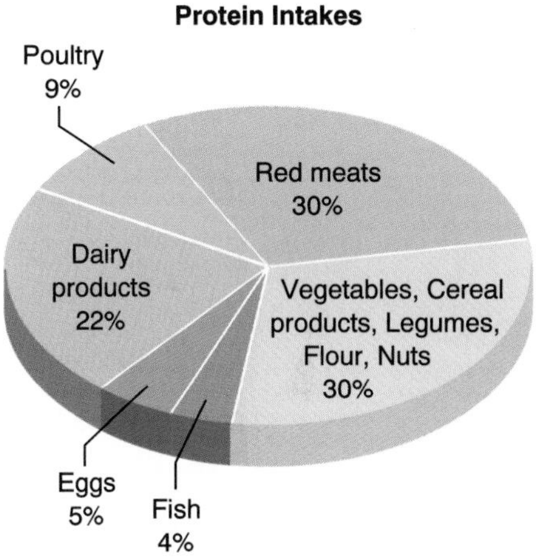

Figure 5–9

Protein in Foods

ONE EXCHANGE	GRAMS OF PROTEIN
Milk (1 c)	8
Vegetable (½ c)	2
Fruit (1 portion)	0
Bread and starchy vegetable (1 slice or ½ c)	3
Sugar	0
Meat (1 oz)	7
Fat	0

Protein Scorecard

How to Estimate Protein Intake

The values presented in Figure 5–9 provide a way to estimate the amount of protein eaten at a meal or in a day. Using those values, let us estimate the amounts of protein in the meals shown here. (These are similar to the meals used in Chapter 4's Fat Scorecard.) The fruits and fats (butter) can be assumed to contain no protein; so the only foods to inspect are the meats, milks, starch/grains, and vegetables. Peas and beans (members of the legume family) contain more protein than other vegetables do. A one-cup portion of legumes, when used as a meat alternate, is treated as having 13 grams of protein (2 portions of starch and one portion of lean meat).

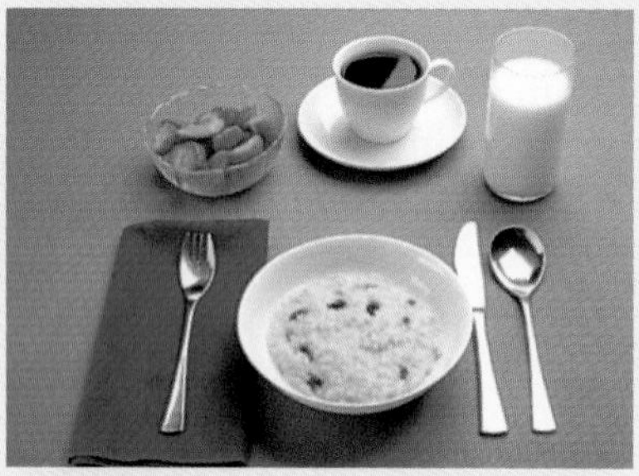

BREAKFAST	PROTEIN (g)
1 c oatmeal = 2 starch/grains	6
¼ c raisins = 2 fruits	—
1 c nonfat milk = 1 milk	8
1¼ c strawberries = 1 fruit	0

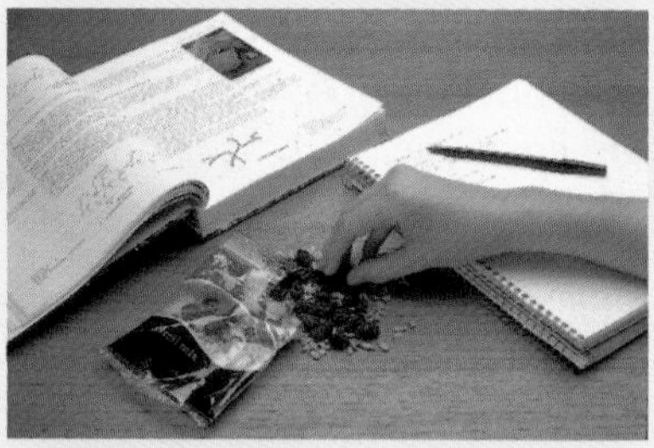

MORNING SNACK	
2 tbsp raisins = 1 fruit	—
2 tbsp sunflower seeds = 2 fats	—

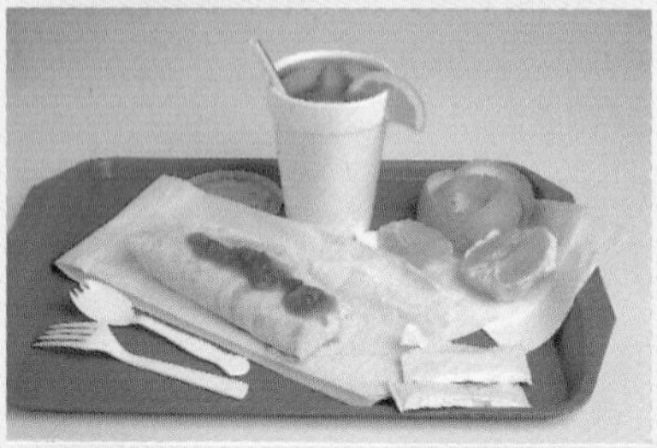

LUNCH	
1 beef and bean burrito	
(1 large tortilla = 2 starch/grains	6
⅓ c beans = 1 starch/grain	3
and ½ high-fat meat)	3½
1 packet sugar	—
1 orange = 1 fruit	—

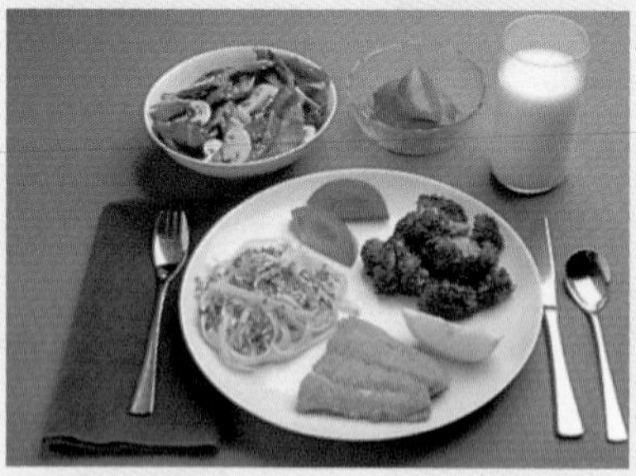

DINNER	
4 oz broiled salmon = 4 lean meat	28
1 c broccoli = 2 vegetable	4
½ c noodles = 1 starch/grain	3
2 tsp butter = 2 fats	—
¼ c parsley = ¼ vegetable	½
¼ tomato = ¼ vegetable	½
¼ c mushrooms = ¼ vegetable	½
¼ c water chestnuts = ¼ vegetable	½
1 c fresh spinach = 1 vegetable	2
1 tbsp sesame seeds = 1 fat	—
⅓ c garbanzo beans = 1 starch/grain	3
1 tbsp vinaigrette dressing = 1 fat	—
1 c nonfat milk = 1 milk	8
½ c sherbet = 2 starch/grains	6
Day's totals	82.5 grams

A total of 82.5 grams of protein times 4 calories per gram is 330 calories from protein, about 19 percent of the day's total 1,750 calories. This 82.5 grams is well above most people's RDA for protein but is not more than double that amount, and so meets the recommendation to hold protein to less than twice the RDA.

Table 5–4 **Protein Sources**

Food	Amount	Grams of Protein	Calories
These are the usual foods people think of when they think of protein:			
Cheese:			
Cheddar	1 oz	7	115
Cottage	½ c	12 to 15	85 to 130
Egg	1 large	7	80
Fish, light and dark, cooked	3 oz	20 to 25	125 to 175
Meat, cooked:			
Ground beef	3 oz	20 to 23	185 to 235
Heart, kidney, liver	3 oz	23 to 28	160 to 215
Pork	3 oz	23 to 28	310
Poultry (without skin), light and dark, cooked	3 oz	25	145 to 175
Milk:			
Nonfat	1 c	9	90
Whole	1 c	9	160
These are other good sources of protein that you could use instead:			
Vegetables, cooked:			
Broccoli	1 medium stalk	6	45
Brussels sprouts	1 c	7	55
Cauliflower	1 c	3	30
Greens	1 c	3 to 7	30 to 65
Legumes:			
Cooked	½ c	7 to 8	90 to 115
Mung sprouts, raw	½ c	2	20
Tofu (soybean curd)	4 oz	9	85
You can also get significant quantities of protein from these foods (if you can afford the calories):			
Cereal grain products:			
Barley, whole grain, cooked	½ c	4	135
Bran, unprocessed	½ c	4	55
Bran cereal (100% bran), uncooked	½ c	5	90
Breads	1 slice	2 to 3	60 to 80
Cornmeal, unrefined ground, uncooked	½ c	5	215
Millet, whole grain, cooked	½ c	3	95
Oatmeal, cooked	1 c	5	130
Pasta, enriched, cooked	1 c	5 to 7	155 to 200
Rice, cooked	1 c	4 to 5	225 to 230
Wheat, bulgur, cooked	½ c	7	225
Wheat, cracked, cooked	½ c	4	110
Wheat berries, cooked	½ c	5	110
Starchy vegetables:			
Corn	½ c	3	70
Peas	1 c	9	115
Baked potato	1 large	4	145
Winter squash, baked	1 c	4	130
Miscellaneous:			
Nut butters[a]	1 tbsp	4	95
Nuts[a]	2 tbsp	2 to 5	80 to 115
Seeds[a]	2 tbsp	3 to 5	95 to 100
Brewer's yeast	2 tbsp	6	40 to 45

[a]These items are high in fat and should be used in moderation.

Source: Adapted from Society for Nutrition Education materials.

● *Figure 5–10*

Legumes

Legumes have long been scorned by the middle class as "the poor man's meat," but they are an inexpensive, health-promoting, land-sparing, nutritious food. Bacteria in the *root nodules* can "fix" nitrogen, contributing it to the *beans*. Ultimately, thanks to these bacteria, the plant leaves in the soil more nitrogen than it takes out. So efficient at trapping nitrogen are the legumes that farmers often grow them in rotation with other crops to fertilize fields. For a variety of legumes used in cooking, see the photographs in Figure 2–8 of Chapter 2.

Legumes include:
black, Cuban, or turtle beans
black-eyed peas
garbanzo beans (chickpeas)
great northern beans
kidney beans
lentils
lima or butter beans
navy beans
peanuts
pinto beans
red beans
soybeans
split peas (green or yellow)

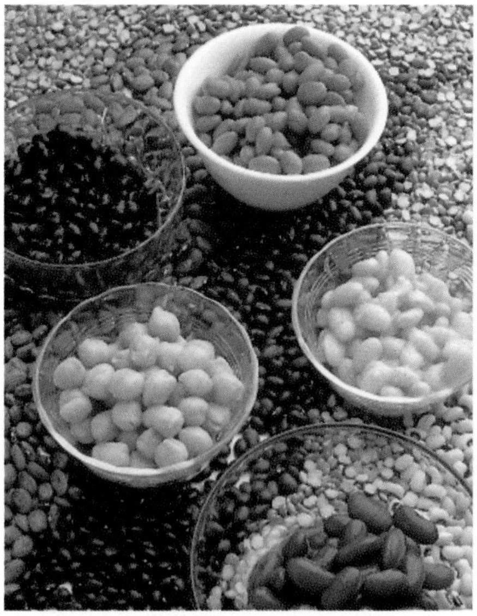

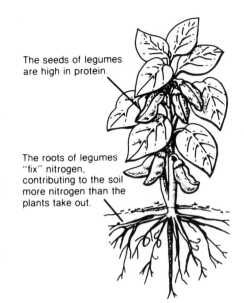

Legumes (leg-GYOOMS) plants of the bean and pea family having roots with nodules that contain bacteria that can trap nitrogen from the air in the soil and make it into compounds that become part of the seed. The seeds are rich in high-quality protein compared with those of most other plant foods.

Tofu (TOE-foo) a curd made from soybeans, rich in protein and calcium, used in many Asian and vegetarian dishes in place of meat.

grain products also contribute significant amounts of protein to the diet. As the vegetarian knows, one can easily design a perfectly adequate diet using plant foods alone by combining a variety of them appropriately. Plant foods taken together will almost inevitably supply the complete spectrum of needed amino acids as long as energy intake is also adequate and not too many nutrient-empty foods are eaten.

Adequate protein in the diet is easy to obtain, as Table 5–4 on page 141 illustrates. A breakfast of one egg, two slices of wheat bread, and a glass of milk provides close to 20 grams of protein. This meets about a third of an average man's recommended protein intake of 63 grams and almost half of an average woman's RDA for protein of 50 grams. The Protein Scorecard on page 140 shows you how to estimate your protein intake.

Many interesting sources of protein are available (see Table 5–4 on page 141). One class of protein-rich foods other than meats has already been mentioned many times: the plant family known as the **legumes** (see Figure 5–10). The protein of legumes is of a quality almost comparable to that of meat. Legumes are also excellent sources of fiber, many B vitamins, iron, calcium, and other minerals. A cup of cooked legumes contains 31 percent of the protein and 42 percent of the iron recommended daily for an adult male. Like meats, though, legumes do not offer every nutrient, and they do not make a complete meal by themselves. They contain no vitamin A, vitamin C, or vitamin B_{12}, and their balance of amino acids needs to be improved by using grains with them. This chapter's Spotlight feature discusses this concept further.

Another form in which the nutrients of soybeans are available is as bean curd, or **tofu**, a staple used in many Asian and vegetarian dishes. Thanks to the way tofu is made, it is high in calcium and can serve as a milk substitute for people who are allergic to or cannot tolerate milk.

The protein-rich, high-fiber, nutrient-dense foods from plants are most often lower in fat than animal-derived foods. People who eat mostly the former can therefore enjoy a nutritious diet that is low in fat, but only if other high-fat foods like nuts, olives, and butter are limited, too. The key to getting enough, but not too much, protein seems to be to use a variety of foods in ample quantities; to deemphasize meats; and to emphasize vegetables, grains, and nonfat milk and nonfat milk products. The Consumer Tips feature shows how to do this with various international cuisines.

Consumer Tips

Choosing Healthful International Cuisine

Every culture has its own typical foods and ways of combining foods into meals. The challenge for healthful ethnic dining is in learning to choose foods for good health without sacrificing good taste. The following tips guide you through a variety of international cuisines with this challenge in mind.

Chinese

Many Chinese dishes are based on an abundance of rice and vegetables, small portions of meat, and low-fat preparation methods, making them quite healthful. Here are a few things to look for when you buy or prepare Chinese food.

LIMIT:	TRY INSTEAD:
1. Foods prepared with whole eggs, such as lobster sauce, egg drop soup, and egg foo yung.	1. Dishes made with low-fat, cholesterol-free egg whites.
2. Fried foods, such as egg rolls, fried noodles, fried rice, "crispy" meat, poultry or fish, and fried dumplings.	2. Foods cooked using the stir-fry method with a small amount of unsaturated oil, such as chicken with broccoli, and shrimp with Chinese vegetables; or by steaming, such as dim-sum selections, and steamed dumplings.
3. Fatty foods, such as duck, goose, poultry with skin, and spare ribs.	3. Lean cuts of meat, skinless poultry, all types of fish, and shellfish—also try bean curd (tofu) to replace or enhance meat.
4. Regular soy sauce, duck sauce, plum sauce, and MSG—they are high in sodium.	4. Reduced-sodium soy sauce. Also, most Chinese restaurants will prepare food without MSG, if requested.

Japanese

Most Japanese cuisine fits into a healthful lifestyle with its emphasis on fresh fish and vegetables prepared with little fat. The basis for much of its flavor, however, is soy sauce (shoyu). This salty condiment may be a problem if you are watching your sodium intake.

LIMIT:	TRY INSTEAD:
1. Deep-fried foods, such as fish, meat, or vegetable tempura.	1. Steamed or grilled (Kushiyaki) vegetable, fish, shellfish, or skinless poultry dishes with a little tempura dipping sauce on the side.
2. Bottled prepared sauces, such as soy sauce, teriyaki, or tempura. They can be high in sodium.	2. Reducing the amount you use, switching to a reduced-sodium soy sauce, or preparing 'daikon' sauce. To make this sauce, grate fresh daikon radish, and add lemon juice, chopped green onions, and a little reduced-sodium soy (optional).
3. Commercial miso soups.	3. Preparing miso soup at home with a lower-salt miso paste.

Continued

Consumer Tips

Choosing Healthful International Cuisine

Continued

African-American

The typical African-American diet has copious amounts of healthful vegetables and whole-grain foods. Many dishes, though, also call for fatty meats and a fair amount of fat added during preparation. Try some of these alternatives.

LIMIT:	TRY INSTEAD:
1. Fried foods, such as fried chicken, fried fish, or beef livers with onions.	1. Baked, broiled, or stewed chicken (no skin); baked, broiled, or steamed fish. Eat liver (chicken or beef) only occasionally and bake or broil instead of frying.
2. High-fat cuts of meat, such as pig feet, chitterlings and hogmaws, pig tails, spare ribs, sausage, regular bacon, oxtails, goat, and ham hocks.	2. Lower-fat meats, such as skinless chicken or turkey, fish, lean stew beef, beef tenderloin, center-cut ham, Canadian bacon, pork tenderloin, and pork loin chops.
3. Vegetables and beans prepared with fat back, neck bones, salt pork, ham hocks, or coconut oil.	3. Vegetables and beans prepared with turkey parts (no skin) and selected herbs for seasoning.
4. Hominy grits with butter, baked macaroni and cheese, and home fries.	4. Hominy grits with a little margarine, baked macaroni and low-fat cheese (5 or fewer grams of fat per ounce), or baked or boiled potatoes.
5. Ice cream, frosted cake, and fruit cobbler made with lard or shortening.	5. Low-fat frozen yogurt, ice milk, fruit ice, angel food cake with fruit instead of icing, or fruit cobbler made with a small amount of liquid vegetable oil or margarine.

Hispanic

Traditionally, Hispanic foods are hearty fare, relying heavily on rice, meat, tortillas, beans, salted fish, and fats. By making some simple ingredient and preparation changes, traditional Hispanic cuisine can be more healthful as well.

LIMIT:	TRY INSTEAD:
1. Corn chips, pork skins (chicharron), and guacamole.	1. Baked tortillas, popcorn, regular salsa, or sauce made from low-fat or plain yogurt with tabasco and coriander.
2. Butter, lard, shortening, coconut oil, palm oil, and salt pork.	2. Small amounts of corn, olive, safflower, canola, sunflower, soybean, cottonseed oils, or margarine/spreads made from these oils.
3. Prepared sauces, such as sofrito and mojo criollo.	3. Homemade sofrito with a little liquid oil instead of lard. For mojo criollo, use garlic powder and seasonings, but no meat drippings.
4. Fried foods, such as fried tortillas, fried vegetable fritters (alcapurrias), banana slices (tostones), fried pork or chicken with skin, and refried beans.	4. Baked tortillas, boiled dumplings (pasteles), boiled bananas (guineo, platano), baked or broiled lean meat or chicken without skin, and boiled beans.
5. High-fat meats and salad dishes, such as roast pork (lechon asado), shrimp, tuna and lobster salads made with mayonnaise, picadillo with ground beef, and chicken stew (pollo asopao).	5. Well-trimmed roast pork, salads with reduced-calorie mayonnaise or low-fat or nonfat plain yogurt, picadillo with lean ground turkey, or chicken stew with skinless chicken.
6. Higher-fat ground beef-filled tacos, burritos, and enchiladas.	6. Lean beef-, chicken-, or bean-filled soft burritos, enchiladas, or tacos.
7. Malt beer and egg yolk (malta), coffee with cream or evaporated whole milk, and blender drinks with whole milk (batidas).	7. Plain malt beer, juice, coffee with nonfat or low-fat milk, and blender drinks with nonfat yogurt or nonfat milk.

Source: Adapted from Ethnic and Healthful, *Nutrition Counselor,* Volume VII, 1990.

Spotlight

The Vegetarian Diet

More and more people are following vegetarian diets. Their reasons for becoming vegetarian vary widely. Some have religious reasons while others have ethical reasons. Some believe that vegetarianism is ecologically sound and others, that it is less costly than the meat-eating alternative. In addition to the traditional types of vegetarians described in Chapter 2 (see page 43 for vegetarian terms), there are people who eat seafood but not other meats, and those who include chicken and other poultry but not red meat. Whatever the particular reasons, the vegetarian needs to be aware of the nutrition and health implications of the vegetarian diet.

• I've been thinking about becoming a vegetarian myself, but I'm still not sure whether vegetarianism is nutritionally sound. Is it?

The answer is yes if the vegetarian carefully plans his or her diet. Specifically, the goals for a vegetarian diet planner include the following:

- To obtain neither too few nor too many calories—that is, to maintain a healthful weight.
- To obtain adequate quantities of complete protein.
- To obtain the needed vitamins and minerals.

• Balancing calories: that sounds familiar. How can the vegetarian adjust calories to maintain a healthful weight?

The idea of balancing calories to maintain a healthful weight should be a familiar one. You may recall from Chapters 1 and 2 that balancing calories is important in everyone's diet. The vegetarian can use the special food group plan (Table 2–7 on page 46) to balance his or her diet.

• Isn't it important, too, to obtain adequate amounts of complete protein?

Yes, obtaining adequate amounts of all the essential amino acids is essential to life. Proteins from animals contain ample amounts of the essential amino acids, so the lacto-ovo vegetarian can get a head start on meeting protein needs by drinking two cups of milk daily, or by consuming the equivalent in milk products in the day's diet.

Adequate amounts of amino acids can be obtained from a plant-based diet when a varied diet is routinely consumed on a daily basis. Mixtures of proteins from unrefined grains, vegetables, legumes, seeds, and nuts eaten over the course of a day complement one another in their amino acid profiles so that deficits in one are made up by another. Since the body is able to compensate for variations in amino acid intakes from day-to-day, researchers now believe that it is not necessary to include **complementary proteins** within each meal, as proposed by the popular theory of **mutual supplementation.**[20] Table 5–5 on page 146 gives examples of how such mixtures of foods can be combined to form complete proteins.

Vegetarians should adopt a strategy of eating a wide variety of protein sources in generous servings. In so doing, they can be virtually assured of an adequate protein intake.

• If I go on a vegetarian diet, will I need to take vitamin supplements?

That depends on the kind of vegetarian diet you follow. The lacto-ovo vegetarian diet can be adequate in all vitamins, but several vitamins may be a problem for the vegan. One such vitamin is vitamin B_{12}, which doesn't occur in plant foods except in fortified foods, such as breakfast cereals or **nutritional yeast,** grown in a vitamin B_{12}-enriched environment. Brewer's yeast, baker's yeast, and live yeast are not good sources of this vitamin. The vegan needs a reliable B_{12} source, such as vitamin B_{12}-fortified soy milk or **meat replacements.** Some vegetarians use seaweeds, fermented soy, and other products in the belief that they provide vitamin B_{12} in adequate amounts, but these products are not currently recommended as reliable sources. A pregnant or lactating woman who is eating a vegan diet should be aware that her infant can develop a vitamin B_{12} deficiency that can damage the baby's nervous system, even if the mother remains healthy. The mother can remain healthy because vitamin B_{12} is stored in the body, and it may take years for a deficiency to develop.

• What other vitamins might vegans lack?

Another vitamin of concern is vitamin D. The milk drinker is protected, provided the milk is fortified with vitamin D, but there is no practical source of vitamin D in plant foods. Fortified margarines and fortified breakfast cereals can supply some vitamin D. Regular exposure to the sun will prevent a deficiency, but a person confined indoors or a vegan living in a northern climate or smoggy city probably should take vitamin D supplements. Excesses of vitamin D are toxic; don't exceed the recommended daily amount of 5 micrograms.

Riboflavin, another B vitamin obtained from milk, is present in the diet of the vegan who eats ample servings of dark greens, whole and enriched grains, mushrooms, legumes, nuts, and seeds. The vegan who doesn't eat these foods, however, may not meet riboflavin needs. Nutritional yeast is a rich source of riboflavin for the vegetarian.

Table 5–5 Nonmeat Mixtures That Provide High-Quality Protein

For the Strict Vegetarian

COMBINE			EXAMPLE
Cereal grains Barley Bulgur Oats Rice Whole-grain breads Pasta Cornmeal	+	Legumes Dried beans Dried lentils Dried peas Peanuts Soy products	Bean taco Chili and corn bread Lentils and rice Peanut butter sandwich Tofu with rice
Legumes Dried beans Dried lentils Dried peas Peanuts Soy products	+	Seeds and nuts Sesame seeds Sunflower seeds Walnuts Cashews Nut butters	Hummus (chickpea and sesame paste) Split pea soup and sesame crackers

Examples:

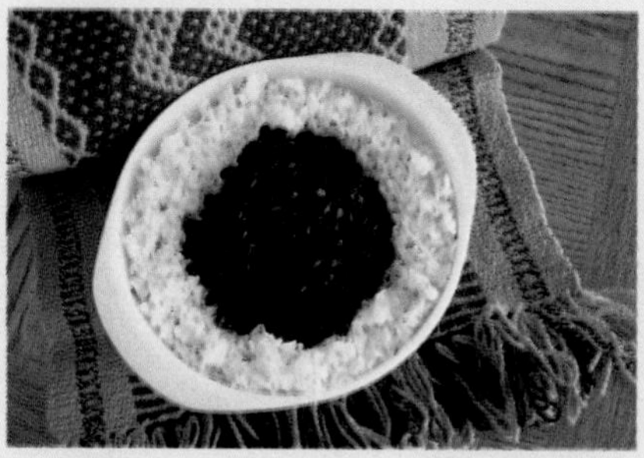
Black beans and rice.

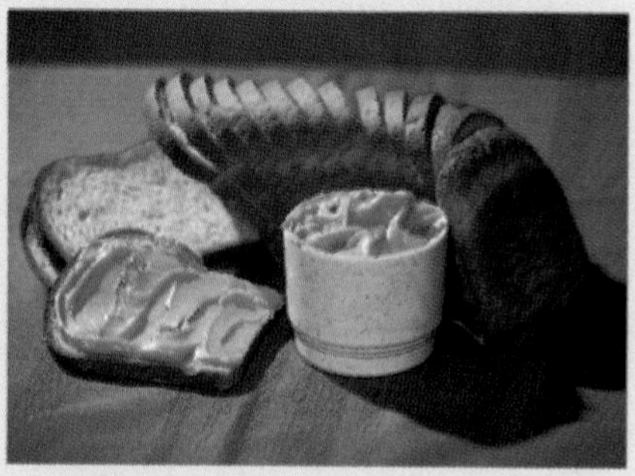
Peanut butter and wheat bread.

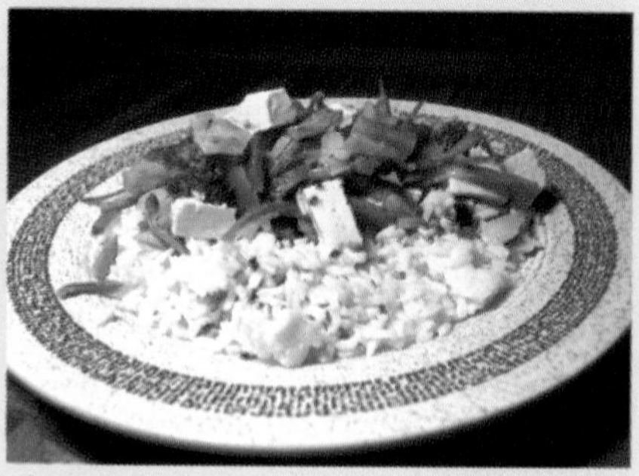
Tofu and stir-fried vegetables with rice.

For the Lacto-ovo Vegetarian

COMBINE			EXAMPLE
Eggs or milk products[a] Eggs Milk Yogurt Cheese Cottage cheese	+	Vegetable protein foods Legumes Nuts Seeds Whole grains Vegetables	Macaroni and cheese Vegetable omelet Eggplant Parmesan Broccoli with cheese sauce French toast Cereal with milk

Examples:

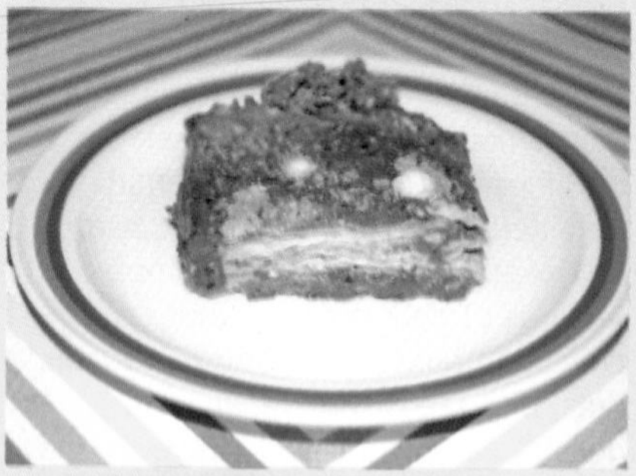
Eggplant Parmesan.

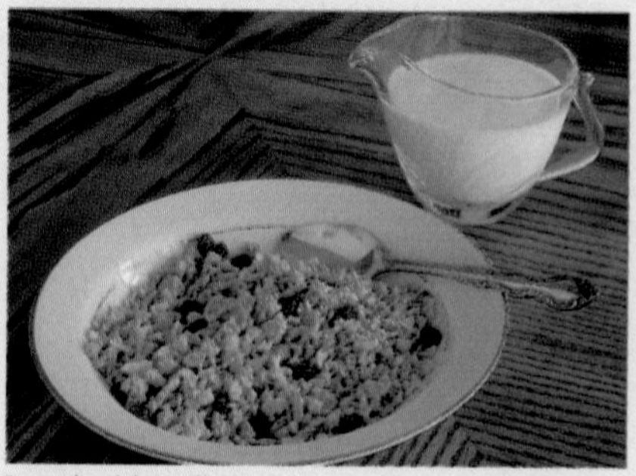
Cereal with milk.

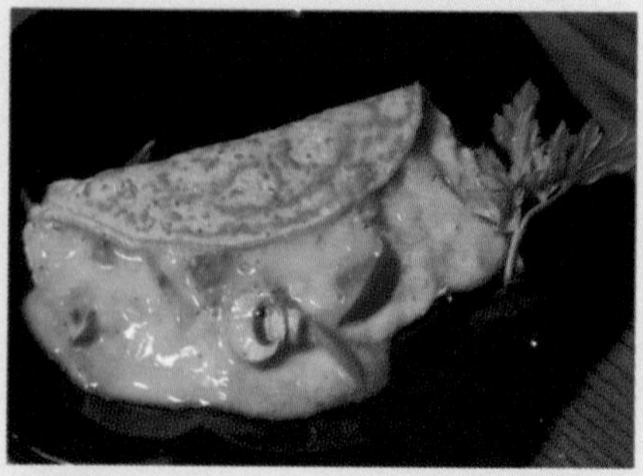
Vegetable omelet.

[a]Choose low-fat or nonfat varieties of milk and other dairy products whenever possible.

Miniglossary

Complementary proteins two or more proteins whose amino acids complement one another in such a way that the essential amino acids missing from each are supplied by the others.

Meat replacement a textured vegetable protein product formulated to look and taste like meat, fish, or poultry. Many of these are designed to match the known nutrient contents of animal protein foods.

Mutual supplementation the strategy of combining two protein foods in a meal so that each food provides the essential amino acid(s) lacking in the other.

Nutritional yeast a fortified food supplement containing B vitamins, iron, and protein that can be used to improve the quality of a vegetarian diet.

• So on a vegan diet, vitamin B_{12}, vitamin D, and riboflavin can be lacking if you're not careful. What about minerals?

Two minerals may be of concern for all vegetarians, not just for vegans: iron and zinc. Legumes, whole grains, dried fruits, nuts, and seeds are important sources of iron in the vegetarian diet. The iron in these foods, however, is not as easily absorbed by the body as that in meat. In fact, people absorb three times as much iron from a meal that includes meat as from one that does not (see Chapter 7). Because vitamin C in fruits and vegetables can triple iron absorption from other foods eaten at the same meal, vegetarian meals should be rich in foods offering vitamin C.

Zinc, too, may be a problem nutrient for vegetarians. It is widespread in plant foods, but its availability may be hindered by the fibers and other binders found in fruits, vegetables, and whole grains. The zinc needs of vegetarians and the effects of mineral binders are subjects of intensive study at the present time. While research continues, vegetarians are advised to eat varied diets that include wheat germ, legumes, nuts, seeds, and whole-grain breads well leavened with yeast. Yeast improves the availability of the minerals in the breads.

• What about minerals for the vegan? Would low intakes of calcium be a problem?

Yes, special efforts are necessary to meet calcium needs. While the milk-drinking vegetarian is protected from calcium deficiency, the vegan must find other sources of calcium. Some good sources of calcium are *regular* servings of stone-ground meal; self-rising flour and meal; some fortified breakfast cereals, flours, and brands of orange juice; legumes; tofu, calcium-fortified soy milk; some nuts, such as almonds; certain seeds, such as sesame seeds; and some vegetables, such as broccoli, collards, kale, mustard greens, turnip greens, okra, rutabaga, and Chinese cabbage (bok choy). The choices should be varied because the absorption of calcium from some of these foods is hindered by binders in them. The strict vegetarian is urged to use *calcium-fortified* soy milk *in ample quantities, regularly.* This is especially important for children. Infant formula based on soy is fortified with calcium, and adults can easily use it in cooking their foods.

• Are there any nutritional advantages to the vegetarian diet?

Yes. Vegetarian protein foods are higher in fiber, richer in certain vitamins and minerals, and lower in fat as compared to meats. Vegetarians can enjoy a nutritious diet very low in fat, provided that they eat in moderation high-fat foods like butter, oil, cheese, sour cream, and nuts. Vegetarians who follow the guidelines presented here and plan carefully can support their health as well as—or perhaps better than—nonvegetarians.

• Are you saying that vegetarians may actually be healthier than meat eaters?

Yes, abundant evidence supports that idea. Informed vegetarians are more likely to be at the desired weights for their heights and to have lower blood cholesterol levels, lower blood pressure, lower rates of certain kinds of cancer, better digestive function, and better health in other ways. Even compared with people who are health conscious, vegetarians experience fewer deaths from cardiovascular disease. Often vegetarianism goes with a healthful life-style (no smoking, abstinence from alcohol, emphasis on supportive family life, etc.), so it is unlikely that dietary practices *alone* account for all the aspects of improved health. Clearly, however, they contribute significantly to it.

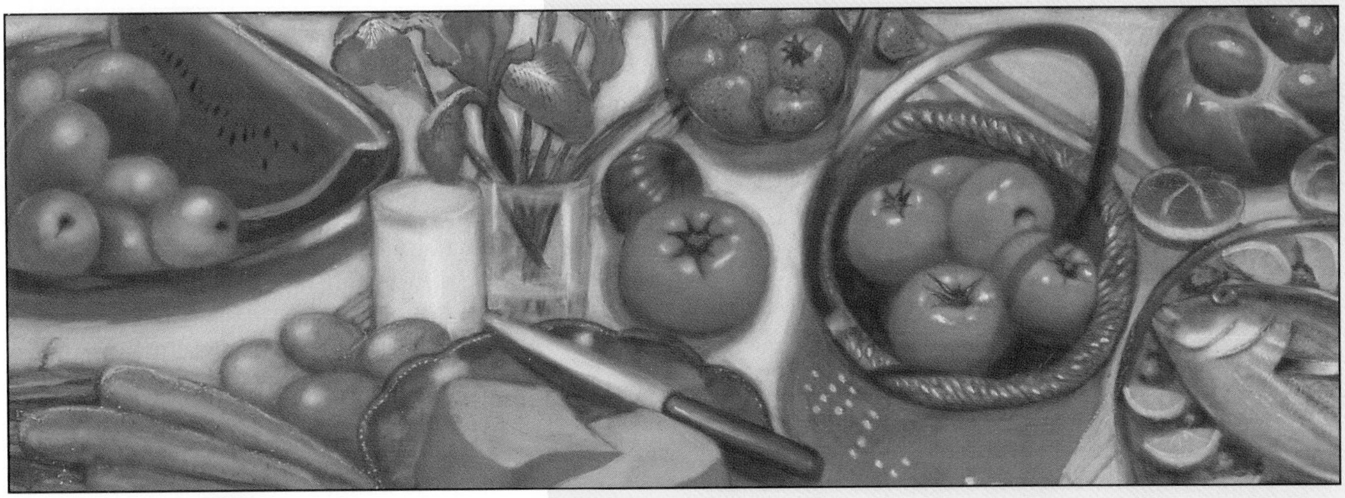

© Deborah Healy

CHAPTER 6
The Vitamins

> *The pleasure of eating . . . is of all times, all ages, all conditions. . . . Because it may be enjoyed with other enjoyments, and even console us for their absence. . . . Because its impressions are more durable and more dependent on our will. . . . Because in eating we experience a certain indescribably keen sensation of pleasure, by what we eat we repair the losses we have sustained, and prolong life.*
>
> A. Brillat-Savarin

Contents

Ask Yourself . . . ?

Which of these statements about nutrition are true, and which are false? For the false statements, what *is* true?

1. The most important role that vitamins play in the body is to provide energy.
2. There is no such thing as a diet too high in vitamins.
3. Now that science has identified all of the vitamins, it is possible to define the perfect vitamin supplement.
4. The richest sources of most vitamins, at least on a per calorie basis, are vegetables.
5. You can't overdose on water-soluble vitamins, because the body excretes excesses of them in the urine.
6. A deficiency of vitamin A can cause blindness.
7. A deficiency of vitamin E can cause heart trouble.
8. Synthetic vitamins are inferior to natural vitamins.
9. A woman who suffers pain before each menstrual period probably has a deficiency of vitamin B_6.
10. Given the choice between fresh and frozen foods, the consumer should be aware that the fresh ones are always more nutritious.

Answers: 1. False. Vitamins do not provide energy, but they enable the body to extract energy from energy-yielding nutrients. 2. False. There is such a thing as a diet too high in vitamins, especially when purified vitamins in supplements are part of it. 3. False. Even if the vitamins are all identified, it is impossible to define the perfect vitamin supplement. 4. True. 5. False. You can overdose on the water-soluble vitamins; all are toxic, at least in some people, when taken in excess. 6. True. 7. False. Research has revealed no connection between vitamin E deficiency and heart trouble. 8. False. Synthetic and natural vitamins are chemically identical, and the body cannot tell the difference between them. 9. False. Premenstrual pain is probably not nutritionally caused. 10. False. Fresh foods are not always more nutritious than frozen foods; it depends on how fresh the fresh foods are.

Since the time of the Greeks and Romans, the relationship between diet and diseases of **alimentary** origin has been recognized. Hippocrates, a Greek physician known today as the father of medicine, described a gangrene of the gums and loss of teeth among military men, a symptom of **scurvy.** This terrible disease was the scourge of traveling armies, sailors, and migrating people for many centuries.[1] Not until the sixteenth century was a cure for scurvy recorded: a beverage made from spruce needles or oranges and lemons. In 1753, James Lind, a British physician, published his famous monograph on scurvy in which he recommended eating herbs, lettuce, endive, watercress, and summer fruits to prevent bleeding gums, tooth loss, and death. By the early 1800s, sailors in the British navy were required to consume lemon or lime juice daily to avoid scurvy, earning them the nickname "limeys."[2] No one knew what caused scurvy, but they knew that consuming certain foods and beverages prevented and cured it. The foods and beverages consumed contained vitamin C.

Alimentary pertaining to food or nutrition.
alimentum = nourishment

Scurvy the vitamin C deficiency disease.

Rickets the vitamin D deficiency disease in children characterized by abnormal growth of bone and manifested in bowed legs and outward-bowed chest.

Pellagra (pell-AY-gra) the niacin-deficiency disease. Symptoms include the 4 D's—diarrhea, dermatitis, dementia, and, ultimately, death.

Rickets was likewise known to result from a poor dietary intake and has been recognized since Roman times, when physicians pondered how to prevent skeletal deformities among children. In the 1600s, the disease was so widespread among English children that it became known as the English disease. By the mid-1800s, cod liver oil was recognized as the well-known and perfect cure for rickets. The "wonder substance" contained in cod liver oil was vitamin D.

By comparison, **pellagra** has been described as a new disease, appearing in several European countries since the eighteenth century. This disease is

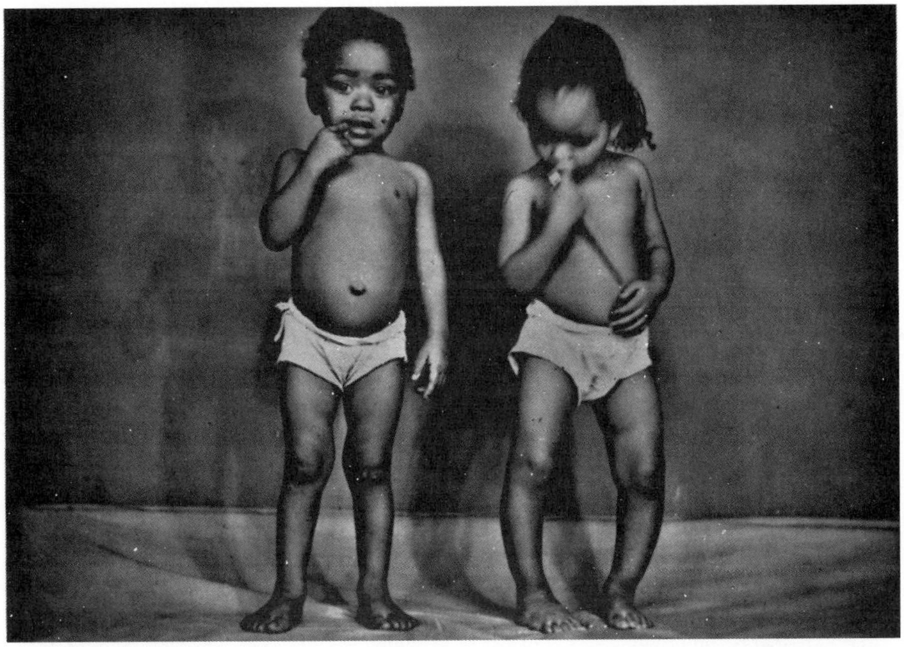

The child on the left has the characteristic protruding belly; the child on the right has the bowed legs seen in rickets.

characterized by crusty, dry, scabby, blackish patches of skin and was first described by a Spanish physician, Gaspar Casal, in 1730. Called *mal de la rosa,* it was believed to be resistant to all treatments and to be incurable. Dr. Casal observed that the peasants who developed this disease had a diet consisting primarily of corn, with very little meat. He correctly determined that the disease was the result of an inadequate diet associated with poverty. In Italy, the disease was called pellagra—from the Italian *pelle agra,* meaning sour skin—and was later determined to be the same disease as the Spanish *mal de la rosa.* The first recorded epidemic of pellagra in the United States occurred in 1906 and created considerable alarm.[3]

For centuries there was no knowledge of how dietary factors were involved in these and other diseases, although in some cases, the appropriate prevention or cure was known. By the middle of the nineteenth century, the science of chemistry had advanced to a point where foodstuffs could be analyzed with accuracy. Chemists believed that foodstuffs consisted of three main classes of organic compounds—proteins, fats, and carbohydrates—and various mineral salts, plus water. These components were shown to account for nearly 100 percent of the chemical analyses of foodstuffs, thus leading scientists to conclude that all compounds with nutritional significance had been identified.

Then in the early twentieth century, it became apparent that there were other components of foods that had nutritional significance. These newly detected substances were found in minute quantities in foods and were shown to be essential to prevent diseases and maintain health. They were called *vitamines,* a term coined in 1912 by Dr. Casimir Funk, who was attempting to identify a substance in rice bran known to cure **beriberi.** He invented this word to indicate first that these ingredients were *vital* for the survival of the organism and second that they contained nitrogen (*amines*).

Beriberi the thiamin deficiency disease characterized by loss of sensation in the hands and feet, muscular weakness, paralysis, and abnormal heart action.

Table 6–1

A Guide to the Vitamins

VITAMIN	BEST SOURCES	CHIEF ROLES	DEFICIENCY SYMPTOMS	TOXICITY SYMPTOMS
Water-soluble Vitamins				
Thiamin	Meat, pork, liver, fish, poultry, whole-grain and enriched breads, cereals, pasta, nuts, legumes, wheat germ, oats.	Helps enzymes release energy from carbohydrate; supports normal appetite and nervous system function.	Beriberi: edema, heart irregularity, mental confusion, muscle weakness, low morale, impaired growth.	Rapid pulse, weakness, headaches, insomnia, irritability.
Riboflavin	Milk, dark-green vegetables, yogurt, cottage cheese, liver, meat, whole-grain or enriched breads and cereals.	Helps enzymes release energy from carbohydrate, fat, and protein; promotes healthy skin and normal vision.	Eye problems, skin disorders around nose and mouth.	None reported, but an excess of any of the B vitamins could cause a deficiency of the others.
Niacin	Meat, eggs, poultry, fish, milk, whole-grain and enriched breads and cereals, nuts, legumes, peanuts, nutritional yeast, all protein foods.	Helps enzymes release energy from energy nutrients; promotes health of skin, nerves, and digestive system.	Pellagra: skin rash on parts exposed to sun, loss of appetite, dizziness, weakness, irritability, fatigue, mental confusion, indigestion.	Flushing, nausea, headaches, cramps, ulcer irritation, heartburn, abnormal liver function, low blood pressure.
Vitamin B_6	Meat, poultry, fish, shellfish, legumes, whole-grain products, green, leafy vegetables, bananas.	Protein and fat metabolism; formation of antibodies and red blood cells; helps convert tryptophan to niacin.	Nervous disorders, skin rash, muscle weakness, anemia, convulsions, kidney stones.	Depression, fatigue, irritability, headaches, numbness, damage to nerves, difficulty walking.
Folate	Green, leafy vegetables, liver, legumes, seeds.	Red blood cell formation; protein metabolism; new cell division.	Anemia, heartburn, diarrhea, smooth tongue, depression, poor growth.	Diarrhea, insomnia, irritability, may mask a vitamin B_{12} deficiency.
Vitamin B_{12}	Animal products: meat, fish, poultry, shellfish, milk, cheese, eggs; nutritional yeast.	Helps maintain nerve cells; red blood cell formation; synthesis of genetic material.	Anemia, smooth tongue, fatigue, nerve degeneration progressing to paralysis.	None reported.
Pantothenic acid	Widespread in foods.	Coenzyme in energy metabolism.	Rare; sleep disturbances, nausea, fatigue.	Occasional diarrhea.
Biotin	Widespread in foods.	Coenzyme in energy metabolism; fat synthesis; glycogen formation.	Loss of appetite, nausea, depression, muscle pain, weakness, fatigue, rash.	None reported.

Thus, the age of the vitamins can be said to have begun in 1912. Over the next few decades, scientists would isolate these vitamins (the *e* was dropped when it was discovered that not all of these compounds were amines). Scientists worked to establish their chemical formulas, synthesize them in the laboratory, define their biological modes of action, measure their levels in

Table 6–1
A Guide to the Vitamins—*Continued*

VITAMIN	BEST SOURCES	CHIEF ROLES	DEFICIENCY SYMPTOMS	TOXICITY SYMPTOMS
Water-soluble Vitamins				
Vitamin C	Citrus fruits, cabbage-type vegetables, tomatoes, potatoes, dark-green vegetables, peppers, lettuce, cantaloupe, strawberries, mangos, papayas.	Synthesis of collagen (helps heal wounds, maintains bone and teeth, strengthens blood vessels); antioxidant; strengthens resistance to infection; helps body's absorption of iron.	Scurvy: anemia, atherosclerotic plaques, depression, frequent infections, bleeding gums, loosened teeth, pinpoint hemorrhages, muscle degeneration, rough skin, bone fragility, poor wound healing, hysteria.	Nausea, abdominal cramps, diarrhea, breakdown of red blood cells in persons with certain genetic disorders, deficiency symptoms may appear at first on withdrawal of high doses.
Fat-soluble Vitamins				
Vitamin A	*Retinal:* fortified milk and margarine, cream, cheese, butter, eggs, liver. *Carotene:* Spinach and other dark, leafy greens, broccoli, deep-orange fruits (apricots, peaches, cantaloupe), and vegetables (squash, carrots, sweet potatoes, pumpkin).	Vision; growth and repair of body tissues; reproduction; bone and tooth formation; immunity; cancer protection; hormone synthesis.	Night blindness, rough skin, susceptibility to infection, impaired bone growth, abnormal tooth and jaw alignment, eye problems leading to blindness, impaired growth.	Red blood cell breakage, nosebleeds, abdominal cramps, nausea, diarrhea, weight loss, blurred vision, irritability, loss of appetite, bone pain, dry skin, rashes, hair loss, cessation of menstruation, growth retardation.
Vitamin D	Self-synthesis with sunlight, fortified milk, fortified margarine, eggs, liver, fish.	Calcium and phosphorus metabolism (bone and tooth formation); aids body's absorption of calcium.	Rickets in children; osteomalacia in adults; abnormal growth, joint pain, soft bones.	Raised blood calcium, constipation, weight loss, irritability, weakness, nausea, kidney stones, mental and physical retardation.
Vitamin E	Vegetable oils, green, leafy vegetables, wheat germ, whole-grain products, butter, liver, egg yolk, milk fat, nuts, seeds.	Protects red blood cells; antioxidant (protects fat-soluble vitamins); stabilization of cell membranes.	Muscle wasting, weakness, red blood cell breakage, anemia, hemorrhaging, fibrocystic breast disease.	Interference with anticlotting medication, general discomfort.
Vitamin K	Bacterial synthesis in digestive tract, liver, green, leafy and cabbage-type vegetables, milk.	Synthesis of blood-clotting proteins and a blood protein that regulates blood calcium.	Hemorrhaging.	Interference with anticlotting medication; may cause jaundice.

various foods, and determine human and animal requirements for these compounds. It is a process that continues today.

To the modern biologist, then, a **vitamin** is a potent, indispensable, noncaloric **organic** compound that performs specific and individual functions to promote growth or reproduction or to maintain health and life. Every minute

Vitamin a potent, indispensable, noncaloric organic compound that performs specific and individual functions to promote growth or reproduction or to maintain health and life.
Organic of, related to, or containing carbon compounds.

vitamins are hard at work in your body, keeping nerves and skin healthy; contributing to growth; building blood, bones, and teeth; healing wounds; and converting food energy to body energy. They make no contribution of energy (calories) themselves, nor do they contribute building material. They do, however, enable energy metabolism and the building of body structures to go on. In short, they serve as helpers, or facilitators, of body processes.

Various amounts of vitamins and minerals are needed in the diet for health and well-being. Generally, a balanced diet of ordinary foods supplies enough, but not too much, of each of the vitamins and minerals. An unbalanced diet can be lacking in several of these nutrients, and the person who takes supplements can easily overdose. A goal for the wise eater is to learn enough about food composition to be able to select the full range of these nutrients.

Based on solubility, vitamins fall into two categories: those dissolving in water (water-soluble) and those dissolving in fat or oil (fat-soluble). To date there are thirteen recognized vitamins, each with its own special roles to play (see Table 6–1 on page 152). Nine are water-soluble, and four are fat-soluble. This distinction has many implications for the kinds of foods they are found in as well as for the way the body absorbs, transports, stores, and excretes them. The water-soluble vitamins are the more fragile of the vitamins, and large proportions of these vitamins naturally present in foods may be washed out or destroyed during food storage, processing, or preparation (see tips for preserving nutrients in foods later in this chapter).

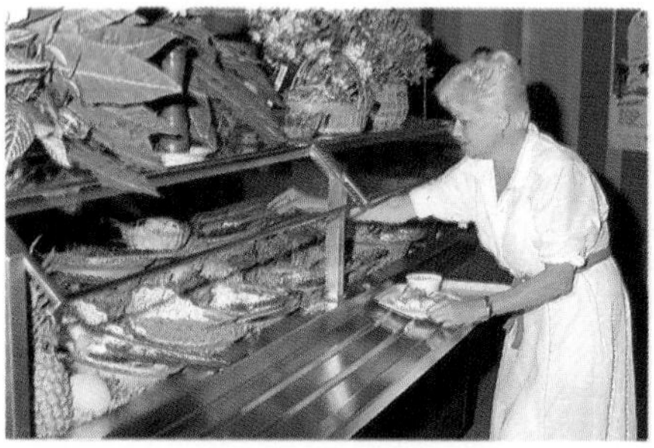

To achieve superb nutritional health, you need much more than a vitamin tablet. You need nutritious foods in variety and abundance.

Water-soluble Vitamins

The B vitamins and vitamin C are water-soluble vitamins. These vitamins are found in the watery compartments of foods, and they are distributed into water-filled compartments of the body. They can be excreted if their blood concentrations rise too high. As a consequence, they are unlikely to reach toxic levels in the body. This is not to say, however, that they cannot have negative effects. Most water-soluble vitamins have now been shown to have toxic effects, at least in some people, when taken in extremely large doses.

The water-soluble vitamins act as **coenzymes**—that is, they assist enzymes in doing their metabolic work within the body. Figure 6–1 shows how a coenzyme works.

Coenzymes enzyme helpers, small molecules that work with enzymes and enable them to do their work. Many coenzymes are made from water-soluble vitamins.

Thiamin

The principal function of thiamin is to act as a coenzyme in the reactions that release energy from carbohydrate. Thiamin is a typical vitamin in that its presence is not felt, but its absence makes itself known all over the body—in the nerves, muscles, heart, and other organs. A severe thiamin deficiency, called beriberi, causes extreme wasting and loss of muscle tissue, swelling all over the body, enlargement of the heart, irregular heartbeat, and paralysis. Ultimately, the victim dies from heart failure. A mild thiamin deficiency can mimic other conditions and typically manifests itself as vague, general symptoms: stomach aches, headaches, fatigue, restlessness, disturbances of sleep, chest pains, fevers, personality changes (aggressiveness and hostility), and a group of symptoms often classed as neurosis. What is especially interesting about a mild thiamin deficiency is that it is most likely to be seen in con-

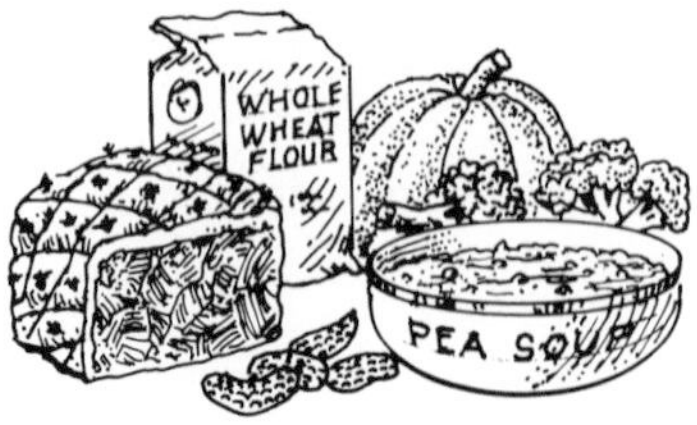

Thiamin: most nutritious foods contribute about 10 percent of daily thiamin need per serving.

sumers of diets containing large amounts of foods low in nutrients and high in calories, sugar, fat, and salt. Research has shown that a group of people who snacked heavily on empty-calorie foods had a thiamin-requiring enzyme in their blood that was not functioning normally. When these people took thiamin supplements for a month or more, the blood enzyme activity returned to normal.[4]

Thiamin is unique among the vitamins in that there is almost no one food that will supply your daily need in a single serving. For example, to meet your daily vitamin C need, you can include a serving of citrus fruit in your diet. But thiamin is evenly distributed in foods, is easily lost during food processing, and so is delivered in adequate amounts only to people who eat *ten or more servings of nutritious foods each day.* To add up your intake of thiamin or any other nutrient mentioned here, turn to Appendix F. To compare your total with the amount recommended, turn to the inside front cover.

Table 6–2 (page 170) shows the thiamin content of foods commonly eaten. Those richest in thiamin per serving are pork, ham, bacon, and legumes (peas and beans). Large servings of these contribute large amounts of food energy. However, thiamin doesn't come at a low calorie cost in these foods. A food is a thiamin bargain if it contributes more thiamin relative to your need for this vitamin than it contributes calories relative to your need for them. By this definition, many vegetables are thiamin bargains. Because thiamin cannot be stored and is used up in the metabolism of energy nutrients, foods that provide it should be eaten every day.

Riboflavin

Like thiamin, riboflavin acts as a coenzyme in energy-releasing reactions. Riboflavin also helps prepare fatty acids and amino acids for breakdown. Riboflavin deficiencies are rare and are characterized by severe skin problems, including painful cracks at the corners of the mouth; a red, swollen tongue; and teary or bloodshot eyes.

Table 6–3 (page 170) shows the riboflavin content of foods. Milk, milk products such as cheese, and organ meats dominate the list, with a few meats and vegetables scattered among them. Dark-green vegetables such as broccoli, spinach, and asparagus are good riboflavin bargains because they are low in calories. For adequate intakes of riboflavin, people can depend on generous servings of many different kinds of vegetables. Two cups of cooked broccoli, for example, offer 0.64 milligram of riboflavin at a calorie cost of 92 calories, whereas an 8-ounce sirloin steak offers 0.70 milligram, but at a calorie cost of 480. Clearly, for most people, broccoli is the better riboflavin buy. Most people derive about one third of their riboflavin from milk and milk products, about a fourth from meats, and most of the rest from leafy green vegetables and whole-grain or enriched bread and cereal products.

Riboflavin is light sensitive; it can be destroyed by the ultraviolet rays of the sun or fluorescent lamps. For this reason, milk is seldom sold in transparent glass containers and should not be stored in them. Cardboard or plastic containers protect the riboflavin in the milk from ultraviolet rays.

Niacin

Like thiamin and riboflavin, niacin is part of a coenzyme vital to obtaining energy. Without niacin to form this coenzyme, energy-yielding reactions

● *Figure 6–1*

How a Coenzyme Works

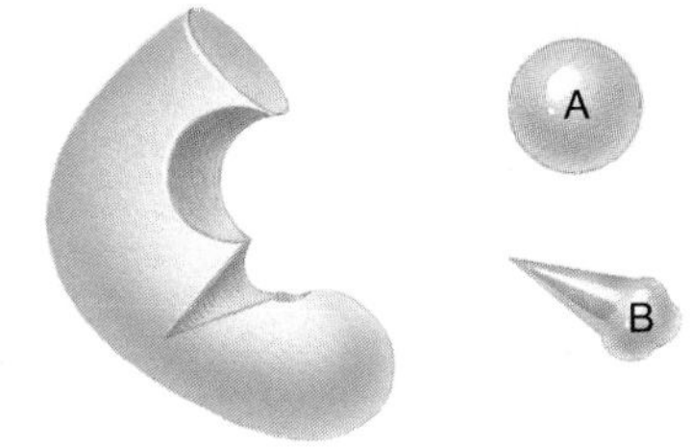

Without the coenzyme, compounds A and B don't respond to the enzyme.

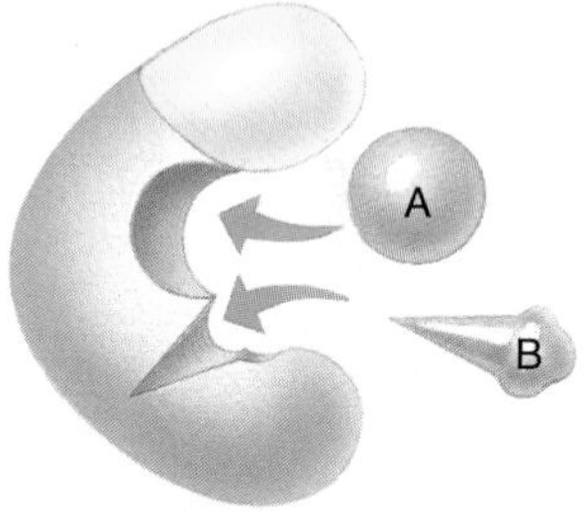

With the coenzyme in place, A and B are attracted to the active site on the enzyme, and they react.

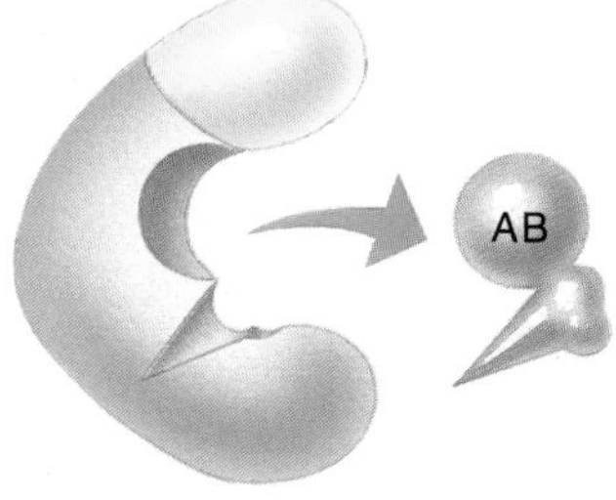

The reaction is completed.

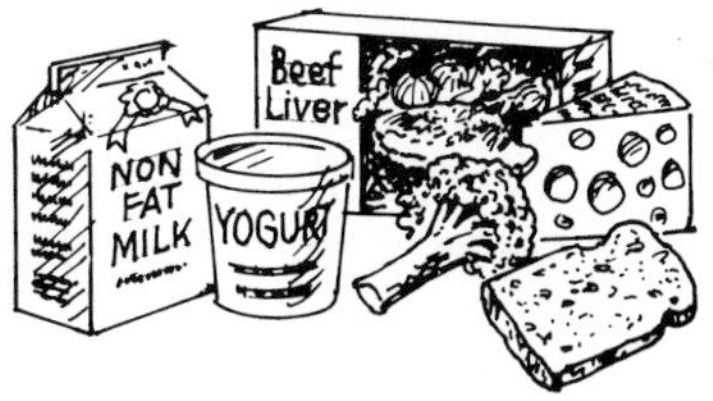

Riboflavin: milk contributes about 33 percent; meat, about 25 percent; and whole-grain or enriched breads and cereals, additional amounts. The person who does not drink milk should substitute large amounts of dark-green vegetables.

come to a halt. A deficiency of niacin is called pellagra and results, as discussed previously, in diarrhea, dermatitis, and, in severe cases, dementia. The dementia of pellagra can be described as a progressive mental deterioration resulting in delirium, mania, or depression.

Niacin equivalents the amount of niacin present in food, including the niacin that can theoretically be made from its precursor tryptophan present in the food.

Recommended niacin intakes are stated in **niacin equivalents**, a term that requires explanation. Niacin is unique among the B vitamins in that it can be obtained both as niacin itself and from another nutrient source—protein. The essential amino acid tryptophan can be converted to niacin in the body; 60 milligrams of tryptophan yield 1 milligram of niacin. Niacin equivalents are the amounts of niacin present in food, including the niacin that can theoretically be made from the tryptophan present in the food. Thus, the RDA for niacin is expressed as milligrams of niacin equivalents (NEs) required in the diet.

Milk, eggs, meat, poultry, and fish contribute about half the niacin equivalents consumed by most people, and about one third comes from enriched breads and cereals. Table 6–4 (page 170) shows that fish and poultry are at the top of the list of niacin sources. Broccoli and other greens are among the richest vegetable sources (per calorie).

Folate

Anemia any condition in which the blood is unable to deliver oxygen to the body cells, such as a shortage or abnormality of the red blood cells. Many nutrient deficiencies and diseases can cause it.

Folate (also called folic acid or folacin*) is a coenzyme with many functions in the body. It is particularly important in the metabolism of amino acids. A deficiency affects the red blood cells, making them misshapen and unable to carry sufficient oxygen to all the body's other cells, a kind of **anemia.** Thus, the effects of folate deficiency are felt as a generalized misery with many symptoms, including fatigue, diarrhea, irritability, forgetfulness, lack of appetite, and headache. Folate deficiency can easily be confused with general ill health, depressed mood, and senility in the elderly. It is most likely to occur in pregnant women and those between 20 and 44 years of age.

One reason that folate deficiency is so widespread is that folate is found predominantly in fresh foods, especially vegetables. It is easily lost when foods are overcooked, canned, dehydrated, or otherwise processed. Moreover, anyone who is growing has extremely high folate requirements. The need for folate rises dramatically during pregnancy, for example. The RDA table doubles the daily folate recommendation during pregnancy.† Pregnant teenagers, who are themselves still growing, need even more folate than pregnant adults.

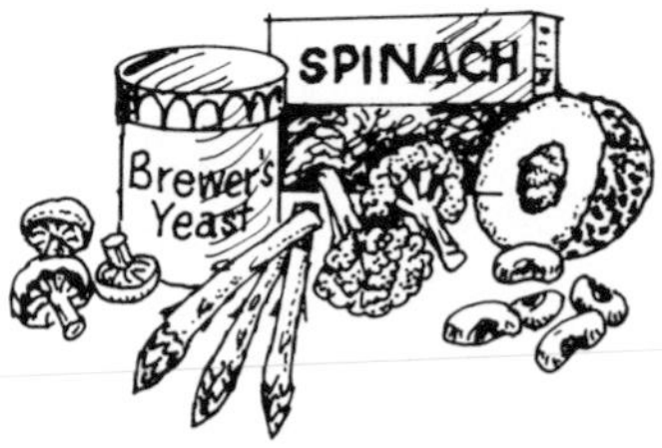

Folate is most abundant in fresh foods.

Folate is abundant in vegetables, legumes, and seeds, as shown in Table 6–5 (page 170). Milk, milk products, and meats are not outstanding sources of this vitamin. On a per calorie basis, leafy vegetables stand out as good sources of folate.

Vitamin B_6

Vitamin B_6, which also functions as a coenzyme, is an indispensable cog in the body's machinery. For example, vitamin B_6 plays many roles in protein

*The folates are a group of chemically related compounds; folic acid is the biologically active form of the molecule. The term folacin is no longer widely used.

†Recommended folate intakes are stated in micrograms (μg). A microgram is a thousandth of a milligram, or a millionth of a gram. The RDA for folate, 200 μg, can also be stated as 0.2 mg.

metabolism. In fact, if a diet is high in protein, additional vitamin B_6 is needed to process that protein. Older people may have an increased need for vitamin B_6 because of their slower synthesis of some key enzymes. Because vitamin B_6 performs so many tasks, the price of a deficiency is a multitude of symptoms. True vitamin B_6 deficiencies occur in some people who eat inadequate diets and whose nutrient needs are higher than usual due to pregnancy, alcohol abuse, some disease conditions, the use of certain prescription medications, or other unusual circumstances.

People who take large amounts of vitamin B_6 are at risk for developing signs of toxicity. Whenever people start taking **megadoses** of a nutrient—believing that if a little of the nutrient is good, more must be better—it is only a matter of time before effects of toxic overdosing occur. This happened in the 1970s with vitamin C after the publication of the popular book *Vitamin C and the Common Cold.*[5] In the 1980s it happened with vitamin B_6.

The first major report of toxic effects of vitamin B_6 appeared in 1983, when physicians reported the stories of seven individuals who had been taking more than 2 grams—more than 2,000 times the RDA—of vitamin B_6 daily for two months or more, most of them attempting to cure the edema of **premenstrual syndrome (PMS)**.[6]* All seven cases were similar. They started with numb feet, then lost sensation in their hands, then became unable to work. Later, in some cases, their mouths became numb. They may have suffered irreversible nerve damage. At the last report, although the symptoms had been clearing up after withdrawal of the supplements, they had not completely disappeared. Since then, controlled studies have failed to demonstrate any benefit of vitamin B_6 in relieving the symptoms of PMS.[7] Other reports have shown nervous system damage from more moderate doses of vitamin B_6.[8]

Not everyone is likely to suffer toxicity symptoms with a vitamin B_6 megadose. Because it is excreted in the urine, vitamin B_6 is a relatively nontoxic nutrient, but individual tolerances vary, and megadoses are therefore not safe. This holds true for every vitamin.

Table 6–6 (page 170) shows the vitamin B_6 content of foods. Meats, legumes, vegetables, fruits, and grains all offer vitamin B_6, but the foods richest in the vitamin on a per calorie basis are clearly the vegetables. The generalization is gaining strength that vegetables, if eaten in sufficient quantities, can provide significant amounts of many nutrients.

Megadoses doses ten or more times higher than the amounts normally recommended (see RDA, inside front cover). An overdose is an amount high enough to cause toxicity symptoms. Megadoses taken over long periods are often overdoses.

Premenstrual syndrome (PMS) a cluster of physical, emotional, and psychological symptoms that some women experience seven to ten days prior to menstruation. Symptoms may include acne, anxiety, appetite changes, back pain, breast tenderness, cramps in the abdomen, depression, fatigue, food cravings, especially for sweets, headaches, irritability, mood changes, water retention, and weight gain.

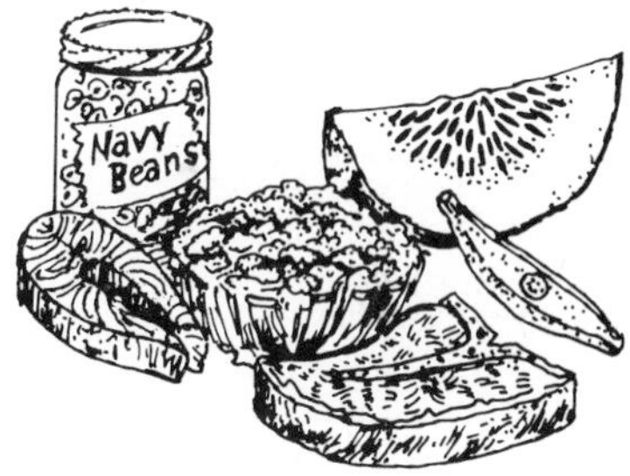

Vitamin B_6 is found in meats, vegetables, and whole-grain (but not enriched) cereals.

Vitamin B_{12}

Two of vitamin B_{12}'s functions are well known. Vitamin B_{12} enables folate to help manufacture red blood cells and it maintains the sheaths that surround and protect nerve fibers. A deficiency of vitamin B_{12} results in an anemia that is not easily distinguished from that of a folate deficiency. The anemia is characterized by large, immature red blood cells; either folate or vitamin B_{12} will clear up this condition. However, a deficiency of vitamin B_{12} causes not

*The exact cause of PMS is not known. Perhaps for this reason, the field is ripe for the sale of vitamin/mineral supplements designed to relieve premenstrual symptoms. In a study of the nutritional status of 38 women suffering from PMS compared with 23 control subjects, there was no evidence that premenstrual syndrome was caused by nutritional deficiencies of vitamins or minerals. M. Mira and coauthors, Vitamin and trace element status in premenstrual syndrome, *American Journal of Clinical Nutrition* 47 (1988): 636–641.

only anemia but also a creeping paralysis of the nerves and muscles due to the vitamin's role in nerve cell growth and maintenance. This latter symptom is not detectable from a blood test, and the paralysis cannot be remedied by administering folate. Early detection and correction are necessary to prevent permanent nerve damage and paralysis. Because excess folate can mask the lack of vitamin B_{12}, the amount of folate in over-the-counter preparations is limited by law to an amount that is too low to mask vitamin B_{12} deficiency.

Vitamin B_{12} is unique among the nutrients in being found almost exclusively in animal flesh and animal products. Anyone who eats meat, milk, cheese, and eggs is guaranteed an adequate intake. Microorganisms make their own vitamin B_{12}, so yeast grown in a vitamin B_{12}-enriched environment is also a good source. Strict vegetarians who do not eat meat, eggs, or dairy products must use vitamin B_{12}-fortified soy milk or other such products or take vitamin B_{12} supplements to avoid deficiency.

Pantothenic Acid and Biotin

Two other B vitamins—pantothenic acid and biotin—are needed for the synthesis of coenzymes that are active in a multitude of body systems. Biotin is also required for cell growth, DNA synthesis, and maintenance of blood glucose levels. Since both pantothenic acid and biotin are widespread in foods, people who consume a variety of foods are not at risk for deficiencies. Claims that pantothenic acid and biotin are needed in pill form to prevent or cure disease conditions are at best unfounded and at worst intentionally misleading.

Vitamin C

Collagen the characteristic protein of connective tissue.
kolla = glue
gennan = to produce

Vitamin C is required for the production and maintenance of **collagen**, the protein foundation material for connective tissues in the body such as bones, teeth, skin, and tendons. Vitamin C also protects against infections, and some research suggests that it may protect against cancer of the stomach and esophagus as well.[9] In addition, the vitamin promotes the absorption of iron. In fact, eating foods containing vitamin C at the same meal with foods containing iron can double or triple the absorption of iron from those foods.

Despite the widespread availability of vitamin C-rich foods, a deficiency of vitamin C is occasionally seen in the United States in bottle-fed infants receiving no vitamin C in formula or fruit juice and in the elderly. Surveys have shown that cigarette smokers and persons with an inadequate food supply due to low income are at increased risk of having a poor vitamin C status. Table 6–7 (page 170) shows the amounts of vitamin C in various common foods. The citrus fruits are rightly famous for their vitamin C content, but many vegetables and some other fruits are in the same league: broccoli, Brussels sprouts, greens, cabbage, cantaloupe, and strawberries. A single serving of any of these foods provides more than 30 milligrams, a half a day's supply, of the vitamin.

The humble potato is an important source of vitamin C in Western countries, not because a potato by itself meets the daily needs, but because potatoes are such a popular food and are eaten so frequently that overall they make substantial contributions to vitamin C levels. Potatoes provide about 20 percent of all the vitamin C in the U.S. diet.

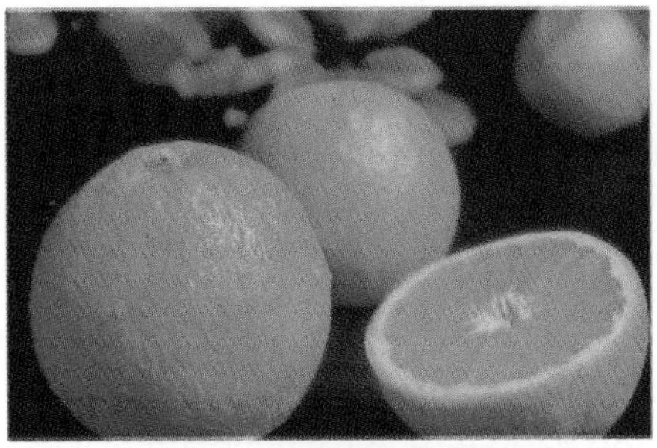

When nutritionists say "vitamin C," people think "oranges" . . .

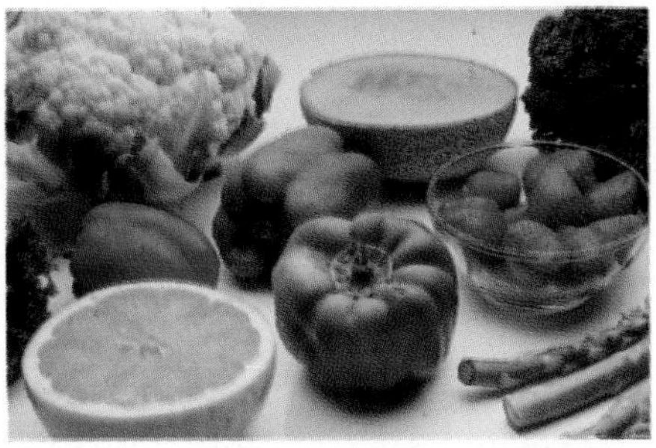

But these foods are just as rich in vitamin C for their calorie cost.

Some people believe that large intakes of vitamin C will help the body cope with stress and prevent or cure the common cold. Is there any truth to this? It's true that in times of stress, the body uses more vitamin C, mainly because the vitamin is involved in the release of the stress hormones from the adrenal gland. Even so, the amount of extra vitamin C used up during stress is very small and well within the safety margin of the RDA. Generous servings of vitamin C-rich fruits and vegetables will more than cover your needs during high-stress periods.

Interest in vitamin C as a cure for the common cold grew with the publication of Linus Pauling's controversial book, *Vitamin C and the Common Cold* (referenced in footnote 5). Some individuals were motivated to take megadoses exceeding 2 grams—or 30 times the RDA—of vitamin C a day. Well-designed clinical experiments have not shown a benefit to taking vitamin C to prevent or cure the common cold. In addition, large intakes of the vitamin can affect the accuracy of some medical tests for detecting diabetes or colon cancer. Excessive amounts of vitamin C can result in side effects such as nausea, abdominal cramps, and diarrhea, and can increase your risk for gout (a condition in which uric acid is deposited in the joints).

Fat-soluble Vitamins

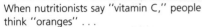

Vitamins A, D, E, and K are generally found in the fats and oils of foods and are absorbed from the digestive tract with the aid of fats in the diet and bile produced by the liver. Therefore, any disorder that interferes with fat digestion or absorption can precipitate a deficiency of the fat-soluble vitamins. Once in the bloodstream, these vitamins are escorted by protein carriers because they are insoluble in water. Since they are stored in the liver and in body fat, you need not consume them daily unless your intakes are typically marginal. Consider the RDA an *average* amount needed per day. However, it is possible for megadoses of the fat-soluble vitamins to build up to toxic levels in the body and cause undesirable side effects.

Vitamin A

Vitamin A has the distinction of being the first fat-soluble vitamin to be identified. It is one of the most versatile vitamins, playing roles in several important body processes.

The best known function of vitamin A is in vision. For a person to see, light reaching the eye must be transformed into nerve impulses that the brain

Pigment a molecule capable of absorbing certain wavelengths of light. Pigments in the eye permit us to perceive different colors.

Retina (RET-in-uh) the layer of light-sensitive cells lining the back of the inside of the eye.

Retinal (RET-in-al) the form of vitamin A that is active in the pigments of the eye.

Night blindness slow recovery of vision after flashes of bright light at night; an early symptom of vitamin A deficiency.

Epithelial (ep-ih-THEE-lee-ull) tissue those cells that form the outer surface of the body and line the body cavities and the principal passageways leading to the exterior. Examples include the cornea, digestive tract lining, respiratory tract lining, and skin.

Preformed vitamin A vitamin A in its active form.

Precursor a compound that can be converted into another compound. For example, carotene is a precursor of vitamin A.
pre = before
cursor = runner, forerunner

Beta-carotene an orange pigment found in plants.

Chlorophyll the green pigment of plants which traps energy from sunlight and uses this energy in photosynthesis (the synthesis of carbohydrate by green plants).

interprets to produce visual images. The transformers are molecules of **pigment** in the cells of the **retina.** A portion of each pigment molecule is **retinal,** a compound the body can synthesize only if vitamin A is supplied by the diet in some form. When vitamin A is deficient, the eye has difficulty in adapting to changing light levels. A flash of bright light at night (after the eye has adapted to darkness) will be followed by a prolonged spell of **night blindness.** Because night blindness is easy to test, it aids in the diagnosis of vitamin A deficiency. Night blindness is only a symptom, however, and may indicate a condition other than vitamin A deficiency.

Vitamin A serves other roles in the body as well. It helps maintain healthy skin and **epithelial tissue**—that is, the cells (called epithelial cells) lining such body cavities as the small intestine. It is also involved in the production of sperm, the normal development of fetuses, the immune response, hearing, taste, and growth.

Up to a year's supply of vitamin A can be stored in the body, 90 percent of it in the liver. If you stop eating good food sources of vitamin A, deficiency symptoms will not begin to appear until after your stores are depleted. Then, however, the consequences are profound and severe.

Because vitamin A is stored in the body, toxicity can also occur. Symptoms include joint pain, dryness of skin, hair loss, bleeding, loss of appetite, irritability, fatigue, headaches, weakness, nausea, and liver damage. That's why it's especially important not to take megadoses of this nutrient.

Normally, it is possible to suffer toxicity symptoms only when excess amounts of **preformed vitamin A** from supplements are taken. The **precursor, beta-carotene,** available from plant foods, does not convert to vitamin A rapidly enough to cause toxicity, but is instead stored in fat depots as carotene.

Table 6–8 shows the vitamin A content of various kinds of foods. The major vitamin A contributors are almost all brightly colored—green, yellow, orange, and red. Any plant food with significant vitamin A activity must have some color, since the vitamin and its plant precursor carotene are colored compounds themselves (vitamin A is a pale yellow; carotene is a rich, deep yellow, almost orange). The dark-green, leafy vegetables contain large amounts of the green pigment **chlorophyll,** which masks the carotene in them.

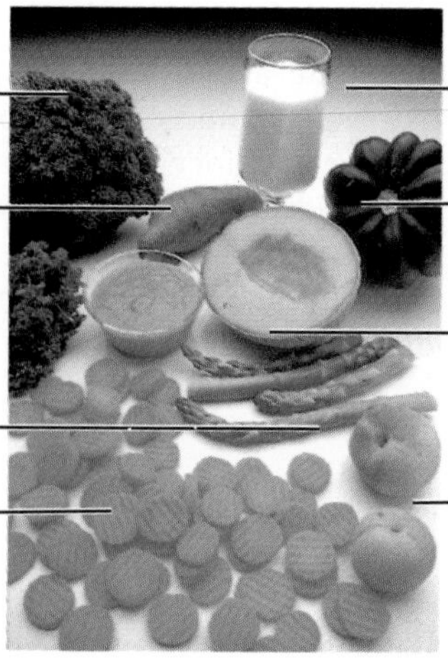
Broccoli 220 RE per cup
Sweet potato 2488 RE per potato
Asparagus 150 RE per cup
Carrots 3830 RE per cup
Fortified milk 149 RE per cup
Butternut squash 1435 RE per cup
Cantaloupe 861 RE per ½ melon
Apricots 280 RE per 3 apricots

Some foods rich in vitamin A: broccoli, sweet potato, fortified milk, butternut squash, cantaloupe, apricots, carrots, and asparagus. A man's RDA for vitamin A is 1,000 RE; a woman's is 800 RE.

About half of the vitamin A in foods consumed in the United States comes from fruits and vegetables, and half of this comes from the *dark* leafy greens (such as broccoli and spinach, but not iceberg lettuce or green beans) and the *rich*-yellow or *deep*-orange vegetables (such as winter squash, carrots, and sweet potatoes, but not corn or bananas). The other half of the vitamin A activity comes from milk, cheese, butter, and other dairy products, eggs, and a few meats, such as liver. When whole milk is processed to produce nonfat milk, the vitamin is lost, since vitamin A is fat-soluble. Thus, nonfat milk is fortified to supply about 40 percent of the RDA per quart to compensate.* The butter substitute margarine is fortified to provide vitamin A equivalent to that in butter.

The safest and easiest way to meet your vitamin A needs, then, is to consume generous servings of a variety of dark-green and deep-orange vegetables and fruits (see Table 6–8). The fruit and vegetable family's importance for meeting vitamin A needs is reflected in the recommendation that adults have at least four servings a day, including at least one dark-green or deep-orange item every other day. Recall that folate and vitamin C, too, are found most abundantly in fruits and vegetables, so these foods meet more than one need.

Traditional fast foods are notable for their *lack* of vitamins A, C, and folate. Anyone who dines frequently on hamburgers, French fries, shakes, and the like is advised to emphasize vegetables heavily (but not just salads) at other meals. However, consumer demand for salad bars in fast-food places has made vitamin A, folate, and vitamin C available where they once were lacking.

Table 6–8

Vitamin A in Foods

Adult RDA is 800 to 1,000 RE.

(mg)	SOURCES
9,120	Beef liver (3 oz)
2,488	Sweet potato (1)
2,025	Carrot, fresh (1)
1,474	Spinach, cooked (1 c)
1,435	Butternut squash (1 c)
872	Winter squash (1 c)
861	Cantaloupe (½)
806	Mango (1)
792	Turnip greens, cooked (1 c)
612	Papaya (1)
437	Bok choy, cooked (1 c)
325	Tomatoes, cooked (1 c)
253	Apricot halves, dried (10)
220	Broccoli, cooked (1 c)
176	Watermelon (1 slice)
150	Asparagus, cooked (1 c)
149	Nonfat milk or yogurt (1 c)
146	Romaine (1 c)
139	Tomato, fresh (1)
86	Cheddar cheese (1 oz)
54	Sole/flounder (3 oz)

Vitamin D

Vitamin D is a member of a large bone-making and maintenance team composed of several nutrients and other compounds, including vitamin C; hormones; the protein collagen; and the minerals calcium, phosphorus, magnesium, fluoride, and others. The special function of vitamin D is to assist in the absorption of dietary calcium and to help make calcium and phosphorus available in the blood that bathes the bones so that these minerals can be deposited as the bones harden.

Vitamin D is different from other nutrients in that the body can synthesize the amount it needs with the help of sunlight. In a sense, therefore, it is not essential to obtain vitamin D from the diet. Another unique feature of vitamin D is that it acts very much like a hormone—a compound manufactured by one organ of the body that has effects on another.

The liver manufactures a vitamin D precursor, which is converted to vitamin D with the help of the sun's ultraviolet rays. The liver alters the molecule, and the kidney alters it further to produce the active vitamin. This is why diseases affecting either the liver or the kidney may lead to bone deterioration.

The precursor of vitamin D is made from cholesterol in the liver. This is one of the body's many "good" uses for cholesterol.

The symptoms of an inadequate intake of vitamin D are those of calcium deficiency. The bones fail to gain normal strength and may be so weak that

*Fortification of milk in Canada follows a similar standard. Milks and margarines must also be fortified with vitamin D.

they bend when they have to support the body's weight. A child with insufficient vitamin D characteristically develops bowed legs, which are often the most obvious sign of the deficiency disease rickets (refer to the photograph on page 151). Worldwide, rickets afflicts many children.

> **Osteomalacia (os-tee-o-mal-AY-shuh)** the vitamin D deficiency disease in adults.
> *osteo* = bone
> *mal* = bad (soft)
> Osteomalacia may also occur in calcium deficiency (see Chapter 7).

Adult rickets, or **osteomalacia**, occurs most often in women who have low calcium intakes and little exposure to sun and who go through several pregnancies and periods of lactation.

Vitamin D deficiency depresses calcium absorption and results in low blood calcium levels and abnormal maturation of bone. An excess of vitamin D does the opposite. It increases calcium absorption, causing abnormally high concentrations of the mineral in the blood, and promotes the return of bone calcium into the blood as well. Excess calcium in the blood tends to precipitate in the soft tissue, forming stones. This is especially likely to happen in the kidneys, which concentrate calcium as they excrete it.

Exposure to sun should be moderate. Excessive exposure may cause skin cancer.

There are two ways to meet your vitamin D needs. You can synthesize it yourself with the help of sunlight, or you can eat foods containing the preformed vitamin. Only a few animal foods supply significant amounts of the vitamin—notably eggs, liver, and some fish. Even in these, the vitamin D content varies greatly. Neither cow's milk nor human breast milk supplies enough vitamin D to meet human needs reliably. Hence, cow's milk is fortified, and infants must be given either fortified formula or supplements.

Most adults, especially in the sunnier regions, need not make special efforts to obtain vitamin D in food. People who are not outdoors much or who live in northern or predominantly cloudy or smoggy areas, however, are advised to make sure their milk is fortified with vitamin D, to drink at least two cups a day, and to occasionally make use of eggs and fortified products such as breakfast cereals and margarine in menu planning.

Cholecalciferol on an ingredients list refers to vitamin D.

Daily doses of vitamin D are not necessary, because excesses are stored. Extreme care in supplementation is called for, since vitamin D is the most toxic of all vitamins. As little as four to five times the recommended daily intake can create an overdose. Fish liver oil, taken by some people for its vitamin or fatty acid content, can deliver an overdose of vitamin D.

Vitamin E

> **Antioxidant** a compound that protects others from attack by oxygen by itself reacting with the oxygen.

Many substances found in foods and important in the body can be destroyed by oxygen. An example is the fat in vegetable oil, which can turn rancid when exposed to air (oxygen). Vitamin E is an **antioxidant**—that is, it reacts with oxygen and so prevents other substances, such as vegetable oil, from doing so. Vitamin E in cell membranes protects the lipids in the membranes; it is especially effective in preventing the destruction of polyunsaturated fatty acids (PUFA), but it protects other lipids as well. One of the most important places in the body in which vitamin E exerts its antioxidant effect is in the lungs, because the exposure of cells to oxygen is maximal there. Vitamin E also protects the lungs from oxidizing air pollutants.

In the rare situation when vitamin E intake is deficient and the blood concentration falls below a certain critical level, the red blood cells tend to break open and spill their contents, probably because of oxidation of the PUFA in their membranes. Abnormal environmental conditions, such as air pollution, may increase human vitamin E needs. A great many diseases can affect people's vitamin E needs also. Among individuals who benefit from vitamin E supplementation are premature infants; infants, children, or adults who cannot absorb fats and oils because of diseases of the intestinal tract or other conditions; and individuals with certain blood disorders, including sickle cell anemia. Two other human conditions appear to be lessened by supplemental vitamin E. One, a benign but uncomfortable disorder, is characterized by painful lumps in the breasts. The other, a leg problem, causes pain on walking and cramps in the calves at night. In each of these situations, need for supplemental vitamin E should be diagnosed and recommended by a physician.

Many extravagant claims were made for vitamin E during the 1960s and 1970s. Vitamin E was said to improve athletic endurance and skill, to increase sexual potency and enhance sexual performance, to prolong the life of the heart, and to reverse the damage caused by atherosclerosis and heart attacks. Vitamin E was also thought to prevent or cure hereditary muscular dystrophy. It was said to have an effect on other processes of aging, such as graying of the hair, wrinkling of the skin, development of "age spots," and reduced activity of body organs. An immense amount of experimentation has discredited these and many similar claims.

Despite these facts, many people take vitamin E supplements. As a result, numerous signs of toxicity are now known or suspected, including interference with the action of vitamin K and some hormones, alteration of the mechanism of blood clotting, alteration of blood lipid levels, and impairment of white blood cell activity.

Vitamin E is widespread in foods. About 60 percent of the vitamin E in the diet comes from vegetable oils and products such as margarine, salad dressings, and shortenings. Another 10 percent comes from fruits and vegetables; smaller percentages come from grains and other products. Soybean oil and wheat germ have especially high concentrations of vitamin E. Cottonseed, corn, and safflower oils rank second, with a tablespoon of any of these supplying more than 10 milligrams (more than the RDA) of the vitamin. Animal fats, such as butter and milk fat, have negligible amounts of vitamin E. Vitamin E is readily destroyed by heat processing and oxidation, so fresh or lightly processed foods are preferable as sources of this vitamin.

Vitamin K

Vitamin K acts primarily in the blood-clotting system, where its presence can mean the difference between life and death. At least 13 different proteins and the mineral calcium are involved in making blood clot. Vitamin K is essential for the synthesis of at least four of these proteins. When *any* of the blood-clotting factors is lacking, blood cannot clot, and hemorrhagic disease and excessive bleeding upon injury result. (Hemorrhaging is not always the result of vitamin K deficiency.) Vitamin K also participates with vitamin D in synthesizing a bone protein that helps to regulate blood calcium levels.

K stands for the Danish word *koagulation* ("coagulation" or "clotting").

Toxicity is not common but can result when water-soluble forms of vitamin K are given, especially to infants or pregnant women. Toxicity symptoms include red cell breakage, jaundice, and brain damage.

Vitamin K can be made within your digestive tract but not by your body. Bacteria in the digestive tract can synthesize vitamin K which is then absorbed. You are not dependent on bacterial synthesis for your vitamin K, however, because many foods also contain ample amounts of the vitamin. Green, leafy vegetables, members of the cabbage family, and milk are notable sources of vitamin K.

The bacterial inhabitants of the digestive tract are known as the **intestinal flora.**
flora = plant inhabitants

Vitamin K deficiency seldom occurs except when unusual combinations of circumstances bring it about. People taking sulfa drugs or other antibiotics for a long period of time may become deficient in vitamin K, for instance, because these drugs destroy some intestinal bacteria. When vitamin K deficiency does occur, however, it can be fatal. This is one reason why a person's clotting time is checked before surgery is performed.

New babies, incidentally, are commonly susceptible to a vitamin K deficiency for two reasons. First, a baby's digestive tract is sterile until birth and then gradually becomes populated by the normal intestinal bacteria. Second, a baby may not be fed adequate amounts of vitamin K at the outset. Breast milk is a poorer source of vitamin K than fortified infant formula. A dose of vitamin K, usually in a water-soluble form, is therefore given at birth to prevent hemorrhagic disease of the newborn.

A very high intake of vitamin K can reduce the effectiveness of drugs used to prevent the blood from clotting. People taking anticoagulants should therefore use moderation in eating foods high in vitamin K, especially liver, lettuce, broccoli, and other leafy vegetables.

With the publication of the 10th edition of the *Recommended Dietary Allowances,* an RDA for vitamin K was established for the first time. Based on

Vegetable Variety Scorecard

The more varied the kinds of vegetables you eat, the better nourished you are likely to be—and because vegetables are, on the whole, much lower in calories for their bulk than are meats, cheeses, and other animal foods, the less likely you are to have a weight problem.

Put a check mark by each vegetable that you have eaten within the past year. Then add up your check marks. A score of 60 or more is excellent and 45 to 60 is good. Any score below that leaves room for improvement.

Acorn squash
Alfalfa sprouts
Asparagus
Beet greens
Beets
Black-eyed peas
Broccoli
Brussels sprouts
Butternut squash
Cabbage
Carrots
Cauliflower
Celery
Chinese cabbage (Bok choy)
Collard greens
Corn
Cucumbers
Dandelion greens
Eggplant
Endive
Escarole
Garbanzo beans (chickpeas)
Green peas
Green peppers
Kale
Kidney beans
Kohlrabi
Lentils
Lettuce
Lima beans
Lotus root
Mung bean sprouts
Mushrooms
Mustard greens
Navy beans
Okra
Onions
Parsley
Parsnips
Pinto beans
Pumpkin
Radishes
Rhubarb
Romaine lettuce
Rutabaga
Soybean sprouts
Spinach
Split peas
String beans
Summer squash
Sweet potato
Swiss chard
Tomatoes
Turnip greens
Turnips
Turtle beans
Vegetable juices
Water chestnuts
Watercress
Wax beans
White potato
Winter squash
Yam
Yam bean root
Zucchini
Lotus root
Other: ______
______

Is there such a thing as eating too many vegetables? Yes, but in our society such a thing is so rare as to be hardly worth mentioning. Children in developing countries, and even vegan children in this country, may receive so many bulky plant foods that they suffer a calorie deficit. Even then, it may not be necessary or desirable to reduce the vegetable intake. Probably a better solution to this problem is to add a small amount of a high-calorie food such as oil to the diet.

the results of recent research, the RDA for vitamin K was set at 1 microgram per kilogram of body weight. This level of intake should be adequate to maintain normal blood clotting in adults.

Nonvitamins

A variety of substances have been mistaken for essential nutrients for human beings because they are needed for growth by bacteria or other forms of life. Among them are PABA (para-aminobenzoic acid), the bioflavonoids (vitamin P or hesperidin), and ubiquinone. Other nonvitamins include vitamin B_{15} (a hoax),[10] vitamin B_{17} (laetrile, a fake cancer cure and not a vitamin by any stretch of the imagination), and vitamin B_T (carnitine, an important piece of cell machinery, but not a vitamin). Three other such compounds, sometimes called B vitamins, are inositol, lipoic acid, and choline, all of which are essential nutrients for animals. Inositol and lipoic acid are not required in the human diet, but some researchers have suggested that choline is actually an essential nutrient for adult humans, especially when the availability of the amino acid methionine and the vitamin folate in the diet is low.[11] More research is needed to fully establish choline's role as an essential nutrient for humans.

Non-B Vitamins

Bioflavonoids
Hesperidin
Laetrile
PABA (para-aminobenzoic acid)
Pangamic acid
Ubiquinone
Vitamin B_5
Vitamin B_{15}
Vitamin B_{17}
Vitamin B_T
Vitamin P

Consumer Tips

Eleven Steps to Preserving Vitamins

Getting the most vitamin nutrition from foods is neither difficult nor time consuming, but it does require knowledge of proper food-handling procedures to preserve the vitamin content. Here are a few tips about fresh foods—particularly fruits and vegetables—to keep in mind:

At the supermarket—purchasing foods

- Choose the freshest fruits and vegetables available.
- Discard produce that is bruised or otherwise damaged.
- Skip over the precut fruits and vegetables.
- Shop as frequently for fresh produce as is reasonable. And buy only as much as you can eat in a few days.

At home—storing foods

- When you get home, immediately store fruits and vegetables in the refrigerator to slow down the enzymatic degradation of the vitamins in these foods.
- If you slice or cut a fruit or vegetable, cover it with an airtight wrapper and store it in the refrigerator to help prevent oxidation and deterioration.
- If you elect to freeze fresh vegetables, dip them first in boiling water for a minute to destroy enzymes that would otherwise remain to attack nutrients. When they cool down, freeze them in plastic containers or freezer bags. Meats should be wrapped to exclude air before freezing.

At home—cooking for maximum nutrition

- When cooking vegetables, use a minimum amount of water. Remember that water-soluble vitamins readily dissolve into the water in which cut vegetables are washed, boiled, or canned.
- To minimize vitamin loss, steam vegetables over water rather than in it or boil them in a very small amount of water.
- Reserve the liquid in canned vegetables for use in making soups, rice, or casseroles.
- During cooking, minimize the destruction of vitamins by avoiding high temperatures and long cooking times.

NUTRITION ACTION

Selecting a Vitamin-Mineral Supplement

Media advertisements would have you believe that you can transform yourself from a tired and overstressed person to a trim and vibrant picture of health with only a little effort. How? Just take Super-Premium Vitamin-Mineral Supplement. If only life were so simple. As you might have surmised by reading this chapter, vitamins are key contributors to physical fitness, but they are not miracle workers—and neither are the minerals which are discussed in the next chapter. Achieving and enjoying health and well-being require much more than a supplement. You need adequate amounts of other nutrients—energy-yielding nutrients, minerals, and water—as well as adequate sleep, exercise, and a positive attitude, to name only a few other necessary elements of a healthful lifestyle.

Considering that a balanced, nutritious diet is the cornerstone for health, it's surprising to learn that many people are confused about how to go about constructing an ideal diet. Is it enough to eat the RDA of all nutrients? If the RDA amounts are good, is more better? Given that billions of dollars are spent on vitamin-mineral supplements in the United States each year, it's clear that many people believe that more *is* better. Some people take a single, daily vitamin-mineral pill as a kind of nutrition insurance—just in case they get overstressed during the day or start to feel ill. Other people take huge stock-piles of nutrient supplements. (See the accompanying miniglossary for a description of foods or food components consumed regularly as supplements by some individuals.)

Seek the advice of a physician if you think you might be at risk for developing a vitamin deficiency. Don't self-diagnose.

The arguments in favor of taking supplements are very persuasive: (1) the RDA aren't enough, because not everyone is "normal"; (2) no one is perfectly healthy all of the time; people are sometimes sick or getting sick; (3) the RDA don't cover *all* normal, healthy people—only most of them.

What should you make of these arguments? First, recall that the RDA were formulated after reviewing the results of many studies, some conducted in animals and others in humans. A built-in safety factor ensures that the RDA will cover the nutrient needs of virtually all healthy people. Moreover, the RDAs are designed as standards for evaluating the diets of populations, not individuals. Second, consider that vitamin-mineral supplements provide only the nutrients (or even nonnutrients) printed on the product label. They do not provide all of the components found in foods that contribute to good health. Consuming nutrients in foods is clearly sufficient, since for centuries our ancestors survived without nutrient supplements. Third, the bioavailability of vitamins and minerals from supplements may differ from that of the vitamins and minerals found in foods. (Bioavailability refers to the amount of a nutrient that is absorbed and utilized. Food processing and some compounds naturally occurring in foods can decrease or increase a nutrient's bioavailability.) Fourth, the indiscriminate use of supplements could result in nutrient imbalances. And finally, consuming high doses of vitamins and minerals may be toxic and produce serious side effects. Nutrients consumed at levels found in foods are considered to be safe.[12]

In view of this, there is little to be said *for* vitamin-mineral supplements. Most people can get all the nutrients they need by eating a reasonably varied diet of whole foods—that is, foods that all naturally contain significant amounts of most nutrients in relation to their energy content. No single whole food is well balanced; 2,100 calories of oranges, milk, salmon, or broccoli, for example, supply much more than the RDA-prescribed amounts of some nutrients and little of others. But look at the diagrams in Figure 6–2. If combined into a 2,100-calorie diet offering one-fourth of the calories each, these four foods would supply a much better balance—at least RDA amounts of nearly all nutrients, and well over RDA amounts for many. This illustrates the value of a balanced assortment of whole foods.

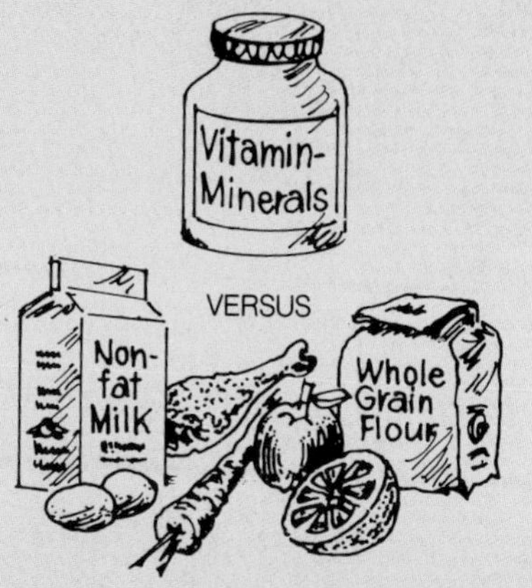

Vitamin-mineral pills cannot do the job that foods can.

Unfortunately, many people simply do not know what a well-balanced, varied, nutritious diet really is, or they know, but for one reason or another still don't eat that way. In addition, government surveys indicate that some people take in suboptimal levels of certain nutrients.

Some individuals who may be at risk for nutrient deficiencies and who may benefit from supplement use include those whose health is compromised by disease or poor nutrition. For example, the nutritional status of chronic alcoholics is often marginal because they tend to substitute alcohol for food. Likewise, some people with severe illnesses such as AIDS or cancer, who have undergone major surgery, or who have been hospitalized for a long period of

Miniglossary of Nutrient Supplements

Cell salts a mineral preparation sold in health food stores that is supposed to have been prepared from living, healthy cells. It is not necessary to take such preparations, and it may be dangerous.

Desiccated liver dehydrated liver, a powder sold in health food stores and supposed to contain in concentrated form all the nutrients found in liver. Possibly not dangerous, this supplement has no particular nutritional merit, and grocery store liver is much less expensive. *Desiccated* means "totally dried."

Garlic oil an extract of garlic.

Granola a cereal mixed from rolled oats and other grains.

Green pills pills containing dehydrated, crushed vegetable matter. One pill contains nutrients equal to those in one small forkful of fresh vegetables—minus losses incurred in processing. Sixty pills costing $15 deliver vegetable matter worth about $1.50.

Kelp a kind of seaweed used by many Asians as a foodstuff. Kelp tablets are made from dehydrated kelp.

Nutritional yeast a preparation of yeast cells, often praised as a concentrated source of B vitamins.

Powdered bone, bonemeal two among many nutrient supplements intended to supply calcium and other bone minerals.

Spirulina a kind of alga ("blue-green manna") said to contain large amounts of vitamin B_{12} and to suppress appetite. It does neither.

Wheat germ the oily embryo of the wheat kernel, rich in nutrients.

Suppose you needed 2,100 calories a day and the U.S. RDA of all nutrients. There is no perfect food, but if there were and if you ate 2,100 calories of it, you would receive 100% or more of the RDA for all these nutrients (and some 35 others):

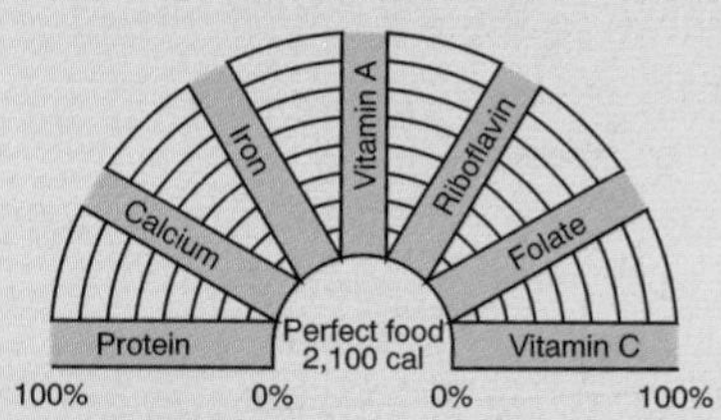

Now, suppose you ate nothing but oranges. To get 2,100 calories, you'd have to eat 35 oranges (!), and you would receive an unbalanced assortment of nutrients as follows:

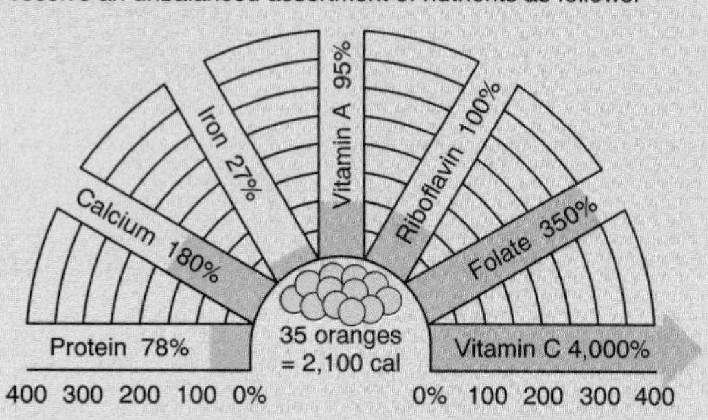

If you chose nonfat milk instead of oranges, you'd have to drink 24 1/2 cups to get 2,100 calories, and you would receive nutrients as follows:

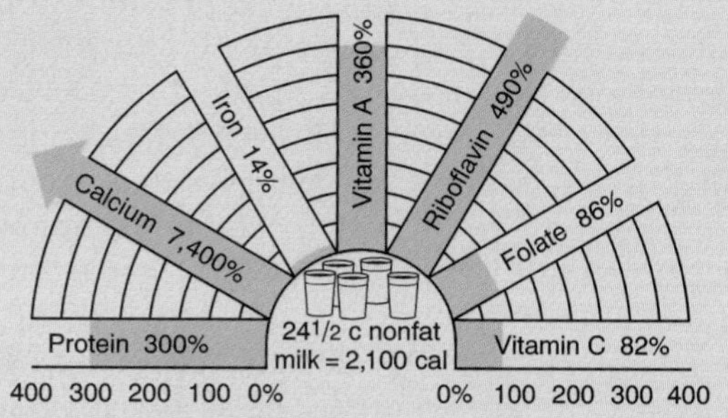

If you ate 2,100 calories of salmon, you'd have to eat 3 1/3 pounds, and you would receive:

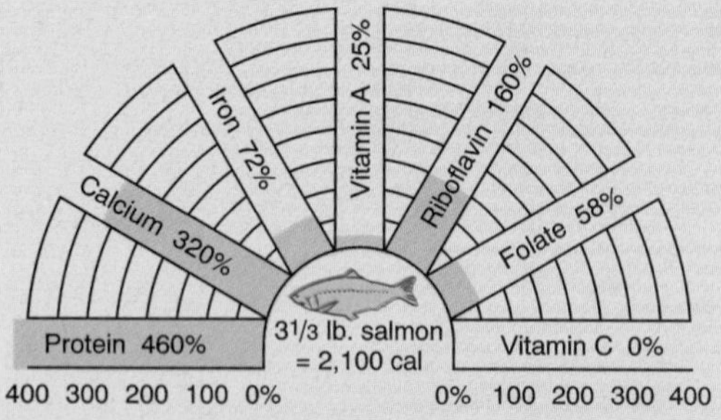

To get 2,100 calories from broccoli, you'd have to eat 40 stalks—but you'd receive:

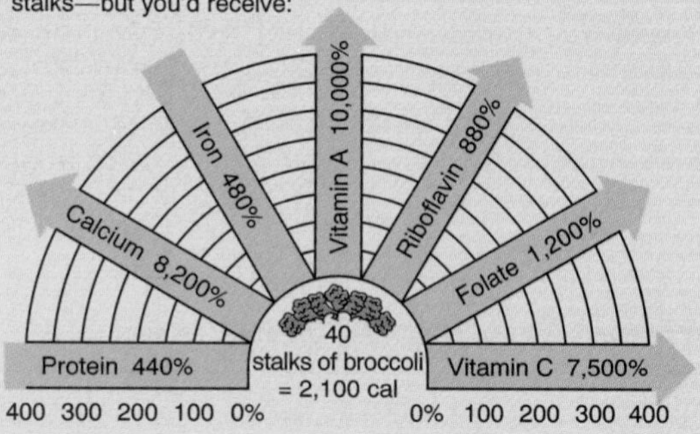

Now, if you mixed all four foods together, using equal-calorie amounts of each, you'd begin to get a balanced diet:

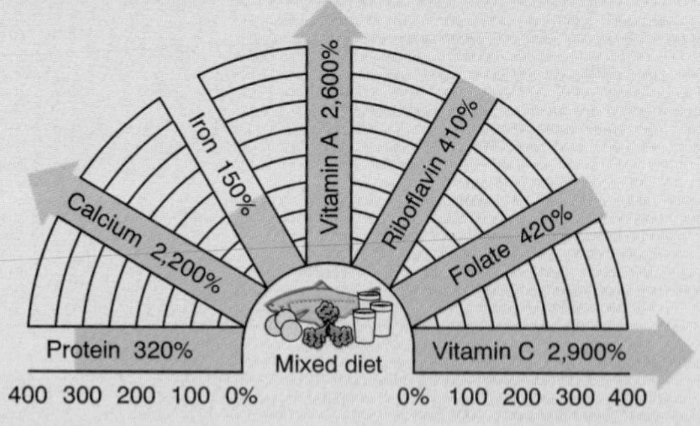

● *Figure 6–2* **How to Mix and Match Foods to Meet Nutrient Needs**
The figure shows how a balanced assortment of foods does a better job of meeting nutrient needs than any single food can possibly do. The extraordinarily high nutrient density of broccoli illustrates a characteristic of vegetables in general and suggests not that you should eat broccoli every day, but that a wide variety of vegetables can help improve your nutrition immensely while staying within your calorie allowance.

time may benefit from temporary supplement use. Strict vegetarians typically require vitamin B_{12} supplementation because their diets lack the meat and dairy products that supply this vitamin.

Many older individuals perceive a need to take vitamin-mineral supplements. But is there merit in doing so? For some elderly people, the use of supplements may be warranted. Particularly at risk of inadequate vitamin and mineral intakes are older individuals living in social isolation or in poor health. One study found that independently living senior citizens aged 60 to 94 years had low intakes of energy and calcium; those in poor health had low intakes of vitamins A and C.[13] Loneliness was cited as a primary factor contributing to dietary inadequacies.

A vitamin-mineral supplement may help improve the nutritional status of some elderly people, particularly those who abuse alcohol, have undiagnosed or untreated diseases, have anorexia due to medication use or depression, or who simply eat poorly because of loneliness or poverty.[14] However, for those who are otherwise healthy and active, a balanced, varied diet—the same as that required for other family members—is believed to provide the proper nutrition for this age group.[15]

For most individuals, a single, balanced vitamin-mineral supplement should do the job. If you decide to take a vitamin-mineral supplement, you may find yourself bewildered by the selection available at the supermarket or drugstore counter. Here are a few pointers to help you make a rational, informed choice:

1. Choose a supplement that provides **no more than** the RDA for essential vitamins and minerals. Read the label carefully and compare the amounts provided in the supplement with the RDA for each nutrient given in the table on the inside front cover of this book. Avoid megadoses, or "high potency" pills, unless prescribed by a physician. Remember, you are also obtaining nutrients from your diet.
2. Don't select "organic" or "natural" preparations over standard pharmacy types. The word *synthetic* may sound like *fake,* but to synthesize just means to put together. The synthetic supplement is identical to the vitamins that are synthesized by plants and animals. Your body can't tell the difference, but your pocketbook can.
3. Avoid preparations containing items that are not needed in human nutrition, such as inositol, as well as pills containing ground parsley, alfalfa, and other vegetable components. They merely add expense but not any nutritional value to the supplements.

In conclusion, it's best to get your nutrients from foods, such as vegetables, which are carriers of important vitamins and minerals. How well are you presently doing in the produce aisle? Try scoring yourself on the Vegetable Variety Scorecard on page 164.

Table 6–2

Thiamin in Foods

Adult RDA is 1.0 to 1.5 mg.

(mg)	SOURCES
0.87	Pork chop (3 oz)
0.82	Ham, canned roasted (3 oz)
0.82	Sunflower seeds (¼ c)
0.46	Green peas (1 c)
0.43	Black beans (1 c)
0.40	Black-eyed peas (1 c)
0.39	Watermelon (1 slice)
0.38	Canadian bacon (2 pieces)
0.29	Sirloin steak (8 oz)
0.26	Oatmeal, cooked (1 c)
0.22	Baked potato (1)
0.19	Peanuts (1 oz)
0.18	Asparagus, cooked (1 c)
0.18	Brown rice, cooked (1 c)
0.18	Tofu (soybean curd) (½ c)
0.13	Broccoli, cooked (1 c)
0.13	Kidney beans (1 c)
0.11	Orange (1)
0.10	Cantaloupe (½)
0.10	Whole-wheat bread (1 oz)
0.09	Nonfat milk or yogurt (1 c)

Table 6–3

Riboflavin in Foods

Adult RDA is 1.2 to 1.7 mg.

(mg)	SOURCES
3.52	Beef liver (3 oz)
0.70	Sirloin steak (8 oz)
0.46	Mushroom pieces, ckd, (1 c)
0.46	Ricotta cheese, skim (1 c)
0.42	Lowfat cottage cheese (1 c)
0.42	Beet greens, cooked (1 c)
0.42	Spinach, cooked (1 c)
0.34	Nonfat milk or yogurt (1 c)
0.32	Broccoli, cooked (1 c)
0.30	Pork roast (3 oz)
0.22	Almonds (1 oz)
0.22	Asparagus, cooked (1 c)
0.18	Ground beef (3 oz)
0.17	Smoked salmon (3 oz)
0.15	Turkey (3 oz)
0.13	Poached egg (1)
0.11	Cheddar cheese (1 oz)
0.10	Strawberries (1 c)
0.10	Chicken breast (½)
0.10	Black-eyed peas (1 c)
0.06	Whole-wheat bread (1 oz)

Table 6–4

Niacin in Foods

Adult RDA is 13 to 19 mg NE.

(mg)	SOURCES
13.20	Tuna (3 oz)
11.80	Chicken breast (½)
9.92	Sirloin steak (8 oz)
7.70	Halibut (3 oz)
6.80	Pink salmon (3 oz)
4.90	Ground beef (3 oz)
4.63	Turkey (3 oz)
4.35	Pork chop (3 oz)
4.02	Peanuts (1 oz)
3.70	Shrimp (3.5 oz)
3.32	Baked potato (1)
2.73	Brown rice, cooked (1 c)
1.90	Asparagus, cooked (1 c)
1.60	Sole/flounder (3 oz)
1.53	Cantaloupe (½)
1.50	Kidney beans (1 c)
1.18	Broccoli, cooked (1 c)
1.07	Whole-wheat bread (1 oz)
0.88	Spinach, cooked (1 c)
0.86	Peach (1)
0.30	Oatmeal, cooked (1 c)

Table 6–5

Folate in Foods

Adult RDA is 180 to 200 μg.

(μg)	SOURCES
262	Spinach, cooked (1 c)
176	Asparagus, cooked (1 c)
171	Turnip greens, cooked (1 c)
170	Lima beans (1 c)
142	Black-eyed peas (1 c)
137	Pinto beans (1 c)
109	Fresh spinach (1 c)
107	Broccoli, cooked (1 c)
85	Sunflower seeds (¼ c)
85	Kidney beans (1 c)
80	Cantaloupe (½)
76	Romaine (1 c)
64	Cauliflower, cooked (1 c)
55	Tofu (soybean curd) (½ c)
40	Orange (1)
30	Peanuts (1 oz)
28	Strawberries (1 c)
19	Sirloin steak (8 oz)
16	Whole-wheat bread (1 oz)
14	Nonfat milk or yogurt (1 c)
10	Oatmeal, cooked (1 c)

Table 6–6

Vitamin B_6 in Foods

Adult RDA is 1.6 to 2.0 mg.

(mg)	SOURCES
0.77	Sirloin steak (8 oz)
0.72	Navy beans (1 c)
0.70	Baked potato (1)
0.69	Watermelon (1 slice)
0.68	Salmon (3 oz)
0.66	Banana (1)
0.52	Chicken breast (½)
0.50	Soybeans (1 c)
0.46	Sunflower seeds (¼ c)
0.44	Spinach, cooked (1 c)
0.42	Tuna (3 oz)
0.42	Figs, dried (10)
0.39	Ground beef (3 oz)
0.35	Pork chop (3 oz)
0.31	Cantaloupe (½)
0.31	Broccoli, cooked (1 c)
0.29	Brown rice, cooked (1 c)
0.28	Sole/flounder (3 oz)
0.26	Asparagus, cooked (1 c)
0.14	Zucchini, cooked (1 c)
0.10	Nonfat milk or yogurt (1 c)

Table 6–7

Vitamin C in Foods

Adult RDA is 60 mg.

(mg)	SOURCES
188	Papaya (1)
124	Orange juice, fresh (1 c)
113	Cantaloupe (½)
98	Broccoli, cooked (1 c)
97	Brussels sprouts, ckd (1 c)
95	Green pepper (1)
94	Grapefruit juice (1 c)
85	Strawberries (1 c)
70	Orange (1)
69	Cauliflower, cooked (1 c)
57	Mango (1)
50	Asparagus, cooked (1 c)
47	Watermelon, (1 slice)
47	Grapefruit (½)
44	Bok choy, cooked (1 c)
40	Spinach, cooked (1 c)
33	Cabbage, raw (1 c)
31	Raspberries (1 c)
26	Baked potato (1)
24	Pineapple, fresh (1 c)
22	Tomato, fresh (1)

Spotlight

Nutrition Savvy—Effects of Cooking and Processing on Food's Nutrient Content

Buying nutrient-rich food at the market is the first step to eating well. The second step is knowing how to store, prepare, and cook food to minimize nutrient losses. In commercial processing such as canning and freezing, losses of vitamins seldom exceed 25 percent. In contrast, losses in food preparation at home can be 100 percent, and it is not unusual to see losses in the 60 percent to 75 percent range. As you can see, while the kinds of foods you buy certainly make a difference, what you do with them in your kitchen makes a major difference. This feature offers advice on food storage, preparation, and cooking so you don't throw valuable vitamins and minerals down the drain with the leftover cooking water and peels.

• Where and how should I store fresh fruits and vegetables?

Two easy rules of thumb are to (1) keep fresh fruits and vegetables (other than potatoes) cold and (2) store them whole. While a basket of fresh fruits and vegetables may make an appealing centerpiece, the nutrient value is slowly disappearing before your eyes. While on the vine, enzymes in fruits and vegetables continuously manufacture and, interestingly, destroy vitamins. After picking, vitamin manufacturing stops, and only vitamin destruction continues. These vitamin wrecking crews work best at the temperature at which the plants grow—room temperature in most homes. Store fruits and vegetables in your refrigerator. Chilling them slows vitamin destruction. Pull out only enough to eat and return any leftovers to the refrigerator soon after you are finished.

As long as the skin is uncut, vitamins inside the fruit and vegetable flesh remain protected from air. Air oxidizes—rusts—vitamins and so destroys them. Vitamin C is a good example. Recall that vitamin C is an antioxidant or acid, hence the name ascorbic acid. As long as the acidic flesh of the fruit or vegetable surrounds the vitamin, the vitamin remains stable. Once cut open and exposed to air, the vitamin C content of, say, citrus fruits, tomatoes, and strawberries begins to decline. Even opened cans of juice are susceptible to rapid vitamin loss. Buy whole fruits and vegetables and peel and cut only what you need immediately before cooking. Wrap any leftovers in airtight plastic or store them in airtight containers inside the refrigerator. Keep any leftover juice in containers with tight-fitting lids.

In an attempt to appeal to the nutrition-conscious but time-pressed shopper, many produce sections sell precut and peeled vegetables and fruits. Convenient? Yes. Nutritious? Probably—depending on how long ago the vegetable was cut. Your best nutritional bet, though, is to routinely purchase whole fruits and vegetables and reserve buying fresh, precut veggies and prechunked fruit for those times when you absolutely can't do it yourself. Table 6–9 compares the nutrient content of fresh and processed forms of peaches.

• Which is more nutritious—Canned or frozen vegetables and fruits?

In general, the nutrient content of frozen foods is similar to that of fresh foods; losses are minimal. The freezing process itself does not destroy any nutrients, but some losses may occur during the steps taken in preparation for freezing, such as blanching, washing, trimming, or grinding. If you are preparing your own frozen vegetables, dip them in boiling water for a minute to destroy the enzymes that will otherwise remain to attack nutrients. When the foods have cooled, freeze them in plastic containers with tight-fitting lids. Most fruits can be sliced and frozen in containers or freezer bags without any special preparation. Meat should be wrapped to exclude all possible air before freezing.

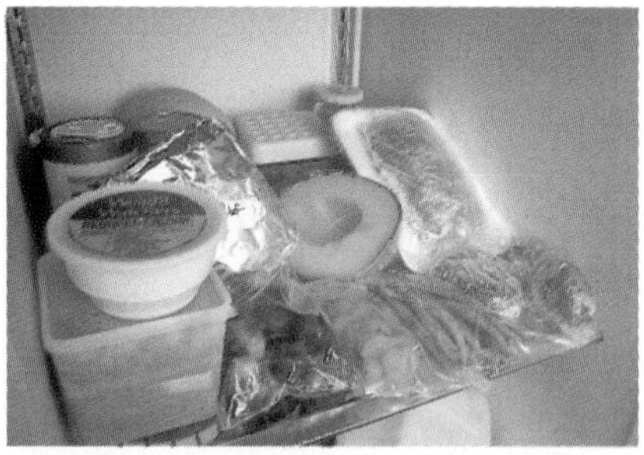
Wrap foods tightly.

It's also important to keep frozen foods *solidly* frozen. To be solidly frozen, a food has to be kept colder than 32 degrees Fahrenheit, or 0 degrees centigrade. Food may seem frozen at 35 degrees Fahrenheit, but much of it is actually partially thawed on the inside. In this unfrozen state, vitamin C is quickly converted to its inactive form. In as little as two months, all of the vitamin C in an improperly frozen food can be destroyed.

Invest in a freezer thermometer and monitor the temperature of your frozen-food storage place. Keep the temperature below 32 degrees Fahrenheit (0 degrees centigrade). Overall, freezing is an excellent way to preserve nutrients; and if foods are frozen and stored under proper conditions, they will often contain more nutrients when served at the table than fresh fruits and vegetables that have stayed in the produce department of the grocery store even for a day.

But what about canned foods? Although canning is one of the better methods of protecting food against food-spoiling bacteria and yeast, the heat treatment process used during

Table 6–9

Comparison of Fresh Versus Processed Forms of Peaches[a]

Type of Peach	Calories	Fiber (grams)	Vitamin C (mg)	Vitamin A (RE)
Fresh (1)	37	2	6	47
Canned (2 halves):				
juice pack	68	2	6	58
heavy syrup pack	120	2	4	54
Frozen, sweetened, sliced (½ cup)	117	2	118[b]	36
Dried (2 halves)	62	2	1	56
Nectar (1 cup)	134	1	13	64

[a]Look for fresh, seasonal fruit in the produce section of your supermarket. Unsweetened canned, frozen, and dried fruits are nutritious alternatives when fresh fruit is out of season. But watch out for added sugars! Processing can reduce vitamin, mineral, and fiber levels of fruit and may add unwanted calories from syrup, sugar, or other sweeteners.
[b]With added vitamin C (ascorbic acid).

canning, unfortunately, destroys some vulnerable vitamins—thiamin and folate, for example. Like other heat treatments, the canning process is based on time and temperature. Fortunately, each small increase in temperature has a major killing effect on microbes, with only a minor effect on nutrients. Therefore the canning industry chooses a process based on the high-temperature/short-time (HTST) principle.

To determine how much a food's nutrient value is lost in canning, food scientists have compared canned foods to fresh. Heat rapidly destroys thiamin—one of the B vitamins; acid, however, stabilizes it. Thus, foods that lose the most thiamin during canning are the low-acid foods like lima beans, corn, and meat. Up to half, or even more, of the thiamin in these foods can be lost during canning. Examining the folate content of spinach cooked in a variety of ways, researchers found that folate destruction was greatest in canned products (see Table 6–10).[16] As for the fat-soluble vitamins, they are relatively stable and are not affected much by canning. The HTST process actually aids in preserving vitamin C. By destroying ascorbic acid oxidase (an enzymatic enemy of vitamin C), the HTST process helps ensure a longer life for the vitamin C in the food. Minerals are unaffected by heat processing because they—unlike vitamins—cannot be destroyed.

The nutrient content of canned foods is usually shown as "solids and liquids." Both minerals and vitamins leak from the cut vegetables into the water they are canned in. If you throw away the liquid from a canned food, you are throwing away all the nutrients that have leaked into that liquid—up to half the amount in the original product.

Table 6–10

Effects of Processing on the Folate Content of Spinach[a]

TYPE OF SPINACH	TOTAL FOLATE (μg/100 g)
Raw	251
Water blanched	43
Steam blanched	147
Canned	21
Canned (stored 3 months)	17
Frozen (stored 3 months)	31

[a]From S. C. DeSouza and R. R. Eitenmiller, Effects of processing and storage on the folate content of spinach and broccoli, *Journal of Food Science* 51 (1986): 626–628.

A bit of Southern folk wisdom is to serve the cooking liquid with the vegetable rather than throwing it away; this liquid is known as the pot liquor. The user of canned vegetables who can think of a way to use the "liquor"—for example, by saving it to make soups, cook rice or stuffing, and moisten casseroles—displays similar wisdom.

Keep in mind, too, that some minerals are added to canned foods. Sodium chloride—salt—is important in this regard. In general, the more highly a food is processed, the more sodium chloride and the less potassium it is likely to contain. Rinsing the canned vegetables under running tap water for one minute will reduce the sodium content by up to 50 percent. Or,

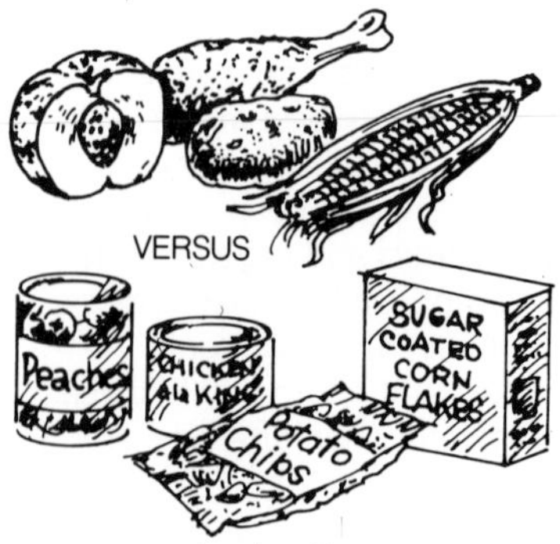

You can often tell two things from the potassium content of a food—how nutritious it is and how processed it is.

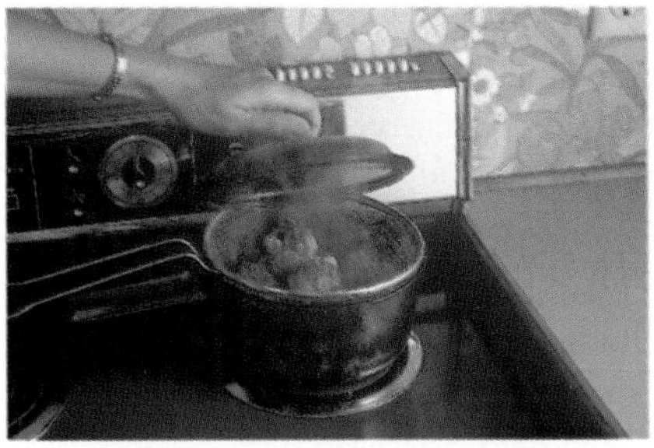

Steam vegetables over water.

manufacturers now make available ''No Added Salt'' versions of many vegetables.

Miniglossary

Canning preservation by killing all microorganisms present in food and sealing out air. The food, its container, and its lid are heated until sterile; as the food cools, the lid makes an airtight seal, preventing contamination.

Freezing preservation by lowering food temperature to the point at which life processes cease. Microorganisms are not destroyed but are held dormant as long as the food is frozen.

Drying preservation by removing sufficient water from food to inhibit microbial growth.

HTST (high-temperature/short-time) principle every 18° F (10° C) rise in processing temperature gives approximately a tenfold increase in microbial destruction, while it only doubles nutrient losses.

● Do these results mean I should stop buying canned foods?

No. When eaten as part of a balanced, varied diet, canned vegetables and other canned foods provide essential nutrients. Their convenience and year-round availability also make them a good pantry stocker. Consider the case of orange juice and vitamin C. The fresh-squeezed juice, per 100 calories, contains 111 milligrams of vitamin C. If the juice were canned, 100 calories of it would supply 82 milligrams of vitamin C. These figures indicate that the fresh-squeezed juice is superior to the canned. That's true, but consider that the U.S. RDA for vitamin C is only 60 milligrams. One serving of either juice would single-handedly meet this vitamin need for a healthy person. In this case, at least for vitamin C, the losses due to the processing can be called negligible, and there is an enormous convenience and distribution

Table 6–11
Comparing Cooking Methods

METHOD	COMMENTS	EXAMPLES
Microwaving	Usually best at retaining nutrients, since it cooks so fast and without any added water.	Cabbage and broccoli lose only 10 percent to 20 percent of vitamin C when microwaved compared to 27 percent to 62 percent when boiled in lots of water.
	Little nutrient loss when reheating leftovers or frozen vegetables.	Microwaved spinach loses only minimal amounts of folate versus 23 percent loss when boiled.
Steaming	Uses little water and requires short cooking time, so good for retaining nutrients.	Generally, vegetables lose 50 percent less in minerals during steaming than during boiling.
Boiling	Done incorrectly, can rob food of nutrients. To boil: Bring water to boil before adding food.	French-cut green beans lose 72 percent of vitamin C, compared to 46 percent when beans are cooked whole.
	Use minimal amount of water and save water for other cooking needs. Cover the pot to speed cooking time. Leave vegetables in the largest pieces possible.	Unpeeled potatoes lose little vitamin C and folate during boiling, compared to up to 25 percent lost if peeled.
		Broccoli boiled for 2 minutes loses 25 percent of vitamin C; 33 percent if boiled for 11 minutes.
Baking/Roasting	The higher the cooking temperature and the longer the cooking time, the more nutrients lost.	Baked potatoes lose 3 times as much vitamin C if they stand for an hour after baking as they do when served immediately after baking.
Frying	Conventional frying in large amounts of hot oil destroys heat-sensitive nutrients.	Fried potatoes lose up to 90 percent of vitamin C.
	Stir-frying should destroy less, since cooking time is shorter.	Most fried vegetables lose 25 percent to 85 percent of folate.

Source: Adapted from *University of California-Berkeley Wellness Letter,* May 1991.

advantage to the processed juice. Fresh orange juice spoils. Shipping it to distant points makes it much more expensive than frozen or canned juice. The fresh product cannot be stored indefinitely without compromising nutrient quality. Without canned or frozen juice, people who have no access to the fresh juice would be deprived of this excellent food.

Which cooking methods keep the most nutrients in the food?

Table 6–11 summarizes the effects of five methods of cooking. In general, cook unpeeled, minimally cut fruits and vegetables for the shortest amount of time in the least amount of water. Covering a pot will reduce cooking time. Microwaving, steaming, and stir-frying (in small amounts of oil) are the quickest, most nutrient retaining cooking options.

The implications for food choices are clear: for an optimally nutritious diet, choose whole foods to the greatest extent possible. Being realistic, few people have the time to bake all their own bread from scratch; shop every few days for fresh meats; or wash, peel, chop, and cook fresh fruits and vegetables at each meal. This is where food processing comes in—commercially prepared whole-grain breads, frozen cuts of meats, bags of frozen vegetables, and prepared fruit juices do little disservice to nutrition and enable the consumer to eat a wide variety of lightly processed foods. The nutrient content of processed foods exists on a continuum:

Whole-grain bread > Refined white bread > Sugared doughnuts

Milk > Fruit-flavored yogurt > Canned chocolate pudding

Corn on the cob > Canned creamed corn > Caramel popcorn

Oranges > Orange juice > Orange-flavored drink

Baked ham > Deviled ham > Fried pork rind

Another continuum parallels it—that of the nutrition status of the consumer. Generally, the closer to the farm the foods you eat, the better nourished you are.

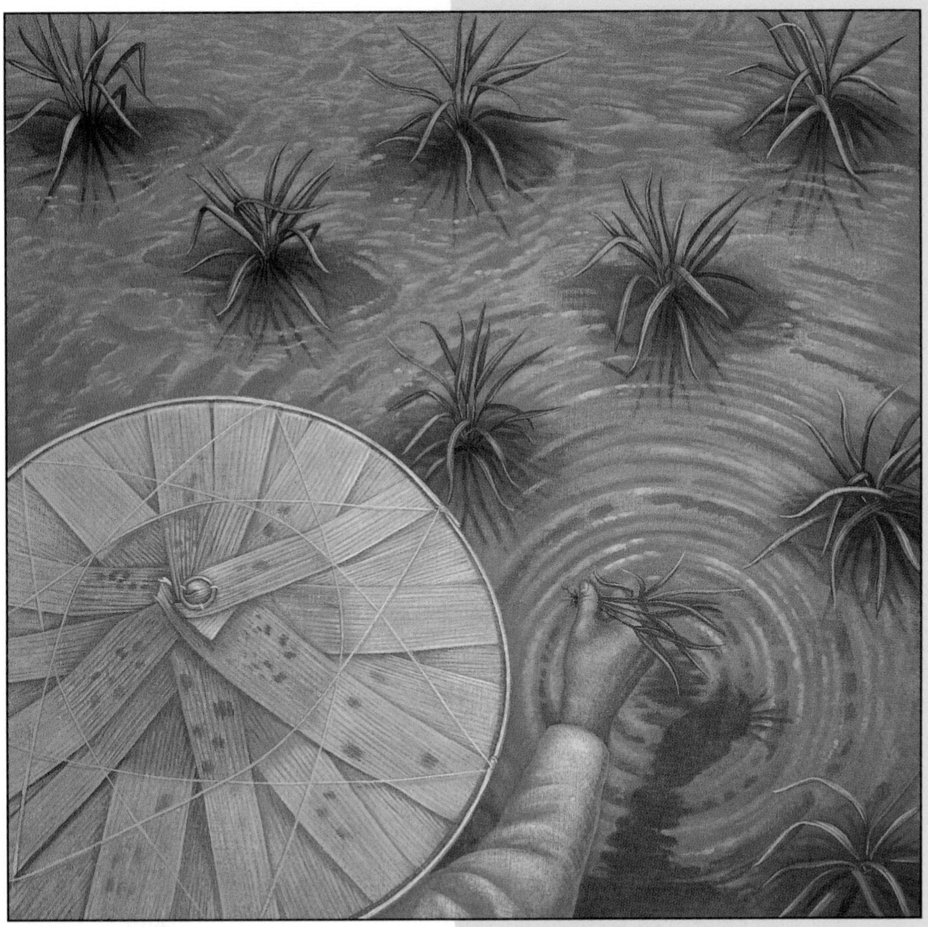

© Teresa Fasolino/Jacqueline Dedell, Inc.

CHAPTER 7
The Minerals

> *All interest in disease and death is only another expression of interest in life.*
> —Thomas Mann

Contents

Ask Yourself . . . ?

Which of these statements about nutrition are true, and which are false? For the false statements, what *is* true?

1. Calcium is the most important mineral in human nutrition.
2. Milk is nature's most nearly perfect food because it is rich in every nutrient.
3. It is harder for women than for men to obtain diets that are adequate in calcium.
4. Milk is necessary for children, but adults can find replacements for it.
5. Sodium is bad for the body and should be avoided.
6. When a person becomes deficient in iron, the first symptom to appear is anemia.
7. Zinc is toxic in excess.
8. Both too little and too much iodine in the diet can cause swelling of the thyroid gland, known as goiter.
9. A diet high in salt is associated with high blood pressure.
10. Adequate calcium intakes help prevent high blood pressure.

Answers: 1. False. No one essential mineral is more important than any other. 2. False. Milk is an excellent food, but it is poor in iron. 3. True. 4. False. Strictly speaking, milk is not absolutely necessary in anyone's diet, but its nutrients are hard to obtain from other foods, and it is recommended for both children and adults. 5. False. Sodium is an essential nutrient, but excesses should be avoided. 6. False. When a person becomes deficient in iron, one of the last symptoms to appear is anemia; fatigue and weakness appear first. 7. True. 8. True. 9. True. 10. True.

For hundreds, if not thousands, of years, the physical and chemical properties of minerals such as gold, silver, lead, and copper were known to metallurgists and alchemists. Even so, the role of some minerals in biological processes was recognized only within the past few hundred years. The discovery of iron in blood, for example, occurred in 1713. The identification of calcium in bone was made in 1771.[1] Not until the late nineteenth century was the role of minerals in human nutrition fully appreciated.

The previous chapter described the water-soluble and fat-soluble vitamins, their biological roles, food sources, and human requirements. This chapter discusses the minerals known to be important in human nutrition. In some respects, minerals are similar to vitamins. Like the vitamins, minerals do not themselves contribute energy to the diet. Of those known to be important in human nutrition, most minerals have diverse functions within the body and work with enzymes to facilitate chemical reactions. As with the vitamins, most minerals are required in the diet in very small amounts.

In other respects, however, minerals are different from vitamins. Whereas vitamins are organic compounds, **minerals** are **inorganic** compounds that occur naturally in the earth's crust. And unlike the vitamins, some minerals (such as calcium) contribute to the building of body structures (such as bone).

Minerals small, naturally occurring, inorganic chemical elements; the minerals serve as structural components and in many vital processes in the body.
Inorganic being or composed of matter other than plant or animal.

As with other areas of research in human nutrition, there are many unanswered questions related to mineral metabolism. Scientists are studying the biochemical functions of minerals, the mechanisms by which they activate enzymes, the factors that control their blood and tissue levels, and how the composition of the diet affects the bioavailability of these dietary components. The many complex metabolic interactions of minerals make this a challenging area of research.

The Major Minerals

The minerals are traditionally divided into two large classes: the **major minerals** and the **trace minerals.** The distinction between them is that the major minerals occur in relatively large quantities in the body and are needed daily in relatively large quantities—on the order of a gram or so each. The trace minerals occur in the body in minute quantities and are needed only in trace amounts in the diet. Table 7–1 lists the minerals known to be essential in human nutrition. The discussions that follow focus on the minerals that are of particular interest in human nutrition, primarily because people are known to suffer deficiencies of them.

Major mineral an essential mineral nutrient found in the human body in amounts larger than 5 grams.

Trace mineral an essential mineral nutrient found in the human body in amounts less than 5 grams.

Calcium

Calcium is the most abundant mineral in the body. Ninety-nine percent of the body's calcium is stored in the bones, which play two important roles. First, they support and protect the body's soft tissues. Second, they serve as a calcium bank, providing calcium to the body fluids whenever the supply is running low.

Although only a small part (about one percent) of the body's calcium is in the fluids, circulating calcium is vital to life. Calcium is required for the transmission of nerve impulses. It is essential for muscle action and so helps maintain the heartbeat. It appears to be essential for the integrity of cell membranes. Calcium must also be present if blood clotting is to occur, and it is a **cofactor** for several enzymes.

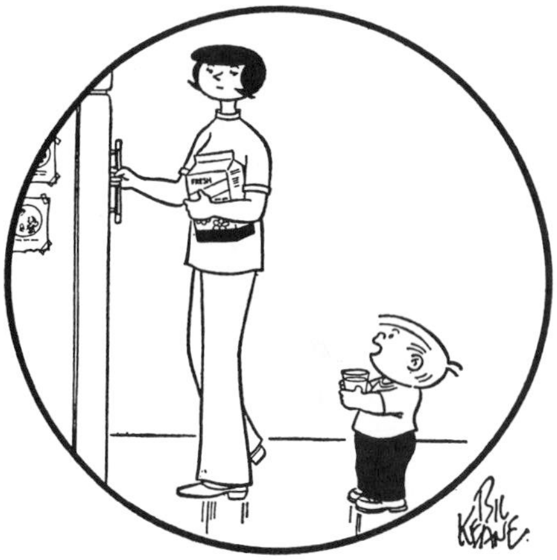

"Guess what, Mommy—you were right! My teacher says milk is good for us."

Reprinted with special permission of King Features Syndicate, Inc.

Everyone knows that children need calcium daily to support the growth of their bones and teeth, but not everyone is aware of adults' needs for daily intakes of calcium. Abundant evidence now supports the importance of calcium for adults, especially women, who need at least as much calcium in their later years as they did when they were adolescents and young adults. A deficit of calcium during the growing years and in adulthood contributes to gradual bone loss, **osteoporosis**, which can totally cripple a person in later life.

Adult bone loss threatens the integrity of the skeleton in at least one out of every three people over the age of 65. It strikes both sexes, although it is eight times more prevalent in women than in men after age 50, for several reasons:

- Women generally have less bone mass than men.
- Women typically have lower calcium intakes than men.
- Women more often use weight-reducing diets, which tend to be low in calcium.
- Bone loss begins earlier in women because of women's different hormonal makeup, and the loss is accelerated at **menopause**, when their protective **estrogen** secretion declines.
- Exercise maintains bones, and until recently women have generally been less active than men.
- Pregnancy and lactation decrease the calcium reserves in bones whenever calcium intake is inadequate.
- Women live longer than men, and bone loss continues with aging.

Cofactor a mineral element that, like a coenzyme, works with an enzyme to facilitate a chemical reaction.

Osteoporosis (OSS-tee-oh-pore-OH-sis), also known as adult bone loss; a disease of older persons in which the bone becomes porous.

osteo = bones
poros = porous

Menopause the time of life at which a woman's menstrual cycling ceases, usually at about 45 to 50 years of age.

Estrogen a major female hormone—important in connection with nutrition because it maintains calcium balance and because its secretion declines at menopause.

Table 7–1

A Guide to the Minerals

Mineral	Significant Sources	Chief Functions In the Body	Deficiency Symptoms	Toxicity Symptoms
Calcium	Milk and milk products, small fish (with bones), tofu, greens, legumes.	Principal mineral of bones and teeth; involved in muscle contraction and relaxation, nerve function, blood clotting, blood pressure.	Stunted growth in children; bone loss (osteoporosis) in adults.	Excess calcium is excreted except in hormonal imbalance states.
Phosphorus	All animal tissues.	Part of every cell; involved in acid-base balance.	Unknown.	Can create relative deficiency of calcium.
Magnesium	Nuts, legumes, whole grains, dark-green vegetables, seafoods, chocolate, cocoa.	Involved in bone mineralization, protein synthesis, enzyme action, normal muscular contraction, nerve transmission.	Weakness, confusion, depressed pancreatic hormone secretion, growth failure, behavioral disturbances, muscle spasms.	Not known.
Sodium	Salt, soy sauce; processed foods: cured, canned, pickled, and many boxed foods.	Helps maintain normal fluid and acid-base balance.	Muscle cramps, mental apathy, loss of appetite.	Hypertension (in salt-sensitive persons).
Chloride	Salt, soy sauce; processed foods.	Part of stomach acid, necessary for proper digestion, fluid balance.	Growth failure in children, muscle cramps, mental apathy, loss of appetite.	Normally harmless (the gas chlorine is a poison but evaporates from water); disturbed acid-base balance; vomiting.
Potassium	All whole foods: meats, milk, fruits, vegetables, grains, legumes.	Facilitates many reactions, including protein synthesis, fluid balance, nerve transmission, and contraction of muscles.	Muscle weakness, paralysis, confusion; can cause death; accompanies dehydration.	Causes muscular weakness; triggers vomiting; if given into a vein, can stop the heart.
Sulfur	All protein-containing foods.	Component of certain amino acids; part of biotin, thiamin, and insulin.	None known; protein deficiency would occur first.	Would occur only if sulfur amino acids were eaten in excess; this (in animals) depresses growth.
Iodine	Iodized salt, seafood.	Part of thyroxine, which regulates metabolism.	Goiter, cretinism.	Very high intakes depress thyroid activity.

Bone loss affects the entire skeleton, but it occurs first in the pelvis and the spine. Often, it first becomes apparent when someone's hip suddenly gives way. People say, "She fell and broke her hip." The fact of the matter is often that the hip was so fragile that it broke and caused the fall. Figure 7–1 shows the effect of the loss of spinal bone on a woman's height and posture.

Table 7–1

A Guide to the Minerals—*Continued*

Mineral	Significant Sources	Chief Functions In the Body	Deficiency Symptoms	Toxicity Symptoms
Iron	Beef, fish, poultry, shellfish, eggs, legumes, dried fruits.	Hemoglobin formation; part of myoglobin; energy utilization.	Anemia: weakness, pallor, headaches, reduced resistance to infection, inability to concentrate.	Iron overload: infections, liver injury.
Zinc	Protein-containing foods: meats, fish, poultry, grains, vegetables.	Part of many enzymes; present in insulin; involved in making genetic material and proteins, immunity, vitamin A transport, taste, wound healing, making sperm, normal fetal development.	Growth failure in children, delayed development of sexual organs, loss of taste, poor wound healing.	Fever, nausea, vomiting, diarrhea.
Copper	Meats, drinking water.	Absorption of iron; part of several enzymes.	Anemia, bone changes (rare in human beings).	Unknown except as part of a rare hereditary disease (Wilson's disease).
Fluoride	Drinking water (if naturally fluoride containing or fluoridated), tea, seafood.	Formation of bones and teeth; helps make teeth resistant to decay and bones resistant to mineral loss.	Susceptibility to tooth decay and bone loss.	Fluorosis (discoloration of teeth).
Selenium	Seafood, meats, grains.	Helps protect body compounds from oxidation.	Anemia (rare).	Digestive system disorders.
Chromium	Meats, unrefined foods, fats, vegetable oils.	Associated with insulin and required for the release of energy from glucose.	Diabetes-like condition marked by inability to use glucose normally.	Unknown as a nutrition disorder. Occupational exposures damage skin and kidneys.
Molybdenum	Legumes, cereals, organ meats.	Facilitates, with enzymes, many cell processes.	Unknown.	Enzyme inhibition.
Manganese	Widely distributed in foods.	Facilitates, with enzymes, many cell processes.	In animals: poor growth, nervous system disorders, abnormal reproduction.	Poisoning, nervous system disorders.
Cobalt	Meats, milk, and milk products.	As part of vitamin B_{12}, involved in nerve function and blood formation.	Unknown except in vitamin B_{12} deficiency.	Unknown as a nutrition disorder.

It is not inevitable that people "grow shorter" as they age, but it does happen if they don't take the measures necessary to prevent bone loss.

Other nutrients are also important to bone growth and maintenance. Fluoride and vitamin D deficiencies, like calcium deficiencies, can cause loss of bone density. So can heredity, abnormal hormone levels, alcohol (even in

Figure 7–1 Bone Loss in Women

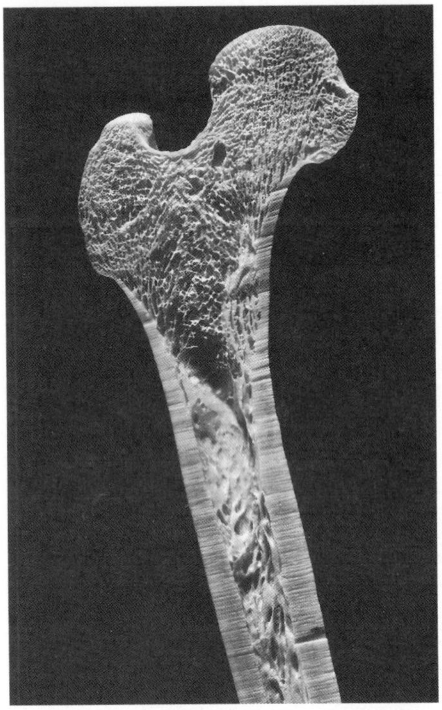

A. Cross section of bone. The lacy structural elements are **trabeculae** (tra-BECK-you-le), which can be drawn on to replenish blood calcium.

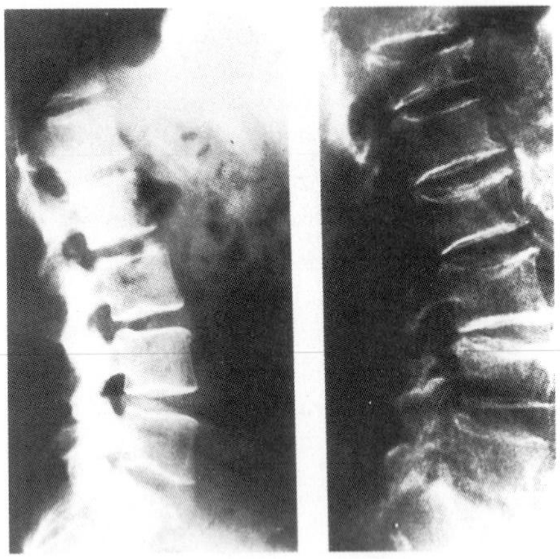

B. A healthy spine (*left*) and one that has deteriorated from adult bone loss, or osteoporosis (*right*). Notice how the vertebrae are being compressed by the weight of the head and shoulders.

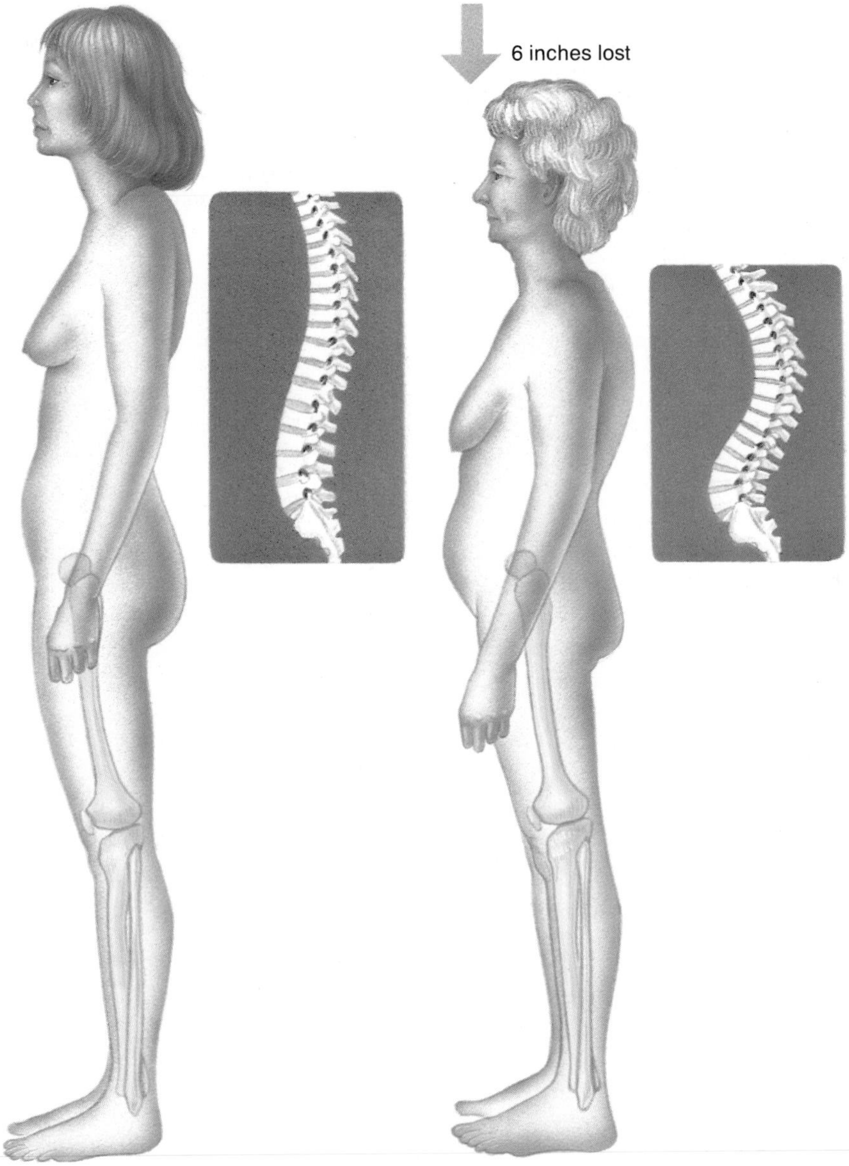

C. Loss of height in a woman caused by adult bone loss. The woman on the left is about 50 years old. On the right, she is 80 years old. Her legs have not grown shorter; only her back has lost length, due to collapse of her spinal bones (vertebrae). Collapsed vertebrae cannot protect the spinal nerves from pressure that causes excruciating pain.

moderate use), prescription medications, other drugs, lack of exercise (especially weight-bearing exercises), and the stress response, but calcium is usually the most important factor.

Table 7–2 shows that calcium appears almost exclusively in three classes of foods—milk/milk products, green vegetables, and a few fish and shellfish. The green vegetables look best in terms of calcium on a per-calorie basis, but milk products contain more calcium per serving. Nonfat milk offers about 300 milligrams of calcium in a 90-calorie cup, for example, while greens (depending on the variety chosen) offer 100 or more milligrams in a 20-calorie cup. The greens would therefore seem to be a good choice, but a complication enters in—absorption. It is not clear to what extent calcium is absorbed from green vegetables, while calcium *is* known to be very well absorbed from milk.[2] Milk contains both vitamin D and lactose, which enhance calcium absorption. Thus, experts recommend that everyone consume milk and milk products daily.

Milk and milk products need not be taken as such; there are ways to include them in other foods. For children and adults who can afford the calories, ice cream, ice milk, and yogurt are acceptable substitutes for regular milk. Puddings, custards, and baked goods can be prepared in such a way that they also contain appreciable amounts of milk. Powdered nonfat milk, which is an excellent and inexpensive source of protein, calcium, and other nutrients, can be added to many foods (such as cookies, soups, casseroles, and meatloaf) during preparation. Nonfat yogurt fortified with extra milk solids is another excellent calcium source. Equal to milk and milk products in calcium richness are small fish such as sardines or herring (if the bones are consumed), salmon (with the bones), or oysters. In some areas, calcium-fortified orange juice and other fortified products are available; a ½-cup serving of fortified orange juice provides about 110 milligrams of calcium.

The word *daily* should be stressed with respect to food sources of calcium. Because of the body's limited ability to absorb calcium, it cannot handle massive doses periodically but needs frequent opportunities to take in small amounts. The word *milk* products should also be stressed, rather than *dairy* products. Butter and cream contain negligible calcium because calcium is not soluble in fat.

Some foods contain **binders** that combine chemically with calcium and other minerals such as iron and zinc to prevent their absorption, carrying them out of the body with other wastes. For example, **phytic acid** renders the calcium, iron, and zinc in certain foods less available than they might be otherwise; **oxalic acid** also binds calcium and iron. Phytic acid is found in oatmeal and other whole-grain cereals; oxalic acid is found in beets, rhubarb, and spinach, among other foods. Fiber in general seems to hinder calcium absorption, so the higher the diet is in fiber, the higher it should be in calcium. This fact doesn't diminish the overall value of high-fiber foods; they are nutritious for many reasons, but they are not useful as calcium sources.

Protein also affects calcium status by affecting excretion, not absorption. The higher the diet is in protein, the greater the amount of calcium excreted. This is why people in the United States are told to consume more calcium than people in countries whose protein intakes are lower. Another piece of advice: Eat less protein.

Milk Substitutes Some people have a **milk allergy** or **lactose intolerance** and can't drink milk. For them, and especially the children among them,

Table 7–2
Calcium in Foods

Adult RDA is 800 to 1,200 mg.

(mg)	SOURCES
371	Sardines, with bones (3 oz)
326	Goat's milk (1 c)
320	Shrimp (3.5 oz)
302	Romano cheese (1 oz)
302	Nonfat milk or yogurt (1 c)
280	Chocolate milk (1 c)
272	Swiss cheese (1 oz)
244	Spinach, cooked (1 c)
204	Cheddar cheese (1 oz)
198	Turnip greens, cooked (1 c)
178	Broccoli, cooked (1 c)
167	Salmon, with bones (3 oz)
165	Beet greens, cooked (1 c)
160	Instant oatmeal, fortified (1 packet)
158	Bok choy, cooked (1 c)
155	Low-fat cottage cheese (1 c)
113	Collards, cooked (1 c)
108	Tofu (soybean curd) (4 oz)
75	Almonds (1 oz)
69	Parmesan cheese (1 tbsp)
52	Orange (1)

The Four Food Group Plan recommends daily milk servings:

Children under 9: 2 to 3 c.
Children 9 to 12: 3+ c.
Teenagers: 4+ c.
Adults: 2 c.
Pregnant women: 3+ c.
Lactating women: 4+ c.
Women over 50: 3 c.

Binders: in foods, chemical compounds that can combine with nutrients (especially minerals) to form complexes the body cannot absorb. Examples of such binders are **phytic** (FIGHT-ic) **acid** and **oxalic** (ox-AL-ic) **acid.**

Milk allergy the most common food allergy, caused by the protein in raw milk. Milk allergy is sometimes overcome by cooking the milk to denature the protein; it is sometimes "cured" by an abstinence from and a gradual reintroduction to milk.
Lactose intolerance as described in Chapter 3, an inherited or acquired inability to digest lactose due to failure to produce the enzyme lactase. Lactose intolerance is prevalent in the majority of adult human population groups.
Milk intolerance digestive or other system symptoms, experienced subjectively after consuming milk. It can be due to the lactose content of the milk, but other chemical substances or contaminating toxins can also produce intolerance to milk in individuals capable of efficient digestion of lactose.

calcium-rich substitutes must be found.[3] Among the possible substitutes are boiled milk, milk of goats or other species, enzyme-treated milk, calcium-fortified soy milk, milk products such as plain yogurt and cheese, nondairy foods containing the nutrients of milk, imitation milk, and calcium supplements.

In theory, it should be easy to choose the appropriate milk substitute. If the person is allergic to milk, in theory, the milk protein is the offending substance and a substitute with altered or different proteins must be found. If the person is intolerant to lactose, a lactose-free substitute is needed. It is often difficult, however, to determine why someone tolerates milk poorly. A **milk intolerance** can occur for reasons other than allergy or lactose intolerance.[4] Both the kinds and amounts of milk any given person can tolerate can be determined only by experimenting. The selection of a substitute may have to proceed by trial and error.

Milk protein is denatured when milk is boiled. Some cases of milk allergy can be solved by this simple means. Preboiled liquid or powdered milk can be cooked into foods such as custards and baked goods. Another alternative is goat's milk. The proteins in goat's milk differ somewhat from the proteins in cow's milk; thus, goat's milk may be tolerated by the person who can't tolerate cow's milk. Nutritionally, the two milks are similar in most respects. Both should be fortified with vitamins A and D, however, to properly complement the standard diet.

The treatment of milk with enzymes to digest its lactose offers a possible solution to the problem of lactose intolerance. The enzyme preparation (Lact-Aid) can be purchased over the counter and mixed with the milk before it's served. Another possible alternative is low-lactose milk. Fermented dairy products, such as yogurt, offer the same nutrients as milk but with a lower lactose content, because in fermenting the milk, bacteria use the lactose as an energy source to do their work. Table 7–3 shows the lactose content of fermented dairy products compared with the lactose content of milk.

Table 7–3 Lactose Content of Dairy Products[a]

Dairy Products	Serving Size to Equal Protein in 1 c Milk	Amount of Lactose Compared with that in 1 c Milk
Plain yogurt	1 c	75%[b]
Strawberry yogurt	1 c	39%[c]
Pasteurized processed cheese food	3 tbsp	33%[c]
Grated American cheese	¾ oz	25%[c]
Cottage cheese	¼ c	14%[b]
Aged cheddar cheese	2 in. cube	6%[b]
Swiss cheese	1 oz	Trace[c]
Extra sharp cheddar cheese	2 in. cube	Trace[c]

[a]Note that these are all fermented dairy products. A nonfermented milk product like ice cream has about the same amount of lactose per protein as milk (1½ cups have 93 percent of the lactose in 1 cup of milk).
[b]Calculated from A. D. Newcomer, Lactase deficiency, *Contemporary Nutrition,* April 1979.
[c]Calculated from D. E. Lee and C. B. Lillibridge, A method for qualitative identification of sugars and semiquantitative determination of lactose content suitable for a variety of foods, *American Journal of Clinical Nutrition* 29 (1976): 428–440.

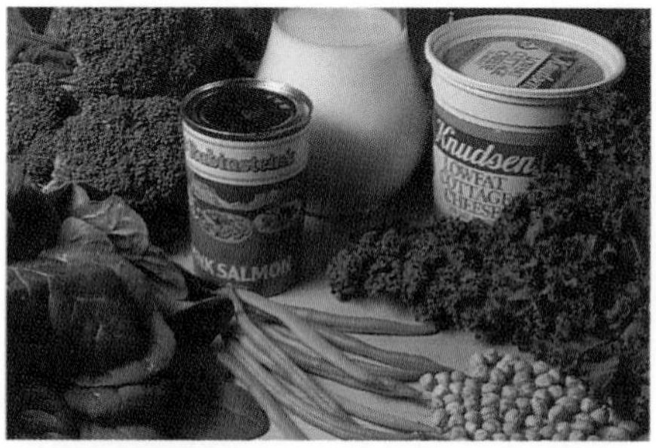

Food sources of calcium.

If foods are to be chosen to help replace milk in the diet, their calcium and riboflavin content should be the basis for making the choice, because milk and milk products normally supply about 75 percent of people's intake of calcium and about 40 percent of their riboflavin. Foods to emphasize could be selected from Table 7–2. Many of these foods supply ample amounts of vitamin A as well, but their vitamin D content is variable.

The alternatives offered for milk so far have been superior in the sense that they are whole milk dairy products or foods that offer many nutrients besides the ones listed in the tables. An inferior alternative is imitation milk. Since a milk substitute is satisfactory only if it provides high-quality protein, calcium, phosphorus, riboflavin, and vitamins A and D in quantities comparable to those in fortified fresh milk, the use of imitation milk in the diets of infants and children is generally undesirable.

Figure 7–2 presents a decision tree for people seeking a milk substitute. Note that it recommends calcium supplements only as a last resort. The reason is simply that such supplements are not foods. They do not offer the variety of nutrients foods do, and their calcium is not, for the most part, absorbed as well as that from milk. Whenever possible, a person would do better to obtain calcium from suitable substitutes in some kind of food form.

Calcium Supplements Calcium comes in a number of different salts. The organic salts include calcium lactate, calcium gluconate, and calcium citrate; the inorganic salts include calcium carbonate, calcium phosphate, and others. Since calcium carbonate is 40 percent calcium and calcium gluconate is only 9 percent, fewer pills are necessary to get the needed calcium from calcium carbonate. On the other hand, the organic salts are probably better absorbed, especially by older people, whose secretion of stomach acid—a factor known to enhance calcium absorption—tends to be reduced. A strategy to overcome this problem is to take calcium carbonate with a full breakfast.[5]

Many women wonder whether they can meet their calcium needs by taking calcium supplements instead of using milk and milk products. Supplements have the advantage of being easy to take, but they have the disadvantage of containing only calcium. They do not offer the other nutrients such as thiamin, riboflavin, niacin, potassium, phosphorus, and vitamin A found in milk. The person who omits milk and attempts to make up for it by taking supplements is still left with the task of obtaining these other nutrients. Milk drinking squares with the philosophy that using whole foods is preferable to taking supplements. In the final analysis, nutrition experts, including scientists participating in the Consensus Conference on Osteoporosis and members of the American Society for Bone and Mineral Research, strongly recommend that women consume milk and milk products daily as a source of calcium.[6] There's an easy way to do this: include them in meals.

If supplements must be used, here are some guidelines. Regular vitamin-mineral pills contain only small amounts of calcium, so read the label carefully. A 1-gram pill does not offer 1 gram of calcium; it offers 1 gram of a calcium salt, of which calcium is a part. Do not take dolomite, bone meal, or oyster shell, as their composition varies from one source to another, and some have been found to be contaminated with heavy metal poisons such as arsenic and lead. Take the supplement several times a day in divided doses, with meals, to improve absorption.

We cannot close this section without a brief word about osteoporosis risk factors other than low calcium in the diet. All persons should cut out bone

● *Figure 7–2* **Choosing a Milk Substitute**

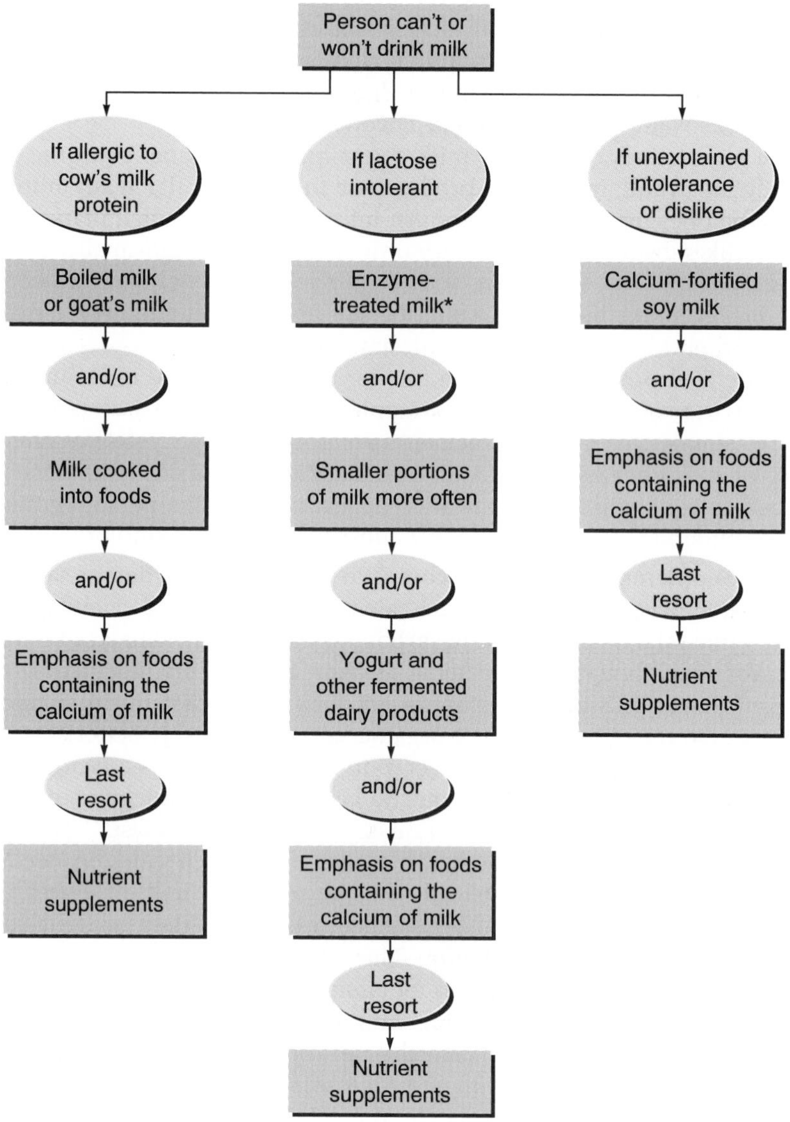

*You can buy milk already treated or add the enzyme (LactAid) yourself. Enzyme treatment may not reduce lactose content sufficiently to relieve symptoms, and you may have to try the other alternatives.

For more about exercise, see Chapter 9.

toxins such as cigarettes and large amounts of alcohol. And everyone should increase his or her activity level since exercise can reduce the risk of developing osteoporosis by making bones stronger and increasing their ability to absorb calcium.

Phosphorus

Phosphorus is second to calcium in abundance in the body. About 85 percent of it is found combined with calcium in the crystals of the bones and teeth as calcium phosphate, the chief compound that gives them strength and rigidity. Phosphorus is also a part of DNA and RNA, the genetic code material present in every cell. Thus, phosphorus is necessary for all growth because DNA and RNA provide the instructions for new cells to be formed.

Phosphorus plays many key roles in the cells' use of energy nutrients. Many enzymes and the B vitamins become active only when a phosphate group is attached. The B vitamins, you will recall, play major roles in energy metabolism. Phosphorus is critical in energy exchange.

Some lipids (phospholipids) contain phosphorus as part of their structure. They help to transport other lipids in the blood; they also form part of the structure of cell membranes, where they affect the transport of nutrients and wastes into and out of the cells.

Animal protein is the best source of phosphorus because phosphorus is so abundant in the energetic cells of animals. People who eat large amounts of animal protein have high phosphorus intakes. The recommended intakes of phosphorus are the same as those for calcium to maintain a one-to-one ratio, a level believed to provide a sufficient intake of phosphorus and ensure adequate absorption and retention of calcium. People need make no special effort to eat foods containing phosphorus, since phosphorus is present in virtually all foods.

Sodium and Potassium

Special conditions are needed to regulate the amounts of water inside and outside the cells so that the cells do not collapse from water leaving them or swell up under the stress of too much water entering them. The cells cannot manage this by pumping water across their membranes, because water slips back and forth freely. However, they can pump minerals across their membranes, and these minerals attract the water to come along with them. This is how the cells maintain water balance. Minerals are used for this purpose in a special form: as **ions** or **electrolytes.** In this form, as single, electrically charged particles, the minerals help maintain water balance and acid-base balance as well as play many other roles.

About 40 percent of the body's water weight is inside the cells, and about 15 percent bathes the outsides of the cells. The remainder is in the blood vessels.

Ions (EYE-ons) electrically charged particles, such as sodium (positively charged) or chloride (negatively charged).

Electrolytes compounds that partially dissociate in water to form ions; examples are sodium, potassium, and chloride.

Sodium and potassium are examples of electrolytes—dissolved substances in blood and body fluids that carry electric charges. Sodium is the main electrolyte found in extracellular fluids; potassium is the chief intracellular electrolyte. Electrolytes influence the distribution of fluids among the various body compartments. As an example of how electrolytes affect fluid volume, let's consider the hypothetical case of a man given one tablespoon of sodium chloride to eat and no water (NOT something we recommend trying!). The salt would become distributed in the man's body's extracellular compartment and would be excluded from his body's cells. To counterbalance this sudden change in electrolyte concentration, water would move from the cells into the extracellular space. The result would be an increase in the man's extracellular fluid volume and a decrease in intracellular volume. Under normal circumstances, many factors work together to keep the extracellular fluid volume fairly constant.

Electrolytes also provide the environment in which the cells' work takes place—work such as nerve-to-nerve communication, heartbeats, and contraction of muscles. When a person's body loses fluid—whether it be sweat, blood, or urine—the person also loses electrolytes. The concentrations of electrolytes are crucial to the life-sustaining activities of the vital organs. When large amounts of body fluid are lost, as in heat stroke, infant diarrhea, or injury, their replacement is a task for a medical team.

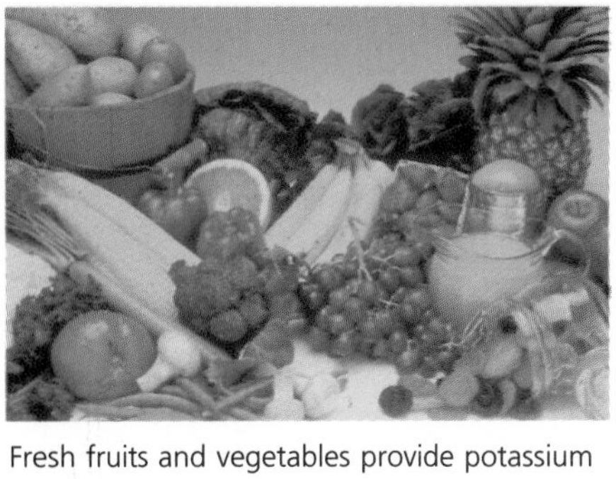

Fresh fruits and vegetables provide potassium in abundance.

Table 7–4

Whole Unprocessed Foods Versus Processed Foods—Potassium and Sodium Content

FOOD	POTASSIUM (mg)[a]	SODIUM (mg)[a]	POTASSIUM-TO-SODIUM RATIO
Milk Foods			
Milk, 1 c	370	120	3:1
Chocolate pudding (homemade), 1 c	445	146	3:1
Chocolate pudding (instant), 1 c	352	880	1:2
Meats			
Beef roast, 3 oz	254	54	5:1
Corned beef (canned), 3 oz	116	855	1:7
Chipped beef, 3 oz	377	2,946	1:8
Vegetables			
Corn, 1 c	408	28	15:1
Creamed corn, 1 c	344	730	1:2
Sugar-coated cornflakes, 1 c	17	103	1:6
Fruits			
Peaches (fresh), 1	171	1	171:1
Peaches (canned), 1	150	10	15:1
Peach pie, 1 piece	235	423	1:2
Grains			
Whole-wheat flour, 1 c	486	6	81:1
Whole-wheat bread, 1 slice	62	222	1:4
Wheat crackers, 4	62	118	1:2

[a]Data are taken from Appendix F.

Salt a pair of charged mineral particles, such as sodium (Na+) and chloride (Cl-), that associate together. In water, they dissociate and help to carry electric current—that is, they become electrolytes.

Hypertension sustained high blood pressure.
hyper = too much
tension = pressure

See Consumer Tips on page 188 for a list of foods that are high in sodium.

Sodium is part of sodium chloride, ordinary table **salt**, a food seasoning and preservative. No recommendation is necessary for a minimum intake of sodium, since sodium is so abundant in the U.S. diet. For some people, however, a ceiling is suggested (see inside front cover), because the use of highly salted foods can contribute to high blood pressure (**hypertension**) in those who are genetically susceptible. (A discussion of the causes, treatment, and prevention of hypertension appears in the Nutrition Action feature of this chapter.)

If some people in your family have high blood pressure (and this is more likely if you are black than if you are white), you are advised to curtail your sodium consumption and make sure that your potassium and calcium intakes are ample. Table 7–4 shows a sampling of the sodium content of common foods and reveals that generally, the more processed a food is, the more sodium and the less potassium it contains. Whole, unprocessed foods, on the other hand, tend to be high in potassium and low in sodium.

Persons who wish to avoid salt need to know that what they pour from the salt shaker may be only a third of the total salt they consume. Up to half of the salt in the diet is that added to foods by food processors. Processed foods don't always taste salty. This makes eating something of a guessing game. The serious sodium avoider must eat fresh rather than processed foods and choose sit-down and Western restaurants rather than fast-food places and Asian restaurants. An even simpler strategy is to stop salting foods at the table. Reducing your salt intake doesn't have to be unpleasant. Many sodium-free flavoring agents such as lemons, onions, chilies, curries, and other spices excite the tastebuds and enhance the flavors of traditional foods.

Potassium is critical to maintaining the heartbeat. The sudden deaths that occur during fasting, severe diarrhea, or severe vomiting are thought to be due to heart failure caused by potassium loss. As the principal positively charged ion inside body cells, potassium plays a major role in maintaining water balance and cell integrity.

When sodium is lost with water from the body, the ultimate damage comes when potassium moves out of the cells with cell water and is excreted. This is especially dangerous because potassium deficiency affects the brain cells, making the victim unaware of the need for water. Adults are warned not to take **diuretics** (water pills) except under the direction of a physician, because some of them cause potassium excretion. Physicians prescribing such diuretics will tell their patients to eat potassium-rich foods to compensate for the losses and, depending on the diuretic, may advise a lowered sodium intake, too.

Diuretics (dye-you-RET-ics) medications causing increased water excretion.
dia = through
ouron = urine

The relationship of potassium and sodium in maintaining the blood pressure is not entirely clear. Abundant evidence supports the simple view that the two minerals have opposite effects, but an occasional experiment produces contradictory findings.[7] In any case, it is clear that increasing the potassium in the diet can promote sodium excretion under most circumstances and thereby lower the blood pressure.[8] A lifelong intake of foods low in sodium and high in potassium protects against hypertension and is thought to account for the low blood pressure seen in vegetarians.[9]

A dietary deficiency of potassium is unlikely, but high-sodium diets low in fresh fruits and vegetables can make it a possibility. Whole foods of all kinds, including fruits, vegetables, grains, meats, fish, and poultry, are among the richest sources of potassium. Potassium is also abundant in milk. Table 7–5 shows the potassium content of foods.

It is hardly ever necessary to take potassium supplements, even with diuretic use, because food sources are so rich in this mineral. Among healthy people, only two groups risk depletion. One group is people who eat diets composed of heavily processed, heavily salted foods. These people might fail to get enough potassium. Of course, rather than take supplements, they need to change their eating habits. The other group is people who ingest fewer than 800 calories a day—for example, people on semifasts to lose weight. A physician must monitor the potassium status of these people and order supplements commensurate with the degree of depletion.[10]

Potassium toxicity is a greater concern than potassium deficiency. The body protects itself from this eventuality as best it can. If you consume more than you need, the kidneys accelerate their excretion and so maintain control. Should their limit be exceeded (if you ingest too much potassium too fast), a vomiting reflex is triggered. However, if the digestive tract is bypassed and potassium is injected into a vein at a high rate, it can stop the heart.

Table 7–5

Potassium in Foods

Suggested intakes: 1,875 to 5,625 mg.

(mg)	SOURCES
1,295	Peach halves, dried (10)
1,163	Lima beans (1 c)
1,071	Winter squash (1 c)
928	Sirloin steak (8 oz)
882	Pinto beans (1 c)
844	Baked potato (1)
838	Spinach, cooked (1 c)
825	Cantaloupe (½)
673	Kidney beans (1 c)
630	Bok choy, cooked (1 c)
626	Prunes, dried (10)
583	Butternut squash (1 c)
573	Black-eyed peas (1 c)
560	Watermelon (1 slice)
558	Asparagus, cooked (1 c)
532	Beets, cooked (1 c)
529	Tomatoes, canned (1 c)
496	Orange juice (1 c)
482	Apricot halves, dried (10)
451	Banana (1)
406	Nonfat milk or yogurt (1 c)

Chloride, Sulfur, and Magnesium

The chloride ion is the major negatively charged ion of the fluids outside the cells, where it is found mostly in association with sodium. Chloride can move freely across membranes and so is also found inside the cells in association

Consumer Tips

Seasoning Foods Without Excess Salt

You've decided to cut your salt intake. How do you know which foods to buy? How can you cook foods with less salt and good flavor? Fortunately, cutting some of the salt out of your diet isn't difficult. Here are a few basic principles.

At the supermarket

- Read labels! Look for the key words *salt* and *sodium* in the ingredients list. These are signals that the foods contain added sodium. Here is a short list of a few sodium-containing ingredients used in food processing:[11] baking powder, baking soda, disodium phosphate, monosodium glutamate (MSG), salt, sodium alginate, sodium benzoate, sodium hydroxide, sodium nitrite, sodium propionate, and sodium sulfite.
- Choose reduced-sodium food products when possible. Many commercially prepared products are now available in sodium-reduced versions. For example, most supermarkets carry reduced-sodium soy sauce, canned tuna, soups, and canned vegetables.
- Buy fresh, natural foods more frequently than processed foods, which tend to be high in salt. Here is a list of processed and convenience foods that are typically high in salt:

Meat, Poultry, Fish

- Cured meats: ham, bacon, luncheon meats
- Sausages
- Hot dogs
- Fish: commercially frozen, prebreaded
- Fish: canned in oil or brine
- Canned shellfish

Meat Substitutes

- Salted nuts or seeds
- Canned beans and peas
- Soy protein products

Main Dish Items

- Pizza, lasagna, macaroni and cheese
- Commercially prepared main course foods (e.g., TV dinners)
- Tacos, enchiladas, burritos
- Canned or dehydrated soups or chowders

Canned Vegetables and Vegetable Juices

Dairy Products

- Cheeses
- Buttermilk
- Instant cocoa mixes
- Dutch process cocoa

Bread Products

- Salted snack foods (e.g., crackers, potato chips)
- Commercially baked goods (e.g., cakes, cookies)

Miscellaneous Products

- Catsup, chili sauce
- Salted gravies and sauces
- Olives, pickles, pickle relish
- Commercial salad dressings
- Seasoning salts
- Bouillon cubes
- Meat tenderizers (e.g., MSG, Accent)

At home—in the kitchen and at the table

- Put the salt shaker in the kitchen cabinet, not on the table, and use it only on rare occasions. It's surprising how much additional sodium is added to foods with just a few shakes of the salt shaker. Here's a handy guide for the sodium content of common kitchen measures of salt:

1/8 tsp of salt	=	288 mg of sodium
1/4 tsp of salt	=	575 mg of sodium
1/2 tsp of salt	=	1,150 mg of sodium
3/4 tsp of salt	=	1,725 mg of sodium
1 tsp of salt	=	2,300 mg of sodium

- Flavor your foods with seasonings and spices, most of which are virtually salt and sodium free. Try some of the seasonings listed in your favorite dishes:

allspice	lemon juice
almond extract	mace
basil	mustard (dry)
bay leaves	nutmeg
caraway seeds	onion (not onion salt)
chives	paprika
cider vinegar	parsley
cinnamon	pimiento
curry powder	rosemary
dill	sage
garlic (not garlic salt)	thyme
ginger	turmeric

- Salt substitutes can be used as a means of reducing sodium intake. They usually consist of a mineral base other than sodium and are compounded to give a taste sensation similar to sodium chloride. The most common components are potassium chloride, calcium chloride, and ammonium chloride. [**Caution:** Before using salt substitutes, check with your doctor. Some people, especially those with kidney problems or liver disease, should *not* use these products.] A few salt substitutes are Adolph's Salt Substitute, Diamond Crystal, Featherweight K Salt Substitute, Morton's Lite Salt, Morton's Salt Substitute, No Salt, and Nu-Salt.[12]

with potassium. In the blood, chloride helps in maintaining the acid-base balance. In the stomach, the chloride ion is part of hydrochloric acid, which maintains the strong acidity of the stomach. Nearly all dietary chloride comes from sodium chloride or salt.

Sulfur is present in some amino acids and in all proteins. Its most important role is in helping strands of protein to assume and hold a particular shape, and so to do their specific jobs, such as enzyme work. Skin, hair, and nails contain some of the body's more rigid proteins, and these have a high sulfur content. There is no recommended intake for sulfur, and no deficiencies are known. Only a person who lacks protein to the point of severe deficiency will lack the sulfur-containing amino acids.

Magnesium acts in all the cells of the soft tissues, where it forms part of the protein-making machinery and where it is necessary for the release of energy. Magnesium also helps relax muscles after contraction and promotes resistance to tooth decay by helping to hold calcium in tooth enamel. Bone magnesium seems to be a reservoir to ensure that some will be on hand for vital reactions regardless of recent dietary intake. A dietary deficiency of magnesium is not likely but may occur as a result of vomiting, diarrhea, alcohol abuse, or protein malnutrition; in people who have been fed incomplete fluids into a vein for too long; or in people using diuretics. Good food sources of magnesium include nuts, legumes, cereal grains, dark-green vegetables, seafoods, chocolate, and cocoa.

The Trace Minerals

If you could extract all of the trace minerals from the body, you would obtain only a bit of dust, hardly enough to fill a teaspoon. As tiny as their quantities are, though, each of the trace minerals performs some vital role for which no substitute will do. A deficiency of any of them may be fatal, and an excess of many is equally deadly.

Iron

Iron is the body's oxygen carrier. Bound into the protein **hemoglobin** in the red blood cells, it helps transport oxygen from lungs to tissues and so permits the release of energy from fuels to do the cells' work. When the iron supply is too low, **iron-deficiency anemia** occurs, characterized by weakness, tiredness, apathy, headaches, and a paleness that reflects the reduction in the number and size of red blood cells. A person with this anemia can do very little muscular work without disabling fatigue but can replenish iron status by eating iron-rich foods for a few weeks.

Hemoglobin (HEEM-oh-globe-in) the oxygen-carrying protein of the blood; found in the red blood cells.
hemo = blood
globin = spherical protein
Iron-deficiency anemia a reduction of the number and size of red blood cells and a loss of their color because of iron deficiency.

It is difficult to convey the extent and severity of iron deficiency among the world's people. Iron deficiency occurs in as many as half of all persons in some settings, even in developed countries—most predictably in inner-city and rural poor. People begin to feel iron deficiency's impact long before anemia is diagnosed. They don't appear to have an obvious deficiency disease; they just appear unmotivated and apathetic. Because they work and play less, they are less physically fit. Prevalence rates for iron-deficiency anemia in developed countries range from 10 to 20 percent. Rates are higher in

[Continued on page 192]

NUTRITION ACTION

Diet and Blood Pressure: The Salt Shaker and Beyond

Think "diet" and "blood pressure," and the first thing that comes to mind is salt. Small wonder, given that experts have long emphasized that a diet high in salt—or more specifically, the sodium it contains—contributes to a public health problem known as hypertension (or high blood pressure).[13] Nevertheless, a number of other, albeit less notorious, dietary factors play roles in the unhealthful rises in blood pressure that afflict some 60 million Americans.

Obesity, for instance, inarguably ranks as the number one dietary culprit linked to hypertension. That's because excess weight forces the heart to work harder to supply the extra pounds of tissue with blood. High blood pressure occurs about twice as often among obese people as it does in thinner people. Fortunately, losing as little as 5 percent of the excess weight has been shown, in some cases, to lower blood pressure to a point at which taking antihypertensive medications becomes unnecessary.[14] In other words, a little weight loss, regardless of sodium intake, can be enough to get a high blood pressure level back under control.

Another dietary factor that may lead to high blood pressure (not to mention poor compliance with drug regimens and other treatments for the problem) is drinking excessive amounts of alcohol. In fact, consuming more than a couple of ounces of alcohol daily has been blamed for leading to 5 to 11 percent of cases of hypertension among men.[15] That's why the Joint National Committee on Detection, Evaluation, and Treatment of High Blood Pressure recommends that to control high pressure, those who drink should limit themselves to no more than 1 ounce of alcohol a day—an amount found in 2 ounces of 100-proof whiskey, an 8-ounce glass of wine, or two 12-ounce cans of beer.[16]

In addition to losing weight and drinking alcohol in moderation, the Committee advises those with hypertension to limit the amount of sodium in their diets. Whether such advice is appropriate for the public at large, however, has been widely debated. Some experts argue against the necessity of doing so in all but a few select cases. The controversy revolves around a growing body of evidence suggesting that not everyone's blood pressure rises as a result of eating a high-sodium diet. Only certain people, presumably because of their genetic makeup, appear to be **salt sensitive**, meaning that their blood pressure rises in proportion to the amount of sodium they eat. For

Salt sensitive the tendency for blood pressure to rise in proportion to salt consumption that certain people seem to have from birth.

them, of course, keeping dietary sodium to a minimum can help lower elevated blood pressure.

The problem is that it is difficult to identify who is salt sensitive and who is not. Thus, some experts argue that a call to the general public to reduce sodium consumption is unwarranted because it recommends that even people who are not salt sensitive avoid the seasoning. On the other side of the fence are experts and organizations, the National Research Council among them, whose position is that because lowering the amount of sodium in the diet does not pose any health hazard and may be beneficial to some people, it is still prudent for the public as a whole to keep sodium intake in check.[17] And for those who take medication to control their blood pressure, the argument in favor of adhering to a low-sodium diet is stronger; eating too much salt can limit the effectiveness of some antihypertensive medications.

In any case, it is clear that modest changes in lifestyle can add up to significant gains in controlling high blood pressure. In addition, it appears that attention to a healthful lifestyle can help prevent the problem from arising in the first place. Consider that researchers at Northwestern University Medical School in Chicago put one group of adults prone to elevations in blood pressure on a preventive program that included losing weight, lowering sodium intake, cutting down on alcohol, and exercising more and compared them to a similar group left to their own devices. They found that over the course of 5 years only one in eleven persons who changed their lifestyles wound up with full-blown hypertension. But of those who didn't alter their habits, one in five became hypertensive.[18]

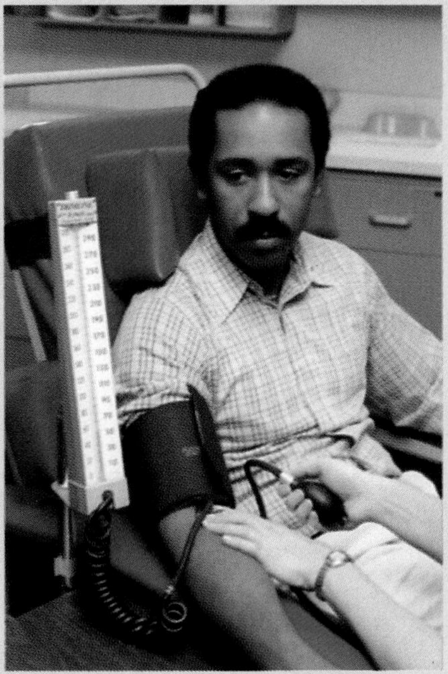

The most effective single measure you can take to protect yourself against high blood pressure is to know what your blood pressure is.

Along with the factors explained above, scientists are exploring other nutrients that may influence blood pressure. Some researchers believe, for instance, that it is not dietary sodium *per se* that alters blood pressure, but rather the ratio between it and potassium, sodium's partner in regulating the body's water balance. In other words, the more potassium and less sodium in the diet, the greater the likelihood that the body will maintain a normal blood pressure. While the evidence is not strong enough to imply that people with high blood pressure need to take potassium supplements (such a practice can be dangerous), it's worth keeping in mind, particularly because diets rich in high-potassium foods such as fresh fruits and vegetables tend to go hand-in-hand with low sodium consumption.[19]

In addition, some studies indicate that people who eat high-calcium diets are less likely to have high blood pressure; conversely, people with inadequate calcium intakes are more likely to have hypertension. The jury is still out on that relationship, however. Until more evidence comes in, simply eating a diet that contains two to three servings daily of calcium-rich foods such as dairy products remains the best advice.[20]

Another nutrient under investigation for contributing to hypertension is chloride, the mineral found along with sodium in salt. (Salt is about 40 percent sodium and 60 percent chloride.) Some evidence has come to light that dietary sodium raises blood pressure only when accompanied by chloride. In other words, it may not be sodium in and of itself, but rather salt, that contributes to elevations in blood pressure. In the United States, incidentally, about 95 percent of sodium consumed comes from salt.[21]

Finally, some evidence suggests that eating a diet low in saturated fat and high in polyunsaturated fat helps lower blood pressure. Though the relation-

Risk Factors for High Blood Pressure

Obesity

Family history of high blood pressure

Race (Black people are more likely than whites to develop hypertension.)

Age (In the U. S., blood pressure tends to rise with age.)

Excess alcohol consumption

ship remains tenuous, it certainly makes sense for those with high blood pressure to eat such a diet, if for no other reason than to help prevent heart disease, a condition that hypertensives run a high risk of developing (refer to the Spotlight feature in Chapter 4).[22]

Are Your Numbers Up?

One of the characteristics of hypertension is that it has been called a silent killer that cannot be felt and may go undetected for years. That's why it is crucial to have your blood pressure checked on a regular basis. Diagnosis of hypertension requires at least two elevated readings. The first of the two numbers in a blood pressure reading—systolic pressure—represents the force exerted by the heart as it contracts to pump blood throughout the body, as measured by the number of millimeters that the pressure pushes a column of mercury up a tube. The second number—diastolic pressure—is a measure of the pressure the blood exerts on artery walls between heart beats. A reading of up to 120 over 80 millimeters of mercury is considered normal for people aged 18 or under. Over the age of 18, measurements as high as 140 over 90 are normal. Beyond those levels, the risks of heart attacks and strokes rise in direct proportion to increasing blood pressure.[23]

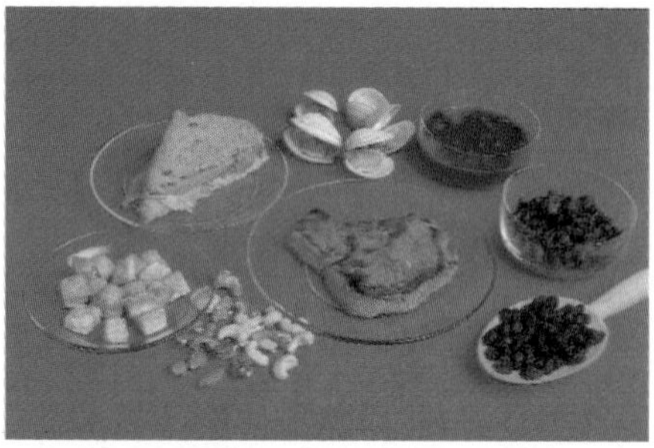

Food sources of iron: liverwurst, steamed clams, black beans, spinach, raisins, beef sirloin, nuts, and tofu.

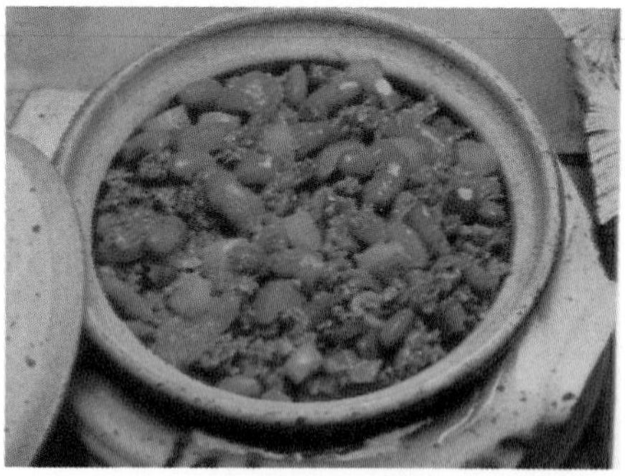

You can combine foods to achieve maximum iron absorption—the meat and tomatoes in this chili help you absorb iron from the beans.

the developing countries, and therefore the incidence of iron deficiency less severe than anemia must be higher still.[24] If this one worldwide malnutrition problem could be alleviated, millions of people would benefit.

The cause of iron deficiency is usually malnutrition—that is, inadequate intake, either from limited access to food or from high consumption of foods low in iron. In the Western world, high sugar and fat intakes are often contributing factors. Among causes other than malnutrition, blood loss is the primary one, caused in many countries by parasitic infections of the digestive tract.

The subject of marginal deficiencies—deficiencies that exhibit few or none of the classic symptoms of severe deficiencies—is a touchy one with reputable dietitians, because it is the stuff of which quackery is made. On the pretext that you have "subclinical deficiencies," quacks will try to sell you an arsenal of expensive and unneeded nutrition nostrums. The majority of subclinical deficiencies are fantasies created by such tricksters, who are clever at stating their claims in such a way that they are hard to either prove or disprove. This is one reason why they are so often successful. Another reason, unfortunately, is that sometimes they are right. Subclinical deficiencies do exist, they do make people miserable, and the relief that can be gained by having them properly diagnosed and treated can be enormous. The case of iron is a case in point. Published scientific research provides massive amounts of evidence that subclinical deficiencies are real and widespread. (Review Chapter 1 for approaches to evaluating nutrition and health claims.)

The usual Western mixed diet provides only about 5 to 6 milligrams of iron in every 1,000 calories. The recommended daily intake for an adult man is 10 milligrams. Because most men easily eat more than 2,000 calories, they can meet their iron needs without special effort.

The situation for women is different. Women may have normal blood cell counts or hemoglobin levels, and yet they may need more iron because their body stores may be depleted, a factor that doesn't show up in standard tests. Because most women typically eat less food than men, their iron intakes are lower. And because women menstruate, their iron losses are greater. These two factors may put women much closer to the borderline of deficiency.

The recommended intake for a woman before menopause is 15 milligrams per day; pregnant women need 30 milligrams daily. To get this much iron from the average U.S. diet, a woman would have to eat 3,000 calories a day (or 6,000 calories if pregnant). Because women typically consume fewer than 2,000 calories per day, they understandably have trouble achieving adequate iron intakes. A woman who wants to meet her iron needs from foods must increase the iron-to-calorie ratio of her diet so that she will receive about double the average amount of iron—about 10 milligrams per 1,000 calories. This means she must emphasize iron-rich foods in her daily diet.

Table 7–6 shows the amounts of iron in foods. Meats, fish, and poultry are superior sources on a per-serving basis, but vegetables compare favorably with all other foods on a per-calorie basis. People must select foods carefully to obtain enough iron because it is present in such small quantities in most foods. The best meat sources are liver and other organ meats, red meats, poultry, fish, oysters, and clams. Among the grains, whole grains and enriched and fortified breads and cereals are best; and dried beans are a good source. Some fruits and vegetables contain appreciable amounts of iron, as shown in the table. Foods in the milk group are notoriously poor iron sources.

Ways to Enhance Iron Absorption Iron occurs in two forms in foods—as **heme** iron, bound into the iron-carrying proteins such as hemoglobin in meats, poultry, and fish, and as **nonheme** iron in plant foods. Heme iron contributes only 1 to 2 milligrams of the 10 to 20 milligrams of iron the average person consumes in a day; nonheme iron makes up the majority of dietary iron. Heme iron is absorbed at a relatively constant rate of about 23 percent over a wide range of meat intakes, but nonheme iron's absorption is affected by many factors, including the amount of vitamin C consumed with meals. The Iron Absorption Scorecard shows you how to estimate the iron you absorb from a meal.[25]

Contamination iron—that is, iron obtained from cookware or soil—can also increase iron intake significantly. Consumers who cook their foods in iron cookware can contribute to their iron intakes. For example, the iron content of a half-cup of spaghetti sauce simmered in a glass dish is 3 milligrams, but it is 87 milligrams when the sauce is cooked in an iron skillet. Similarly, the reason why dried apricots or raisins contain more iron than the fresh fruit is because they are dried in iron pans. Admittedly, this form of iron is not as well absorbed as the iron from meat, but every little bit helps.

Some food components interfere with iron absorption. Phytic acid is one example; it occurs in some fruits, vegetables, and whole grains, as mentioned earlier, as well as in tea. Another example is tannic acid, which occurs in commercial black and pekoe teas, coffee, cola drinks, chocolate, and red

Table 7–6 Iron in Foods

Adult RDA is 10 to 15 mg.

(mg)	SOURCES
7.68	Sirloin steak (8 oz)
6.42	Spinach, cooked (1 c)
5.90	Lima beans (1 c)
5.30	Beef liver (3 oz)
5.28	Peach halves, dried (10)
5.10	Navy beans (1 c)
4.60	Kidney beans (1 c)
3.40	Peas, dry split (1 c)
3.30	Black-eyed peas (1 c)
3.15	Green peas (1 c)
3.14	Beef pot roast (3 oz)
3.02	Prune juice (1 c)
2.75	Baked potato (1)
2.74	Beet greens, cooked (1 c)
2.60	Sardines (3 oz)
2.23	Tofu (soybean curd) (4 oz)
2.20	Shrimp (3.5 oz)
1.78	Broccoli, cooked (1 c)
1.65	Apricot halves, dried (10)
1.59	Oatmeal, cooked (1 c)
0.96	Whole-wheat bread (1 oz)

Heme (HEEM) iron the iron-holding part of the hemoglobin protein, found in meat, fish, and poultry. About 40% of the iron in meat, fish, and poultry is bound into heme. Meat, fish, and poultry also contain a factor (MFP factor) other than heme that promotes the absorption of iron, even of the iron from other foods eaten at the same time as the meat.

Nonheme iron the iron found in plant foods.

Contamination iron iron found in foods as the result of contamination by inorganic iron salts from iron cookware, iron-containing soils, and the like.

Iron Absorption Scorecard

Three factors go into the calculation of how much iron you absorb from a meal—first, how much of the iron in the meal was heme versus nonheme iron; second, how much vitamin C was in the meal; and third, how much total meat, fish, and poultry (MFP) you consumed. (It is assumed that your iron stores are moderate; otherwise, you would have to take this into consideration, too.) Here is how it works. First, answer these six questions:

1. How much iron was from animal tissues (MFP)? _______ mg.
2. Forty percent of this is heme iron. _______mg heme iron.
3. How much iron was from other sources? _______mg.
4. This, plus 60 percent of (1), is nonheme iron. _______mg nonheme iron.
5. How much vitamin C was in the meal? Less than 25 milligrams is low; 25 to 75 milligrams is medium; more than 75 milligrams is high. Check one: ___low ___medium ___high.
6. How much MFP was in the meal? Less than 1 ounce lean MFP is low; 1 to 3 ounces is medium; more than 3 ounces is high.[a] Check one: ___low ___medium ___high.

Now you are ready to calculate.
You absorbed 23 percent of your heme iron, so take the number you wrote in number 2 and multiply it by 0.23. Enter the result in A, below.

Now, look at numbers 5 and 6. If you recorded one "high" or two "mediums," check *high availability* below. If you recorded no "highs" and only one "medium," check *medium availability.* If you recorded two "lows," check *low availability.* Check one: ____low availability ____medium availability ____high availability.

Now multiply your nonheme iron (from number 4) by one of the following:

- If you checked *high availability:* multiply by 0.08.
- If you checked *medium availability:* multiply by 0.05.
- If you checked *low availability:* multiply by 0.03.

Enter the result in B below.
Finally, add A and B together:

A. _______ mg heme iron absorbed.
B. _______ mg nonheme iron absorbed.
Total = _______ mg iron absorbed.

Now, was that enough?[b] If you are a man of any age or a woman over 50 years old, you need to absorb 1 milligram per day. If you are a woman 11 to 50 years old, you need to absorb 1.8 milligrams. If you have higher menstrual losses than the average woman, you may need still more.

[a]We have adapted the calculations of Monsen and coauthors, stating them in ounces. Their actual numbers are 69 grams cooked meat (high); 23 to 46 grams (medium); less than 23 grams (low). E. R. Monsen and coauthors, Estimation of available dietary iron, *American Journal of Clinical Nutrition* 31 (1978): 134–141.
[b]The RDA assumes you will absorb 10 percent of the iron you ingest.

wines. Fiber can also reduce iron absorption, because it speeds up the transit of materials through the intestine.

Zinc

Zinc plays roles of major importance in association with the cellular machinery in every body organ. It is necessary for the normal metabolism of protein, carbohydrate, fat, and alcohol. Zinc is associated with the hormone insulin, which regulates the body's fuel supply. It is involved in cell multiplication, immune reactions, the utilization of vitamin A, taste perception, wound healing, the synthesis of sperm, and the development of the fetus. Zinc is lost from the body daily in much the same way as protein is, and so it must be replenished daily.

Zinc deficiencies were first reported in the 1960s in the Middle East, where studies on adolescent boys revealed severe growth retardation and delayed sexual maturation—symptoms responsive to zinc supplementation. The native diets were typically low in animal protein and zinc and high in fiber and other compounds that bind minerals. The researchers learned that

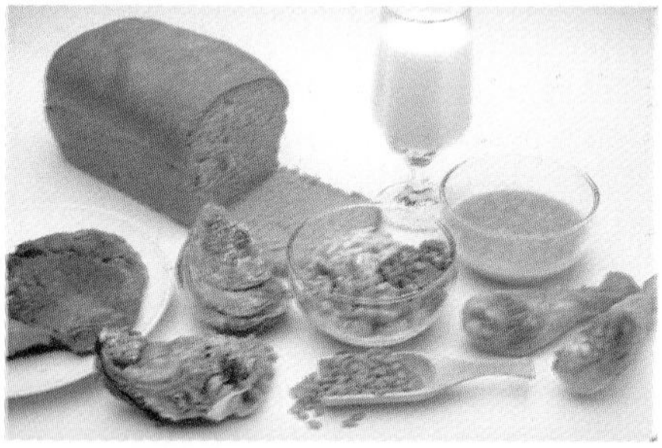
Food sources of zinc: whole-wheat bread, milk, pea soup, chicken, peanuts, legumes, oysters, and pork chops.

the binders were carrying zinc out of the boys' bodies, thus causing the deficiency.

Since then, cases of zinc deficiency have been discovered closer to home.[26] A number of Denver schoolchildren had poor growth, poor appetite, and decreased taste sensitivity due to zinc deficiency. The children were described as picky eaters and ate less than an ounce of meat per day.

People who are building new tissue have the highest zinc needs—infants, children, teenagers and pregnant women. The pregnant teenager is at particular risk because she needs zinc for her own growth as well as for her fetus's growth. Pregnant vegetarians are at risk, too, because their diets are high in zinc-binding fibers. Dieters also need to be reminded that very-low-calorie diets cause not only a low zinc intake but also a loss of zinc from body tissues as they break down to release fuel.

Zinc is a relatively nontoxic element. However, it can be toxic if consumed in large enough quantities. Consumption of high levels of zinc may cause vomiting, diarrhea, fever, exhaustion, and a host of other symptoms.[27] The hazards of overconsumption are greatest when consumers dose themselves with supplements. Chronic consumption of zinc exceeding 15 milligrams per day is not recommended without close medical supervision.

Table 7–7 shows the zinc amounts in foods. An average 1,500-calorie diet provides about 6.3 milligrams of zinc per day, or about 40 percent to 50 percent of the RDA. Zinc is highest in foods of high protein content, such as shellfish (especially oysters), meats, and liver. As a rule of thumb, two ordinary servings a day of animal protein will provide most of the zinc a healthy person needs. Eggs and whole-grain products are good sources of zinc if large quantities are eaten (the phytate in grains does not inhibit the absorption of zinc in people consuming ordinary diets). Cow's milk protein (casein) binds zinc avidly and seems to prevent its absorption somewhat; infants absorb zinc better from human breast milk. Fresh or canned vegetables vary in zinc content, depending on the soil in which they are grown. The zinc content of cooking water varies from region to region as well.

Table 7–7

Zinc in Foods

Adult RDA is 12 to 15 mg.

(mg)	SOURCES
76.70	Oysters, cooked (6)
13.38	Sirloin steak (8 oz)
5.13	Crabmeat (1 c)
5.09	Beef pot roast (3 oz)
4.34	Beef liver (3 oz)
3.99	Lamb chop (3 oz)
3.74	Ground beef (3 oz)
3.70	Shrimp (3.5 oz)
3.22	Black-eyed peas (1 c)
2.64	Turkey (3 oz)
2.40	Pinto beans (1 c)
2.00	Kidney beans (1 c)
1.37	Spinach, cooked (1 c)
1.10	Swiss cheese (1 oz)
0.93	Collards, cooked (1 c)
0.93	Peanuts (1 oz)
0.92	Nonfat milk or yogurt (1 c)
0.92	Cheddar cheese (1 oz)
0.88	Tofu (soybean curd) (4 oz)
0.86	Asparagus, cooked (1 c)
0.50	Whole-wheat bread (1 oz)

Iodine

Iodine occurs in the body in an infinitesimally small quantity, but its principal role in human nutrition is well-known. It is part of the thyroid hormones, which regulate body temperature, metabolic rate, reproduction, and growth. The hormones enter every cell of the body to control the rate at which the cells use oxygen and release energy.

When the iodine level of the blood is low, the thyroid gland may enlarge until it causes swelling in the throat area—a condition called **goiter.** Goiter is estimated to affect 200 million people the world over.

Goiter (GOY-ter) enlargement of the thyroid gland due to iodine deficiency.

Cretinism (CREE-tin-ism) severe mental and physical retardation of an infant caused by iodine deficiency during pregnancy.

In addition to causing sluggishness and weight gain, an iodine deficiency may have serious effects on fetal development. Severe thyroid undersecretion of a women during pregnancy causes the extreme and irreversible mental and physical retardation of the child known as **cretinism.** A person with this condition has a face and body with many abnormalities including mental retardation. Much of the mental retardation associated with cretinism can be averted by early diagnosis and treatment of the mother's iodine deficiency.

The amount of iodine in foods reflects the amount present in the soil in which plants are grown or on which animals graze. In the United States, in areas where the soil is low in iodine (most notably around the Great Lakes and in the Willamette Valley of Oregon), widespread goiter and cretinism appeared in the local people during the 1930s. Iodized salt was introduced as a preventive measure, and these scourges disappeared.

Excessive intakes of iodine can cause an enlargement of the thyroid gland resembling goiter; in infants it can be so severe as to block the airways and cause suffocation. A dramatic increase in iodine intakes in the United States has occurred recently. The toxic level at which detectable harm results is thought to be only a few times higher than current average consumption levels.[28] Most of the excess iodine seems to be coming from iodates (dough conditioners used in the baking industry) and from milk produced by cows exposed to iodine-containing medications and disinfectants. Now that the problem has been identified, both the baking and the dairy industries have reduced their use of these compounds, but the sudden emergence of this problem points to a need for continued surveillance of the food supply.

Fluoride

Only a trace of fluoride occurs in the human body, but studies have demonstrated that where diets are high in fluoride, the crystalline deposits in teeth and bones are larger and more perfectly formed than where diets are low in it. Fluoride not only protects children's teeth from decay, but also makes the bones of older people resistant to adult bone loss (osteoporosis). Its continuous presence in body fluids is desirable.

Alternatives to water fluoridation:

- Fluoride toothpastes
- Fluoride treatments for teeth
- Fluoride tablets and drops

Fluorosis (floor-OH-sis) discoloration of the teeth due to ingestion of too much fluoride during tooth development.

Drinking water is the usual source of fluoride. Where fluoride is lacking in the water supply, the incidence of dental decay is very high. Fluoridation of community water where needed to raise its fluoride concentration to one part per million (ppm) is thus an important public health measure (see Figure 7–3).

In some communities, the natural fluoride concentration in water is high (2–8 ppm), and children's teeth develop with mottled enamel. This condition, called **fluorosis**, may not be harmful (in fact, these children's teeth may be extraordinarily decay resistant), but it violates the prejudice that teeth should be white. Fluorosis does not occur in communities where fluoride is added to the water supply.

True toxicity from fluoride overdoses can occur, but only after chronic daily intakes, for years, of 20 to 80 times the amounts normally consumed from fluoridated water. Despite the value of fluoride, violent disagreement often surrounds the introduction of fluoridation to a community's water. Additional coverage of the debate about the health effects of fluoride is given in the Spotlight feature at the end of this chapter.

Copper, Manganese, Chromium, Selenium, and Molybdenum

Several trace minerals have been found to play important roles in a variety of metabolic and physiologic processes. Copper, for example, is involved in making red blood cells, manufacturing collagen, healing wounds, and maintaining the sheaths around nerve fibers. Chromium works closely with the hormone insulin to help the cells take up glucose and break it down for energy. Selenium functions as part of an antioxidant enzyme and can substitute for vitamin E in some of that vitamin's antioxidant activities. Manganese

● *Figure 7–3* **Fluoridation in the United States**

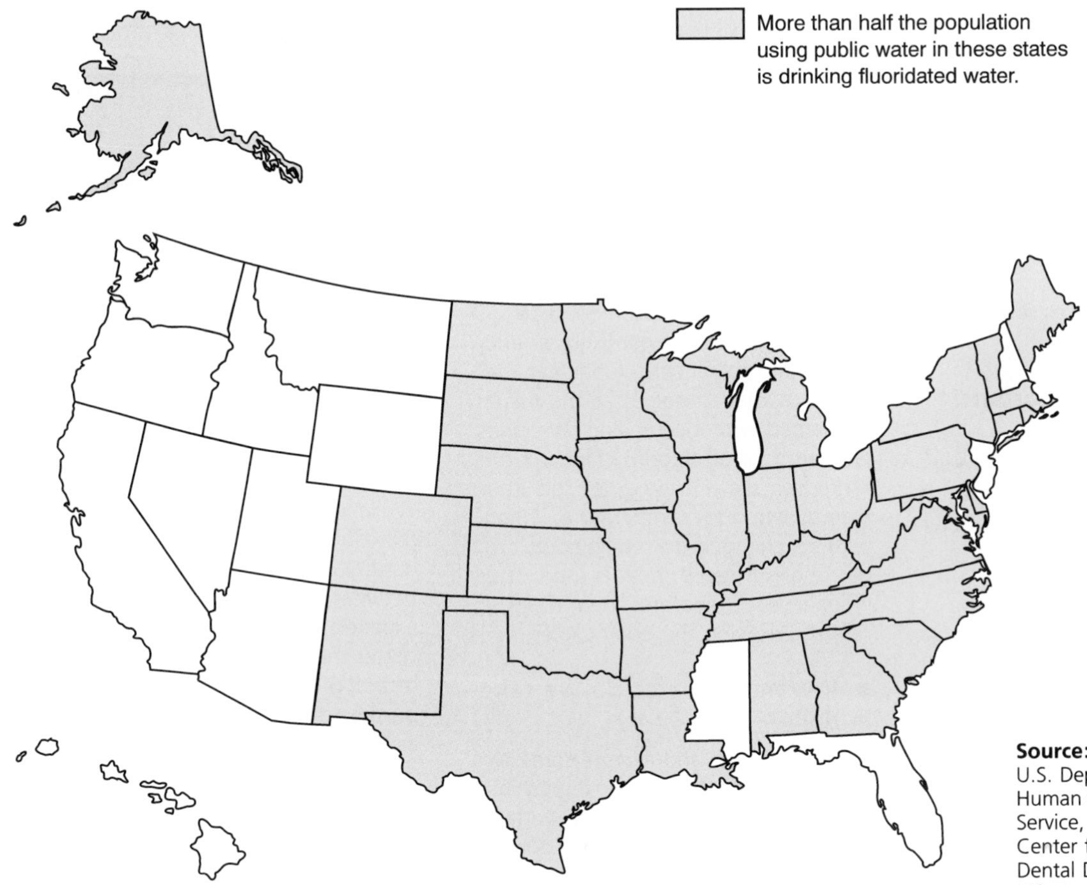
More than half the population using public water in these states is drinking fluoridated water.

Source: Fluoridation Census—1985. U.S. Department of Health and Human Services, Public Health Service, Centers for Disease Control, Center for Prevention Services, Dental Disease Prevention Activity. Atlanta, GA 30333, July 1988.

and molybdenum both function as working parts of several enzymes. (Refer to Table 7–1 for a brief description and common food sources of each of these minerals.)

Trace Minerals of Uncertain Status

None of the trace minerals has been known for very long, and some are extremely recent newcomers. Nickel is now recognized as important for the health of many body tissues; deficiencies harm the liver and other organs. Silicon is known to be involved in bone calcification, at least in animals. Tin is necessary for growth in animals and probably in humans. Vanadium, too, is necessary for growth and bone development as well as for normal reproduction. Cobalt is recognized as the mineral in the large vitamin B_{12} molecule; the alternative name for this vitamin—cobalamin—reflects the presence of cobalt. In the future we may discover that many other trace minerals—for example, silver, mercury, lead, barium, and cadmium—also play key roles in human nutrition. Even arsenic, famous as the poisonous instrument of death in many murder mysteries and known to be a carcinogen, may turn out to be an essential nutrient in tiny quantities.

Spotlight

Water—The Most Essential Nutrient

We often take it for granted, yet water is by far the nutrient most needed by the body. While we can survive for months or even years without some vitamins and minerals, we can last only a few days without water. The discussion that follows will help you understand why water is so vital as well as how the various sources of the nutrient may differ.

• Why is water so important?

A combination of hydrogen and oxygen, water makes up part of every cell, tissue, and organ in the body and accounts for about 60 percent of body weight (see Figure 7–4), even contributing to body parts thought of as "dry." For example, bone is more than 20 percent water, muscle is three-quarters water, and teeth are about 10 percent water.[29]

Inside the body, water performs many tasks vital to life. It helps transport the nutrients needed to nourish the cells, for example. The blood is a river of water that flows through the arteries, capillaries, and veins, bringing each cell the exact substances and particles it requires. The same river carries away waste products formed during the reactions that take place in the cells. In addition, water acts as a shock absorber in joints and around the spinal cord, lubricates the digestive tract as well as all the tissues moistened with mucus, and surrounds and cushions an unborn child. Moreover, water plays a key role in maintaining body temperature. When water is changed from a liquid to a gas, a great deal of heat is used. Thus, when sweat evaporates, heat is released, leaving the body cooler.

• *Figure 7–4*

Water—The Number One Nutrient

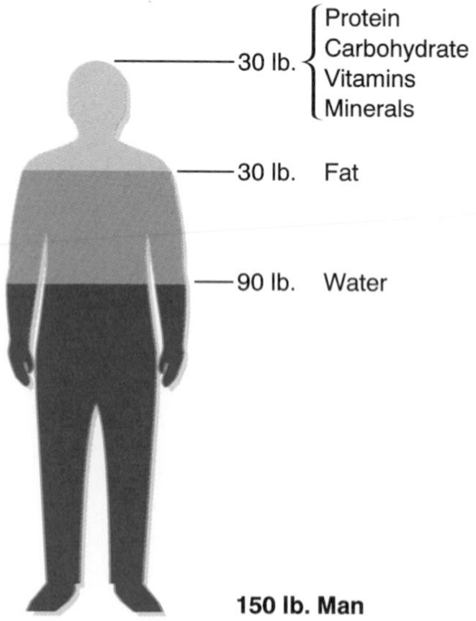

Source: C. Lecos, Water: The Number One Nutrient, *FDA Consumer,* November 1983.

• How much water do we take in daily?

Adults consume and excrete some two and a half to three quarts of water a day. While most of the water we take in comes from juice, milk, soft drinks, and other beverages, foods also add considerable amounts of water to the diet. Water makes up 85 percent to 95 percent of fruits and vegetables, for instance.[30]

• I often hear people talk about hard water and soft water. What do they mean?

The makeup of water differs depending on where the water comes from and how it is processed, and these variations can have significant health implications. One of the most basic distinctions—hard versus soft water—is based on the concentrations of three minerals: calcium, magnesium, and sodium. Hard water usually comes from shallow ground and contains relatively high levels of minerals, primarily calcium and magnesium. Soft water, on the other hand, generally flows from deep in the earth and has a higher concentration of sodium.

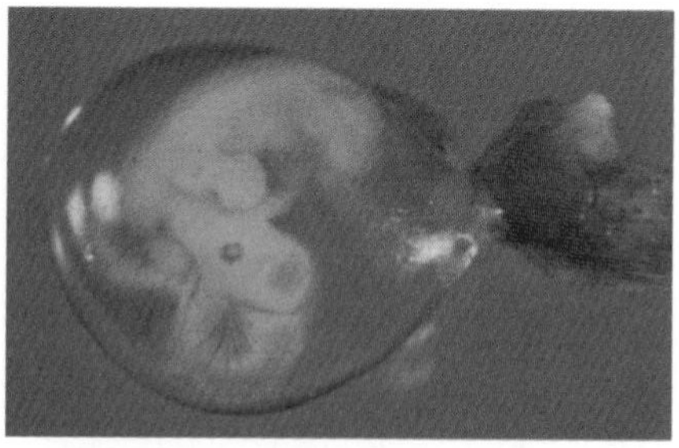

Life begins in water.

• How can I figure out which type of water I have in my home?

While your water utility company can tell you whether your water is soft or hard, you can probably distinguish between the two based on your own experience. Soft water helps soap lather better than hard water and leaves less of a ring on the bathtub. Hard water, on the contrary, doesn't clean clothes as thoroughly as soft water and leaves a residue of rocklike crystals on the inside of the teakettle over time. That's why many consumers prefer soft water to hard water.

• Which one is better to drink?

From a health standpoint hard water seems to be the better alternative. One reason is that the excess sodium carried in soft water, even in small amounts, adds more of the mineral to our already sodium-laden diets. More importantly, soft water can dissolve potentially toxic substances such as lead from pipes into the water. Thus, people who install water softeners in their homes for the purpose of getting cleaner laundry and better mileage from soap would do well to connect them only to their hot water lines for washing and bathing and use cold, hard water for drinking and cooking.

• What about contamination? I've heard that some people's tap water isn't safe to drink.

It's true that water taken from the earth contains different levels of bacteria, microorganisms, and heavy metals such as lead. Still, to ensure that the water that flows from the tap is safe to drink, the Environmental Protection Agency (EPA), the arm of the government responsible for monitoring municipal water supplies, sets limits for potential contaminants such as mercury, nitrate, and silver in drinking water. The EPA also mandates that tap water be disinfected if bacteria levels run high in order to prevent the spread of water-borne diseases such as typhoid and dysentery. Such precautionary measures go a long way in keeping our water supply one of the safest in the world.[31]

One potential health threat over which the EPA has little control, however, is the level of lead that comes out of your faucet. Although the EPA has put a ceiling on the concentration of lead allowed in public water supplies, once the water leaves a reservoir, unhealthfully high levels of the metal may be dissolved into it (see Figure 7–5). That's because it may flow through pipes made of lead or joined by lead solder, which then can leach the metal into the water as it passes through. Granted, the government banned the use of lead-containing plumbing systems back in 1986, but dwellings built before that time may not have lead-free pipes.

The issue has generated a good deal of publicity and concern of late. Certainly attention to the matter is warranted given that once lead accumulates in the body, it begins to damage the nerves, kidneys, and liver along with the cardiovascular, reproductive, immunologic, and gastrointestinal systems. The metal is especially toxic to children and fetuses, in whom it can cause neurologic problems as severe as brain damage.

Figure 7–5

Lead in Drinking Water

Lead usually gets into water after the water leaves the local drinking water treatment plant and makes its way through lead-containing plumbing systems.

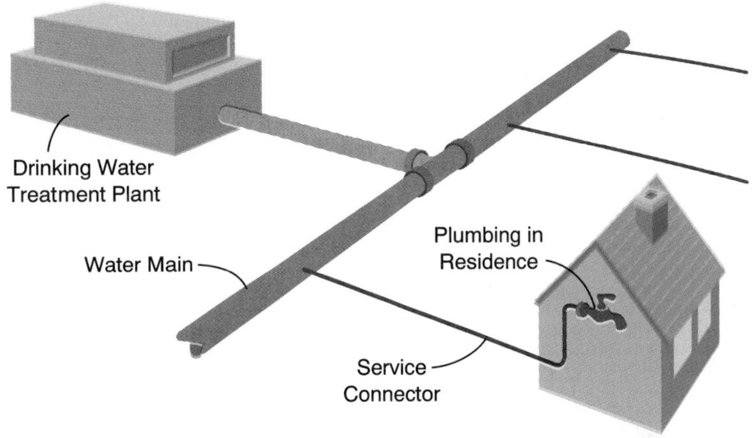

How can I make sure that my water doesn't contain too much lead?

Lead levels can usually be kept to a minimum simply by flushing the tap, that is, letting the water run until it becomes as cold as possible, thereby ridding it of water that has been sitting in pipes and dissolving lead for any length of time. Pipes should be flushed with cold water only, because cold water is less likely to dissolve lead as it flows through them than warm or hot water. To be sure, in some instances flushing is not enough to reduce harmful lead levels. Some homes or apartments may need special water treatment systems, the necessity of which can be determined only by subjecting tap water to a lead test. Most cost between \$20 and \$100; names of certified laboratories that analyze water can be obtained from a local branch of the EPA or by calling the EPA's Safe Drinking Water Hotline (800–426–4791).[32]

Another mineral in water that worries me is fluoride. A friend of mine told me not to drink water that contains fluoride, because it can cause cancer. What do you think about that?

As explained earlier in the chapter, drinking fluoridated water ranks as one of the most effective ways to prevent cavities. But despite the clear-cut benefits of fluoridation, at least 40 percent of Americans continue to drink water not treated with the mineral, putting them at a high risk of developing tooth decay. Part of the problem is that the practice has been the subject of bitter controversy over the years. Antifluoridation groups claim that drinking fluoride-containing water can cause everything from AIDS to cancer to sickle cell anemia, despite reports to the contrary issued from major health organizations such as the American Dietetic Association.[33] In fact, according to *The Surgeon General's Report on Nutrition and Health,* conclusive evidence demonstrates that the levels of fluoride added to public water supplies to protect dental health are safe.[34]

Nevertheless, the debate rages on. The latest wave of antifluoridationist publicity hit the media in 1990. A government study of rats and mice suggested, by some accounts, that fluoridated water may cause cancer. Truth be told, not a trace of cancer surfaced in any of the female rats or mice of either gender studied. And only one out of 50 male rats developed a rare bone cancer after two years of drinking an amount of water containing about 45 times the level of fluoride allowed in home drinking supplies. Four out of 80 rats suffered the same after drinking water treated with almost 80 times the allowable human limit for fluoride. In other words, an adult would have to swallow

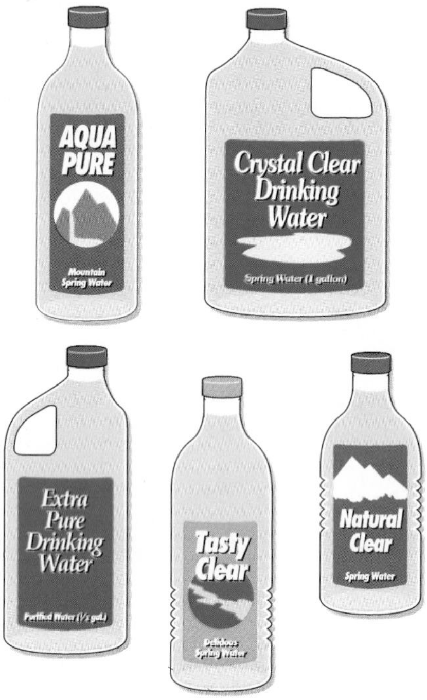

700 cups of fluoridated water daily for 70 years to obtain the amount of fluoride the rats received. Thus, if anything, the report underscores the practically imperceptible risk to health posed by drinking fluoridated water.[35]

• You seem to be saying that our water supply is fine. Nevertheless, wouldn't it be better to play it safe and drink bottled water?

Not necessarily. Granted, Americans drink nearly four times as much bottled water these days as a decade ago, totaling about 1.7 billion gallons annually. And while the reasons for the trend are many, bottled water's perceived health benefits fall near the top of the list. Surveys have found that about 25 percent of bottled water drinkers choose the beverage for health and safety reasons; another quarter believe it is pure and free of contaminants.[36]

Regardless of its pristine image, bottled water is not necessarily any purer or more healthful than what flows right out of the tap. Consider that the Food and Drug Administration (FDA)—the bottled-water industry watchdog—does not require that bottled water meet higher standards for quality, such as the maximum level of contaminants, than public water supplies regulated by the EPA. For the most part, the FDA simply follows EPA's regulatory lead. Granted, bottled water is often filtered to remove chemicals such as chlorine that may impart a certain taste. But that doesn't make it any safer. In fact, about 25 percent of bottled water comes from the same municipal water supplies as tap water.[37] Furthermore, some bottled waters do not contain any or enough of the fluoride needed to fight cavities.[38] The only way to determine whether a certain water contains the mineral is to check with the company that bottles it.

This is not to say that bottled water is necessarily any better or worse, from a health standpoint, than tap water. It's certainly preferable to tap water for those who like its taste. The problem is that many consumers pay 300 to 1,200 times more per gallon for bottled than tap water because they think bottled water is the more healthful of the two. Bottlers add to the confusion by sprinkling terms such as *pure, crystal pure,* and *premium* on labels illustrated with pictures of glaciers, mountain streams, and waterfalls, even when the water inside comes from a public reservoir. The Miniglossary of Bottled Waters explains what some of the terms used on bottles actually mean.

Miniglossary of Bottled Waters[39]

Natural water water that does not come from a municipal system or public supply and is not changed by blending with water from another source or the addition or subtraction of minerals.

Naturally sparkling water water whose carbon dioxide (the ingredient that makes soda pop bubbly) is from the same or an adjacent source as the water.

Sparkling water water to which carbon dioxide has been injected. In other words, artificially carbonated water.

Spring water water derived from an underground formation from which water flows naturally to the surface of the earth and to which minerals have not been added or taken away.

Purified water (also known as distilled) water from which all the minerals have been removed, thereby eliminating the possibility that the minerals might corrode, say, a steam iron.

Mineral water legally, this term is meaningless; all water (except purified) contains minerals. Moreover, the FDA has never set forth a legal definition that mandates just how many minerals mineral water must contain to be identified as such. The International Bottled Water Association, however, defines it as water containing not less than 500 parts per million total dissolved solids. The minerals, incidentally, give the water its taste.

Seltzer* tap water injected with carbon dioxide and containing no added salts.

Club soda* artificially carbonated water containing added salts and minerals.

*These are not considered bottled water in government parlance. The FDA defines bottled water as water that is sealed in bottles or other containers and is intended for human consumption, excluding soda, seltzer, flavored, and vended water products.

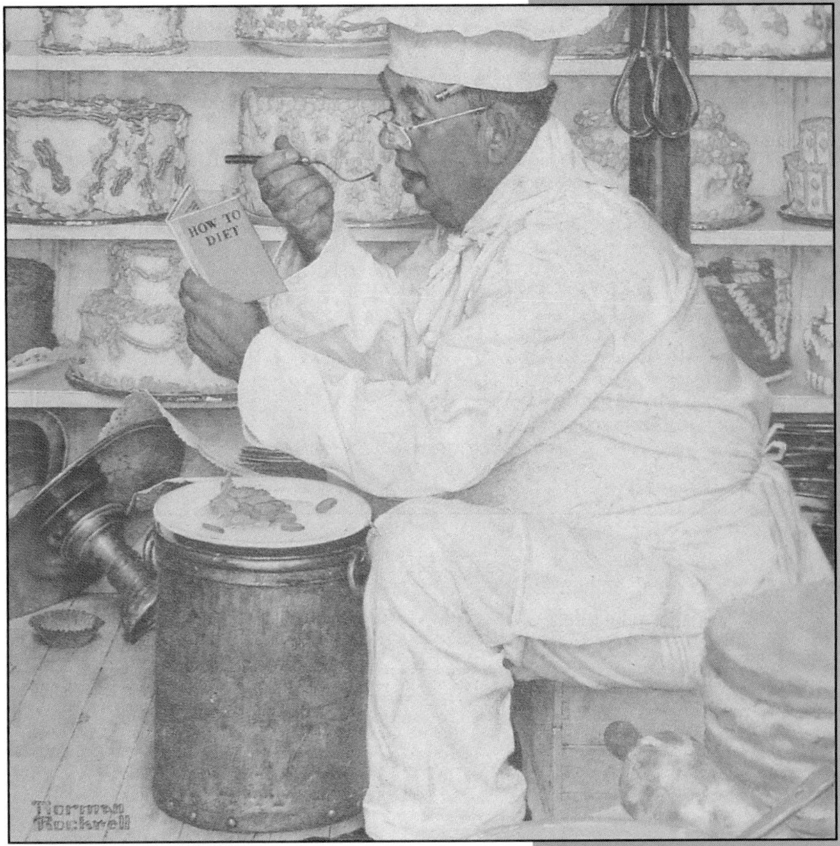

Printed by permission of the Norman Rockwell Family Trust. Copyright © 1942 the Norman Rockwell Family Trust.

> *Before you begin a thing, remind yourself that difficulties and delays quite impossible to foresee are ahead . . . You can see only one thing clearly, and that is your goal. Form a mental vision of that and cling to it through thick and thin.*
>
> K. Norris

CHAPTER 8
Weight Control

Contents

Ask Yourself . . . ?

Which of these statements about nutrition are true, and which are false? For the false statements, what *is* true?

1. The less you weigh, the better it is for your health.
2. Fat people pay higher insurance premiums than thin people.
3. If you weigh too much according to the scales and the so-called ideal weight tables, you are too fat.
4. If you are too fat, it is because you eat too much.
5. Basal metabolism contributes only a small percentage of a person's daily energy output.
6. It is probable that the most important single contributor to the obesity problem in our country is underactivity.
7. Any food can make you fat, even carrot sticks, if you eat enough of them.
8. A properly designed diet and exercise program can make you lose weight faster than a total fast.
9. To gain weight, you should learn to eat faster.
10. Anorexia nervosa is a disease in which a person has no appetite.

Answers: 1. False. Being thin is good for health only to a point; being too thin is as risky as being too fat. 2. True. 3. False. A high weight according to the scales and the so-called ideal weight tables may reflect heavy bones and muscles rather than overfatness. 4. False. If you are too fat, it may be because you exercise too little. 5. False. Basal metabolism contributes about 60 percent or more of the average person's daily energy output. 6. True. 7. True. 8. True. 9. True. 10. False. Anorexia nervosa is misnamed; the person with anorexia nervosa is constantly hungry, but controls it.

Overweight conventionally defined as weight between 10% and 20% above the desirable weight for height.
Underweight weight 10% or more below the desirable weight for height.
Obese conventionally defined as weight 20% or more above the desirable weight for height, but see *body mass index (BMI)* on page 206 for a more accurate definition. Morbid obesity is a weight of at least 100 pounds above "ideal" weight for height.

How much should you weigh? At one time, you could look up the answer in the so-called ideal weight tables. Defining **overweight** and **underweight** was simple: if a person's weight was 10 percent or more above the ideal weight, the person was overweight; 20 percent or more meant the person was **obese.** If the person's weight was 10 percent or more below the ideal weight, the person was underweight. Now the term *ideal weight* is no longer in use, and defining overweight and underweight is no longer simple.

Regardless of how you define it, obesity has become a major public health problem for both young and old in the United States today. Some 10 percent to 25 percent of all teenagers and some 25 percent to 50 percent of all adults are obese.

There is clearly such a thing for each individual as a weight too low or a weight too high to be healthful. The too-thin person has minimal body fat stores with which to meet prolonged starvation and will be the first to die during a siege or in a famine. A fact not always recognized, even by health care providers, is that thin people are also at a disadvantage when hospitalized, where they may have to go for days without food while undergoing tests or surgery. Underweight also increases the risk for any person fighting a wasting disease such as cancer or tuberculosis. In fact, people with cancer die as often from starvation as from the cancer itself. Thus, underweight people are urged to learn how to nourish themselves optimally, not just to gain body fat—although even that is desirable—but to acquire healthful reserves of all the nutrients that can be stored.[1]

The physical risks of obesity are greater for some people than for others, depending on inherited susceptibilities to conditions such as high blood pressure, high blood cholesterol, and diabetes. High blood pressure is made worse by obesity and can often be normalized merely by weight loss. Some people with high blood pressure can tell you exactly at what weight their blood pressure begins to rise. Diabetes can be precipitated in genetically

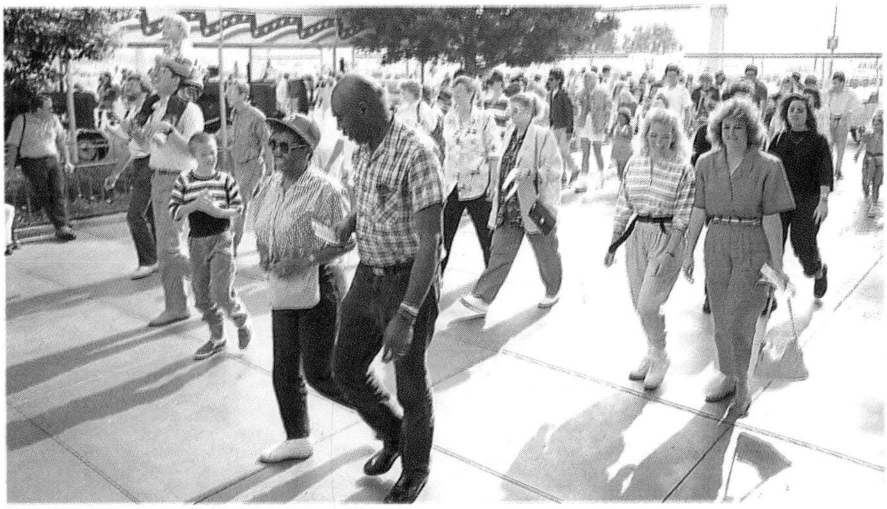

Bodies come in many shapes and sizes. Which are healthy?

susceptible people if they become overweight. If any of these conditions run in your family, you are urgently in need of a sensible weight-control program before you become obese.

Obesity also increases the risk of heart disease because excess fat pads crowd the heart muscle and the lungs within the body cavity. These fat pads encumber the heart as it beats, making it work hard to deliver oxygen and nutrients. The lungs, too, cannot expand fully, and this limits the oxygen intake of each breath, causing the heart to work even harder to pump the needed amount of oxygen to other parts of the body. Furthermore, since each extra pound of fat tissue demands to be fed by way of miles of capillaries, the heart in a fat person labors to pump its blood through a network of blood vessels vastly larger than that of a thin person. Even a healthy heart is strained by excess fatness. If a diseased heart finds itself in this bind, a sudden burst of exercise may be more of a workload than it can handle. Chapter 9 discusses precautions relevant to exercise.

Gallbladder disease, too, can be brought on in susceptible people merely by excess weight. Similarly, women with a family history of breast cancer are warned that to become obese is to increase their risk. Table 8–1 lists other conditions brought on or made worse by obesity.

Besides being at risk for these health hazards, millions of obese people throughout much of their lives incur risks from ill-advised, misguided dieting. Some fad diets are more hazardous to health than is obesity itself. One survey of 29,000 claims, treatments, and theories for losing weight found fewer than 6 percent of them effective—and 13 percent were dangerous.[2] Over the centuries, "magical" weight-loss plans have been offered time and again, the success of which is in their popularity, not in their achievement.

Some people can be obese and suffer none of the risks of these physical health hazards, but there is one disadvantage of obesity that no one in our society quite escapes. Obesity in many parts of North America is a social and economic handicap. Fat people are less sought after for romance, are less often admitted to college, pay higher insurance premiums, pay more for clothes, and suffer job discrimination and even ridicule. Psychologically, a body size that embarrasses or shames a person confers severe disadvantages. For people who cannot talk freely about their own self-doubt, a less-than-

Table 8–1

Problems Associated with Obesity

- Abdominal hernias
- Accidents
- Arthritis (knees, hips, lower spine)
- Certain cancers
  In men: colon, rectum, prostate gland
  In women: breast, uterus, ovaries, gallbladder
- Complications during pregnancy
- Complications after surgery
- Decreased longevity
- Decreased quality of life
- Depression
- Diabetes
- Gallbladder and liver disease
- Gout
- Heart disease
- High blood cholesterol levels
- Hypertension
- Injury to weight-bearing joints
- Poor self-esteem
- Respiratory problems
- Varicose veins

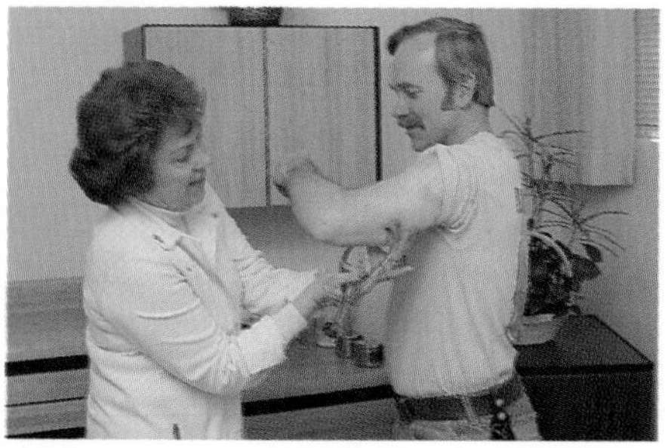

The fatfold test gives a fair approximation of total body fat.

ideal body image becomes a private anguish. For people who perceive themselves as fat in a society that prizes thinness, real or imagined obesity can thrust them into withdrawal, shame, humiliation, and isolation.

How thin, then, is too thin—and how fat is too fat? Because the term *ideal weight* cannot be defined, the following section discusses the concept of a healthful weight.

What Is a Healthful Weight?

The problems of defining a healthful weight are many. Consider the question, Healthful for what? For long-distance runners, every unneeded pound is a disadvantage; the lowest amount of body fat that doesn't compromise hormonal balance and fuel availability is desirable. For swimmers, weight matters less, and fat contributes to their buoyancy and insulates them against the cold. In this case, to a point, more is desirable. Dancers or models may value thinness so highly that to attain it, they must compromise their health. For women who want to conceive a child, considerably higher than the so-called appropriate body weight predicts a successful pregnancy.

Some societies value fatness, equating it with prosperity; others value thinness to the point of obsession (our own being an example). This chapter first asks what range of weights is compatible with wellness and long life and then suggests that personal preferences dictate the choice of a weight within that range.

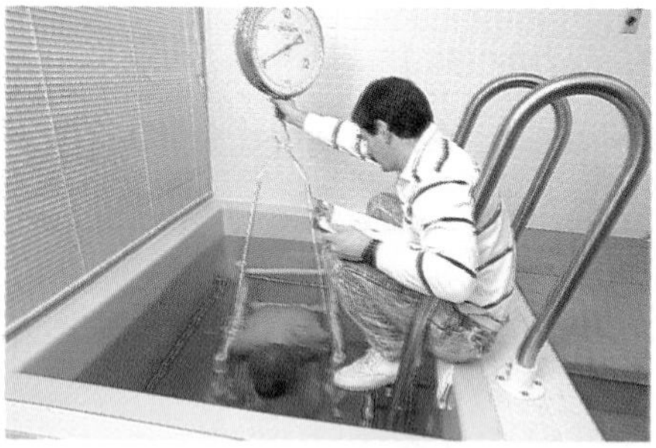

Hydrostatic (underwater) weighing.

Body Weight Versus Body Fat

The question of what weight is healthful is harder to answer than you might at first think. In 1959, insurance companies published the "ideal weight tables" referred to earlier, but the tables were really not ideal *for* anything. They were, simply, the weight ranges that correlated with longer-than-average life expectancy in the population studied—people who bought life insurance. But people who buy life insurance may be unlike others in terms of their health, and such tables thus may not be applicable to everyone. The weights reflected in the tables were measured only once, if ever, when young buyers purchased insurance. Some people merely reported their weights verbally, without being weighed. Insurance table weights are thus by no means an ideal to compare with your own weight, but are simply an average found among insurance buyers long ago who ended up living the longest. The weight tables currently in use were published in 1983 (see the inside back cover). The basis for the 1983 weights has now been challenged.[3]

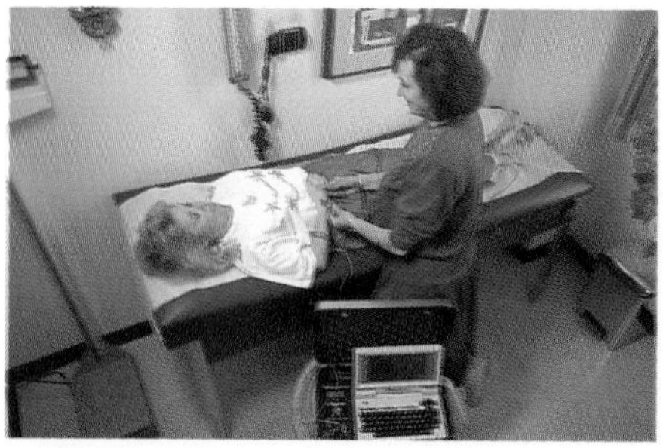

Electrical impedence measurement of body fat content.

Not only are valid standards unavailable, but to think merely in terms of weight oversimplifies the issue of body fatness and health. Two people of the same sex, age, and height may both weigh the same, yet one may be too fat and the other too thin. The difference lies in their body composition. One may have small, light bones and minimally developed muscles, while the other has big, heavy bones and well-developed muscles. The first person could have too much body fat and the second person too little. For example, football players, dancers, bodybuilders, and other athletes may weigh in as overweight for their height, according to the weight tables. However, they probably will have less body fat than the amount that poses a risk to health.

Likewise, many sedentary persons may weigh in as normal weight but be overly fat. This comparison points to the need to define obesity in terms of people's body fatness rather than in terms of their weight. The health risks of obesity and overweight refer to people who are overfat. On the average, men having over 25 percent body fat and women having over 30 percent body fat are considered obese. More desirable measures are 12 percent to 18 percent body fat for most men and 20 percent to 28 percent body fat for most women (see Table 8–2 on page 206).[4]

Hydrostatic weighing or underwater weighing the less a person weighs under water compared to the person's out-of-water weight the greater the proportion of body fat (fat is less dense or more buoyant than lean tissue).
Fatfold test a clinical test of body fatness in which the thickness of a fold of skin on the back of the arm (on the triceps), below the shoulder blade (subscapular), or in other places is measured with an instrument called a caliper. Obesity is defined by triceps skinfold thickness equal to or greater than 18–19 mm in adult men, 25–26 mm or more in women.
Bioelectrical impedance estimation of body fat content made by measuring how quickly electrical current is conducted through the body.
Central obesity excess fat on the abdomen and around the trunk. Peripheral obesity is excess fat on the arms, thighs, hips, and buttocks.

Measuring Body Fat

Body fatness is hard to measure. The only accurate way is to obtain a measure of the body's density—that is, weight divided by volume. Weight is easy enough; just step on an accurate scale. But to obtain the body's volume, you have to immerse the whole body in a tank of water. Not many health professionals have space in their offices for the equipment needed for this procedure, known as **hydrostatic weighing** or **underwater weighing.** Most employ the **fatfold test**, using a caliper—a pinching device that measures the thickness of a fold of fat on the back of the arm, below the shoulder blade, on the side of the waist, or elsewhere. About 50 percent of the body's fat lies beneath the skin, and its thickness at these locations can be compared with standard tables to give a fair approximation of total body fat, at least for most people.

A relatively new method for assessing body fatness is **bioelectrical impedance**, in which electrodes are attached to a person's hand and foot. This provides an estimate of how much fat a person has by measuring the speed at which electrical current is conducted through the body (from the ankle to the wrist). Since fat is a poor conductor of electricity, the more fat one has, the more resistance this current encounters in the body.

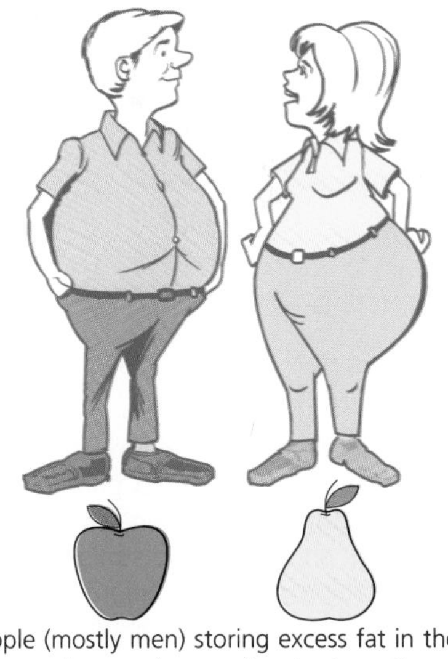

People (mostly men) storing excess fat in the chest and stomach areas (apple-shaped) are at a higher risk for diabetes, heart disease, and hypertension than people storing excess fat in the hips, thighs, and buttocks (pear-shaped). Find the waist-to-hip ratio by measuring the waist's circumference, then the widest part of the hip, and divide the first number by the second. The average healthy ratio is below 1.0 for men and below 0.8 for women. People with values greater than these are apple-shaped.

Distribution of Fat

Not everyone carries his or her body fat distributed in the same way. To complicate matters still further, the distribution itself turns out to have health implications. Excess fat around the middle—**central obesity**—is associated with increased health hazards. Body types are compared as being either apple-shaped or pear-shaped. One theory proposes that people who store most of their excess fat around the abdomen (typically men) are at a greater risk for developing diabetes, hypertension, elevated levels of blood cholesterol, and heart disease than are people who store excess fat elsewhere on the body—notably, hips, thighs, and buttocks (typically women).[5] A simple comparison of a person's waist-to-hip measurement can be used to assess abdominal fat.[6]

Body Weight and Frame Size

Although the problem of how to define obesity has not been solved, everyone agrees that obesity presents one of the most serious health risks that people face—and one that people should, theoretically, be able to control. While the experts argue, medical professionals are making do with a definition of obesity based temporarily on two measures. The first is the body weight taken on an accurate scale and compared with **frame size**, determined by measuring

Table 8–2
Body Fat Standards

	MEN	WOMEN
Normal	15%–18%	20%–28%
Athletes	12%–15%	20%–25%
Elite athletes	7%–10%	12%–18%
Obesity	25% +	30% +

Source: Adapted from S. Escott-Stump, *Nutrition and Diagnosis-Related Care* (Philadelphia: Lea & Febiger, 1988), p. 19.

Frame size the size of a person's bones and musculature. A person with a large frame can weigh more than a person the same height with a small frame without increased risks.

Body mass index (BMI) an index of degree of obesity derived from one's height and weight.

the breadth of the elbow. The weight tables (inside back cover) and Table 8–3 provide the information you need to compare your body weight and frame size with the set standards. The second measure is the **body mass index (BMI)**, which you can obtain by drawing a line from your height to your weight on the nomogram in Figure 8–1.[7] The standards are shown in the figure. The boxed feature "What Is a Healthful Weight for You?" guides your use of both the standard weight tables and the body mass index to help you answer the question for yourself.

Other Ways to Measure Body Fat

There are other ways to answer the question of what weight is desirable for you (these are just for fun):

- A crude measure of body fatness is the pinch test (this is a fatfold measure without the equipment to make it accurate). Pinch the skin and fat at the back of either arm with the thumb and forefinger of the other hand. Keep your fingers still, so as not to lose the "measurement" when you pull them away from your arm. Measure the thickness on a ruler. A fatfold over an inch thick reflects obesity; less than half an inch thick, underweight.

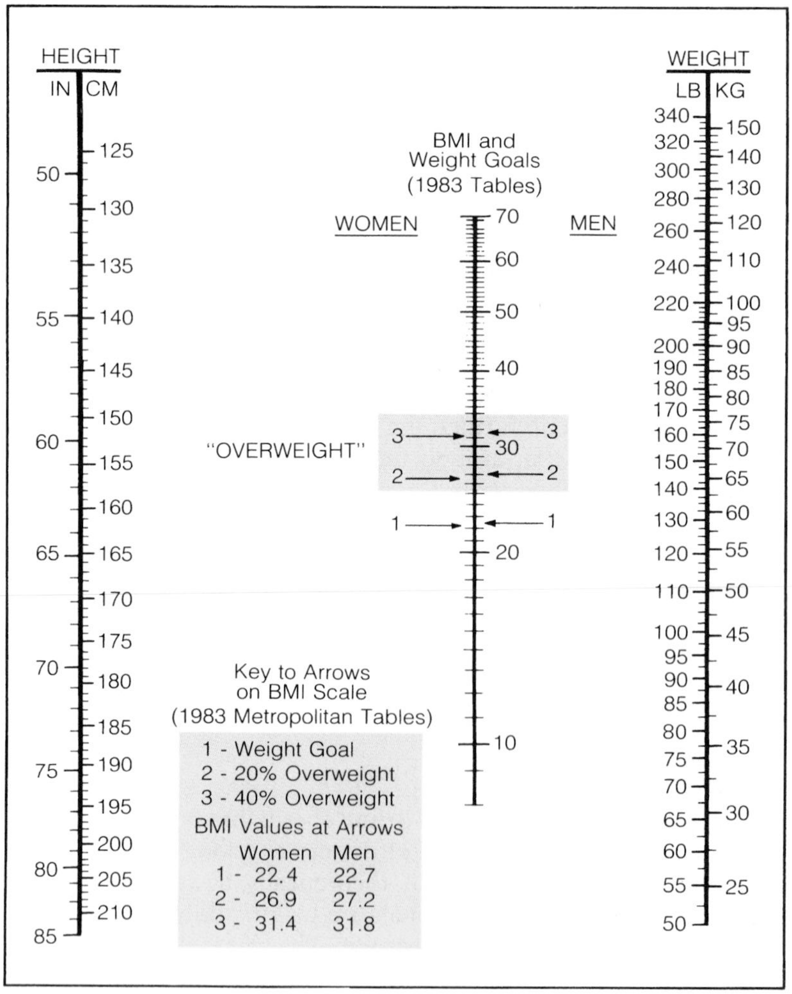

Figure 8–1
Nomogram for Body Mass Index

Weights and heights are without clothing. With clothes, add 5 pounds for men or 3 pounds for women, and 1 inch in height for shoes. Draw a straight line or place a ruler from your height (left) to your weight (right). At the point where the line or ruler crosses the BMI line, read your body mass index. A body mass index greater than 27.2 for men or 26.9 for women indicates obesity.

Source: From the 1983 Metropolitan Life Insurance Company tables, designed by B. T. Burton and W. R. Foster, Health implications of obesity, an NIH Consensus Development Conference, *Journal of the American Dietetic Association* 85 (1985): 1117–1121.

What Is a Healthful Weight For You?

A wide range of weights is compatible with good health. Within this range, the definition of desirable or healthful weight is up to the individual, depending on such factors as family history, occupation, physical and recreational activities, and personal preferences. To find a healthful weight for you:

1. Determine the safe range for a person of your height and sex:
   - Record your height: __________ feet __________ inches.
   - Determine your frame size, using Table 8–3. Record whether you have a small, medium, or large frame: __________ frame.
   - Look up the appropriate weight for a person of your height, sex, and frame size on the inside back cover of this book. Note that the weight tables assume you measured your height in shoes with one-inch heels. If you measured your height barefoot or if you wore shoes with heels higher or lower than an inch, adjust accordingly. Record the entire range: __________ to __________ pounds.
     Example: For a man 5 feet 7 inches tall (in shoes) with a small frame, the range of weights is 138 to 145 pounds.
   - Determine the bottom end of the safe range. A person who is more than 10 percent below the indicated weight for height is considered underweight to a degree that might compromise health. Take 10 percent off the bottom end of the range of weights for a person of your height and frame size. Bottom end of range: __________ pounds.
     Example: Ten percent of 138 pounds is 13.8 pounds (rounded off to 14 pounds). The bottom end of the range is 138 minus 14, or 124 pounds.
   - Determine the top end of the safe range. A person who is more than 20 percent above the indicated weight for height is considered obese—and obesity is a risk factor for many harmful health conditions. Add 20 percent to the top end of your range: __________ pounds.
     Example: Twenty percent of 145 pounds is 29 pounds. The top end of the range is 145 plus 29, or 174 pounds.
   - Record your safe range here: __________ to __________ pounds.
     Example: 124 to 174 pounds.
2. If your weight is below the bottom end of this safe range, you need to gain weight for your health's sake. You can also refer to the BMI nomogram in Figure 8–1 to check on your weight status. If your weight is above the top end of the range, determine your body mass index to obtain confirmation that you need to lose weight.
3. Check your health history for further confirmation. A family or personal medical history of diabetes (non-insulin-dependent type), hypertension, or high blood cholesterol indicates a need to lose weight.
4. Choose a goal weight within the safe range. Answering the following questions should help you to determine where, within the safe range, your personal desirable weight may be:
   - Does your occupation demand that you have a certain body shape? Record the weight, within the safe range, that would most nearly approximate this body shape: ________ pounds.
   - Do you engage in a sport or other physical activity that requires a particular body weight for optimal performance? Consult your instructor or other expert in that sport or activity and record the weight recommended on that basis: __________ pounds.
   - Do you hope to start a pregnancy soon? If so, consult your health care provider as to the ideal weight with which to begin a pregnancy: __________ pounds.
   - Undress and stand before a mirror. Do you think you need to gain or lose weight? Add or subtract pounds from your current weight to arrive at a personal goal weight (but be sure to stay within the safe range): __________ pounds.

Now choose a goal weight, giving consideration to each of the weights you just listed. No formula exists for this estimate: you decide, but don't choose a weight outside the safe range.

Your goal weight: __________ pounds.

Table 8–3 **Frame Size**

To make a simple approximation of your frame size:
Extend your arm, and bend the forearm upward at a 90-degree angle. Keep the fingers straight and turn the inside of your wrist away from your body. Place the thumb and index finger of your other hand on the two prominent bones on *either side* of your elbow. Measure the space between your fingers against a ruler or a tape measure.[a] Compare the measurements with the following standards. (These standards represent the elbow measurements for medium-framed men and women of various heights. Measurements smaller than those listed indicate you have a small frame, and larger measurements indicate a large frame.)[b]

MEN	
Height in 1-in. Heels	**Elbow Breadth**
5 ft 2 in. to 5 ft 3 in.	2½ to 2⅞ in.
5 ft 4 in. to 5 ft 7 in.	2⅝ to 2⅞ in.
5 ft 8 in. to 5 ft 11 in.	2¾ to 3 in.
6 ft 0 in. to 6 ft 3 in.	2¾ to 3⅛ in.
6 ft 4 in. and over	2⅞ to 3¼ in.

WOMEN	
Height in 1-in. Heels	**Elbow Breadth**
4 ft 10 in. to 4 ft 11 in.	2¼ to 2½ in.
5 ft 0 in. to 5 ft 3 in.	2¼ to 2½ in.
5 ft 4 in. to 5 ft 7 in.	2⅜ to 2⅝ in.
5 ft 8 in. to 5 ft 11 in.	2⅜ to 2⅝ in.
6 ft 0 in. and over	2½ to 2¾ in.

[a]For the most accurate measurement, have your health care provider measure your elbow breadth with a caliper.
[b]A simple estimate of frame size can be derived by circling your wrist with the thumb and middle finger of your other hand. If the thumb and finger do not meet, you most likely have a large frame. If the thumb and finger just meet, you most likely have a medium frame, and if the fingers overlap greatly, you may have a small frame.

Source: Metropolitan Life Insurance Company.

Target Weight Scorecard

For a female:

Start with 100 lb	100 lb
For every inch above 5 ft (barefoot), add 5 lb	___ lb
Total	___ lb

Thus, a woman who is 5 ft 4 in. tall would have an ideal weight of 120 lb: 100 + (4 × 5).

For a male:

Start with 110 lb	110 lb
For every in. above 5 ft (barefoot), add 5 lb	___ lb
Total	___ lb

Thus, a 6-ft man would have an ideal weight of 170 lb: 110 + (12 × 5).

- Another shortcut method is to measure your waist compared with your chest (not bust). Every inch by which your waist measurement exceeds your chest measurement is said to take two years off your life.
- Another crude measure: lie down, relax, and place a ruler across your abdomen from one hipbone to the other. If the ruler doesn't easily touch both bones while you're relaxing, you're too fat.
- You can also use the Target Weight Scorecard.

Energy Balance

Suppose you decide that you are too fat or too thin. You got that way by having an unbalanced energy budget—that is, by eating either more or less food energy than you spent. Fatness and thinness are reflections of excessive or deficient energy stores. You store extra energy as fat only if you eat more food energy in a day than you use to fuel your metabolic and other activities. Similarly, you lose stored fat only if you eat *less* food energy in a day than you use as fuel. A day's energy balance can be stated like this:

Change in energy stores (calories) = Food energy taken in (calories) − Energy spent on metabolism and muscle activities (calories)

Weight loss: Calories eaten are less than calories burned.
Weight gain: Calories eaten are greater than calories burned.

More simply stated:

Change in energy stores = Energy in − Energy out

You know about the "energy in" side of this equation. An apple brings you 100 calories; a candy bar, 290 calories. (Calorie amounts for several hundred foods are listed in Appendix F.) You probably also know that for each 3,500 calories you eat in excess of need, you store one pound of body fat.

As for the "energy out" side, the body spends energy in two major ways: to fuel its metabolic activities and to fuel its muscle activities. You can change your activity level to spend more or less energy in a day, and if you do so consistently, your metabolic activities will ultimately speed up somewhat, too.

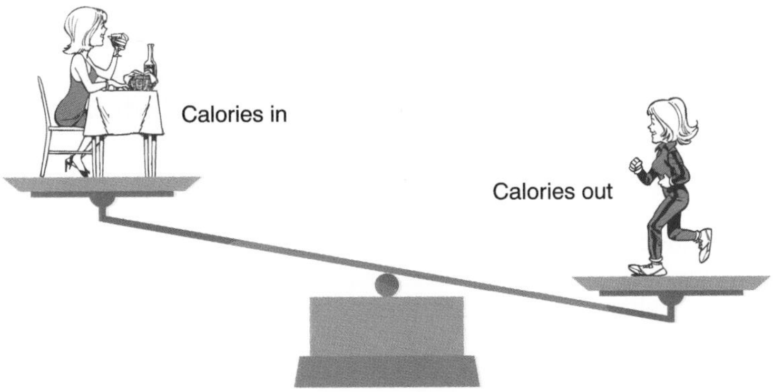

The balance between energy in and energy out determines whether a person stores or uses body fat.

Still another way energy is used in the body is called diet-induced thermogenesis—the rise in metabolic rate that occurs as a result of eating a meal due to the energy used by the body to fuel its digestion, absorption, and transport of nutrients in that meal. It is approximately 10 percent of the food energy one consumes. Therefore, if you eat a sandwich containing 500 calories, the body uses 50 calories (10 percent) to utilize those 500 calories. For the purpose of determining a ballpark figure for your energy expenditure, this factor can be ignored. The following three sections discuss the body's needs for energy.

Basal Metabolism

About 60 percent or more of the energy the average person spends goes to support the ongoing metabolic work of the body's cells, the **basal metabolism.** This is the work that goes on all the time, without conscious awareness. The beating of the heart, the inhaling and exhaling of air, the maintenance of body temperature, and the sending of nerve and hormonal messages to direct these activities are the basal processes that maintain life. Basal metabolic needs are surprisingly large. A person whose total energy expenditure amounts to 2,000 calories a day spends as many as 1,200 to 1,400 of them to support basal metabolism.

Basal metabolism the sum total of all the chemical activities of the cells necessary to sustain life, exclusive of voluntary activities—that is, the ongoing activities of the cells when the body is at rest.

Basal metabolic rate (BMR) the rate at which the body spends energy to support its basal metabolism. The BMR accounts for the largest component of a person's daily energy (calorie) needs.

The **basal metabolic rate** (often abbreviated **BMR**) is influenced by a number of factors (see Table 8–4). In general, the younger a person is, the higher the basal metabolic rate. This is in part due to the increased activity of cells undergoing division. The BMR is most pronounced during the growth spurts that take place during infancy, puberty, and pregnancy. Body composition also influences basal metabolic rate. Muscle tissue is highly active even when it is resting, whereas fat tissue is comparatively inactive. The more lean tissue in a body, the higher the BMR; the more fat tissue, the lower the BMR. Lean body mass decreases with age, and it is estimated that the BMR decreases by about 2 percent every ten years after age 30.

Gender correlates roughly with body composition. Men generally have a faster metabolic rate than women, and researchers believe that this is due to men's greater percentage of lean tissue. (A woman athlete has a greater percentage of lean tissue than a sedentary man of the same weight and so would have a faster metabolic rate.)

Table 8–4

Factors that Influence the Basal Metabolic Rate

Factors That Increase BMR
Fever
Growth (higher in children and pregnant women)
Height (higher in tall, thin people)
Male gender (more lean tissue)
Muscle mass (the more lean tissue, the higher the BMR)
Recent food intake
Recent exercise
Stress
Thyroid hormone
Factors That Decrease BMR
Age (slows down with age)
Reduced energy intake (fasting, starvation, low-calorie diets)

Fever increases the energy needs of cells. Their increased activities to generate heat and fight off infection speed up the metabolic rate.

Fasting and constant malnutrition lower the metabolic rate because of the loss of lean tissue and the slowdown of activities the body can't afford to support fully. This slowing of metabolism seems to be a protective mechanism to conserve energy when there is a shortage, and it hampers weight loss in a person who fasts or undertakes a too-strict diet.

Some hormones—the stress hormones, for example—influence metabolism. They increase the energy demands of every cell and thus raise the metabolic rate. This raised metabolism partly accounts for the weight loss sometimes seen in people experiencing extreme stress in their lives, although other factors, such as upset digestion and loss of appetite, also enter in.

The activity of the thyroid gland influences the basal metabolic rate. The less thyroid hormone secreted, the lower the energy requirement for maintenance of basal functions.

Voluntary Activities

Muscular activity does not make as big a contribution as basal metabolism does to most people's energy outputs. On the average, it amounts to only about 30 percent of the total. But unlike basal metabolism, which cannot be changed immediately, physical activity can be changed at will. If you want to tinker with your energy balance, this is the component—on the output side—that you can alter significantly in the short term. If you increase it consistently, you will also ultimately increase the energy your body spends on metabolic activity.

The energy spent on physical activity is the energy spent moving the body's skeletal muscles—the muscles of the arms, back, abdomen, legs, and so forth—and the extra energy spent to speed up the heartbeat and respiration rate as needed. The number of calories spent depends on three factors: (1) the amount of muscle mass required, (2) the amount of weight being moved, and (3) the amount of time the activity takes. Thus, an activity involving both the arms and legs requires more calories than an activity of the same intensity involving only the legs; an activity performed by a heavier person requires more energy than the same activity performed by a lighter person; and an activity performed for 40 minutes requires twice as much energy as that same activity performed for 20 minutes.

As disheartening as it may be for a college student to discover, mental activity requires little energy, even though it may be tiring. Studying for an exam may be hard work, but it won't burn off body fat. People who are very, very busy—writing letters, making phone calls, riding in their cars from place to place—may wonder why they tend to gain weight, because they think of themselves as active people. They may be socially or intellectually active, but such activity involves few muscles and therefore little energy expenditure.

Total Energy Needs

A typical breakdown of the total energy spent by a lightly active person (for example, a student who walks back and forth to classes) might look like this:

Energy for basal metabolism:	1,400 calories
Energy for physical activity:	560 calories
Total:	1,960 calories

Energy Output Scorecard

A. First figure the energy you spend on BMR.* It's about 10 calories per pound of your body weight if you are a woman or 11 calories per pound if you are a man (men generally have more muscle than women):

A. ________ cal

B. Now figure the energy you spend on activities:

If you are not very active (sedentary)—you sit down most of the day and drive or ride whenever possible—take 25% to 40% (men) or 25% to 35% (women) of your BMR calories in A.

If you are lightly active—you sit most of the day, but you move around two to four hours of the day as a teacher might—take 50% to 70% (men) or 40% to 60% (women) of A.

If you are moderately active—you do some amount of regular exercise four or five times a week, or your job requires some physical labor—take 65% to 80% (men) or 50% to 70% (women) of A.

If you are very physically active—your job requires much physical labor, or you are physically active four or more hours each day—and you do little standing or sitting, take 90% to 120% (men) or 80% to 100% (women) of A.

B. ________ cal

C. Total energy need = A + B = C. ________ cal

*Note: Another way to estimate the energy spent on basal metabolism is to use the factor (for men) 1.0 cal/kg/hour (or for women, 0.9 cal/kg/hr) for a 24-hour period. Then add an increment of this amount depending on how physically active you are.

The first component is larger, and you cannot change it much. You can, however, change the second component—physical activity—and so spend more calories. If you want to increase your basal metabolic output, make exercise a daily habit. Your body composition will change, and your basal energy output will pick up the pace as well. You can figure roughly how much energy you spend in a day by using the Energy Output Scorecard.

In summary, the amount of fat stored in a person's body depends on the balance between the total food energy the person has taken in and the total energy the person has expended. The end of this chapter shows how to alter both—with diet and exercise—to regulate body weight. But first: why do so many people have excessive fat stores?

Causes of Obesity

Some people eat more than they need or exercise less than they need to maintain their body weight, and they get fat. Some eat less or exercise more, and they get thin. Perhaps most amazingly, some people—most people, in fact—eat exactly what they need and stay at the same weight year after year. A single extra pat of butter each day would make them gain 5 pounds in a year, but if they overeat by that much one day, they undereat by the same amount the next. How do they do this—and, in contrast, why do some people fail to maintain their weight?

Genetics versus Environment

In general, two schools of thought address the problem of obesity's causes. One attributes it to inside-the-body causes; the other, to environmental factors. One popular inside-the-body theory is the so-called **set-point theory**. Noting that many people who lose weight on reducing diets subsequently return to their original weight, some researchers have suggested that the body "wants" to maintain a certain amount of fat and regulates eating behaviors and hormonal actions to defend its "set point." The theory implies that science

Set-point theory the theory that the body tends to maintain a certain weight by adjusting hunger, appetite, and food energy intake on the one hand and metabolism (energy output) on the other so that a person's conscious efforts to alter weight may be foiled.

should search inside obese people to find the causes of their problems—perhaps in their hunger-regulating mechanisms.

The other point of view is that obesity is environmentally determined. Proponents of this view hold that people overeat or underexercise because they are pushed to do so by factors in their surroundings—foremost among them, the availability of a multitude of delectable foods and the lack of opportunities for vigorous physical activity. The two views are not mutually exclusive, and they may both be operating, even in the same person.

Perhaps some people have inherited or learned a way of resisting external stimuli to eat, while others have not. Of interest in this connection is the report of an experiment in which lean and fat people were housed in a metabolic ward of a hospital and were offered their meals in monotonous liquid formula from a feeding machine. The lean people ate enough to maintain their weight, but the fat people drastically reduced their food intakes and lost weight. When calories were added to the formula, the lean people adjusted their intakes to continue maintaining weight as if they had internal calorie counters. The obese people were unaware of the change, continued drinking the same amount of formula as before, and stopped losing weight.[8]

External cues were the only signals the obese people had to go by, and the obese people responded the same way to the same environmental situation regardless of how many calories they were getting. This is the basis of the **external cue theory**—the theory that at least in some people, the internal regulatory systems are easily overridden by environmental influences. A question to ponder: Does this make obesity hereditary, environmental, or both?

External cue theory the theory that some people eat in response to such external factors as the presence of food or the time of day rather than to such internal factors as hunger.

Fat cell theory states that during the growing years, fat cells respond to overfeeding by producing additional fat cells (**hyperplastic obesity**); the number of fat cells eventually becomes fixed, and overfeeding from this point on causes the body to enlarge existing fat cells (**hypertrophic obesity**). Hypertrophic obesity is the more common type and is usually seen in adults.

It seems likely that both hereditary and environmental factors influence obesity in human beings. The tendency to obesity is probably inherited, but the environment is probably influential in the sense that it can prevent or permit the development of obesity when the potential is there.

The complexity of the situation is reflected in observations of the ways obesity develops from infancy on. Some fat infants become fat adults, but most grow out of their obesity in childhood. An overweight child, however, is more likely to remain overweight into adulthood. Researchers propose the **fat cell theory**—that childhood obesity is persistent because early overfeeding (in childhood) may cause fat cells to increase abnormally in *number* (**hyperplastic obesity**). The number of fat cells is thought to become fixed by adulthood; afterwards, a gain or loss of weight either increases or diminishes the *size* of the fat cells (**hypertrophic obesity**). Unfortunately, persons with greater than normal numbers of fat cells are least likely to lose weight successfully. Some researchers suggest that the body triggers hunger signals when the fat stored in these cells begins to decrease.

The theory that a hereditary, inside-the-body basis for obesity may exist is supported by the existence of animal strains that are genetically fat; such animals tend to be fat in any environment—that is, they are fat regardless of the kind or variety of food offered. In humans, studies have shown that identical twins—whether raised together or apart—tend to have similar weight gain patterns.[9] Also, twins raised by adoptive parents tend to have body shapes similar to their biological parents. Not all studies confirm this, however.[10] Moreover, pairs of twins purposefully overfed in clinical experiments tend to respond similarly to the extra calories; some sets of twins gain considerable amounts of weight when fed a certain number of calories, whereas other pairs put on relatively few pounds even on the same diet.[11]

Environment and Behavior

The environmental obesity model is supported by experiments with "cafeteria rats." Ordinary rats fed regular rat chow are of normal weight (for rats), but if those very same rats are offered free access to a wide variety of tempting, rich, highly palatable foods, they greatly overeat and become obese.[12]

In human beings, learning plays an important role. We have genetically inborn instincts, but superimposed on these are learnings from our early childhood experiences; and depending on our environments, the two may differ. Thus, **hunger** is a drive programmed into us by our heredity, but learned responses to **appetite** can teach us to ignore or over-respond to our hunger. In contrast, appetite is more influenced by learning. Another way to say this is to say that hunger is physiological, while appetite is psychological, and the two don't always coincide. We have all experienced appetite without hunger: "I'm not hungry, but I'd love to have some." We also often experience the reverse, hunger without appetite: "I know I'm hungry, but I don't feel like eating." Hunger is a negative experience (and we may eat in order to avoid it); appetite is positive.

The ways people respond to hunger and appetite determine whether they eat too much, too little, or just enough to maintain their weights. A third factor enters in, too: **satiety**, which signals that it is time to stop eating. One view holds that eating behavior is turned on all the time, except when the satiety signal turns it off. But the ways in which hunger, appetite, and satiety regulate food intake are unknown.

In human physiology, research is beginning to find possible answers to what regulates food behavior. The stomach's nerves perceive stretching, and you stop eating when your stomach feels stretched full. Blood glucose level is thought to be involved: you get hungry when your blood glucose level falls—or perhaps when your liver glycogen is beginning to be exhausted. Blood lipids, and possibly amino acids and other molecules, also play a role. When you eat, you secrete hormones to regulate digestive activity. These hormones may also convey the message to the brain that it is time to stop eating. When you eat carbohydrate, **endogenous opiates** are made in your brain that have a tranquilizing effect. It is thought that people may eat in order to obtain this effect.

This brings us to the question, Where in the brain are these messages received (whatever they are)? One brain area stands out as a regulator for food behavior—the **hypothalamus**. The hypothalamus is a center that communicates with both the hormonal and the nervous systems. It integrates many kinds of signals received from the rest of the body, including information about the blood's temperature, sodium content, and glucose content. We know it is important in regulating eating, because damage to the hypothalamus produces derangements in eating behavior and body weight—in some cases causing severe weight loss; in others, vast overeating. In the person with a normal hypothalamus, however, appropriate eating behavior seems to be a response not to a single signal arriving at some one location in the hypothalamus, but to a whole host of signals. Somehow these many inputs become integrated into a final common path—the act of eating.

A person who eats inappropriately may have established a habitual behavior pattern that wrongly links many different stimuli to the act of eating. In this connection, the study of behavior offers insight into the problem of

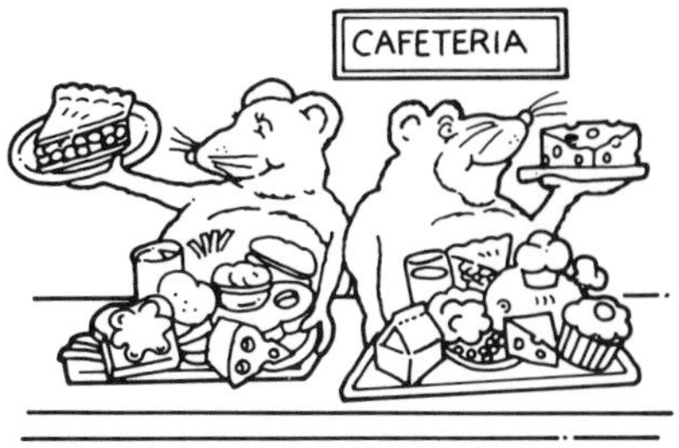

Given a wide variety of tempting foods, these laboratory animals become obese, just as human beings do.

Hunger the physiological drive to find and eat food, experienced as an unpleasant sensation.

Appetite the psychological desire to find and eat food, experienced as a pleasant sensation, often in the absence of hunger.

Satiety the feeling of fullness or satisfaction at the end of a meal that prompts a person to stop eating.

Endogenous opiates morphine-like compounds that act as internal tranquilizers when produced in the brain in response to pain, stress, certain drugs, and other circumstances.

Hypothalamus (high-poh-THALL-ah-mus) a part of the brain that senses a variety of conditions in the blood, such as temperature, salt content, and glucose content, and then signals other parts of the brain or body to change those conditions when necessary.

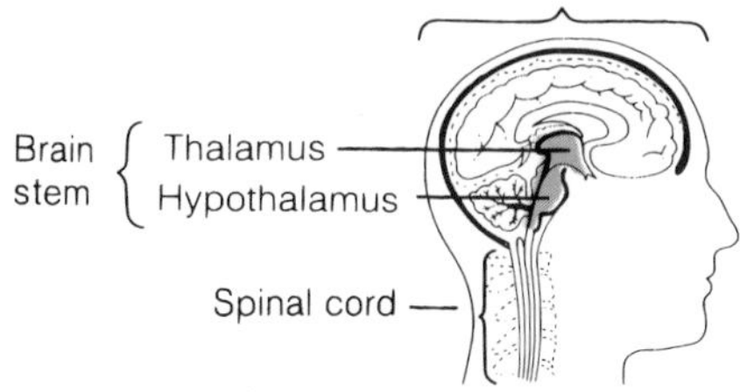

Researchers believe that the hypothalamus controls the sensations of hunger and satiety.

overeating by viewing it as a conditioned response to a variety of stimuli. Sometimes eating behavior tends to get turned on by the wrong triggers. A crying child with a skinned knee who is offered a lollipop to help soothe the hurt may learn to associate food with comfort and so seek food inappropriately when experiencing emotional pain later in life.

Eating behavior, then, may be a response not only to hunger or appetite but also to complex human sensations, such as yearning, craving, addiction, or compulsion.[13] For an emotionally insecure person, eating may be less threatening than calling a friend when lonely and risking rejection. Often, especially in adolescent girls, eating is used to relieve boredom or to ward off depression. Some obese people respond to anxiety—or, in fact, to any kind of **arousal**—by eating. Significantly, however, if they are able to give a name to their aroused condition and thereby gain a feeling that they have some control over it, they are not as likely to overeat.[14]

Arousal as used in this context, heightened activity of certain brain centers associated with excitement and anxiety.

Stress may also directly promote the accumulation of body fat. The stress hormones favor the breakdown of energy stores (glycogen and fat) to glucose and fatty acids, which can be used to fuel the muscular activity of fight or flight. If a person fails to use the fuel in physical exertion, however, the body can't turn these fragments back into glycogen. It has no alternative but to convert them to fat. Each time glucose is pulled out of storage in response to stress and then transformed into fat, the lowered glucose level or exhausted glycogen will signal hunger, and the person will eat again soon after.[15]

Stress eating may appear in different patterns. Some people eat excessively at night, while others characteristically binge during emotional crises. The overly thin often react oppositely. Stress causes them to reject food and thus become thinner. It is not yet known why these behaviors occur, but research continues.

It is probable that the most important single contributor to the obesity problem in our country is underactivity.

The many possible causes of obesity mentioned so far all relate to the input side of the energy equation. What about output? It is probable that the most important single contributor to the obesity problem in our country is underactivity. The control of hunger and appetite works well in active people and fails only when activity falls below a certain minimum level.[16] Some obese people eat less than lean people, but they are so extraordinarily inactive that they still manage to store surplus calories. Some people move more efficiently than others, too. Two people of the same age, height, and weight, walking five miles, might spend different amounts of energy because of the different ways in which they move their muscles.

No two people are alike, either physically or psychologically. No doubt, the causes of obesity are as varied as the obese people themselves. Many causes may contribute to the problem in a single person. Given this complexity, it is obvious that there is no panacea. The top priority should be prevention, but where prevention has failed, the treatment of obesity must involve a simultaneous attack on many fronts.

Weight Gain and Loss

When you step on the scale and note that you weigh a pound more or less than you did the last time you weighed yourself, this doesn't necessarily mean you have gained or lost body fat. Changes in body weight reflect shifts in many different materials—not only fat but also fluid, bone minerals, and lean tissues such as muscles. This means that the loss of a pound does not always reflect the loss of fat. Similarly, the gain of a pound may not reflect gained fat; some of it may reflect gained muscle and bone and an overall shift toward a leaner body type. Because it is so important for people concerned with weight control to realize this, this section discusses the changes that take place with gains and losses of weight.

A healthy man or woman about 5 feet 10 inches tall who weighs 150 pounds carries about 90 of those pounds as water and 30 as fat.* The other 30 pounds are the so-called lean tissues: muscles; organs such as the heart, brain, and liver; and the bones of the skeleton. Stripped of water and fat, then, the person weighs only 30 pounds. This lean tissue is the body's vital machinery that maintains health and life. When a person who is too fat seeks to lose weight, it should be fat—not this precious lean tissue—that is lost. And for someone who wants to gain weight, it is desirable to gain weight in proportion—lean *and* fat, not just fat.

Weight is gained or lost in different body tissues, depending on how a person goes about it. To lose fluid, for example, one can take a diuretic ("water pill"), causing the kidneys to siphon extra water from the blood into the urine. Or one can engage in heavy exercise in the heat, losing abundant fluid in perspiration. (Both practices are dangerous, incidentally, and are not being recommended here.) To gain water weight, a person can overconsume salt and water; for a few hours the body will then retain water, until it manages to excrete the salt. (This, too, is not recommended.) Most quick-weight-loss diet schemes promote large losses of fluid that create large, temporary changes in the scale weight with little or no real loss of body fat. The rest of this chapter underscores this distinction, and a later section on weight-loss strategy stresses exercise as a means of supporting lean tissue during weight loss.

Weight Gain

When you eat more food energy than you need, where does it go in your body? The energy nutrients—carbohydrate, fat, and protein—contribute to body stores as follows:

- Carbohydrate is broken down to small units (sugars) for absorption. Inside the body, these may be built up to glycogen or converted to fat and stored as such.
- Fat is broken down to its component parts (including fatty acids) for absorption. Inside the body, these are most easily converted to storage fat.
- Protein, too, is broken down to its basic units (amino acids) for absorption. Inside the body, these units may be used to replace body proteins. Those amino acids that are not used can't be stored as protein for later use. They lose their nitrogen and are converted to fat.

Notice in Figure 8–2 that although three kinds of materials enter the body, they are stored for later use in only two forms: glycogen and fat. Also notice that when protein is stored in the form of fat, it cannot be recovered later as protein. The amino acids lose their nitrogen—it is actually excreted in the

*For a healthy woman or man 5 ft tall who weighs 100 lb, the comparable figures would be 60 lb of water, 20 lb of fat, and 20 lb of lean tissue.

● *Figure 8–2*

Feasting and Fasting

In A, the person is storing energy. In B, the person is drawing on stored energy. In C, the person is in ketosis.

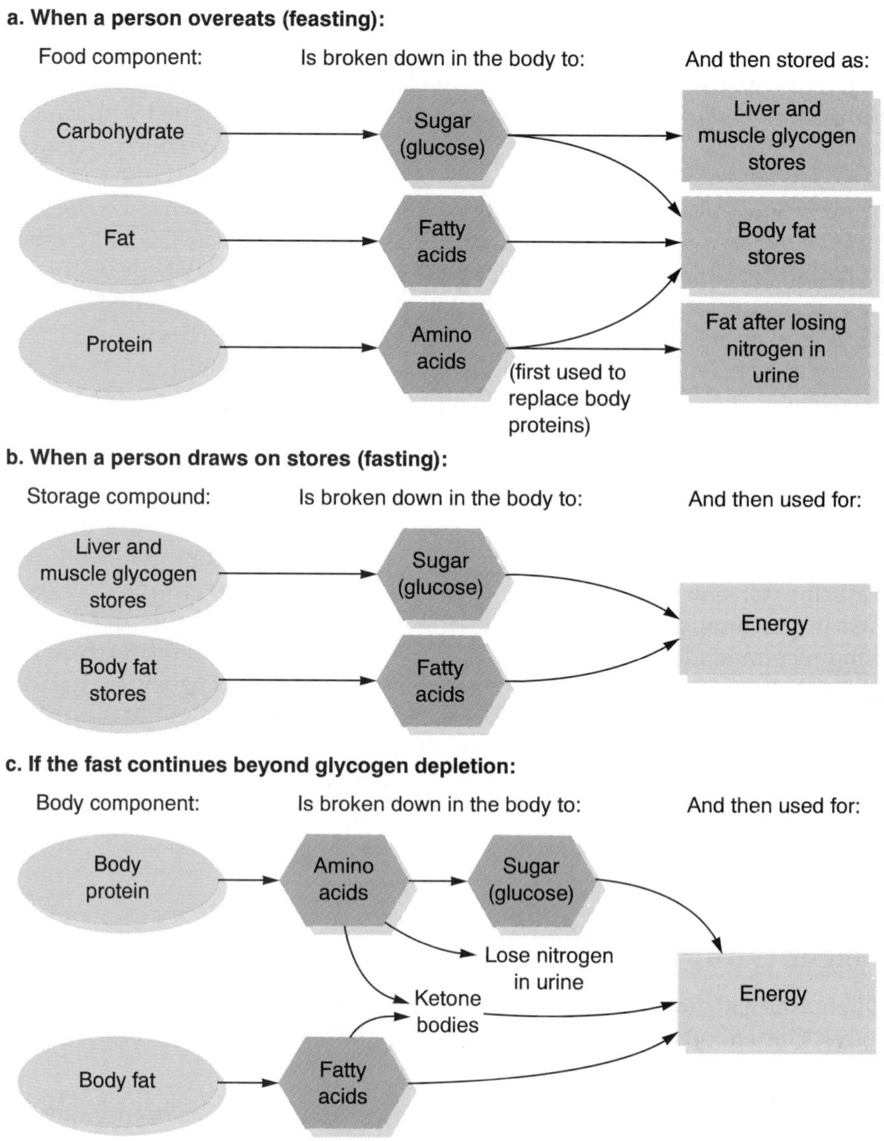

urine. It does not matter whether you are eating hamburgers, brownies, or carrot sticks; if you eat enough of the food, the excess will be turned to fat within hours. (On the other hand, as Chapter 9 will make clear, a judicious program of eating well and exercising will help build muscle.)

Of the three energy nutrients, fat from food is especially easy for the body to store as fat tissue.* This implies, then, that the calories from fat may be more fattening than those from carbohydrate or protein.[17] Researchers have shown in both animals and humans that subjects who ate higher fat diets had higher body fat contents than those who ate diets high in carbohydrate and lower in fat, even though the two diets were similar in terms of total calo-

*Scientists have recently questioned whether fats in foods actually yield 9 or 11 calories per gram when eaten.

ries.[18] This suggests that obesity develops more easily from eating a high-fat diet. If you choose to overeat, therefore, there may be some advantage to overeating carbohydrate-rich bread or potatoes than overeating fat-rich butter or sour cream—you may deposit less fat.

Weight Loss and Fasting

When the tables are turned and you stop eating altogether, your body has to draw on its stored supplies of nutrients to keep going. Nothing is wrong with this; in fact, it is a great advantage to you that you can eat periodically, store fuel, and then use up that fuel between meals. The between-meal interval is ideally about 4 to 6 hours—about the length of time it takes to use up most of the available liver glycogen—or 12 to 14 hours at night, when body systems are slowed down and the need for energy is lower. If a person doesn't eat for, say, three whole days or a week, the body makes one adjustment after another.

The first adjustment is to use the liver's glycogen. (The muscles' glycogen is reserved for the muscles' own use—and they are using it.) The liver's glycogen, remember, is the body's source of blood glucose to fuel the brain's and nerves' activities. Ordinarily, the brain and nerves can use no other fuel. But after about a day, the primary supply is gone. Where, then, does the body turn to keep its nervous system going? Whatever it has to do, it will do, for the nervous system runs the body, and when it stops, the body dies.

An obvious alternative source of energy would be the abundant fat stores most people carry. At first, these are of no use to the nervous system. The muscles and other organs use fat as fuel, but the nervous system ordinarily cannot. Nor can the body convert this fat to glucose, because it possesses no enzymes to do so. It does, however, possess enzymes to convert protein to glucose.

As the fast continues, the body turns to its own lean tissues to keep up the supply of glucose (see Figure 8–2). One reason why people lose weight so dramatically within the first three days of a fast is that they are devouring their own protein tissues as fuel. Since protein contains only half as many calories per pound as fat, it disappears twice as fast. Also, with each pound of body protein, three or four pounds of associated water are lost. As you will see in a moment, the same reasons account for the rapid weight loss seen in the early stages of a low-carbohydrate diet.

If the body were to continue to consume itself at this rate, death would ensue within about ten days. After all, the liver, the heart muscle, the lung tissue, and the blood—all vital tissues—are being burned as fuel. (In fact, fasting or starving people remain alive only until their body fat is gone or until half their lean tissue is gone, whichever comes first.) But now the body plays its last ace: it begins converting fat stores into a form it can use to help feed the nervous system and so forestall the end. This is known as **ketosis.**

Ketosis is an adaptation to prolonged fasting or carbohydrate deprivation. Instead of breaking down fat molecules all the way to carbon dioxide and water, as it normally does, the body takes partially broken down fat fragments, combines them into ketone bodies (compounds that are normally rare in the blood), and lets them circulate in the bloodstream. The advantage is that about half of the brain's cells can use these compounds for energy. Thus, indirectly, the nervous system begins to feed on the body's fat stores. This

Ketosis (kee-TOE-sis) an adaptation of the body to prolonged (several days') fasting or carbohydrate restriction: body fat is converted to ketones, which can be used as fuel for some brain cells.

reduces the nervous system's need for glucose. It spares the muscle and other lean tissue from being devoured so quickly and prolongs the starving person's life. Because of ketosis, an initially healthy person totally deprived of food can live for as long as six to eight weeks.

Fasting has been practiced as a periodic discipline by respected, wise people in many cultures. However, ketosis may be harmful to the body by upsetting the acid-base balance of the blood. For the person who merely wants to lose weight, then, fasting is usually not the best way. For one thing, even in ketosis, the body's lean tissue continues to be lost at a rapid rate to supply glucose to those nervous system cells that cannot use ketones as fuel. For another, the body becomes conservative during a fast and slows its metabolism so as to lose as little energy as it possibly can. A well-designed low-calorie diet, accompanied by the appropriate exercise program, has actually been observed to promote the same rate of *weight* loss and a faster rate of *fat* loss than a total fast.[19] Just how to design a low-calorie diet is the subject of a later section, but first the low-carbohydrate diet—an example of how *not* to design a diet—deserves attention.

The Low-Carbohydrate Diet

People are attracted to low-carbohydrate diets because of the dramatic weight loss that occurs within the first few days. Such people would be disillusioned if they realized that the major part of this weight loss is a loss of body protein, along with quantities of water and important minerals.

The low-carbohydrate diet is designed to make a person go into ketosis. The sales pitch is that "you'll never feel hungry" and that "you'll lose weight fast—faster than you would on any ordinary diet." Both claims are true, but knowledgeable consumers see through them. They know that the loss of appetite is common to any low-calorie diet. To the fast weight loss, they say, "Yes, but what kind of weight loss: water and lean tissue, or fat?"

The body responds to a low-carbohydrate diet as it does to a fast. It is receiving protein and fat (on a fast it draws on its own protein and fat), but it has used up its stored glycogen. It therefore turns to protein to make the needed glucose. Why should you give it protein if it will only convert that protein to glucose? And why *not* give it carbohydrate if that is the very material it needs? Carbohydrate will sustain it and allow it to use up its stored fat at the maximal rate. In fact, traditional religious fasting is more sensible; the "juice fast" is a sort of carbohydrate-only diet that offers the body the one substance it needs most to conserve its vital lean tissue.

Protein, then, is inefficient fuel for a carbohydrate-deprived body. It has another disadvantage as well. On being converted to glucose, protein loses its nitrogen, and that nitrogen has to be excreted. This puts a burden on the kidneys. Advising the low-carbohydrate dieter to drink sufficient water is intended to prevent kidney damage that may result from the large amounts of nitrogen-containing waste material being produced from used-up protein as well as from the ketone bodies circulating in the blood.

A multitude of other physiological hazards accompany low-carbohydrate diets—metabolic abnormalities such as high blood cholesterol, hypoglycemia, and mineral imbalances. Legitimate practitioners never recommend these diets.

Low-carbohydrate diets come in many disguises with many different names: Air Force Diet, the Atkins Diet, the Calories Don't Count Diet, the Drinking Man's Diet, the Herbalife Diet, the Mayo Diet, the Protein-Sparing Fast, the Scarsdale Diet, the HCG Diet, the Ski Team Diet, and the Stillman Diet. Some of these diets involve eating foods that are high in both protein and fat (abundant meats, for example); others allow only protein-rich foods (fish and chicken without the skin); and some offer no foods at all, but only powders or liquids that are supposed to "spare" body protein while the body burns its own fat as fuel. The latter are the most dangerous of all. Numerous deaths have been traced to them, many caused by abnormalities found in the heart muscle, which disintegrates without sufficient nutrients to maintain it.

Low-carbohydrate diets appear every year under new names. Bringing out new diet books and products is a profitable business, and it will continue to be successful as long as people are deceived by the initial rapid weight loss into thinking that the diets work. Before adopting any new diet plan, compare it to the guidelines presented in Table 8–5. To identify fraudulent low-carbohydrate diets for what they are, learn to add up the carbohydrate grams they supply: fewer than 100 to 125 grams a day is inadequate. Appendix F shows the carbohydrate content of foods, and Table 8–6 evaluates popular weight-loss diets and programs by asking several key questions.

Table 8–5 Guidelines for Evaluating Weight-Loss Promotions

Beware of weight-loss programs that:

1. Promise or imply dramatic, rapid weight loss (i.e., substantially more than 1% of total body weight per week).
2. Promote diets that are extremely low in calories (i.e., below 800 cal/day; 1,200 cal/day diets are preferred) unless under the supervision of competent medical experts.
3. Attempt to make clients dependent upon special products rather than teaching how to make good choices from the conventional food supply. (This does not condemn the marketing of low-calorie convenience foods that may be chosen by consumers.)
4. Do not encourage permanent, realistic lifestyle changes, including regular exercise and the behavioral aspects of eating wherein food may be used as a coping device (i.e., programs should focus on changing the causes of overweight rather than simply on the overweight itself).
5. Misrepresent salespeople as "counselors" supposedly qualified to give guidance in nutrition and/or general health. Even if adequately trained, such counselors would still be objectionable because of the obvious conflict of interest that exists when providers profit directly from products they recommend and sell.
6. Require large sums of money at the start or require that clients sign contracts for expensive, long-term programs. Such practices too often have been abused as salespeople focus attention upon signing up new people rather than delivering continuing, satisfactory service.
7. Fail to inform clients about the risks associated with weight loss in general or the specific program being promoted.
8. Promote unproven or spurious weight-loss aids, such as human chorionic gonadotropin (HCG) hormone, starch blockers, diuretics, sauna belts, body wraps, passive exercise, ear stapling, acupuncture, electric muscle stimulating (EMS) devices, spirulina, amino acid supplements (e.g., arginine or ornithine), glucomannan, and so forth.
9. Claim that cellulite exists in the body.
10. Claim that the use of an appetite suppressant or methylcellulose (a bulking agent) enables a person to lose body fat without restricting accustomed caloric intake.

Source: Adapted with permission from *National Council against Health Fraud Newsletter,* March/April 1987.

Table 8–6
Weight-Loss Diets and Programs Compared

With a balanced perspective on foods and a sense of what is important in diet planning and what is not, you can evaluate the many different available diets and decide which might be best for you. Here's a summary of the questions you might ask, followed by a comparison of some of the currently popular diets and programs.

1. Is this a diet you could live with indefinitely?
2. What is the recommended rate of weight loss?
3. Does the program take individual differences into account to determine caloric needs?
4. To what extent does the plan educate the client about nutrition, behavior modification, and the importance of exercise?
5. Does the program put you in contact with professionals such as physicians or registered dietitians?
6. Does the program offer a maintenance plan once the weight is lost?
7. What is the nature of the advertisements and endorsements?
8. How much does it cost (can you afford it)?

Diet Name and Description	Question 1 Can live with diet?	Question 2 Weight loss rate?	Question 3 Individualized?	Question 4 Diet, Exercise, Beh. Mod.?	Question 5 Professionals?	Question 6 Maintenance Plan?	Question 7 Ads/Endorsements?	Question 8 Cost?
Diet Center, real food diet with supplements (vitamins, minerals, and blood sugar stabilizer).	Yes	1½ to 2 pounds per week	Variations within set regimen.	One-to-one brief meetings with staff person daily, if desired.	No—contact is with Diet Center counselor.	Yes	Testimonials.	Initial fee averages \$400–\$700 for 9-week program.
Diet Workshop, real food diet without special products.	Yes	1½ to 2 pounds per week	Variations within set regimen.	1 hour/week in group setting.	No—contact is with trained graduates of program.	Yes	Testimonials.	\$14 membership. \$9/week until maintenance.
Health Management Resources (HMR), medically supervised very-low-calorie diet.	No	3 to 5 pounds per week	Variations within set regimen.	1½ hour/week in group setting.	Yes	Yes	Testimonials plus extensive statistics from company data.	Averages \$2,775 for entire program.
Jenny Craig, real food diet that requires prepackaged meals until maintenance phase.	No	1 to 2 pounds per week	Variations within set regimen.	14 1-hour video classes plus one-to-one sessions with counselor.	No—college graduates implement program.	Yes	Celebrity testimonials and client case studies.	\$185 membership, \$60–\$70/week for food.

Medifast, liquid fast dispensed from individual physician's office; program support varies greatly, depending on intensity of doctor's approach.	No	3 to 5 pounds per week	Variations of set plan left to M.D.'s discretion.	Lifestyles weekly group program and one-to-one counseling.	Yes	Yes	Testimonials plus information about obesity as "disease."	Averages $1,700–$1,900 ($50/week).
Nutri/System, real food diet that requires prepackaged foods until maintenance phase.	No	1½ to 2 pounds per week	Variations within set regimen.	30-minute weekly group classes plus one-to-one sessions with nutrition "specialist."	No—most who implement program are college graduates.	Yes	"Dieting DJ" testimonials.	Ranges from $100–$1,000 plus $48–$58/week for food.
Optifast, medically supervised very-low-calorie diet.	No	Up to 1% to 2% of body weight	Variations within set regimen.	1½ hour/week in group setting; weekly meetings for at least 21 weeks; at least one meeting with an R.D.	Yes	Yes	Show before-and-after pictures, discuss medical team approach, and describe program.	$2,500–$3,500 for 26-week program.
Slim Fast/Ultra Slim Fast, over-the-counter product.	Not without dependence on product.	Up to individual	No—self-regulated.	No	No	No	Celebrity testimonials.	$8–$12/week.
Take Off Pounds Sensibly (TOPS), real food diet that does not require special products.	Yes	Varies	Variations with prescribed ADA exchange plans.	Yes, group meetings.	No—contact is with trained graduates of program.	Yes	Newspaper announcement.	$12 annual fee.
Weight Loss Clinic, real food diet that does not require special products.	Yes	2 to 3 pounds per week	Variations within set regimen.	One-to-one brief meetings with staff person up to 5 days/week.	Yes	Yes	Testimonials.	Averages $60/week.
Weight Watchers, real food diet that does not require special products.	Yes	1 to 2 pounds per week	Variations within set regimen.	45 minute weekly group meeting plus question/answer period.	No—contact is with trained graduates of program.	Yes	Testimonials of "graduates."	$12–$20 membership plus $7–$9/week until maintenance.

Source: Adapted from Smart losers' guide to choosing a weight-loss program, *Tufts University Diet & Nutrition Letter,* August 1990.

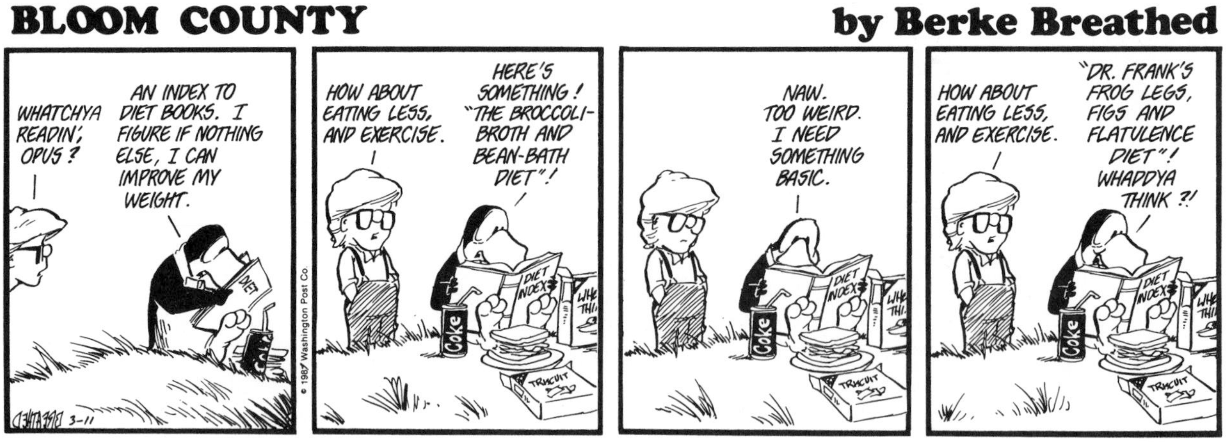
BLOOM COUNTY
by Berke Breathed
WHATCHYA READIN', OPUS ?
AN INDEX TO DIET BOOKS. I FIGURE IF NOTHING ELSE, I CAN IMPROVE MY WEIGHT.
HOW ABOUT EATING LESS, AND EXERCISE.
HERE'S SOMETHING ! "THE BROCCOLI-BROTH AND BEAN-BATH DIET" !
NAW. TOO WEIRD. I NEED SOMETHING BASIC.
HOW ABOUT EATING LESS, AND EXERCISE.
"DR. FRANK'S FROG LEGS, FIGS AND FLATULENCE DIET" ! WHADDYA THINK ?!
DIET
DIET INDEX
Coke
TRACUIT

The Very-Low-Calorie Diets

Very-low-calorie diets (VLCDs) are mostly powdered formulas available by prescription, are usually medically supervised, and provide between 400 and 700 calories. VLCDs consist of about 30 grams of carbohydrate (not enough to spare protein) and high-quality protein equivalent to about twice the RDA. Supplements of vitamins and minerals are provided.

For particular individuals, especially the morbidly obese, these diets may provide some benefit in that they promote rapid weight loss and free the individual from having to make decisions regarding food intake—they simply drink the prescribed formula. Because of the health risks that may accompany these diets, it is recommended that a VLCD be undertaken only when other more traditional approaches have failed and always under the supervision of a health team that includes both a physician and a registered dietitian. A significant loss of heart muscle can occur and lead to sudden death from heart attack if the client loses weight too rapidly on a VLCD.[20] Other risks of VLCDs are listed in Table 8–7. The more valid VLCD programs include exercise, nutrition education, behavior modification, and support groups to improve their long-term effectiveness. (Details about several of the VLCDs can be found in Table 8–6.)

Table 8–7

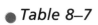

Risks Associated with the Very-Low-Calorie Diets

- Blood sugar imbalance
- Cold intolerance
- Constipation
- Decreased basal metabolic rate
- Dehydration
- Diarrhea
- Emotional problems
- Fatigue
- Headaches
- Heart irregularity
- Ketosis
- Kidney infection
- Loss of lean body tissue
- Weakness
- Weight gain

Source: Adapted from ADA report: Position of American Dietetic Association: Very-low-calorie weight loss diets, *Journal of the American Dietetic Association,* May 1990, p. 722.

Other Options for Weight Loss

Fasting and low-carbohydrate diets are not healthful ways to lose weight. Other ways *not* to choose are water pills, diet pills, health spa regimens, muscle stimulators, hormones, and surgery. Water pills (diuretics) do nothing to solve a fat problem, although they may bring about the loss of a few pounds on the scale for half a day and cause dehydration. Diet pills (stimulants) reduce appetite temporarily by triggering the stress response but leave the dieter with another problem: how to get off them without gaining more weight. Fiber diet pills increase bulk in the stomach and could ideally lead to satiety, but they can also cause intestinal gas and blockage. Moreover, the bran fiber typically found in diet pills does not seem to be effective at producing satiety.[21] Health spas may be a nice place to exercise, but you cannot "jiggle" or "melt" pounds away on their special machines. Muscle stimulators reduce body measurements by making muscles tighter, not by reducing the fat content—and only for an hour or so. Hormones are powerful body chemicals, and many affect fat metabolism, but all have proven ineffective and are often hazardous as weight-loss aids.

Sheer desperation prompts some obese people to request surgery. One operation—bypass surgery—involves removing or disconnecting a portion of the small intestine to reduce absorption. After bypass surgery, the person can continue overeating but will absorb fewer calories. This procedure has many dangerous side effects, including liver failure, massive and frequent diarrhea, urinary stones, intestinal infections, and malnutrition. Such surgery is seldom performed anymore because results have been so disappointing.

Another more common operation—**gastroplasty**—involves stapling the stomach to make it smaller, thus forcing the person to eat less (see Figure 8–3). Nausea and vomiting occur if the person continues to overeat following the procedure. Still, although the theory is pleasingly simple, stapling involves hazards in practice: stomach tissue is damaged, scars are formed, staples pull loose. The person contemplating surgery should think long and hard before submitting to it.

Gastroplasty surgery on the stomach (also called stomach stapling) that reduces its volume to less than 2 ounces (the size of a shot glass) to prevent overeating.

New approaches to limit the stomach's capacity have been developed at intervals. One involved slipping a balloon into the stomach and inflating it. A large number of these balloons were found to spontaneously deflate and pass painfully through the intestinal tract; as a result, this procedure is no longer available. Wiring the jaws closed is still another method of reducing food intake by physical control. This procedure forces the person to consume a liquid diet through a straw. Unfortunately, little attention is given to changing eating or exercise habits. Although the person loses weight while his or her

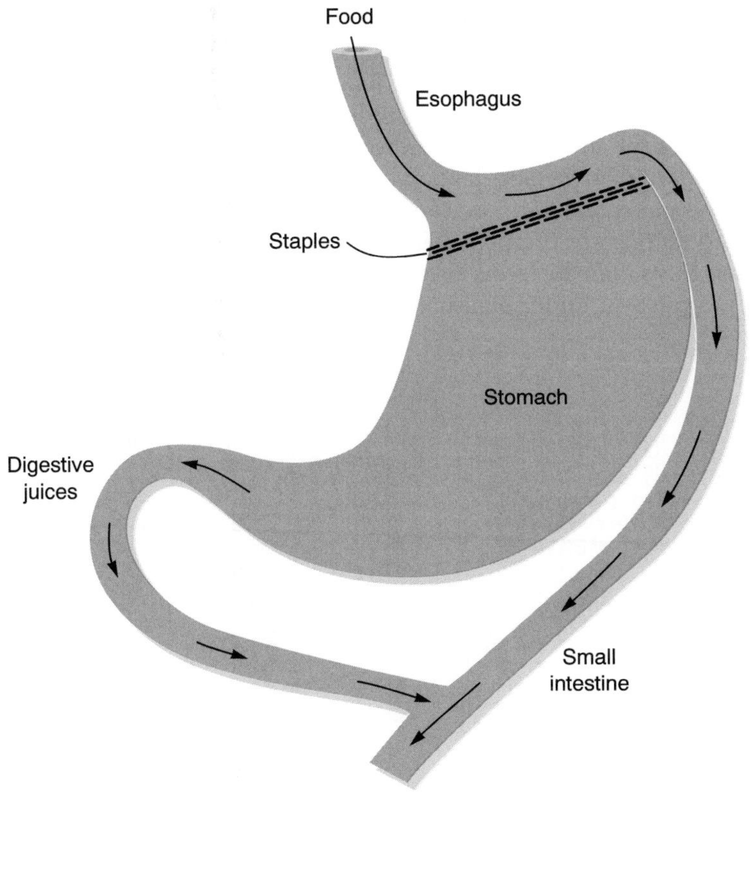

Figure 8–3

Stomach Stapling

The stomach is stapled closed near the top, leaving only a small opening that can be connected directly to the small intestine, as shown in this diagram.

Lipectomy a type of surgery that vacuums out fat cells that have accumulated, typically in the buttocks and thighs. If the person continues to overeat, fat will return to the fat cells that remain in those regions.

jaws are closed, the lost weight is regained when the wires are removed. Success, as measured by long-term weight maintenance, is seldom achieved by either of these methods.

Other approaches involve cosmetic surgery. One is **lipectomy**, a procedure in which the surgeon uses a small hollow tube to suction out fatty tissue from beneath the skin. People who wish to remove the fat from a particular area can elect this procedure, which sometimes brings pleasing results but sometimes produces a figure in which one part is disproportionately thin relative to the others.

Surgery is appropriate in some instances. Cosmetic surgery can minimize disfigurements, improve self-confidence, and ease the way toward concentration on life issues more important than external appearances. But after surgery, the same person resides within the skin as before. A changed appearance does not guarantee changed eating habits, a better personality, reduced interpersonal conflicts, or any other improvements in the quality of one's life. Moreover, surgery involves risks. Of every 10,000 people who go under anesthesia, several become more ill than they were to begin with, and one dies.[22]

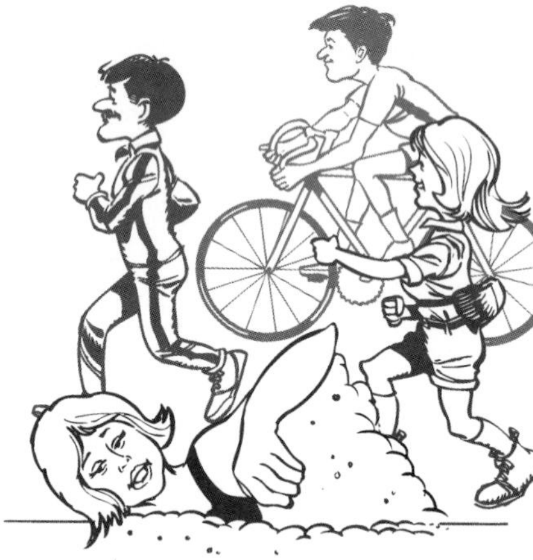

To burn 250 extra calories a day (equal to a half a pound of fat loss per week), you could add one of these activities to your daily routine:

Walk (briskly) for 45 minutes (5.5 cal/min).

Bike (moderate pace) for 36 minutes (7.0 cal/min).

Swim (fast) for 23 minutes (11 cal/min).

Run (moderate pace) for 18 minutes (14 cal/min).

Weight-loss Strategies

Given that so many approaches are guaranteed to fail, what weight-loss strategies work? How can a person lose weight safely and permanently? The secret is a sensible (we didn't say *easy*) approach involving diet, exercise, and behavior modification. It takes tremendous dedication, especially at first, for a fat person whose habits have all promoted obesity to learn and make habits of the hundred or so new behaviors necessary to promote a healthful weight. Even the most effective weight-loss programs can boast of only a one-third success rate: two of every three people who enter them regain whatever weight they lose. But when people succeed, they do so because they have employed many of the techniques described in this chapter.

The way a particular person loses weight is a highly individual matter. Two weight-loss plans may both be successful and yet have little or nothing in common. To emphasize the personal nature of weight-loss plans, the following section is written in terms of diet-planning advice to "you." This is intended not to put you under pressure to take it personally, but to give you

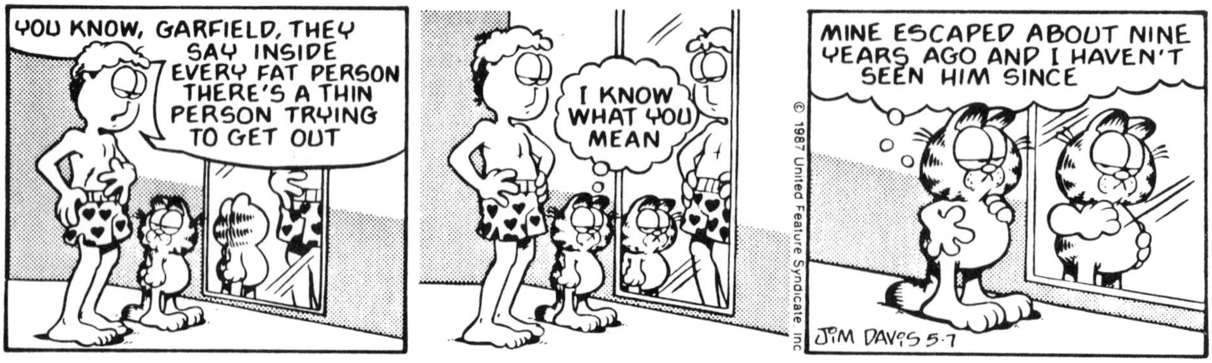
YOU KNOW, GARFIELD, THEY SAY INSIDE EVERY FAT PERSON THERE'S A THIN PERSON TRYING TO GET OUT
I KNOW WHAT YOU MEAN
MINE ESCAPED ABOUT NINE YEARS AGO AND I HAVEN'T SEEN HIM SINCE
© 1987 United Feature Syndicate, Inc
JIM DAVIS 5-7

the illusion of listening in on a conversation in which a person with, say, anywhere from 10 to 200 pounds to lose is being competently counseled by someone familiar with the techniques known to be effective. Notes in the margin on page 227 highlight the principles involved.

Diet Planning

No particular diet is magical, and no particular food must be either included or avoided. Since you are the one who will have to live with the diet, you had better be involved in its planning. Don't think of it as a diet you are going "on"—because then you may be tempted to go "off" it. The diet can be called successful only if the pounds do not return. Think of it as an eating plan that you will adopt for life. It must consist of foods that you like or can learn to like, that are available to you and that are within your means.

For the person wanting to lose weight, a deficit of 500 calories a day for seven days (3,500 calories a week) is enough to lose a pound of body fat a week. If you were to spend an extra 500 calories a day in some form of exercise (see Table 8–8), you could double this energy deficit.

Choose a calorie level you can live with. The ten-calorie rule will enable you to lose a pound or two a week while supporting your basal metabolism: allow 10 calories a day for each pound of your present body weight. As you lose weight, you can gradually adjust calories to keep losing at this rate. Thus, a person who starts at 220 pounds should eat 2,200 calories a day at first; one who starts at 150 should eat 1,500 calories.[23]

Put nutritional adequacy high on your list of priorities. This is a way of putting yourself first. "I like me, and I'm going to take good care of me" is the attitude to adopt. This means including low-calorie foods that are rich in valuable nutrients—vegetables and fruits; whole-grain breads and cereals; and a limited amount of protein-rich foods such as poultry, fish, eggs, low-fat cheeses, and nonfat milk. Within these categories, learn what foods you like and use them often. If you plan resolutely to include a certain number of servings of food from each of these groups each day, you may be so busy making sure you get what you need that you will have little time or appetite left for high-calorie or empty-calorie foods. Foods such as vegetables and whole grains take more time to eat, and crunchy, wholesome foods offer bulk and satiety for far fewer calories than do smooth, refined foods.

Table 8–8

Calories Spent During Various Activities

ACTIVITY	CALORIES EXPENDED PER HOUR[1] Man[2]	Woman[2]
Sitting quietly	100	80
Standing quietly	120	95
Light activity: Cleaning house, Office work, Playing baseball, Playing golf	300	240
Moderate activity: Walking briskly (3.5 mph), Gardening, Cycling (5.5 mph), Dancing, Playing basketball	460	370
Strenuous activity: Jogging (9 min/mile), Playing football, Swimming	730	580
Very strenuous activity: Running (7 min/mile), Racquetball, Skiing	920	740

[1]May vary depending on environmental conditions.
[2]Healthy man, 175 lbs;* healthy woman, 140 lbs*
*To determine caloric expenditure at a different weight, both men and women should divide their body weight by 175, then multiply by the man's caloric expenditure for the activity.

Source: U.S. Department of Agriculture, U.S. Department of Health and Human Services, *Dietary Guidelines for Americans,* 1990.

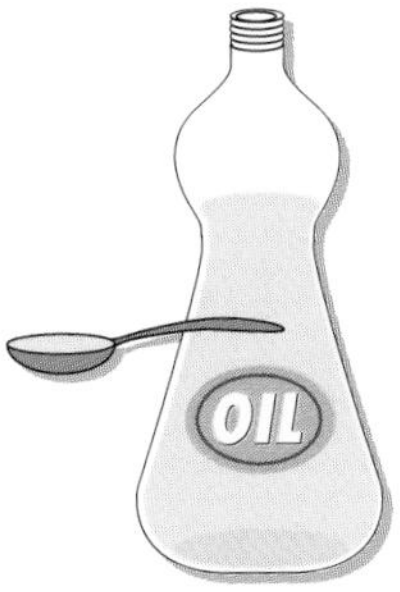

1 teaspoon fat/oil = 40 calories

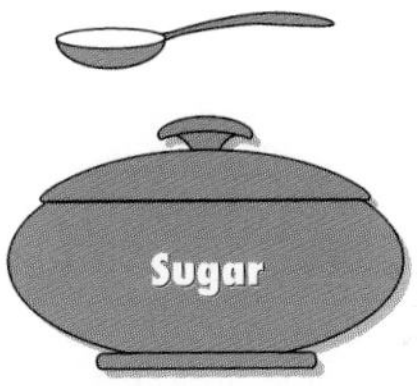

1 teaspoon sugar = 16 calories

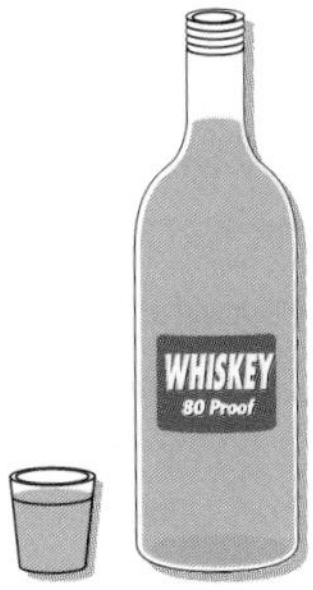

1 fluid ounce alcohol (80 proof) = 65 calories

Watch out for fats, sweets, and alcoholic beverages. They are often the source of extra calories.

Table 8–9 A Sample Balanced Weight-Loss Diet

FOOD GROUP	NUMBER OF PORTIONS	TYPICAL PORTION	CALORIES
Starch/bread	4	1 slice bread ½ c rice 1 small potato	320
Meat (lean)	2	2–3 oz lean meat	250
Vegetables	4	½ c any nonstarchy vegetable (carrots, onions, broccoli, etc.)	100
Fruit	4	1 small orange ½ small banana ⅓–½ c any juice	240
Milk (nonfat)	2	1 c nonfat milk	180
Fat	3	1 tsp butter, margarine, oil, or mayonnaise	135
		Total calories:	1,225

About a teaspoon of fat should be included in each meal to make it satisfying and keep you from getting hungry again too soon. You don't have to use pure fat—butter, margarine, or oil. Rather, most of the fat should come from protein-rich foods, such as lean meats, eggs, poultry, fish, and low-fat cheeses. Add any pure fat with extra caution. A slip of the butter knife adds more calories than a slip of the sugar spoon. Keep concentrated sweets to a minimum and let your carbohydrate come from starchy foods. Table 8–9 shows a suitable pattern for a weight-loss diet, and Table 8–10 offers more tips on cutting back on calories.

Table 8–10 Calorie-Cutting Tips

- Watch out for second helpings of higher calorie foods and gradually cut back on serving size.
- Choose low-calorie versions of foods you like.
- Go easy on foods that are high in fat or sugar.
- Limit alcoholic beverages.
- Roast, broil, boil, steam, or poach foods rather than fry them.
- Select lean cuts of meat and trim visible fat.
- Eat poultry and fish without skin.
- Use spices and herbs instead of sauces, butter, or other fats.
- Consume lowfat or nonfat dairy products.
- Drink coffee or tea without cream or sugar.
- Try fresh fruit for dessert, or baked products made with less fat and sugar (for example, angel food cake).
- Use alternatives to foods as rewards (for example, long walks, relaxing baths, a visit with a friend, a hobby, gardening, a good book).

Source: Adapted from USDA Home and Garden Bulletin Number 232–2, 1986.

Table 8–11 Calories in Alcoholic Beverages and Mixers

BEVERAGE	OUNCES	CALORIES
Beer	12	150
Gin, rum, vodka, whiskey (86 proof)	1½	105
Dessert wine	3½	140
Table wine	3½	85
Tonic, ginger ale, other sweetened carbonated water	8	80
Cola, root beer	8	100
Fruit-flavored soda, Tom Collins mix	8	115
Club soda, diet drinks	8	1

If you include alcohol in your diet plan, limit it strictly to no more than 150 calories a day (see Table 8–11). Add this amount on top of your chosen calorie level and reconcile yourself to a slower rate of weight loss.

Three meals a day is standard for our society, but no law says you shouldn't have four or five meals—only be sure they are smaller, of course. What is important is to eat regularly and, if at all possible, to eat before you become very hungry.

Do not weigh yourself more than once a week or so. Although 3,500 calories roughly equals a pound of body fat, there is no simple relationship between calorie balance and weight loss over short intervals. Gains or losses of a pound or more in a matter of days reverse themselves quickly; the smoothed-out average is what is real. Don't expect to lose continuously as fast as you did at first. A sizable water loss is common during the first week, but it will not happen again.

Many dieters experience a temporary plateau after about three weeks—not because they are slipping, but because they have gained water weight temporarily while they are still losing body fat. The fat they are hoping to lose must be used for energy. To use it, the body must combine it with oxygen (oxidize it) to make carbon dioxide and water. These compounds are heavier than the fat they are made from because oxygen has been added to them.* The carbon dioxide will be exhaled quickly, but the water stays in the body for a longer time. The water takes a while to leave the cells, then makes its way into the spaces between them, and finally enters the bloodstream. Only after the water has arrived in the blood do the kidneys "see" it and send it to the bladder for excretion. Meanwhile, the dieter has a weight gain, but one day the plateau will break. The signal that this is happening is frequent urination.

If you have been working out lately, successive weighings may show an occasional gain when you expect a loss. This may reflect a welcome development: the gain of lean body mass—just what you want if you want to be healthy. In fact, weight loss without exercise can have a negative effect on body composition. No doubt you've heard someone say as a joke, "I've lost 200 pounds, but I was never more than 20 pounds overweight." This person expects to diet, regain weight, and diet again throughout life. People who behave this way may not realize that with each bout of dieting, they trade in small amounts of lean body tissue for a slightly higher body fat content, as explained in the Nutrition Action feature, "The Ups and Downs of Dieting."

*Water weight accumulates during fat oxidation because one fatty acid weighing 284 units leaves behind water weighing 324 units— 14 percent more.

Profile of successful dieters:

They know their weight.

They know what they eat (they keep records).

They engage in regular exercise.

They have social support (relationships/groups).

They control their intake of alcohol.

They follow an individualized diet plan—one that they can enjoy permanently.

Diet-planning strategies:

1. Get involved personally.
2. Adopt a realistic plan and then keep track of calories—especially those from fat.
3. Make the diet adequate.
4. Emphasize high nutrient density.
5. Individualize. Use foods you like.
6. Stress dos, not don'ts.
7. Eat regular meals, at least three a day—no skipping.
8. Take a positive view of yourself.
9. Visualize a changed future self.
10. Take well-spaced weighings to avoid discouragement.

The Ups and Downs of Dieting

Less than a year after Oprah Winfrey proudly announced on her television talk show that she had lost 67 pounds on a liquid fasting diet, she had already regained 17 of those pounds, an upward trend that appears to have continued. Unfortunately, her dieting experience is not unique. Many of the one out of two women and one out of four men who are currently counting calories in an effort to lose weight will lose some pounds quickly, only to gain them back again a few weeks or months later and then start the cycle all over again with yet another diet.[24]

The pattern of losing, gaining, and then losing weight again, however, sets the stage for a lifetime of weight fluctuations that may have a lasting impact on the makeup of the body and the way the body burns calories. Dubbed the **yo-yo effect**, the up and down movement of the needle on the scale can, over time, cause the body to accumulate a greater percentage of fat and less lean muscle with each round of dieting.[25]

Yo-yo effect the effect of repeated rounds of dieting without exercise. The person rebounds to a higher weight (and body fat content) at the end of each round. Also called the ratchet effect.

If you cut back drastically the number of calories you consume without exercising for, say, a month or two, each week you'll probably lose a great deal of weight in the form of not only fat but also lean muscle. The problem is that if you later put the weight back on, the regained pounds will be primarily fat—not muscle. Thus, you may end up weighing the same as you did when you began the diet, but your body will now be composed of more fat and less muscle. Because muscle burns more calories just to sustain itself than fat does, your body will need fewer calories to maintain its weight than it did before. If you go back to eating the way you used to, chances are you will gain even more weight. By the same token, it will be more difficult to lose weight the next time you try.

Consider a hypothetical example of a 22-year-old woman who is 5 feet 5 inches tall and who recently has put on about 15 pounds and wants to lose them before swimsuit season. The woman weighs 140 pounds, 49 of which are fat (35 percent of her total body weight). Instead of cutting back on the amount she eats and exercising to burn calories, she opts for a crash diet that involves a 900-calorie-a-day regimen and includes no exercise. She loses 15 pounds— 8 in the form of fat and the rest muscle and water—leaving her with a body made up of 41 pounds of fat (33 percent of the total).

Satisfied with her new figure, she begins eating the way she had always eaten. Unfortunately, over the course of the next year, the 15 pounds she lost creep back on. Even worse is that the regained weight is all fat and no muscle. While she's back to weighing 140 pounds, she is fatter than before. Her body now carries 56 pounds of fat (40 percent of the total). In other words, even though the scale registers at the same number as it did when she began her weight-loss endeavors, her cycle of yo-yo dieting changed her overall body composition, leaving it fatter, not fitter.

Frustrated, she resolves to start another diet. This time, however, she'll have to eat less to lose the weight again, because her body has less of the muscle that burns more calories than fat. And if her weight fluctuates again, her body's percentage of lean muscle will probably drop even lower, a vicious cycle that will perpetuate itself with each new diet.

In addition to altering the body's overall composition, repeated bouts of weight loss appear to have other equally disturbing consequences. For one, some research indicates that the body responds to weight fluctuations by redistributing more fat around the abdomen.[26] Besides looking unattractive, that repositioning of fat is particularly unhealthful, because excess fat around the abdomen, as discussed earlier, raises the risk of suffering from health problems such as heart disease and diabetes. Another pitfall is that, as experiments in animals and humans suggest, repeated gain-loss cycles may heighten a dieter's preference for fatty—and thereby high-calorie and more fattening—foods, which in turn may contribute to a lifetime weight problem.

Compounding the physical impact of the yo-yo effect is the psychological toll it takes. Consider that each unsuccessful attempt to keep weight off is often viewed by the dieter as a personal failure, which can erode the person's self-esteem and trigger painful feelings of guilt and depression.

Fortunately, the gain-loss cycle can be broken with exercise. Regular, moderate physical activity burns fat and builds muscle, thereby shifting the body's composition in the dieter's favor. A leaner physique looks more at-

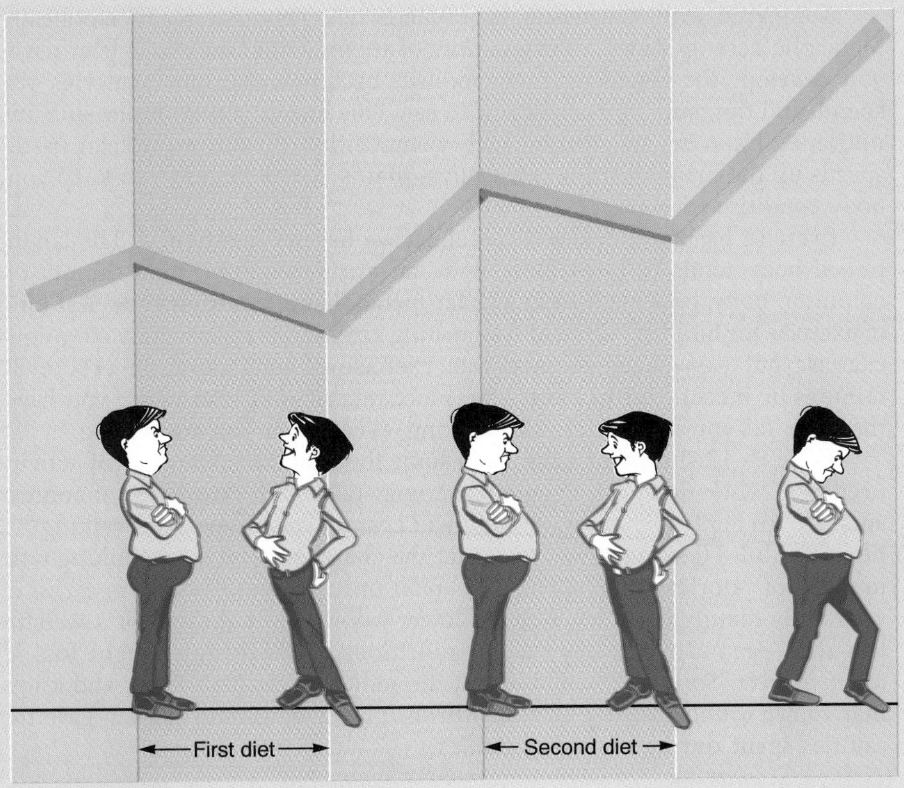

The yo-yo effect of dieting. This person dieted and lost weight, then zoomed up to a higher weight than before the diet. On dieting again, the person did not lose as much, and then zoomed up higher still.

tractive and requires more calories to maintain its muscle mass than a fatter body. In addition, each bout of exercise speeds up the metabolism temporarily, thereby causing the body to burn more calories than usual, even after the workout is finished. Exercise plays a vital role in boosting self-esteem as well, which can enhance the motivation to maintain a healthful lifestyle for the long run.

Exercise

Some people who want to lose weight hate the very idea of exercise. Obese people often—understandably—do not enjoy moving their bodies. They feel heavy, clumsy, even ridiculous. A word of reassurance: weight loss, at least to a point, is possible without exercise. Even if you choose not to alter your exercise habits at first, let your mind be open to the possibility that you will want to take up some kind of activity later on. As the pounds come off, moving your body becomes a pleasure.

The physical contributions exercise makes to a weight-control program are threefold: exercise increases one's energy expenditure, it alters body composition in a desirable direction, and it alters metabolism. It also offers the psychological benefits of looking and feeling healthy and the increased self-esteem that accompanies these benefits.

Compared with lean tissue, fat tissue is relatively inactive metabolically. Metabolic activity burns calories—lots of them. Thus, the more lean tissue you develop, the faster your metabolism becomes, the more calories you spend, and the more you can afford to eat. This brings you both pleasure and nutrients. Exercise, by shifting body composition toward more lean tissue, speeds up the metabolism *permanently*—that is, for as long as you keep your body conditioned.

Exercise has another beneficial effect we haven't mentioned. The conditioned body tends to burn more body fat during exercise than the out-of-condition body, because it has more fat-metabolizing enzymes. The best kind of exercise for building up your fat-burning enzymes is not severely strenuous exercise but easy-paced to moderate exercise of long duration (15 to 30 minutes or more). Furthermore, the more muscle and lean tissue you have, the more fat you will burn—all day long, even when you are resting.

Examples of easy-paced to moderate exercise:

Walking at about 3 mi/hr.

Bicycling on level ground at about 9 mi/hr.

You can tell it's moderate if you are breathing a little faster than normal but can still easily carry on a conversation.

Table 8–12 shows the calories in some foods and the amounts of activity needed to work them off. People sometimes take such charts out of context and say, "An apple and a glass of milk will cost me half an hour of walking . . . hmm, I think I'll skip eating." Don't let the chart fool you into thinking only in terms of calories. First, such charts refer only to calories eaten in *excess* of your daily maintenance level or the lower caloric level chosen for a weight-loss diet. Second, your body needs nutritious foods during weight loss as much as ever. So eat the apple, drink the milk, do your workout, and know that you've found the best of both worlds. (Table 8–8 on page 225 gave the calories spent during various activities.)

Table 8–12

Activity Cost of Eating Foods Beyond Calorie Need[a]

To Work Off the Calories from this Food Eaten beyond your Energy Need	You Have to Walk:	Or Jog:	Or Wait:
Cookie, chocolate chip (50 cal)	10 min	3 min	39 min
Ice cream, ⅔ c (200 cal)	38 min	11 min	2½ hr
T-bone steak, 8 oz (800 cal)	2½ hr	41 min	10¼ hr
Pizza, 1 slice (300 cal)	1 hr	15 min	3¾ hr
Beer or cola beverage, 12 oz (150 cal)	29 min	8 min	2 hr
Caramel candy, 1 oz, or potato chips, 10 (115 cal)	22 min	6 min	1½ hr
Chocolate-coated peanuts, 8 (160 cal)	31 min	8 min	2 hr

[a]For a 150-lb person, the energy cost of walking at 3.5 mph is 5.2 cal/min; of running is 19.4 cal/min; and of reclining is 1.3 cal/min.

The next chapter will give you many pointers about becoming fit, but a few notes on strategy are in order here. For one thing, you must keep in mind that if exercise is to help with weight loss, it must be active exercise—voluntary moving of muscles. Being moved passively, as by a machine at a health spa or by a massage, does not increase calorie expenditure. The more muscles you move, the more calories you spend.

Strategies for using exercise for weight control:

1. Make it active exercise; move muscles.
2. Think in terms of quantity, not speed.
3. Exercise informally, in daily routines.

People sometimes ask about spot reducing. Can you lose fat in particular locations? Unfortunately, muscles don't "own" the fat that surrounds them. Since all body fat is shared by all the muscles and organs, spot-reducing exercises that work only the flabby parts won't help reduce the fat located there. There is some good news, though: tightening muscles in trouble spots by way of a balanced, all-over exercise program will improve the appearance of the fatty areas.

Another thing to keep in mind is that the number of calories spent in an activity depends more upon how much a person weighs than on how fast the person can do the exercise. For example, a person who weighs 120 pounds burns off 83 calories by running a 6-minute mile. That same person, hiking a mile in 10 minutes, burns almost the same amount— 76 calories. Similarly, a 220-pound person spends 148 calories on the 6-minute mile and only a little less— 136 calories—on the 10-minute hike. The rule seems to be that you don't have to work fast to use up calories effectively. If you choose to walk the distance instead of run, you will use up about the same energy; it will just take you longer.

You may have heard the suggestion that you incorporate more exercise into your daily schedule in many simple, small-scale ways. Park the car at the far end of the parking lot; use the stairs instead of the elevator; do a round of sit-ups before you get up in the morning. These strategies don't add up to many calories each, but over a year's time they become significant. If you also incorporate regular aerobic exercise (see Chapter 9) into your schedule, your heart and lungs as well as your skeletal muscles will be fit.

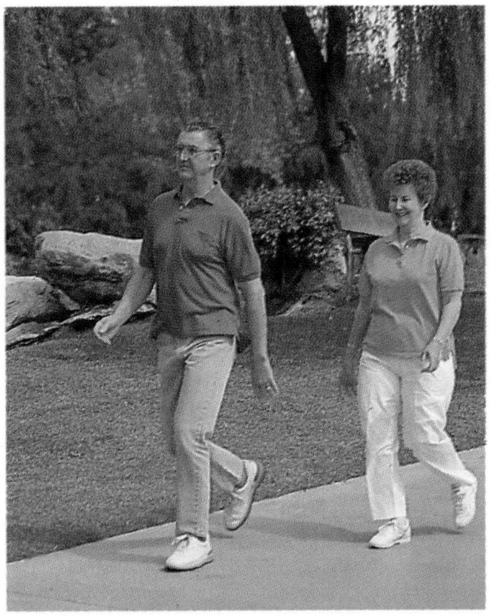

Exercise helps with weight control.

NUTRITION ACTION

Breaking Old Habits

Elements of Behavior Change

1. Awareness: "I could change."
2. Cognition: "I know how to change."
3. Emotion: "I want to change."
4. Decision: "I will change."
5. Action: "I **am** changing."

Behavior modification a process developed by psychologists for making lasting behavior changes.

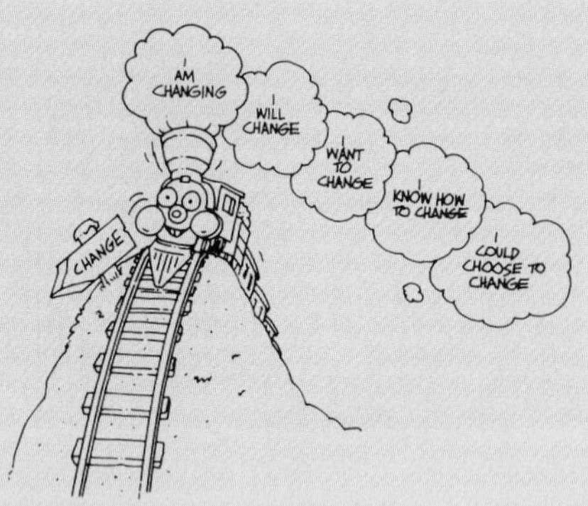

The elements of behavior change.

The makers of Nike sportswear urge, "Just do it," on billboards, in magazines, and wherever else they promote their products, implying that adhering to a fitness program is just a matter of donning sneakers and heading for the track or gym. But as anyone who has ever tried sticking to a regular exercise program for the first time or changing his or her eating habits knows, sometimes it's not that simple. Breaking old patterns of behavior and developing new ones involves going through a number of stages before reaching the point at which you're ready to change.

First, you must be aware that you could change. "I could lose some weight and try to become more physically fit," you might tell yourself. Then you must know how to change by, say, talking to a registered dietitian about strategies for cutting back on fat and calories in your diet and by reading about various forms of exercise. Next, you need a strong desire to start modifying your eating habits and begin exercising, which in turn will help motivate you to make a conscious decision to do so. Finally, after you've gone through those steps, you will be ready to take action—that is, "just do it."

Of course, even after you've gone through those steps, making lasting changes in behavior poses an ongoing challenge. That's where a process known as **behavior modification** can help. Developed by psychologists to help people change their habits, behavior modification uses techniques similar to mapping out a game plan.

To start, identify your goals. You might decide, for example, to try to lower the fat and calorie content of your diet. Once you've chosen your goals, record your present pattern of behavior along with the reasons behind it. Keep a food diary by writing down everything you eat for five days as well as how you feel at the time you eat (see Table 8–13 for a sample food diary). This technique can help you understand why you behave the way you do in certain situations. You might find, for instance, that every time you are angry at your significant other or get a bad grade you eat a candy bar or two to comfort yourself. Or perhaps without even thinking about it you nibble on whatever happens to be handy while watching television.

Once you've identified your goals and current patterns of behavior, determine some new strategies that will help you meet these goals and set yourself some rewards for sticking to them. If you talk to a friend instead of heading to the kitchen cupboard or vending machine when you're angry, for instance, you'll save hundreds of calories and probably feel the relief of getting your feelings off your chest. After you've pinpointed behaviors you want to alter, commit yourself to making the changes and try to envision the healthier, slimmer person you'll become as a result.

The next step is to divide the behavioral goals into small portions that can be achieved one at a time. While you may have come up with 20 behaviors that you want to change in order to meet your overall goals, trying to accomplish all 20 in a week or two is asking a great deal of yourself and may

Table 8–13

Sample Entries in Food Diary

Food Eaten	Time and Place	With Whom	Mood	Other Activity
1 large blueberry muffin 1 cup coffee with 1 oz cream and 1 tsp sugar	7:30 a.m., donut shop	alone	stressed—late for class	skimming notes for upcoming class
1 hot dog with 2 tbsp ketchup 1 small bag potato chips 12-oz can diet soda	12:45 p.m., cafeteria	2 friends	relaxed	talking with friends
1 candy bar	2:35 p.m., bedroom	alone	angry about argument with significant other	watching TV

be setting yourself up for disappointment and failure. Instead, pick one or two, see if you can stick to them for, say, two weeks, and then reward yourself for doing so before going on to try more.

As you meet your goals, remind yourself of the progress you're making as well as the benefits you're gaining—weight loss, increased energy, better health. Give yourself a tangible reward, such as a night out at the movies or a new item of clothing. This step is key, because behavior research indicates that once you have instituted a change in your life, you will maintain it only by positive reinforcement. Along with rewarding yourself, feel free to modify your goals if you think that those you initially set were too difficult or too simple to achieve, and evaluate your progress on a regular basis.

While you're working on modifying your behavior, it is critical to keep in mind that you're only human and there will be days when you slip and revert back to an old pattern of behavior. Instead of dwelling on it or berating yourself, learn to forgive yourself and simply get back on track. In addition, set priorities to ensure that there are one or two behaviors you make it a point to stick to all the time. Furthermore, be aware of how other areas of your life are affecting your readiness to make changes and meet your goals. Many people waste a great deal of time and energy trying to change when the timing isn't right for them. Someone who is going through the breakup of a long-term relationship or having difficulties at work or school, for example, may be under too much stress to deal with making a change in behavior on top of everything else. Realizing that you have limits and waiting until the timing is right can stave off additional frustration and guilt brought about by feeling like a failure if you aren't able to change.

Another point to keep in mind is that you might need to try new behaviors more than once before you begin to like them. Dietitians sometimes use a "rule of three" in counseling. Try nonfat milk once, and you may not like

Behavior Modification Steps

1. Identify the goal.
2. Record your present behavior pattern. Identify the reasons you practice these behaviors.
3. Identify the behaviors that will lead to the goal and the rewards of those behaviors.
4. Commit yourself to changing. Face what you'll have to give up or change to make the desired behavior a reality. Envision your changed future self.
5. Plan. Divide the behavior into manageable portions. Set small, achievable goals and plan periodic rewards.
6. Try out the plan. Modify the plan, if necessary, in ways that will help you succeed.
7. Evaluate your progress on a regular basis.

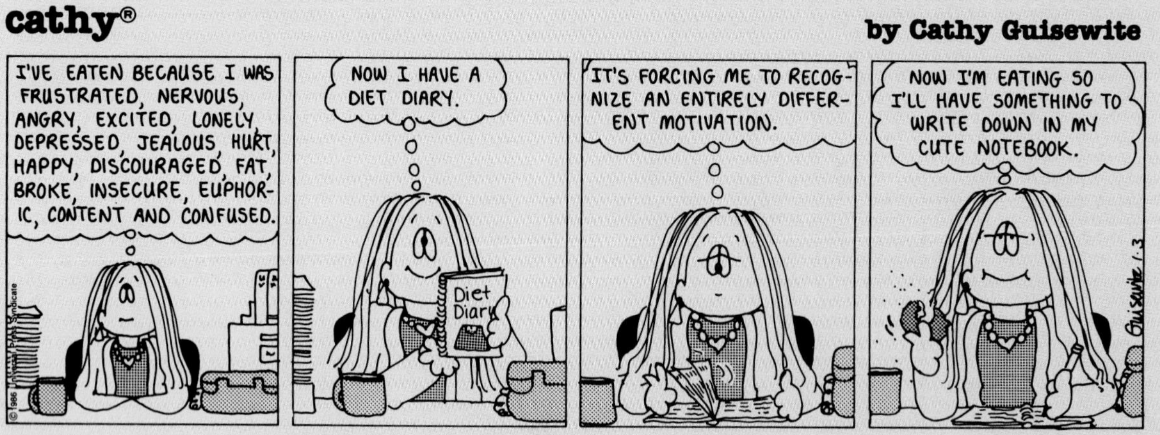
cathy®
by Cathy Guisewite
I'VE EATEN BECAUSE I WAS FRUSTRATED, NERVOUS, ANGRY, EXCITED, LONELY, DEPRESSED, JEALOUS, HURT, HAPPY, DISCOURAGED, FAT, BROKE, INSECURE, EUPHORIC, CONTENT AND CONFUSED.
NOW I HAVE A DIET DIARY.
Diet Diary
IT'S FORCING ME TO RECOGNIZE AN ENTIRELY DIFFERENT MOTIVATION.
NOW I'M EATING SO I'LL HAVE SOMETHING TO WRITE DOWN IN MY CUTE NOTEBOOK.

Continued Motivation

- Persist long enough to experience the rewards, such as improved self-image and enhanced self-esteem.
- Remember the price of the old behavior.
- Keep in mind where you started from.
- Tune in to the benefits of the new behavior.

it. Try it a second time, and you may be able to tolerate drinking it, even though it doesn't taste as good as whole milk. Try it a third time, and you may conclude that while it's not as good as whole milk, you don't really mind drinking it. Then you'll be able to maintain your new habit more easily.

Strategies for Changing the Way You Eat

This section covers the steps designed specifically to help with weight control. (Chapter 9 includes strategies for modifying exercise behavior.) To begin with, keep a record of your present eating behavior that you can compare with your future progress as well as use to determine situations that trigger your reaching for food. In this way you can see how far you've come in changing your eating habits.

Next, try to identify cues that prompt you to eat even when you're not hungry, such as watching television, talking on the telephone, and walking by a convenience store or vending machine. Then resolve to stop responding to those cues, and try to eat only in one place in a certain room, such as the table in the dining room. In addition, try these tips to eliminate the temptation to eat when you really don't want to:

- Don't buy hard-to-resist foods such as cakes, cookies, and ice cream.
- Don't shop when you're hungry and thereby are more likely to buy tempting foods.
- Let the people you live with buy, store, and serve their own sweet foods.
- Clear food from plates directly into the garbage. The calories and fat in a nibble here and a nibble there add up quickly.
- Create obstacles to eating tempting foods. Make it necessary to unwrap, cook, and serve each one separately, for example, or store it in a hard-to-reach cupboard or in the back of the refrigerator.
- Don't leave large amounts of food within easy reach. Keep serving dishes off the table, for instance, and put the cookie jar out of sight.
- Make small portions of food look large by spreading food out and putting it on smaller plates. Garnish empty space with low-calorie vegetables.
- Try to eat regular meals and snacks instead of skipping them, thereby reducing the likelihood of becoming uncomfortably hungry and then overeating later.

- Ask your family and friends to encourage you to eat a healthful diet and not to criticize you if you splurge occasionally.

Third, make it easy for yourself to eat the way you want to eat.

- Keep a variety of nutritious foods such as fruits and vegetables readily available.
- If you like to eat between meals, plan snacks that fit easily into your diet, such as low-fat yogurt and fruit.
- Prepare attractive meals for yourself.

Fourth, take a look at and then, if necessary, alter the manner in which you eat.

- If you eat quickly, slow down by chewing food thoroughly, pausing between bites, putting down your utensils, and swallowing before reloading your fork or spoon. Eating slowly will give your body a chance to feel full and satisfied.

Finally, reward yourself for positive behaviors.

- Plan to buy something new to wear or do something you enjoy, such as attending a favorite sporting event or a concert, each time you meet your goals.
- Ask your friends and family to support and encourage you as you change.

Weight-gain Strategies

It is as hard for a person who tends to be thin to gain a pound as it is for a person who tends to be fat to lose one. The person who wants to gain weight is faced with some of the same challenges as the one who wants to lose weight—learning new habits, learning to like new foods, and establishing discipline related to meals and mealtimes. But there are major differences.

Knowing that vigorous physical activity costs calories, an active person may wonder if it is advisable to curtail activity. The answer is no, not unless the underweight condition is so extreme as to be life-threatening. The healthful way to gain weight is to build yourself up by patient and consistent training and, at the same time, to eat enough calories (of nutritious foods) to support the weight gain. To gain a pound of muscle mass, you have to eat about 2,500 calories more than you expend (muscle is less calorically dense than fat, which requires 3,500 calories per pound). If you add a big snack of high-calorie, nutritious foods (for example, a bowl of chili and rice and a milkshake) between meals, you can eat 700 to 800 extra calories a day, thus achieving a healthful weight gain of 1 to 1½ pounds per week.

A person wanting to gain weight often has to learn to eat different foods. No matter how many helpings of boiled carrots you consume, you won't gain weight very fast, because carrots simply don't offer enough calories. The person who can't eat much volume is encouraged to consume nutritious, calorie-dense foods at meals (the very ones the dieter is trying to stay away from). Choose a milkshake instead of milk, peanut butter instead of lean meat, avocado instead of cucumber, whole-wheat muffin instead of whole-wheat bread. When you do eat carrots, put margarine on them; use creamy dressings on salads, yogurt on fruit, sour cream on potatoes, and the like. (Because fat contains twice as many calories per teaspoon as sugar, it adds calories without adding bulk.) These dietary recommendations may not apply to everyone trying to gain weight. If you have a history of heart disease, a diet low in saturated fat is recommended (consult your physician).

Eat more frequently. Make three sandwiches in the morning and eat them between classes in addition to the day's three regular meals. Spend more time eating each meal: if you fill up fast, eat the highest-calorie items first. Don't start with soup or salad; start with the main course. Always finish with dessert. Many an underweight person has simply been too busy (for months) to eat enough to gain or maintain weight. These strategies will help you change this behavior pattern.

Whether you need to gain, lose, or maintain weight, attention to what you eat can pay off in long-term wellness benefits. This chapter has emphasized the relationship of food and eating to body weight and has come to the same conclusion reached earlier in this book: to support wellness, you should eat regular, balanced meals composed of a wide variety of foods you enjoy.

Consumer Tips

Defensive Dining

Dining out can be a pleasant time to relax, socialize, and provide a break from your usual schedule, and it does not have to involve overindulgence in high-calorie, low-nutrient foods. With practice, you can maximize the benefits of eating out by adopting some of the following strategies.

- Make specific requests: "I'll have this sandwich with only half the cheese and just a teaspoon of mayonnaise served on the side."
- Ask for salad dressings, sauces, or gravies *on the side*. This puts you in control of the portions and cuts down on salt, fat, and calories.
- Request fresh fruit for dessert. It will give you the sweetness you want without the calories of fat and sugar.
- Order low-fat or nonfat milk instead of whole milk. This reduces your fat intake. If a restaurant doesn't have low-fat milk, your suggestions might make a difference.
- At fast-food windows, ask that they hold the sauce on your sandwich and give you extra tomato and lettuce or other vegetables instead.
- Order mineral water or club soda with a twist, alcoholic drinks with just the mix and not the alcohol (e.g. Bloody Marys without the vodka), or a wine spritzer. Remember, alcohol supplies empty calories.
- When ordering, inquire about preparation. Ask for entrees to be broiled, baked, grilled, poached, boiled, or roasted, with only a minimal amount of fat (or none at all).
- Cut down on overall portion sizes. Order à la carte: one or two nutritious low-fat appetizers along with a salad and bread, instead of a huge main meal. This will cut calories and offer you variety.
- Request a plain baked potato or one with cottage cheese and chives instead of butter and sour cream. Order your vegetables steamed or stir-fried without added butter or sauces. This, too, reduces the amount of fat you eat.
- Request a vegetable-based sauce for your pasta rather than the traditional meat sauces. This reduces fat and calories.
- Order a special omelet. Instead of the usual three-egg version, ask for one made with one egg plus extra egg whites with no salt, filled with plenty of vegetables. This will minimize your fat and salt intakes.
- Avoid the all-you-can-eat restaurants and those that specialize in fried foods. Overindulgence is easy at these places, and there aren't enough high-bulk, high-fiber foods on the menu.
- Finally, take time to enjoy your meal, along with the company and conversation. Eating slowly gives your body time to digest the food and feel satisfied.

Spotlight

Anorexia Nervosa and Bulimia

For an estimated 7 million American women, the relentless pursuit of thinness and the fear of being fat are a haunting nightmare that drives them to starve, vomit, or purge. The illness of anorexia nervosa—self-starvation—has been recognized as a psychiatric syndrome since the 1870s. Its companion disease bulimia—gorging on food and then purging—was not recognized as a separate eating disorder until the 1960s and 1970s. Some researchers suspect that a complex interplay between environmental, societal, and perhaps genetic factors triggers the disorder in victims, mostly women. Others question whether or not the fear of fatness isn't a mask for underlying emotional problems. Experts speculate that focusing on the body diverts these women's attention away from and suppresses the painful emotion of anger, feelings of low self-esteem, the inability to express their feelings, or poor family relationships.[26] The acute focus on the body develops into an intense fear of fatness, a characteristic intrinsically linked with food. As a result, food is seen only as a source of body fat and so becomes carefully controlled. But why food? Why not use some other method of coping with stress?

Enter the societal link. In a culture where thinness is equated with material success and self-worth, especially for women, becoming thin appears to be the yellow brick road that leads to happiness. Unfortunately, as victims of eating disorders come to learn, practicing self-starvation or gorging and purging leads, instead, to physical and emotional pain.

• What are the symptoms of anorexia nervosa?

Anorexics deprive themselves of food, except for controlled amounts of very-low-calorie foods such as unbuttered toast or popcorn, apples, and green beans. And even those foods are painstakingly limited. After three to four days of eating very small amounts of food, hunger pangs subside. Once their appetite is suppressed, anorexics report feeling quite energetic, as if on a high, making the strict fast easier to stick to. But the body needs fuel to run. To compensate for the lack of fuel from food, the body turns inward for its fuel and begins to slowly destroy muscle and fat tissue for energy.

The following are some of the physical symptoms associated with starvation seen in anorexics:

- Wasting of the whole body, including muscle tissue.
- Arresting of sexual development and cessation of menstruation.
- Drying and yellowing of the skin due to an accumulation of a stored vitamin A compound released from body fat.
- Growth of hair on the body, perhaps in response to a decrease in body temperature.
- Loss of health and texture of hair.
- Pain on touch.
- Lowered blood pressure and metabolic rate.
- Anemia.
- Severe sleep disturbance.[27]

Simultaneously, bizarre mental symptoms develop. Looking in the mirror, the anorexic does not see the emaciated body others see, but continues to see someone who is too fat. A preoccupation with death develops, accompanied by a frantic pursuit of physical fitness by means of stringent exercise routines. The person deals with parents and family in a manipulative way so as to become the center of attention. Diet becomes so all-engrossing that the person may be quite isolated socially except from friends who stick close by and worry without knowing how to help.

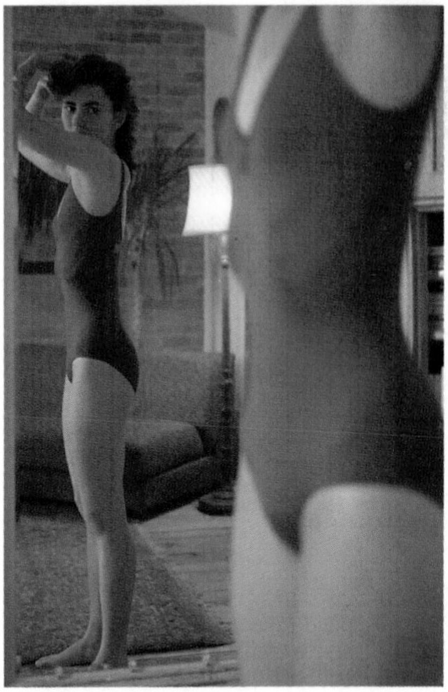

Anorexia nervosa.

By this time, the anorexic has reached absolute minimum body weight—for example, 65 to 70 pounds for a woman of average height. The person is on the verge of incurring permanent brain damage and chronic invalidism or death. The National Association of Anorexia Nervosa and Associated Disorders (ANAD) estimates that of those with severe eating disorders 6 percent die, usually because major organs—heart and kidneys—fail.

• What are the symptoms of bulimia?

Unlike anorexics, bulimics don't shrink to skeleton-like proportions. They usually are of ideal body weight or even slightly overweight. Bulimics also follow rigid rules of dietary restraint, but their rules are not as rigorous as the anorexics' starvation routines.

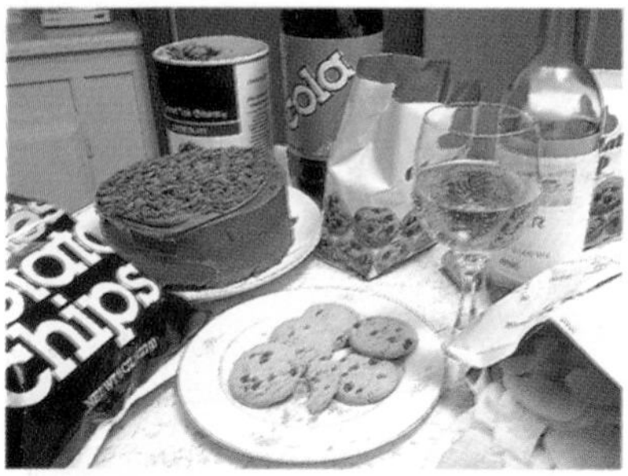

For many people with bulimia, guilt, depression, and self condemnation follow a binge-eating episode.

Occasionally, bulimics break their rigid rules. Quickly, and usually privately, they gorge on foods that are often sweet, starchy, high in fat or calories, and require little chewing. The binge ends when it would hurt to eat any more, when they are interrupted, or when they go to sleep or induce vomiting to expel the food just eaten.

Bulimics often feel controlled by the vicious cycle that develops: anxiety about being "fat" leads to rigid dietary restraint. Mounting hunger from not eating and an increased preoccupation with food leads to a break in the rules—binging. After gorging, an intense fear of fatness overtakes the person, who then vomits to get rid of the food and release the fear of becoming "fatter." Feelings of guilt and shame follow the purge, building a new level of anxiety over the body, and the cycle begins again. Each binge reinforces the idea that additional rigidity of dietary restraint is required to prevent weight gain. Excessive use of laxatives and diuretics or bouts of vigorous exercise replace vomiting in some cases.

Binge eating is seldom life-threatening, but at the extreme it can be physically damaging, causing lacerations of the stomach, irritation of the esophagus (in those who vomit frequently), dental caries (from acidic vomit attacking the teeth), and malnutrition (in vomiters and laxative takers). Bulimics also suffer from distorted body image. They see themselves as fat and needing to restrict food, even though they actually are of ideal body weight. Bulimics prefer a body size somewhat smaller than normal.

How are anorexia nervosa and bulimia treated?

There are several philosophies regarding the treatment of eating disorders. The four major approaches include individual psychotherapy, hospitalization, family therapy, and behavior modification therapy. Some therapists use more than one approach. Most treatment methods focus on identifying the societal and environmental pressures that triggered the eating disorder and on exposing the emotions masked by it. An interdisciplinary team made up of a psychologist, a social worker, a family therapy counselor, and a dietitian work with the family and the patient to reestablish emotional and nutritional health.[28] Length of treatment varies from two months to two to three years, depending on the patient's readiness for change and the type of treatment. American researcher Hilde Bruche, M.D., focuses on the problems of feelings of low self-esteem, guilt, anxiety, and depression and a sense of helplessness. In addition, family therapy focuses on changing patterns of family interaction.

Normal nutrition must be restored in the anorexic. In some cases, tube feeding directly into the stomach is used. In others, the person is expected to eat 2,000 to 2,500 calories per day. After some progress is made in counseling, the dietitian can help the patient gain a new understanding and

Table 8–14 Diagnosis of Eating Disorders

ANOREXIA NERVOSA	BULIMIA
a. Refusal to maintain body weight over a minimal normal weight for age and height (for example, weight loss leading to maintenance of body weight 15% below that expected); or failure to make expected weight gain during period of growth, leading to body weight 15% below that expected. b. Intense fear of gaining weight or becoming fat, even though underweight. c. Disturbance in the way in which one's body weight, size, or shape is experienced. The person claims to "feel fat" even when emaciated, believes that one area of the body is "too fat" even when obviously underweight. d. In females, absence of at least three consecutive menstrual cycles when otherwise expected to occur (primary or secondary amenorrhea). (A woman is considered to have amenorrhea if her periods occur only following administration of hormones, such as estrogen.)	a. Recurrent episodes of binge eating (rapid consumption of a large amount of food in a discrete period of time). b. A feeling of lack of control over eating behavior during the eating binges. c. The person regularly engages in either self-induced vomiting, use of laxatives or diuretics, strict dieting or fasting, or vigorous exercise to prevent weight gain. d. A minimum average of two binge eating episodes a week for at least 3 months. e. Persistent overconcern with body shape and weight.

Source: American Psychiatric Association, *Diagnostic and Statistical Manual of Mental Disorders,* 4th ed. (Washington, D.C. American Psychiatric Association, 1987), p. 67, with permission.

Miniglossary

Anorexia nervosa literally "nervous lack of appetite," a disorder (usually seen in teenage girls) involving self-starvation to the extreme.
an = without *orexis* = appetite

Bulimia, bulimarexia (byoo-LEE-me-uh, byoo-lee-ma-REX-ee-uh) binge eating (literally "eating like an ox"), known popularly as "pigging out." Combined with an intense fear of becoming fat and sometimes followed by self-induced vomiting or the taking of laxatives, this form of eating behavior has also been called the **binge-purge syndrome.**
buli = ox

clear up some earlier misconceptions about nutrition.

● Are there any early warning signs to watch for regarding eating disorders?

Families and friends can be alerted to several key symptoms of eating disorders (see Table 8–14). A diet often precedes the illness. Anorexics develop an exaggerated interest in food, but at the same time deny their hunger and stop eating. A distorted body image makes them feel fat, even as weight loss continues. The anorexic begins to have sleep problems, shows unusual devotion to schoolwork, and often undertakes a program of unrelenting exercise. Bulimics may binge and self-induce vomiting or use excessive amounts of laxatives. Reduced food intake usually causes sufficient weight loss to stop menstrual cycles in women. People with eating disorders were usually good children who did not indulge in rebellion. Not all anorexics and bulimics exhibit all symptoms. Early detection is vital.

For more information regarding anorexia and bulimia and a list of qualified professionals to treat these diseases, write to the National Association of Anorexia Nervosa and Associated Disorders, Box 7, Highland Park, IL 60035 or call (708) 831–3438. Please include one dollar to cover the cost of postage and handling. Other resources are listed in Appendix A.

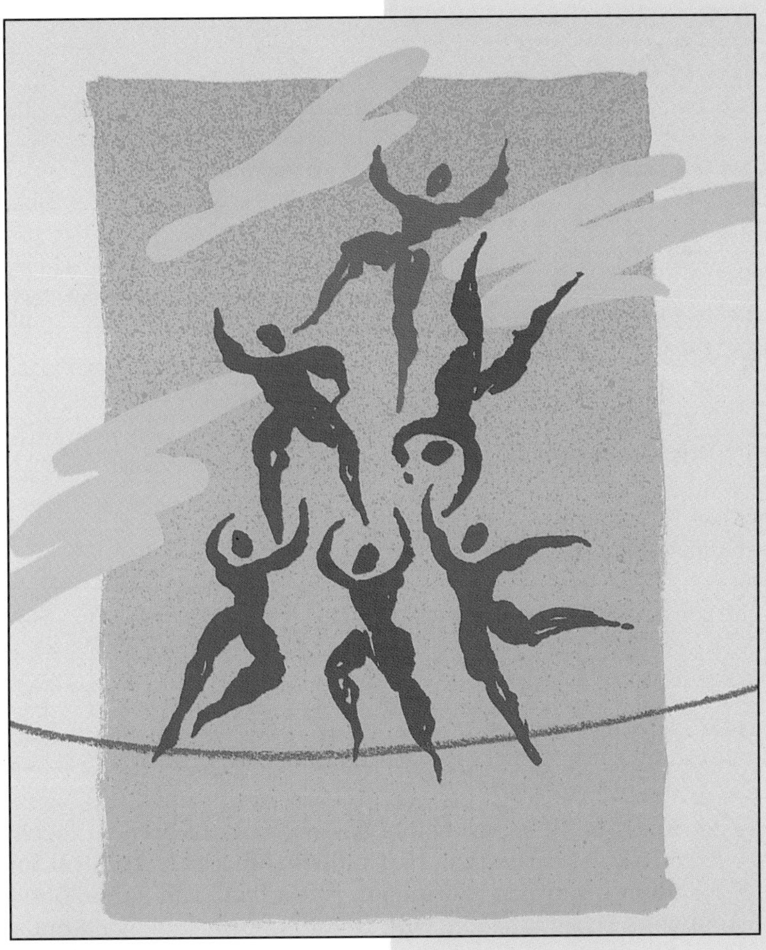

© Don Sibley

> *Get health. No labor, effort, nor exercise that can gain it must be grudged.*
>
> *—R. W. Emerson*

CHAPTER 9
Nutrition and Fitness

Contents

Ask Yourself . . . ?

Which of these statements about fitness are true, and which are false? For the false statements, what *is* true?

1. Regular exercise can help people increase their lean body mass and reduce their fat tissue.
2. Only about half of U.S. adults exercise regularly.
3. People who fail to exercise regularly are likely to fall prey to degenerative diseases such as heart disease, digestive disease, and diabetes.
4. Essentially, to be fit means to be at desirable weight and to have strong muscles.
5. People should never push themselves to exercise longer or harder than they can easily manage to do.
6. Of all the components of fitness, cardiovascular endurance has the most impact on health, disease resistance, and longevity.
7. If you run out of breath, it is a sign that your heart and lungs are not strong enough to perform the tasks you are demanding of them.
8. Active athletes can eat 60,000 calories a day and not gain weight.
9. In a muscular athlete who stops exercising, much of the muscle tissue turns to fat.
10. The use of steroid hormones can cause a disfiguring disease.

Answers: 1. True. 2. True. 3. True. 4. False. To be fit means not only to be at desirable weight and to have strong muscles, but to be flexible, and most importantly, to have muscular and cardiovascular endurance. 5. False. The overload principle states that people *should* push themselves to exercise longer or harder than they can easily manage to do—although not to the point of strain, of course. 6. True. 7. False. If you run out of breath, it is not a sign that your heart and lungs are weak, but that you are going into oxygen debt. 8. False. No one can eat 60,000 calories a day, but many football players can eat 6,000 calories a day and not gain weight. 9. False. Muscle tissue does not turn to fat, but in a muscular athlete who stops exercising, muscle tissue is lost and fat is gained. 10. True.

Fitness is in! Never before has our culture been so focused on fitness. Surveys estimate that 10.3 million Americans perform fitness walking, 8.1 million run or jog, 4.9 million ride a bike, and 2.6 million swim.[1] That's good news because people who are fit not only look good but also feel good. They can do the activities they must do and still have energy left over to do the things they want to do. In a general sense then, fitness is a state of physical well-being that lets you lead a higher quality of life.

In addition, mounting evidence suggests that our bodies need regular, moderate exercise that gets our hearts beating and forces our muscles to work harder than they usually do to stay healthy. Physiologically speaking, then, overall fitness is a balance between different body systems. With respect to the joints, flexibility is important. With respect to muscles, strength and endurance are important. Endurance is also important to the heart and lungs: this type of endurance is called cardiovascular endurance (discussed a little later in the chapter).

This chapter illustrates the effects of nutrition on fitness—and the reverse, for there is a two-way relationship. Optimal nutrition contributes to athletic performance; conversely, regular exercise contributes to a person's ability to use and store nutrients optimally. The two together are indispensable to a high quality of life; **fitness**, like good nutrition, is an essential component of good health.

Fitness the body's ability to meet physical demands, composed of four components: flexibility, strength, muscle endurance, and cardiovascular endurance.

Reasons to Exercise

The benefits of regular exercise make up an impressive list, which is growing longer as new discoveries are made.[2] Through regular exercise, people can gain energy and confidence, increase their lean body tissue, reduce their body fat, improve the health of their skin and their muscle tone, improve their sleeping habits, reduce their risk of heart disease,[3] reduce their blood cholesterol levels, reduce their blood pressure, build bones that remain strong into old age, and live a more enjoyable, perhaps even longer, life.[4]

No one can promise that you will receive all of these benefits if you exercise, but almost everyone who exercises reaps at least some of them. Despite evidence of the benefits, only about half of U.S. adults exercise regularly. Perhaps this is because exercise requires some time—at least 20 to 30 minutes every other day just to maintain a strong, healthy heart. Sometimes it is inconvenient and hard to get started. But once an exercise routine is established, the felt benefits far outweigh the inconveniences. People may begin a fitness program to trim fat or add muscle, but soon they are pleasantly surprised to find that they have more energy, feel less tense, sleep better, and feel healthier, and so they keep it up.

People can get in the habit of doing things that are good for them, just as they can get hooked on alcohol and other drugs, including nicotine and caffeine. You can cultivate the habit of engaging in regular physical activity if you:

Choose an activity that you can do without a great deal of mental effort.

Choose an activity that doesn't depend on other people's presence—that is, one you can do alone when a partner is not available.

Believe it has physical, mental, or spiritual value for you.

Enjoy the activity or some aspect of it (even just enjoying the knowledge that you do it).

Can experience progress through doing it.

Can do the activity without criticizing yourself.[5]

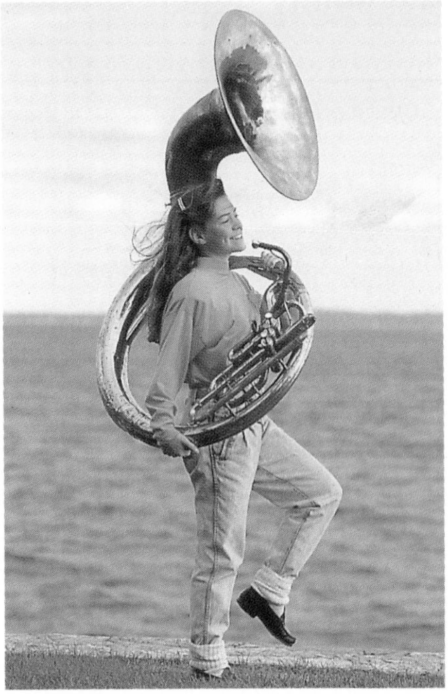

Being fit is more than being free of disease; it is feeling full of vitality and enthusiasm for life.

There is no RDA for exercise, although there probably should be. The notion that a certain minimum daily average amount of exercise is indispensable to health is just now reaching public consciousness. A consequence of not exercising is accelerated development of diseases associated with sedentary life—heart disease, intestinal disorders, and others. Researchers are still searching to find an optimum fitness level and have yet to discover how little exercise is too little and how much might be too much. The minimum amount needed for cardiovascular endurance is thought to be 20 minutes of exercise, at least three times each week, that raises the heart rate. Some state that if you expend 3,500 calories a week in any form of exercise, the heart will benefit. (Refer to Table 8–8 in Chapter 8 for the amount of energy expended during various types of exercise.)

Fitness is not restricted to the seasoned athlete. With a basic understanding of the concept of total fitness and a personal commitment to a physically active lifestyle, anyone can become fit. To be fit, you don't have to be able to finish the local marathon, nor do you have to develop the muscles of a Mr. Universe or Miss Olympia. Rather, what you need is a healthful weight (refer to Chapter 8) and enough flexibility, muscular strength, and endurance to meet the everyday demands life places on you, plus some to spare.

Physical Conditioning

It seems obvious that people's bodies are shaped by what they do, but this fact is often overlooked. Physical conditioning refers to a planned program of

Overload an extra physical demand placed on the body. A principle of training is that for a body system to improve, its workload must be increased by increments over time.

Hypertropy an increase in size in response to use.

Atrophy a decrease in size in response to disuse.

Frequency number of occurrences per unit of time (for example, the number of exercise sessions per week).

Intensity degree (for example, the degree of exertion while exercising).

Duration length of time (for example, the length of time spent in each exercise session).

Strength the ability of muscles to work against resistance.

exercise directed toward improving the function of a particular body system. Placing regular, physical demand on the body and forcing the body to do more than it usually does will cause it to adapt and function more efficiently. This is called **overload.** Muscles respond to the overload of exercise by gaining strength and ability to endure. Strength gains may not be visible in all cases. But in some, such as with male bodybuilders, muscles increase in strength and size, a response called **hypertrophy.** The converse is also true: muscles, if not called on to perform, decrease in size, a response called **atrophy.** For example, an arm that is in a cast for six weeks will gradually become smaller in size because the arm muscles are not being used.

Thus, runners often have well-developed, strong legs; a tennis player may have one arm that is stronger than the other. Swimmers usually develop in a balanced way—all limbs, chest, back, and so forth, are called on to perform and so develop uniformly. This doesn't mean that everyone should give up tennis and running for swimming; it only means that a variety of exercises will produce the most uniform overall fitness. This is why people are told to use different muscle groups in their exercise from day to day.

The overload principle applies equally to all aspects of fitness: flexibility, muscle strength, muscle endurance, and cardiovascular endurance. It also applies to the skeleton. To develop a strong, dense skeletal system, you must start by demanding that the bones bear slightly more stress (through weight-bearing exercises such as walking, running, weightlifting, or aerobic dance) than they are used to. The bones respond by depositing more minerals. Eventually, a maximum is reached. People can develop their fitness to an amazing extent by progressively increasing overload.

You can apply overload in several ways. You can do the activity more often—that is, increase its **frequency**; you can do the activity more strenuously—that is, increase its **intensity**; or you can do it for longer periods of time—that is, increase its **duration.** All three strategies work well, and you can pick one or a combination, depending on your fitness goals.

The Four Components of Fitness

Strength

Strength is the ability of the muscles to work against resistance: pulling yourself up and out of a swimming pool, carrying a backpack full of large books, or opening a jar of pickles. The purpose of strength training is to build well-toned muscles that let you accomplish daily activities at work and during recreation as well as to prevent injury. As muscles get stronger, individual fibers thicken and enlarge. The connective tissues making up muscles, tendons, and ligaments also strengthen and become more efficient at using energy. Strong muscles, tendons, and ligaments play a key role in preventing injury. For example, strong quadriceps—muscles on the front of the thigh—stabilize your knee as you bike. Strong calf muscles and ankle ligaments decrease the risk of an ankle sprain when walking briskly or jogging.

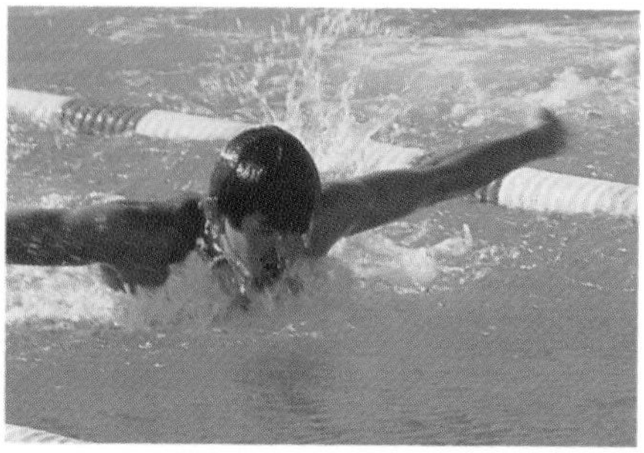

People's bodies are shaped by what they do.

Many of today's mechanical helpers invented to spare effort rob us of the opportunity to develop strength—for example, the strength we would gain from chopping firewood instead of turning up a thermostat. Today, we must put forth conscious effort to develop strength. The kind of equipment you can

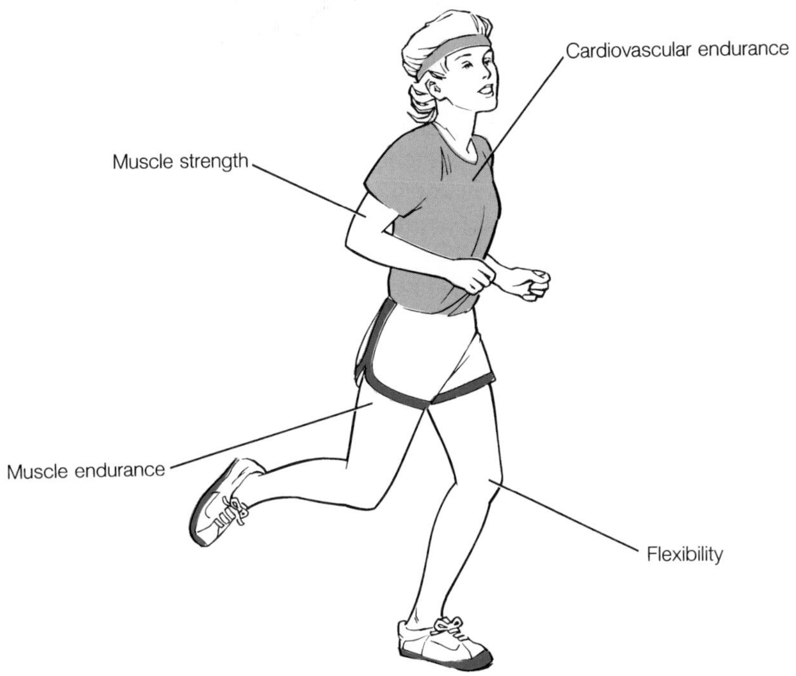

Components of fitness

use is largely a matter of availability and personal preference. If you belong to a health club, you probably have access to weight-training equipment. If not, you can use equipment you have at home, from plastic gallon jugs filled with water or sand to large rubber bands designed for strength training. No matter what method you choose, safety in strength training is essential. Get proper instruction. Before you set up a strength-training program, consult an exercise physiologist or physical therapist or enroll in a college class. Trying to set up your own program is an open invitation to injury.

Because many women mistakenly think they will develop enlarged muscles, which they view as undesirable and unattractive, they don't participate in strength-training programs. Testosterone—a male hormone—is responsible for muscle overdevelopment. Women only have 10 percent of the amount of testosterone that men do. Because of their lower testosterone levels, it is unlikely that women would develop bulging or overdeveloped muscles as a result of three weekly sessions of weight training. What will occur, though, is improved muscle strength, shape, and tone.[6]

A final note: Only muscle can be shaped and toned; skin and fat can't. Even with regular strength training, "flabby" regions may not look toned until the fat is reduced. Aerobic exercise (explained in another section) is the best way to burn excess body fat.

Flexibility

Keeping your muscles and joints pliable is critical for developing a fit body. A flexible body can move as it was designed to move and will bend rather than tear or break in response to sudden stress. **Flexibility** (range of motion)

Components of fitness:
- Flexibility
- Muscle strength
- Muscle endurance
- Cardiovascular endurance

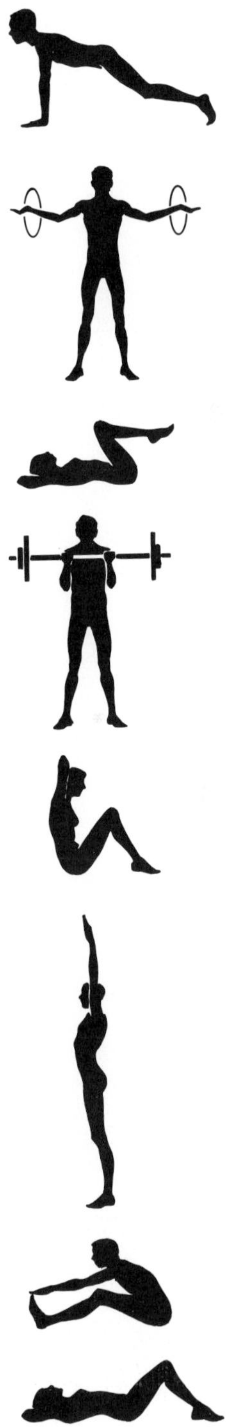

Flexibility and strength.

Flexibility the ability to bend or extend without injury; it depends on the elasticity of the muscles, tendons, and ligaments and on the condition of the joints.

Static stretches stretches that lengthen tissues without injury; characterized by long-lasting, painless, pleasurable stretches.

Ballistic stretches stretches characterized by short, choppy, sometimes painful movements, which often pull connective tissues beyond their elastic limits.

depends upon the condition and interrelationships between bones, ligaments, muscles, and tendons.

Stretching exercises improve flexibility by increasing muscle and tendon elasticity and length. Stretching should be done slowly—called **static stretches.** When you feel a slight strain in the muscle, hold the position for 10 to 30 seconds. Bouncy, rapid stretches—known as **ballistic stretches**—can cause minute tears in the muscle and also set up a reaction in the muscle that makes it resist the stretch. Avoid painful stretches. They are clearly excessive.

Flexibility tends to decrease as you age but improves in response to stretching, and it can be maintained in most people by doing frequent stretching exercises. While regular exercise will increase muscle tone and strength, it can also make muscles stiffer—making them more prone to strain and injury. For example, jogging and dancing can reduce flexibility of the lower back, front of thighs, and calves. Joggers and dancers should emphasize flexibility exercises for these areas. When beginning an exercise program, stretching is especially critical for previously sedentary people whose muscles are short and tight.

Stretching routines are commonly done as part of a warm-up before exercise. Low-intensity preliminary exercise allows your heart—also a muscle—to slowly accelerate and make adjustments in blood flow and oxygen supply, preparing for the work it is about to perform. Using calisthenics as a warm-up in addition to walking, marching in place, or doing some other moderate rhythmic activity prepares your heart muscle for action. After your light warm-up, stretch the muscles that will be used in the activity. Waiting to stretch until after your warm-up allows blood to move into the muscles, making them easier to stretch. Doing stretches after your exercise session gives your heart a chance to gradually slow its pace. It also allows you to lengthen those muscles that have become tight and tense because of the exercise. You can make greater gains in flexibility by stretching after your workout because muscles are warm and easier to stretch.

Muscle Endurance

Endurance the ability to sustain an effort for a long time. One type, **muscle endurance,** is the ability of a muscle to contract repeatedly within a given time without becoming exhausted. Another type, **cardiovascular endurance,** is the ability of the cardiovascular system to sustain effort over a period of time.

Muscle endurance, the third component of fitness, is the power of a muscle to keep on going for long periods. Your muscle endurance influences your performance in the last set of a tennis match, your swing on the 18th hole of a golf game, or your ability to pedal during the last 10 miles of a 100-mile bike tour. Endurance of certain muscles can be tested by the number of situps or pushups you can accomplish in a certain period of time. But remember, these tests evaluate only the abdominal and upper-arm muscles.

Cardiovascular Endurance

Another realm in which endurance is important is the length of time that you can keep going with an elevated heart rate—that is, how long your heart can endure a given demand. This kind of endurance is **cardiovascular endurance.** The heart is a muscle, and it, like your other muscles, can respond to repeated demands by becoming larger and stronger.

Exercises that promote cardiovascular endurance are the best for making short-term fitness gains and long-term health improvements as well as for weight control. The best exercises to develop cardiovascular endurance are those that repetitively use large muscle groups—arms and legs—and that last for a continuous 20 to 30 minutes. Examples include brisk walking, aerobic dance, running, cycling, cross-country skiing, and rowing. Playing such sports as basketball, soccer, downhill skiing, and volleyball adds fun to your exercise routine. Done alone, sports are not good enough to achieve cardiovascular conditioning. Frequent starts and stops and standing around cause benefits to decline quickly. The American College of Sports Medicine recommends that people participate in cardiovascular conditioning activities at least three times a week for a continuous 20 to 30 minutes.[7]

To develop cardiovascular fitness, choose an activity that:

- Is steady and constant.
- Uses large muscle groups, such as the arms, legs, and buttocks. If you move 50 percent of your muscle mass, the activity is aerobic.
- Is uninterrupted, lasts for more than 20 minutes, and is done at least 3 times per week.

Getting Started on Lifetime Fitness

For total fitness, an exercise program that incorporates strength training, stretching, and cardiovascular endurance activity is best. If you are just beginning a fitness program, though, it makes sense to begin with cardiovascular endurance, which is the most basic of all components to health and long life. Cardiovascular fitness is discussed in a separate section of this chapter. You can get an indirect estimate of your current fitness level by answering the questions in the Physical Activity Scorecard on page 248.

The more active you are, the more fit you are likely to be. Tests that measure your ability to perform various physical activities reveal more about your fitness level, and if you were to have an **exercise stress test** or other such measurement taken by a professional, you would obtain an accurate estimate of your fitness.

Exercise stress test a test that monitors heart function during exercise to detect abnormalities that may not show up under ordinary conditions; exercise physiologists and trained physicians or health care professionals can administer the test.

In proceeding with a fitness program, it is important to keep your own goals in mind; they carry you through periods of discouragement and help you choose the activities that best meet your needs. Keep in mind that fitness builds slowly, and so activity should increase gradually. Don't rush things by taking on too much, too soon. View your exercise time as a lifelong commitment.

A few cautions on getting started: If you are an apparently healthy male older than 40 years of age or an apparently healthy woman older than 50 years of age, the American College of Sports Medicine recommends that you have a medical examination and diagnostic exercise test before you start a *vigorous* exercise program. Beginning a *moderate* program, such as walking, however, would not require a physician's exam.[8]

For most people, physical activity should not pose any problem or hazard. The Physical Activity Readiness Questionnaire was designed to identify the small number of adults for whom physical activity might be inappropriate or those who should have medical advice concerning a suitable type of activity.[9] If you answer yes to any of the following questions, seek advice from a health care provider before you begin a *vigorous* exercise program:

1. Has your doctor ever said you have heart trouble?
2. Do you frequently suffer from pains in your chest?
3. Do you often feel faint or have spells of dizziness?
4. Has a doctor ever said your blood pressure was too high?
5. Has a doctor ever told you that you have a bone or joint problem, such as arthritis, that might be made worse with exercise?
6. Is there a good physical reason not mentioned here why you should not follow an activity program even if you wanted to?
7. Are you over age 65 and not accustomed to vigorous exercise?

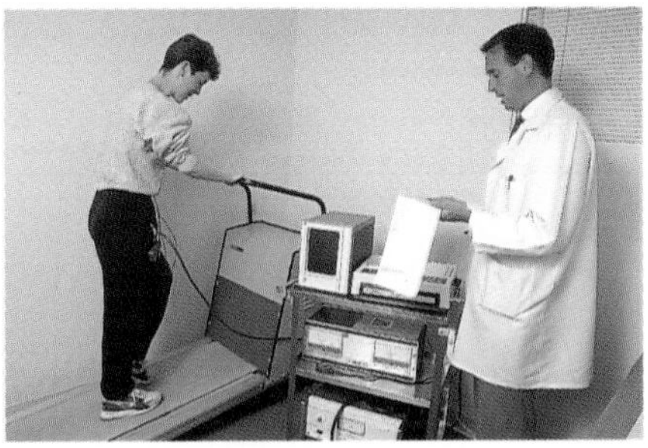

The exercise stress test measures heart function during exercise.

Physical Activity Scorecard

How physically active are you? For each question answered yes, give yourself the number of points indicated. Then total your points to determine your score.

Occupation and Daily Activities

1. I usually walk to and from class, work, or shopping (at least ½ mile each way). 1 point
2. I usually take the stairs rather than use elevators or escalators. 1 point
3. The type of physical activity involved in my job or daily household routine is best described by the following statement (select one):
   a. Most of my day is spent in office work, light physical activity, or household chores. 0 points
   b. Most of my workday is spent in farm activities, moderate physical activity, brisk walking, or comparable activities. 4 points
   c. My typical workday includes several hours of heavy physical activity (shoveling, lifting, etc.). 9 points

Leisure Activities

4. I do several hours of gardening or lawn work each week. 1 point
5. I fish or hunt once a week or more on the average. (Fishing must involve active work, such as rowing a boat. Dock sitting doesn't count.) 1 point
6. At least once a week, I do an hour or more of vigorous dancing, such as square or folk dancing. 1 point
7. In season, I play golf at least once a week, and I do not use a power cart. 2 points
8. I often walk for exercise or recreation. 1 point
9. When I feel bothered by pressures at school, work, or home, I use exercise as a way to relax. 1 point
10. Two or more times a week, I perform calisthenic exercises (situps, pushups) for at least 10 minutes. 3 points
11. I regularly participate in yoga or perform stretching exercises. 2 points
12. I participate in active recreational sports such as tennis or handball:
    a. About once a week. 2 points
    b. About twice a week. 4 points
    c. Three times a week or more. 7 points
13. At least once a week, I participate in vigorous fitness activities like jogging or swimming (at least 20 continuous minutes per session):
    a. About once a week. 3 points
    b. About twice a week. 5 points
    c. Three times a week or more. 10 points

Total points earned:_______

Scoring: 0 to 5 points—inactive. This amount of exercise leads to a steady deterioration in fitness. Improvement needed.
6 to 11 points—moderately active. This amount slows fitness loss but will not maintain adequate fitness in most persons.
12 to 20 points—active. This amount will maintain an acceptable level of physical fitness.
21 points or over—very active. This amount of activity will maintain a high state of physical fitness.

Source: Adapted with permission of Russell Pate (University of South Carolina, Human Performance Laboratory).

Energy for Exercise

Your body runs on water, oxygen, and food—primarily carbohydrate and fat. The chemical reactions that use these substances to make energy are called metabolism. Your body has two interrelated energy-producing systems—one dependent on oxygen—**aerobic** metabolism—and the other able to function without oxygen—**anaerobic** metabolism. An understanding of how the two systems work is important, because it explains why you choose certain exercises over others to strengthen your heart, why you eat what you do, and what factors influence your performance during sporting events.

Aerobic requiring oxygen.
Anaerobic not requiring oxygen.

Aerobic and Anaerobic Metabolism

At rest, your muscles burn mostly fat and some carbohydrate for energy. During exercise, though, the amounts the muscles use depend on an interplay between fuel availability and oxygen availability. To an exercising muscle, oxygen is everything. With ample oxygen, muscles can extract all available energy from carbohydrate and fat by means of aerobic metabolism. During moderate exercise, your lungs and circulatory system have no trouble keeping up with the muscles' need for oxygen. You breathe deeply and easily, and your heart beats steadily—the exercise is aerobic. But the heart and lungs can supply only so much oxygen so fast.

When the muscles' exertion is great enough that their energy demand outstrips their oxygen supply, they must also rely on anaerobic metabolism to make energy. The anaerobic metabolic pathway can burn only carbohydrate for fuel, and so it draws heavily on your limited body stores of carbohydrate. Nevertheless, this system does provide an immediate source of energy without relying on oxygen. Because of this system, you can dash out of the way of an oncoming car or sprint ahead of your competitor at the finish line. Unfortunately, this energy-yielding system is extremely inefficient. Only 5 percent of carbohydrate's energy-producing potential is harnessed by this pathway.[10]

Because the anaerobic metabolic pathway only partially burns your carbohydrate, it litters your muscles with partly broken down portions of glucose. You may have heard the name for these partly broken down products: lactic acid. The buildup of lactic acid causes burning pain in the muscles and can lead to muscle exhaustion within seconds if it is not drained away. A strategy for dealing with lactic acid buildup is to relax the muscles at every opportunity so that the circulating blood can carry it away and bring oxygen to support aerobic metabolism. Fortunately, lactic acid is not a waste product. When oxygen reaches your muscles, lactic acid is ushered to your liver, which converts it back to glucose.

Neither the aerobic nor the anaerobic metabolic pathways functions exclusively to supply energy to your body. The two work together, complementing and supporting each other. Keep in mind, however, that carbohydrate is absolutely essential for exercise. Without it, your muscles can't perform. You want to exercise aerobically because muscles burn fat and extract energy from carbohydrate more efficiently in the presence of oxygen, thereby conserving your body's limited store of carbohydrate. Thus, you want to exercise at an intensity that allows your heart and lungs to keep pace with your working muscles' oxygen needs.

Aerobic Exercise

Aerobic dancing	Rowing
Bicycling	Running
Cross-country skiing	Speed skating
Fast walking	Stair climbing
Jogging	Swimming
Rope jumping	

Sports

Sports add fun to your exercise routine, but because of frequent starts and stops, they don't allow for a continuous 20-minute bout of aerobic exercise. Aerobic training, however, will help you perform these sports:

Baseball	Racquetball
Basketball	Soccer
Fencing	Squash
Golf	Tennis
Ice hockey	Volleyball
Lacrosse	Weightlifting

Aerobic Exercise—Exercise for the Heart

To meet your body's increased oxygen needs during aerobic exercise, your heart must pump oxygen-rich blood to muscles at a faster pace than normal. This increased demand on the heart makes the heart stronger and increases its endurance. In addition, aerobic exercise improves the endurance of the lungs and the muscles along the arteries and in the walls of the digestive tract and, of course, the muscles directly involved in the activity. These all-over improvements are called **cardiovascular conditioning** or the **training effect.** In cardiovascular conditioning, the total blood volume increases, so the blood can carry more oxygen. The heart muscle becomes stronger and larger. Each beat of the heart pumps more blood, so it needs to pump less often. The muscles that work the lungs gain strength and endurance, and breathing becomes more efficient. Circulation through the body's arteries and veins

Cardiovascular conditioning or **training effect** the effect of regular exercise on the cardiovascular system—including improvements in heart, lung, and muscle function and increased blood volume.

Figure 9–1

Delivery of Oxygen by the Heart and Lungs to the Muscles

The more fit a muscle is, the more oxygen it draws from the blood. That oxygen has to be drawn from the lungs, so the person with more fit muscles extracts from the inhaled air more oxygen than a person with less fit muscles. Researchers can measure cardiovascular fitness by measuring the amount of oxygen a person consumes per minute while working out, a measure called the VO_2 *max.*

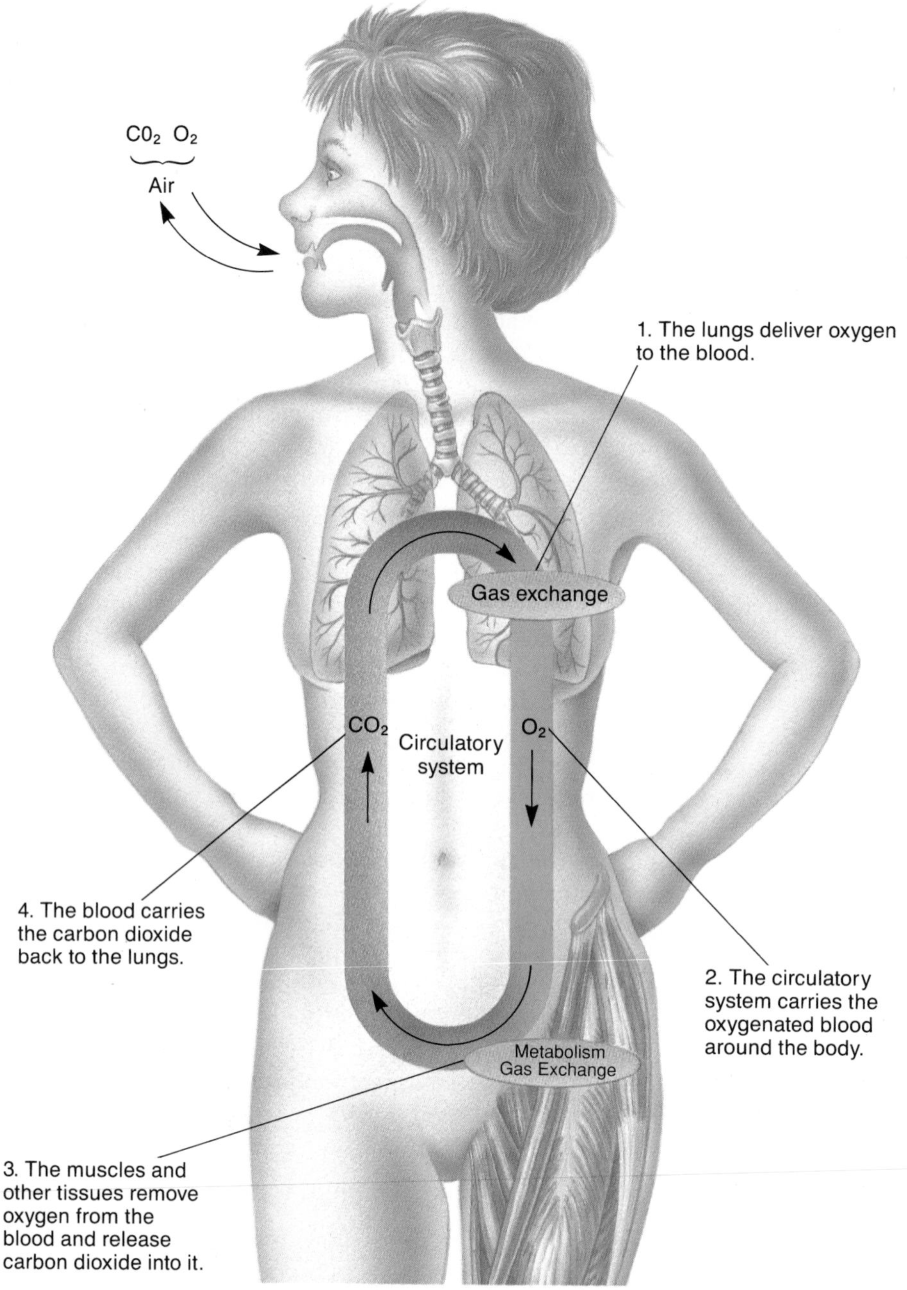

CO2 O2
Air
1. The lungs deliver oxygen to the blood.
Gas exchange
CO2
Circulatory system
O2
4. The blood carries the carbon dioxide back to the lungs.
2. The circulatory system carries the oxygenated blood around the body.
Metabolism Gas Exchange
3. The muscles and other tissues remove oxygen from the blood and release carbon dioxide into it.

improves. Blood moves easily, and the blood pressure falls. Muscles throughout the body become firmer. Figure 9–1 shows the major relationships among the heart, circulatory system, and lungs.

To make these gains in cardiovascular conditioning, you must work up to a point where you can continuously exercise aerobically for 20 minutes or more. This means you must elevate your heart rate (pulse). This heart rate—called your **target heart rate**—must be considerably faster than the resting rate to push (overload) the heart, but not so fast as to strain it.

An informal pulse check can give you some indication of how conditioned your heart is to start with. As a rule of thumb, the average resting pulse

Target heart rate the heartbeat rate that will achieve a cardiovascular conditioning effect for a given person—fast enough to push the heart, but not so fast as to strain it.

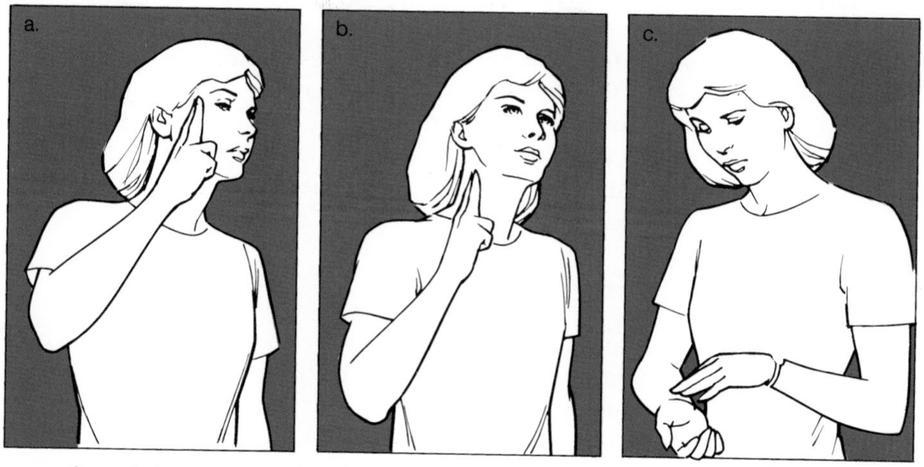

Figure 9–2

How to Take Your Pulse

Use a watch or a clock with a second hand. Rest a few minutes for a resting pulse; for an exercising pulse, take the reading immediately after stopping the workout. Convenient places to feel the pulsations of your heartbeat are (a) the temporal arteries, (b) the carotid arteries, next to your trachea (windpipe), and (c) the radial artery (on the thumb side of the wrist). Start counting your pulse at a convenient second and continue counting for 10 seconds. Multiply by 6 to obtain your heart rate per minute. To ensure a true count:

- Use only fingers, not your thumb, on the pulse point (the thumb has a pulse of its own).
- Press just firmly enough to feel the pulse. Too much pressure can interfere with the pulse rhythm.

rate for adults is around 70 beats per minute, but the rate can be higher or lower. Active people can have resting pulse rates of 50 or even lower. Figure 9–2 gives instructions for taking your pulse.

For cardiovascular conditioning, your target heart rate can be calculated from your age. The older you are, the lower your maximum heart rate. As your heart gets stronger, more intense exercise will be required to reach the same target rate. For example, at first, walking at a pace of 3 miles per hour may cause you to reach your target heart rate. After 6 to 8 weeks of walking at this pace, you may notice you no longer reach your target heart rate. That's because your heart is stronger. It now needs more of a challenge to beat faster. Increasing the intensity of your workout by walking faster can provide this challenge. To calculate your target heart rate range:

1. *Find your resting heart rate.* Take your pulse as shown and described in Figure 9–2.
2. *Estimate your maximum heart rate.* Subtract your age from 220. This provides an estimate of the absolute maximum heart rate possible for a person your age. You should never exercise at this rate, of course.
3. *Determine your target heart rate range.* Subtract your resting heart rate from your maximum heart rate, multiply this figure by 60 percent and 85 percent to find your upper and lower limits, and add these numbers to your resting heart rate.

Example: Ray Oliver, age 35

Resting heart rate:
65 beats per minute

Maximum heart rate:
220 − 35 = 185

Difference: 185 − 65 = 120

60% of difference: 0.60 × 120 = 72

Lower limit of target heart rate range:
72 + 65 = 137

85% of difference: 0.85 × 120 = 102

Upper limit of target heart rate range:
102 + 65 = 167

Target heart rate range: 137 to 167 beats per minute. Therefore, when Ray exercises aerobically, his heart should beat at least as fast as 137 beats per minute but no faster than 167 beats per minute.

When you can work out at your target heart rate for 20 to 30 minutes, you know that you have arrived at your cardiovascular fitness goal. In the building-up stage, a pattern used to make progress is called **fartlek** training. To use it, a jogger might run at the target heart rate for 2 minutes before tiring, then rest by walking until ready to jog again, run another 2 minutes, then rest by walking, and so on for 20 minutes. At each session, the jogger can make the running periods longer and the resting periods shorter. Eventually, in about 2 months or so, the rest periods will no longer be needed at all. Once you have worked up to that, you can maintain your level of fitness by repeating the workout about every other day. The American College of Sports Medicine recommends that to maintain your cardiovascular endurance, you should exercise within your target heart rate range at least three times a week for 20 to 60 minutes. Activities of lower intensity should be performed for longer periods of time.

Fartlek speed play; alternating periods of fast and slow exercise.

Nutrition and Exercise

The person interested in fitness is necessarily interested not only in exercise but also in nutrition, for the two support each other. The following sections discuss each aspect of nutrition: fuels (carbohydrate and fat), protein needs, energy needs and weight control, fluid needs (the most important aspect of nutrition and exercise), and vitamin and mineral needs.

Fuels for Exercise

Most of what we know about fuel use during exercise comes from research on athletes, but you do not have to be an athlete to make use of it. As mentioned before, your energy-producing pathways require oxygen and the two muscle fuels: glucose and fatty acids. As Figure 9–1 showed, the oxygen comes from the lungs, which pass it to the blood, which carries it to the muscles. Your muscles, and to some extent your liver, supply carbohydrate to your muscles from their carbohydrate supply (see Figure 9–3). The fatty acids come mostly from fat inside the muscles, but partly from fat that is released from the body's fat stores, and the blood delivers these fatty acids to the muscles.

Exercise and Glucose

Glucose comes from carbohydrate-rich foods—breads and grains, pasta, rice, fruits, vegetables, milk, and yogurt. Your body stores glucose in your liver and muscles as glycogen, which is a long chain of glucose molecules linked together.

During exercise, the body supplies glucose to the muscles from the stores of glycogen in the muscles themselves. Interestingly, only the glycogen stores of active muscles are reduced. Because the body can't transfer glycogen between muscles, the other muscles not involved in the exercise retain their glycogen stores.[11] The longer the exercise lasts, or the more intense it is, the more glucose a person uses. Recall that exercise done at an intensity that outstrips the ability of the heart and lungs to supply oxygen to working muscles relies primarily on glucose for fuel. Thus, activities such as sprinting quickly deplete the body's stores of glycogen. Other activities, such as jogging or brisk walking, where the body can meet the muscles' oxygen demands, are more conservative of glycogen. Nonetheless, joggers and walkers still use it, and eventually they can run out of it.

When a person begins exercising, for the first 20 minutes or so, about one-fifth of the body's total glycogen store is rapidly used.[12] If you tested the person's blood glucose during this period, you would see it rise for a while. This signals that the liver is pouring out its stored glycogen for the muscles' use. The muscles, ravenous for glucose, increase their uptake twentyfold or more.[13] This keeps blood glucose from rising too high, and indeed, it soon begins to decline.

If exercise continues beyond 20 minutes, glycogen use slows down. The body begins to rely more on fat for fuel to conserve the remaining glycogen supply. It protects its glycogen supply because without it, muscles simply can't run. Also, without glucose, fat can't be used for energy, either. At some point, if exercise continues long enough, glycogen will run out almost com-

Figure 9–3

The Use of Glycogen and Body Fat for Energy During Exercise

Training can increase the amount of glycogen a muscle can store. The more fit a muscle is, the more fat it can burn for energy when oxygen is present—sparing the valuable glycogen.

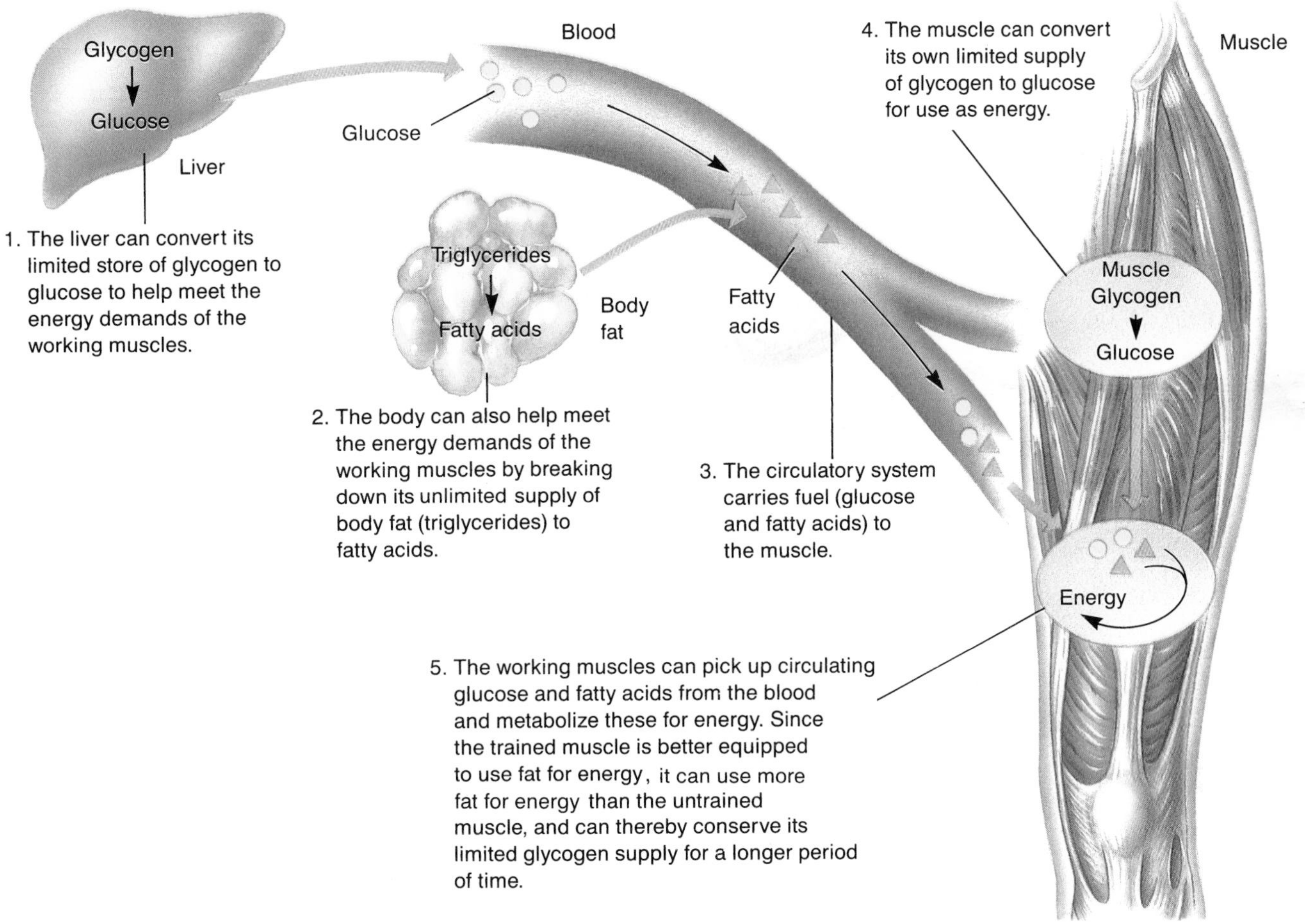
Glycogen
Glucose
Liver
1. The liver can convert its limited store of glycogen to glucose to help meet the energy demands of the working muscles.
Blood
Glucose
Triglycerides
Fatty acids
Body fat
2. The body can also help meet the energy demands of the working muscles by breaking down its unlimited supply of body fat (triglycerides) to fatty acids.
Fatty acids
3. The circulatory system carries fuel (glucose and fatty acids) to the muscle.
4. The muscle can convert its own limited supply of glycogen to glucose for use as energy.
Muscle
Muscle Glycogen
Glucose
Energy
5. The working muscles can pick up circulating glucose and fatty acids from the blood and metabolize these for energy. Since the trained muscle is better equipped to use fat for energy, it can use more fat for energy than the untrained muscle, and can thereby conserve its limited glycogen supply for a longer period of time.

pletely. Exercise can continue for a short time after that, only because the liver scrambles to produce the minimum amount of glucose needed to briefly forestall body shutdown. When blood sugars dip too low, the nervous system function comes almost to a halt, making exercise difficult, if not impossible, although there is still plenty of fat left to burn.

Another factor that influences how much glycogen a person uses during exercise is how well trained the person is to do the particular exercise. When first attempting an activity, a person uses more glucose than a trained athlete. This is because the muscles can quickly and easily extract energy from glucose. Extracting energy from fat takes longer and requires that the muscle cells contain abundant fat-burning metabolic enzymes. Untrained muscle cells rely heavily on the quick energy source glucose; with training, they adapt, packing their cells with more fat-burning enzymes. As a result, trained muscles use more fat and conserve their glucose. Training has another effect: it moderates the initial hormonal response to exercise, so the rate of glucose released from the liver is slower. This, too, conserves glycogen. Finally, the amount of glycogen present in the muscles before exercise influences glycogen use. A later section shows how to store a maximum amount of glycogen in the muscles (see pages 264–265).

Exercise and Fatty Acids

When you exercise, the fat your muscles burn comes from the fatty deposits all over the body, especially from those with the greatest amounts of fat to spare, such as the abdomen and buttocks. That is why physically fit people look trim all over—they reduce their fat stores all over the body, not just those overlaying the working muscles.

The body can store lots of fat but very little carbohydrate. A person who is of desirable body weight may store 25 to 30 pounds of body fat but only about one pound of carbohydrate. Each pound of fat contains about 3,500 calories—more than twice as much as one pound of carbohydrate. So, you may wonder why body fat can't be used exclusively for energy if fat is such a concentrated source of energy and your body has virtually an unlimited amount. Although your supply of fat is almost unlimited, the ability of your muscles to use fat for energy is not. Fat use depends on a simultaneous supply of carbohydrate. The old saying, "Fat burns in the flame of carbohydrate," is true. That's why exercise duration is limited by the supply of carbohydrate, not body fat.

The intensity of the workout also matters. Recall that for a working muscle to burn fat, oxygen must be present. If you work out at a rate that allows your heart to supply ample oxygen to working muscles, the muscles will draw heavily on fat stores for fuel. When exercise intensity outstrips your oxygen supply, fat still contributes as much energy as ever, but glucose pitches in and is burned by the anaerobic pathway. Thus, the percentage of the total energy supplied by fat declines. Your breathing rate can signal which fuel is providing most of the energy. A rule of thumb for gauging exercise intensity for aerobic workouts is this: if you can't talk normally, you are incurring oxygen debt and are burning more glucose than fat (so slow down); if you can sing, you aren't getting a cardiovascular workout or burning much of anything (so speed up).

Athletic training also controls the amount of fat used during a bout of exercise. Exercise training improves the body's ability to deliver fat to working muscles, and trained muscles have an increased ability to use the fat.

Much attention has been focused on the type of fuel used for varying exercise intensities and duration. Research conducted on athletes shows that when they exercise at a moderate intensity, they initially use more carbohydrate than fat for fuel. Gradually, as exercise continues for more than 20 minutes, the fuel ratio shifts, and they use more fat. For athletes participating in endurance sports, such as marathon runners and long-distance bicyclists who want to conserve their limited supply of carbohydrate, switching to a fat-burning energy system is crucial. However, for people who want to lose weight—body fat—it doesn't matter if they burn body fat or carbohydrate for energy during exercise.

A commonly held misbelief is that you must exercise for at least 20 minutes before you will burn body fat. Recall that your body is always using a combination of glucose and fat for fuel. While it's true that glucose is the primary fuel source during the first 20 minutes or so of exercise, body fat is being burned, too. After 20 minutes, your fuel mixture changes, and you burn more fat than glucose. For people trying to lose weight, a calorie burned is a calorie burned, regardless of whether it came from carbohydrate or from fat. Body fat stores will shrink and weight will be lost when you expend more energy than you eat, and body fat must be burned to make up for the lack of energy intake. There appears to be no scientific evidence that the type of fuel used for exercise influences weight loss.[14]

Protein Needs for Fitness

Fit people have more muscle than fat; exercise involves muscles; muscles are made largely of protein. It would seem logical, then, that to become or stay fit, one might need more protein. While it's true that fat and glucose are the primary fuels for working muscles, 5 percent to 15 percent of energy needs of weight lifters or athletes competing in endurance sports comes from muscle protein. So do athletes need more protein?

For athletes, fitness enthusiasts, and sedentary people alike, protein is the body's architect. Protein is used for growth and repair of all tissue. In addition, hormones, enzymes, and your blood transport system are all made of protein. The current recommendation to eat a diet that supplies 0.8 gram of protein per kilogram of ideal body weight calls for enough protein to meet these basic needs in nonathletes. Athletes, however, may need slightly more protein. During the initial stages of training, getting more protein may be more important than getting it later in training. Initial increases in muscle mass, numbers of red blood cells to carry oxygen, and amounts of aerobic enzymes in muscles to use fuel efficiently elevate an athlete's protein needs. Exercise also can promote muscle protein breakdown.

Hormonal changes during exercise can temporarily slow the amount of protein the muscle makes and can encourage the muscle to break down its protein stores.[15] This combination of using fewer amino acids and breaking down muscle, thereby releasing amino acids, builds up a pool of available amino acids. The circulating blood can then transport some liberated amino acids to the liver, where some can be converted into glucose. The blood then ushers the glucose back to working muscles to feed them. How much protein an athlete uses for fuel during hard exercise (endurance exercise and heavy weightlifting) depends on exercise intensity and duration, the athlete's fitness level, and the glycogen stores in the athlete's muscles. When glycogen stores are well stocked, protein contributes only 5 percent of fuel needs.

Although muscle protein breakdown dominates during exercise, muscle growth escalates after exercise. Muscles use the available amino acids to repair and build. The net effect of these changes is muscle protein buildup. Training enhances muscle protein buildup after exercise.

The American Dietetic Association recommends that athletes consume one gram of protein per kilogram of ideal body weight. Some athletes involved in prolonged heavy endurance training may need more than 1.5 grams of protein per kilogram.[16] The recommendation of one gram per kilogram is not much more than the 0.8 gram per kilogram recommended for nonathletes. This is nothing for most athletes to be concerned about, given that the average American eats more than twice the protein needed. You might ask why the athlete doesn't need more protein. To build muscle requires a positive nitrogen balance (explained in Chapter 5), but even that doesn't mean eating more protein. Muscle won't respond to excess protein by helplessly

Example: An athlete with an ideal body weight of 150 pounds can determine protein need by:

1. Changing pounds to kilograms: divide 2.2 into 150 pounds.

   $$\left(\frac{150}{2.2} = 68 \text{ kg}\right)$$

   (Note that 1 kilogram = 2.2 pounds.)
2. Multiply this number by one:
   $68 \times 1 = 68$
   (The protein recommendation for athletes = 1 gram protein per kilogram ideal body weight.)

This athlete needs 68 grams of protein.

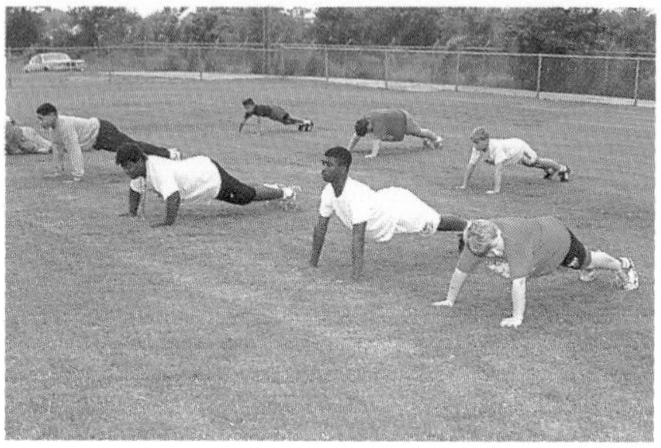

Muscles grow in response to work, not to protein feeding alone.

accepting it. They respond to the hormones that regulate them and to the demands put upon them, and then they select the nutrient they need from what is offered. So the way to make muscle cells grow is to put a demand on them—that is, to make them work. They will respond by taking up nutrients, amino acids included, so that they can grow.

In summary, don't push protein at your muscles. Exercise them so they demand and pull protein in for themselves. Then just eat an ordinary diet. Athletes eat considerably more food than nonathletes eat, and their diets may contain three to four times the recommended amount of protein.

Energy Needs and Weight Control

Depending on the sport or exercise, a person in active training and competition may have extraordinarily high energy needs. Football players, for example, seem to average close to 6,000 calories a day during the football season, with intakes on some days topping 10,000 calories.[17] Along with the increased energy expenditure goes an increased need for the B vitamins used to generate energy in metabolism. The increased intake, therefore, shouldn't be just any high-calorie food but should be food rich in B vitamins—breads, cereals, fruits, and vegetables. It is a rare individual who can eat more than 5,000 calories of nutritious food in only three meals during a day; eating five to six meals makes the task easier. Food sufficient to provide this much energy will also supply the vitamins and minerals needed to go with it—provided the selection is balanced and varied.

Chapter 8 was devoted to weight control for everyone, but a few words especially for the athlete are appropriate here. First of all, the recommended weight for an athlete is whatever weight and body composition lets him or her perform the best. When the muscles are in top condition for performance of the chosen sport, the amount of body fat and total body weight should be whatever the muscles can carry most easily. Too little fat can make the body susceptible to too-rapid heat loss; too much creates a drag on motion. The ideal body composition is considered to be about 15 percent fat for men in most sports and 20 percent or more for women.

Great variation in body composition exists among athletes of various sports (see Table 9–1). Body fat content of world-class male runners ranges from 4 percent to 9 percent—the less fat a runner has, the less he has to transport while running. Some professional football defensive backs have been measured with body fat levels as low as one percent of body weight.

Early research on body composition levels of female athletes suggested that females with body fat levels below a critical fat value—thought to be 17 percent body fat—suffered from amenorrhea—disruption of the normal menstrual cycle. Recent findings, however, dispute this theory. It is now thought that participation in rigorous physical training and perhaps the accompanying psychological stress can affect menstrual patterns independently of body fat levels. Many female athletes with body fat levels in the range of 8 percent to 13 percent have normal menstrual cycles, with no disruption of their cycle during training or competition.[18] To maintain good health, female athletes are advised not to dip below 10 percent to 12 percent body fat.

Sometimes seasonal sports or competitions require that an athlete gain or lose weight. The healthful way to gain weight is to build oneself up by patient

Table 9–1

Average Percentage Body Fat

	MALES	FEMALES
Nonathletes		
Lean	<8%	<13%
Optimal	8–15%	13–20%
Slightly overfat	16–20%	21–25%
Fat	21–24%	26–32%
Obese (overfat)	>25%	>32%
Athletes		
Long-distance runners	4–9%	6–15%
Wrestlers	4–10%	–
Gymnasts	4–10%	10–17%
Elite bodybuilders	6–10%	10–17%
Swimmers	5–11%	14–24%
Basketball players	7–11%	18–27%
Tennis players	14–17%	19–22%

Source: Adapted from D. C. Nieman, *Fitness and Sports Medicine: An Introduction* (Palo Alto, Calif.: Bull, 1990), p. 126.

and consistent training and at the same time eating nutritious foods containing enough extra calories to support the weight gain. A pound of muscle mass contains about 2,500 to 3,000 calories' worth of material. To gain a pound of muscle requires about a week of hard workouts, along with an energy intake that is 3,000 calories above the amount sufficient to support that work. By eating a large snack of complex carbohydrate-rich, lowfat foods between meals, one can add 700 to 800 extra calories to each day's intake. This, together with long, vigorous workouts, will support a weight gain of 1 to 1½ pounds, mostly muscle, in a week. A later section in this chapter, Food for Fitness, illustrates how to plan meals and snacks for exercisers.

Athletes need to remember to cut down on calories between and after training periods. Muscles respond to reduced demand by losing mass. It would be magical thinking to believe that the mass simply disappears. In fact, the cells slowly atrophy, and the materials they are made of (mostly carbohydrate, fat, and protein) become available as potential fuel for other body cells. Of course, this fuel will be stored as fat unless it is expended in activity. It should be no surprise, then, that a heavily muscled 20-year-old who stops working out but keeps on eating like a football player in training can become flabby and obese at age 30. It is not literally true that the person's muscle has turned to fat, but it is true that muscle has been lost and fat has been gained.

Losing weight, like gaining it, can be done wisely or unwisely. The goal is to lose primarily body fat. All people, including athletes, should be wary of techniques such as sauna bathing, exercising in a plastic suit (as if to "sweat off" the fat), using diuretics or cathartics, or inducing vomiting, all of which achieve fast weight loss by causing dehydration. As athletes know, dehydration seriously impairs performance. The hazards of fasts and fad diets have already been described, but a reminder should be repeated here. What is achieved by quick weight-loss dieting is loss of lean tissue, glycogen, bone minerals, and fluids—all materials vital to healthy body functioning. Abnormal heart rhythms have been seen in healthy adults after only ten days of fasting. Weight loss of about 2 pounds per week achieved by calorie control and exercise will encourage fat loss. The American College of Sports Medicine's exercise prescription for weight loss is similar to the one for cardiovascular conditioning. It recommends participating in aerobic exercise (such as brisk walking, jogging, bicycling, swimming, aerobic dance) three to five times per week at a moderate intensity (60 percent to 85 percent of maximum heart rate) for 20 to 60 minutes. Your goal is to expend at least 300 calories per exercise session.[19]

Before leaving the issue of energy expenditure, let's look at the issues surrounding elevated calorie burning after exercise and elevated resting metabolic rate. A common misconception held by fitness enthusiasts is that the body continues to burn large amounts of calories for hours after the exercise is completed. While researchers have documented elevated calorie expenditures for more than eight hours after exercise, the documentation followed exercise of unusual duration and exertion—such as 80 minutes of intense running. Moderate amounts of exercise, such as jogging two miles at a 12-minutes per mile pace causes only an additional 10 calories to be expended in the 30 minutes after exercise. When the pace is increased to 8.5-minutes per mile, an additional 15 calories are expended 30 minutes after jogging.[20] More research must be done on this issue. Although 15 calories may seem insignificant, over the course of a year, the extra 15 calories can add up to a loss of one pound of body fat if exercise is done four times per week. Still, though, the best advice for now remains, if you want to expend more calories, walk or jog longer. Don't count on the afterburn to expend a significant number of calories effortlessly.

Another misconception about energy expenditure and exercise is that regular exercise causes a relatively permanent increase in resting metabolic rate. If proven that fit individuals do expend more calories at rest, it is more likely because of their having a greater portion of muscle than fat; muscle burns more calories than fat. Studies are inconclusive about this point. Once again, the benefits of exercise come from doing it.

Fluid Needs and Exercise

Replenishing fluids lost during exercise is easily accomplished by drinking fluids before, during, and after physical activity. Yet many athletes and fitness enthusiasts either don't drink enough or don't drink at all. Ignoring body fluid needs can hinder performance and increase risk of heat-related injury. This section reviews why your body needs fluids during exercise, how much to drink, and what to drink—either water or fluid-replacement drinks.

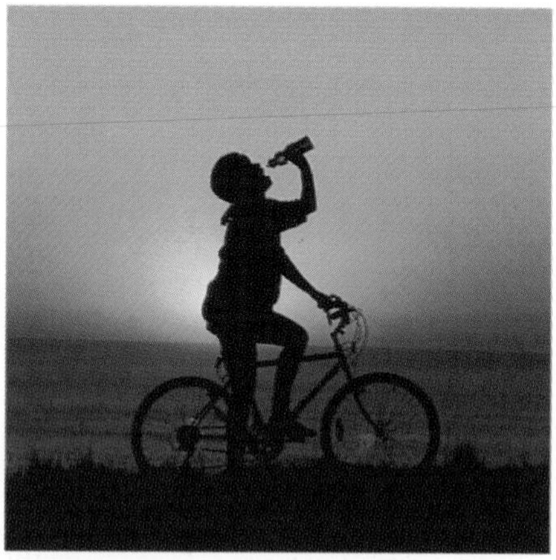

Plan to drink fluids before, during, and after exercise.

Water and Exercise

The water in your blood—known as plasma volume, or just plasma—serves a similar function as the water in the radiator of your car. It continually circulates throughout your body, picking up the tremendous amount of heat generated by working muscles. The plasma then transports this heat to your skin, through which the heat is expelled from the body by conduction, convection, and evaporation of sweat. Think of sweating as your body's air-conditioning system. As sweat evaporates from your skin, it expels large amounts of heat, helping to keep your body cool. Unfortunately, sweating works only when the sweat is evaporated from your skin. If the sweat simply rolls down your face or down your back, body heat is not released. On a humid day, the air is already saturated with water, and this impairs evaporation of sweat from your skin. Hot, humid days, then, are doubly dangerous: you continue to sweat and lose precious body water, but your body temperature doesn't fall. You need to pay particular attention to your fluid needs on humid days.

Sweat is the primary way your body loses water during exercise. How much sweat you lose depends on the intensity and duration of the activity. The more intense the exercise, the more heat you generate and the more sweat you will lose. If you don't replace the water you lose from sweat, your plasma volume decreases. In an attempt to maintain plasma volume, your body will pull water from your muscles and organs. Since approximately 45 percent of total body water is stored in muscle, muscle contributes the greatest amount of water to maintain plasma volume.[21] As water is pulled from muscles, cramps may occur along with premature fatigue. The complex reactions that produce energy in muscles must occur in a water medium. Thus, a lack of water compromises the muscles' ability to fuel the activity and results in a noticeable decline in performance.

Lower plasma levels also force your heart to beat faster. Since the heart pumps less blood with each beat, it must beat more often to supply oxygen to your muscles. Finally, with less plasma available to transport the heat to your skin, the heat builds, and your body's internal temperature continues to rise. All these changes force your body to work at a higher intensity level, leading to early exhaustion. A water loss equal to 5 percent of body weight can reduce muscular work capacity by 20 percent to 30 percent.

The recommended amount of fluid sufficient to prevent dehydration and **heat stroke** can be quite a bit. Athletes can lose 2 to 4 quarts of fluid during every hour of heavy exercise and must rehydrate before, during, and after exercise to replace it all. Even casual exercisers must drink some fluids while exercising. Thirst is unreliable as an indicator of how much to drink—it signals too late, after fluid stores are depleted. If you wait to drink until you are thirsty, you've waited too long! Table 9–2 presents one schedule of hydration before, during, and after exercise. To find out how much water is needed to replenish fluid losses after a workout, weigh yourself before and after—the difference is all water. One pound equals roughly 2 cups of fluid.

Water and Fluid-replacement Drinks

For fitness enthusiasts, the choice between water and a sports drink (a properly balanced carbohydrate-electrolyte fluid-replacement drink) is more a matter of personal taste and desired performance abilities. But for endurance athletes (people in continuous exercise for longer than 90 minutes), mounting evidence indicates that consuming a properly balanced sports drink during exercise enhances energy status and endurance and maintains plasma volume levels better than drinking water does.[22]

How the body manages water and carbohydrate use during exercise determines how well it performs. Sports drinks are designed to enhance the body's use of carbohydrate and water (see Table 9–3). The carbohydrate in a sports beverage serves three purposes during exercise: (1) it becomes an energy source for working muscles; (2) it helps maintain blood glucose at an

Table 9–2

Schedule of Hydration before and during Exercise

WHEN TO DRINK	AMOUNT OF FLUID
2 hours before exercise	About 3 c
10 to 15 minutes before exercise	About 2 c
Every 15 minutes during exercise	1 c (about 1 qt per hour)
After exercise	2 c fluid for each pound of body weight lost

Source: A. L. Hecker, *Nutrition and Physical Performance.* In R. H. Strauss (Ed.), *Drugs and Performance in Sports* (Philadelphia: W. B. Saunders, 1987), pp. 23–52.

Heat stroke an acute and dangerous reaction to heat buildup in the body.

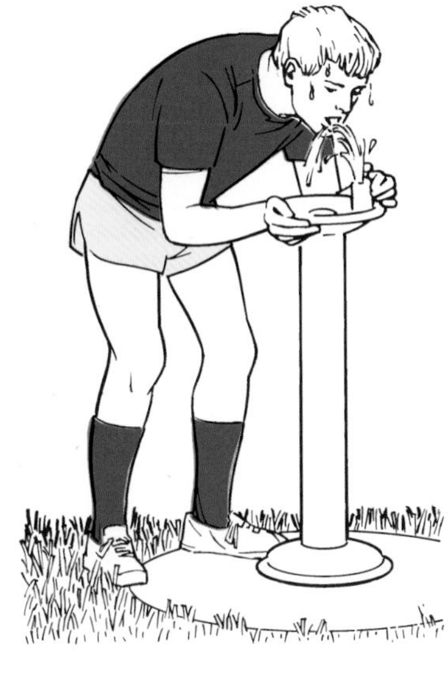

Table 9–3 Fluid-replacement Drinks

SPORTS DRINK	CALORIES/CUP	CARBOHYDRATE PERCENTAGE	CARBOHYDRATE TYPE	SODIUM
Body Fuel	70	7 %	Glucose polymer, fructose	70 mg
Exceed	70	7 %	Glucose polymer, fructose	50 mg
Gatorade	70	6 %	Sucrose, fructose	110 mg
10-K Thirst Quencher	60	6.5%	Sucrose, fructose, and glucose	54 mg

optimum level; and (3) it helps increase the rate of water absorption from the small intestine, helping to better maintain plasma volume. In addition, the drink supplies water and minerals lost from sweating.[23]

There are many factors to consider when choosing a sports drink. The ideal beverage should leave the digestive tract rapidly and enter circulation, where it is needed. Carbohydrate solutions don't all empty from the stomach at the same rate. Drinks containing high concentrations of sucrose, fructose, and glucose (soda pop, fruit juice, Kool-Aid types of products, and some sports drinks) slowly empty from the stomach, delaying working muscles' receipt of water and carbohydrate. Therefore, most sucrose-containing solutions should not be consumed during exercise, especially in the heat. Drinks using a blend of glucose polymers—short chains of carbohydrate—and fructose leave the stomach at the same rate as water, speeding the availability of the carbohydrate and water to working muscles.[24]

Carbohydrate concentration is another factor to consider. The drink should contain at least 5 percent but no more than 7 percent carbohydrate by volume (50 grams of carbohydrate per quart). Drinks containing more than 10 percent carbohydrate, such as soda pop, fruit juice, Kool-Aid types of drinks, and some sports drinks, take longer to absorb. They also can cause cramps, nausea, bloating, and diarrhea. Drinks with less than 5 percent carbohydrate may not offer an endurance-enhancing effect.

Sodium is another ingredient to pay attention to. Since most people eat enough salt in their regular diet to replace the sodium they lose during exercise, it's not essential that the fluid-replacement drink provide large amounts of sodium. In fact, too much sodium can delay muscles' receipt of water, but some is better than none. Research shows about 50 milligrams per cup will help stimulate water absorption from your gut. Other studies have found that people who drink a beverage with some sodium drink more. If the drink tastes good, athletes and exercisers will want to drink it and so meet their fluid needs.[25]

There are several practical considerations to keep in mind when using an energy drink. The drink should be consumed cold, in 4-ounce to 8-ounce portions, and frequently (every 15 to 20 minutes *once exercise begins*). Cooled beverages leave the digestive tract quickly to supply water to muscles and cool the body. Competitive athletes should establish fluid consumption patterns during practice. An event is not the time to try a new product or employ a new system of drinking.

In summary, water is always an adequate fluid-replacement beverage. However, if a sports drink is available, endurance athletes and performance-minded fitness enthusiasts should consider fluid-replacement beverages, particularly if they prefer the taste. For people who are exercising to lose weight, however, drinking a quart of sports drink to meet fluid needs may supply the amount of calories they expended during a 40-minute aerobic class or in 30 minutes of continuous swimming or biking. The choice to drink a sports drink or water is up to the individual.

As for salt loss, when the exercise is over, eating regular food can make it up. Salt tablets are not recommended, because they increase potassium losses and can irritate the stomach. After exercise, the replacement of magnesium and potassium may be more important than the replacement of sodium. Potassium is abundant in fruits, fruit juices, and fresh vegetables; and unprocessed foods of all kinds are especially good sources of both potassium and magnesium.

Vitamins and Minerals for Exercise

Your muscles burn food and oxygen to make energy. How well they burn these fuels depends, however, on your supply of vitamins and minerals. Without small amounts of these potent substances, your muscles' ability to work is compromised.

The Vitamins

Vitamins are the links and regulators of energy-producing and muscle-building pathways. Without them, your muscles' ability to convert food energy to body energy is hindered and muscle protein formation is slowed. Table 9–4 shows a few vitamins and minerals and their exercise-supporting functions.

The B vitamins are of special interest to athletes and exercisers because they govern the energy-producing reactions of metabolism. Needs for these vitamins increase proportionally with energy expenditure. A person who expends 4,000 calories per day needs twice as much of these vitamins as someone who spends 2,000 calories. Many athletes have been falsely led to believe that they can enhance energy production by taking supplements of B vitamins. Little experimental evidence exists to support this theory.[26] Once the system that uses B vitamins is full, generally the extra vitamins will be washed away through the urine. A well-balanced diet that meets athletes'

Table 9–4

Exercise-related Functions of Vitamins and Minerals

VITAMIN OR MINERAL	FUNCTION
Thiamin, riboflavin, niacin, magnesium	Energy-releasing reactions.
Vitamin B_6, zinc	Building of muscle protein.
Folate, vitamin B_{12}	Building of red blood cells to carry oxygen.
Vitamin C	Collagen formation for joint and other tissue integrity; hormone synthesis.
Iron	Transport of oxygen in blood and in muscle tissue; energy transformation reactions.
Calcium, vitamin D, vitamin A, phosphorus	Building of bone structure; muscle contractions; nerve transmissions.
Sodium, potassium, chloride	Maintenance of fluid balance; transmission of nerve impulses for muscle contraction.
Chromium	Assistance in insulin's energy-storage function.
Magnesium	Cardiac and other muscle contraction.

Note: This is just a sampling. All vitamins and minerals play indispensable roles in exercise.

energy needs and that features complex carbohydrate-rich foods will ensure B vitamin intakes proportional to energy intake.

The Minerals

Iron is a core component of the body's oxygen taxi service: hemoglobin and myoglobin. A lack of oxygen compromises the muscles' ability to perform. Iron deficiency has not been reported to be a problem for fitness enthusiasts who exercise moderately.[27] Male and female endurance athletes, though, may be prone to developing mild iron deficiency, diagnosed by low blood ferritin levels, a measure of the body's store of iron. Menstruating female athletes are at particular risk—growth and menstruation combined with strenuous training can take a toll on women's iron stores.[28]

A combination of factors increases an athlete's chances of depleting his or her iron stores. Inadequate dietary intake compounded by decreased iron absorption in people who already have depleted stores compromises iron status. This, coupled with increased iron losses in sweat, feces, and urine, plus increased destruction of red blood cells that occurs during exercise, leaves athletes wanting for this mineral all the more. Preparing meals with adequate iron requires careful planning. Iron-rich meals include meats, legumes, and dark green vegetables combined with absorption-enhancing factors such as (again) meats and foods rich in vitamin C. Chapter 7 contains numerous suggestions for obtaining sufficient iron from foods. Sometimes iron deficiencies can be corrected only with iron supplements. If you are concerned about your iron level, see a physician. Iron supplements should not be taken without medical supervision. High iron intakes can induce deficiencies of trace minerals, such as copper and zinc, and produce an iron overload in some people.

An apparent anemia also can occur in athletes that reflects no reduction in the blood's iron supply, but rather an increase in the blood plasma volume.[29] This occurs because athletic training causes the kidneys to conserve sodium and water. In other words, the extra blood plasma dilutes the concentration of iron, thereby making it seem as if the blood does not contain enough of the mineral. The causes of athletes' anemia have not yet been determined, nor is it agreed whether it is a desirable effect of normal physiology or a pathological change.

Adequate electrolytes are essential for fluid balance, a crucial factor in athletic performance. When sodium is retained, potassium is lost. There has been some concern that potassium depletion might occur in people who engage in vigorous activity day after day, particularly if the activity involves sweating. The ordinary nutritious diet can easily supply enough potassium to cover the athlete's needs if designed according to guidelines similar to those just described for iron. (Chapter 7 offers more on this subject.)

This brief treatment of vitamins and minerals for the athlete is intended to show the importance of nutrition for athletes. It is not meant to imply that special supplements are needed, except for diagnosed medical conditions. A diet composed of a variety of nutritious foods offers the best support for athletic performance.

The Bones and Exercise

Bones absorb great stress during exercise, and like the muscles, they respond by growing thicker and stronger. Weight-bearing exercises, running, walking, dancing, rope skipping, or activities such as resistance exercise training, in which significant muscular force can be generated against the long bones of the body, encourage bone development. A bone not strong enough to withstand the strain placed on it by athletic exertion can break in what has become known as a **stress fracture.** When a person suffers such a break, there are three probable causes. One is unbalanced muscle development, which allows strong muscles to pull against the bone opposed only by weaker, undeveloped muscles, thereby leaving the bone susceptible to fractures. Another is bone weakness caused by inadequate calcium intake during bone remodeling. A possible third cause, which occurs in women, is reduced estrogen concentration, which leads to bone mineral loss, and therefore fragile bones, in women who have ceased menstruating.

Stress fracture bone damage or breakage caused by stress on bone surfaces during exercise.

Balanced muscle development can protect the bones from undue stress. Each set of muscles pulling against bone should be kept in check by an equally strong set of opposing muscles. You should not work a set of muscles in training without working the opposing muscles. So if you work your back and leg muscles a lot (by jogging or walking, for example), work your abdominal muscles too (do situps). If you work your biceps (by weightlifting), work your triceps and deltoids, too. Bones, like muscles, take time to develop strength. Giving bones and muscles plenty of time to build up to one level of performance before moving up to the next level can also prevent stress fractures.

Eating an adequate amount of calcium throughout life may be one of the primary defenses against developing weak bones. The ideal sources of dietary calcium are milk and milk products and other calcium-containing foods, not calcium supplements. (Refer to Chapter 7 for more information.)

Some women who exercise strenuously cease to menstruate, a condition called **athletic amenorrhea.** Such women have lower than normal amounts of estrogen, a hormone essential for maintaining the integrity of the bones. With low estrogen levels, the mineral structures of the bones are rapidly dismantled, weakening the skeleton. Women who have athletic amenorrhea are at risk for stress fractures now and adult bone loss later in life.[30] To reverse the condition, they should not stop exercising altogether, for reasonable amounts of exercise may be a key defense against bone depletion. They should, however, seek evaluation from a health care provider who specializes in sports medicine to find the cause of their amenorrhea and to receive treatment.

Athletic amenorrhea cessation of menstruation associated with strenuous athletic training.

Eating disorders are sometimes related to athletic amenorrhea, and a logical part of diagnosis is to look carefully at the woman's diet for adequacy.[31] It could be that a diet too low in calories, coupled with low body fat stores and strenuous exercise, sets the stage for athletic amenorrhea to develop. In such cases, calcium intakes between 1,000 and 1,500 milligrams per day may help protect the bones somewhat.[32]

Food for Fitness

The best nutrition prescription for peak performance is a well-balanced diet. Although no one diet meets every athlete's needs, certain fundamental components are common to all well-balanced diets. For athletes, the diet should account for increased energy needs, vitamin/mineral needs, the relative efficiency of various foods as fuels, and current knowledge about long-term health. A diet that supplies 60 percent of calories from complex carbohydrate, 12 percent to 15 percent of calories from protein, and less than 30 percent of

Figure 9–4

The Effect of Diet on Physical Endurance

A high-carbohydrate diet can triple an athlete's endurance.

Source: Data from P. Astrand, Something old and something new . . . very new, *Nutrition Today*, June 1968, pp. 9–11.

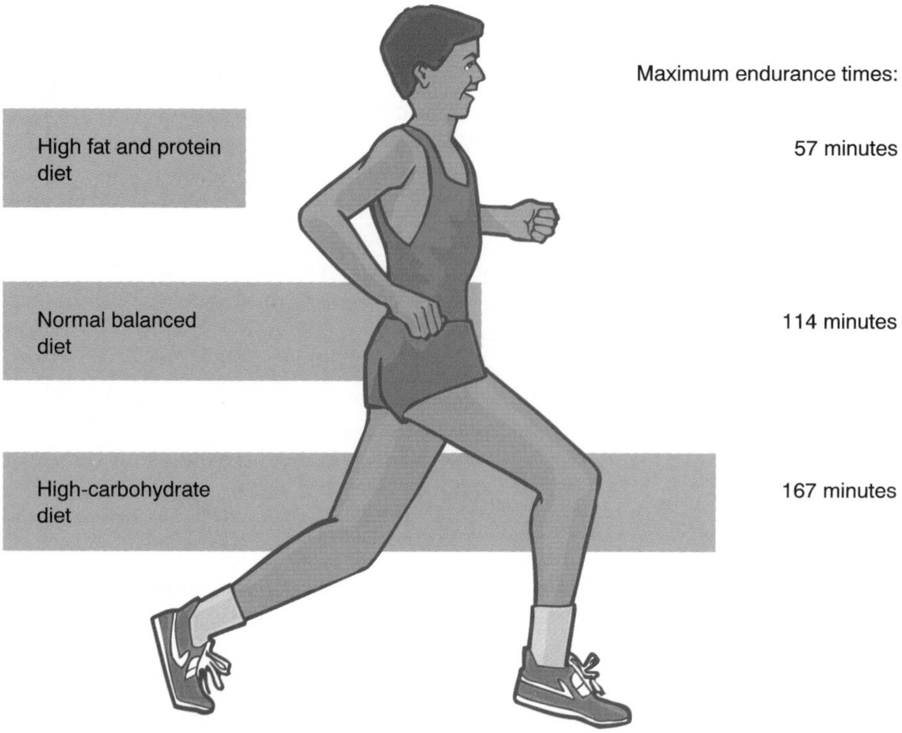

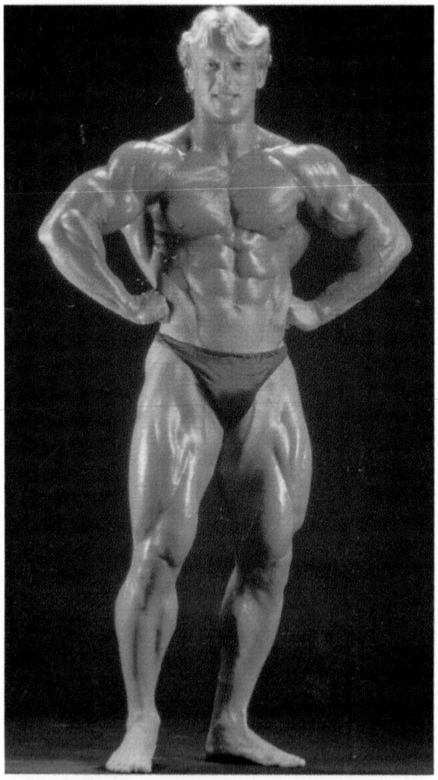

This is a body that vegetable foods maintain: Andreas Cahling, a vegetarian.

calories from fat will enable both athletes and fitness enthusiasts to supply muscles with a proper fuel mix and maintain health. Two critical nutrition periods for the athlete are the training diet and the precompetition diet.

Planning the Diet

A diet rich in complex carbohydrate and low in fat not only provides the best balance of nutrients for health but also supports physical activity best, as Figure 9–4 shows.[33] Athletes should consume a significant proportion of their day's calories before beginning physical activities. This will assure that muscle fuel needs are met during exercise. Eating most of the calories at the end of the day can lead to unwanted fat accumulation.[34]

Following the diet prescription in Figure 9–4 will provide fitness enthusiasts' muscles with enough glycogen to support exercise. For the casual exerciser who participates in low-intensity activities (walking, bicycling, jogging), the activity is rarely sufficient to totally deplete glycogen stores. Carbohydrate loading—a practice competitive athletes follow to trick their muscles into storing extra glycogen—may not be beneficial for people who exercise for less than 90 minutes per workout at a low intensity, although competitive athletes who exercise at a high intensity for more than 90 minutes at a time may benefit from carbohydrate loading. Muscles typically have enough glycogen to fuel one-and-a-half to two-hour bouts of activity.

When carbohydrate loading was first introduced, athletes learned a two-step procedure. First, they reduced their carbohydrate intake for several days by eating meals high in protein and fat. Simultaneously, they exercised heavily to empty their muscles of glycogen. A few days before the event, they reduced the intensity of the exercise and switched abruptly to a high carbo-

Table 9–5

Diet Plans for High-calorie, High-carbohydrate Intakes

Use the number of portions indicated to arrive at the specified energy levels[a]

FOOD GROUP	ENERGY LEVEL				
	3,000 cal	3,300 cal	3,800 cal	4,400 cal	5,400 cal
Nonfat milk	3	4	5	6	8
Vegetable	9	10	11	13	13
Fruit	8	8	10	12	16
Starchy vegetable/grain	16	17	20	22	26
Lean meat	7	8	8	11	15
Fat	8	10	10	10	12

[a]Refer to Chapter 2, Figure 2–8 for portion sizes.

Note: These plans supply 55% to 60% of calories as carbohydrate and less than 30% as fat. To increase the carbohydrate content to over 60%, substitute ⅓-c servings of legumes for the meats. People who cannot eat these quantities of whole foods may have to replace some of them with refined sugars and fats to meet their energy needs.

hydrate diet. Muscle glycogen stores rebounded to about two to four times the normal level.

Glycogen loading practiced this way has side effects, including abnormal heartbeat; swollen, painful muscles (glycogen attracts and holds water); and weight gain immediately before competition. Most exercise physiologists now recommend a modified plan that confers similar benefits but is not so extreme. The athlete exercises intensely without restricting carbohydrates, then gradually cuts back on exercise the week before the competition, rests completely the day before the event, and eats a very high carbohydrate diet for a few days before the competition.[35] Endurance athletes who follow this plan can keep going longer than their competitors without ill effects. In a hot climate, extra glycogen offers an additional advantage. As glycogen breaks down, it releases water, which helps to meet the athlete's fluid needs.[36]

For fitness enthusiasts and people who exercise for less than 90 minutes per session, such extremes in glycogen storage are unnecessary. The feelings of stiffness and heaviness that often accompany carbohydrate loading may hinder the performance of such people. Glycogen isn't likely to run out in a short exercise session, no matter how intense. All that is necessary to provide consistently full glycogen stores for workouts is to eat a high-carbohydrate diet based on whole foods and allow muscle groups to recover fully before working them again. Full recovery of glycogen stores takes from 24 to 48 hours. This doesn't mean you can work out only every other day. It means you should vary your exercise routine from day to day, as suggested earlier, to work different groups of muscles on different days.

Table 9–5 shows some sample diet plans for athletes who wish to increase their carbohydrate intakes along with their calories by using whole foods. These plans are effective only if the user chooses whole foods to provide nutrients as well as calories—extra milk for calcium and riboflavin, many vegetables for B vitamins, meat or alternates for iron and other vitamins and minerals, and whole grains for magnesium and chromium. In addition, these foods provide plenty of sodium, potassium, and chloride.

Up to a point, adding more carbohydrate-rich foods is a sound and reasonable option for increasing calories. The point at which it becomes unreasonable is when the calories needed by the individual outstrip the ability to eat that much food. At that point, the person must find ways of adding calories to the diet. After the athlete has met the required number of servings from fruits, vegetables, grains, and dairy products, refined sugars and even some fat may be used to make up the calorie need. High-carbohydrate liquid nutritional supplements also are available on the market.

A way that an athlete may be able to eat more food is to consume it in six or eight meals each day rather than in three or four meals. Large snacks of milkshakes, dried fruits, peanut butter sandwiches, or cheese and crackers can add substantial calories and nutrients.

In summary, the diet that supports performance is similar to—although higher in calories than—the diet recommended for good health. Think back to the diet recommendations in Chapters 2, 3, 4, and 7—diets designed to minimize risks of the diseases diabetes, heart disease, cancer, and high blood pressure. Both for health promotion and for fitness, the diet should consist of whole, minimally processed foods low in fat, sugar, and salt and high in complex carbohydrates and vitamins and minerals.

The Pregame Meal

The meal before a competitive event can be an issue of heated debate. Many coaches and athletes believe intensely in special food rituals. For example, a football team "can't play without breakfasting first on steak." A swim team is forbidden milk at the meet because it "causes cotton mouth." A bicyclist takes two tablespoons of honey before the race to give her "an energy boost" as she pedals away. Do these rituals work?

Scientifically, no particular food confers a special benefit before an athletic contest. A meal of steak may boost morale, but it is high in fat and may take so long to digest that it might hinder the football team's performance. The swim team's idea that milk causes cotton mouth is pure superstition. Honey demands water from the blood to dilute it and will actually handicap the cyclist during exertion.[37] In short, some rituals have a neutral effect, and some can actually impair performance. However, if neutral practices give competitors a morale boost or extra confidence, they should be respected. People may have special personal meanings associated with certain foods, and their faith in rituals can make the difference between winning and losing a game.

All of this is not to say that it doesn't matter what the meal before an event consists of. The best choices are foods that are high in carbohydrate and low in fat, protein, and fiber. Fat and protein slow the stomach's emptying, and protein's waste products generated during metabolism require that too much water be excreted with them. Fiber is not desirable right before physical exertion either, because it stays in the digestive tract too long and attracts water out of the blood. A high-carbohydrate meal will support blood glucose levels during competition. Olympic training tables are laden with foods such as breads, pasta, rice, potatoes, and fruit juices. Competitors eat as much of these foods as they comfortably can, because they supply energy without burdening the body. And they know it's especially important to include plenty of fluids—one or two 8-ounce glasses of water or juice, per meal—to ensure adequate hydration.

Any meal should be finished a good three or four hours before the event, because digestion requires routing the blood supply to the digestive tract to pick up nutrients. By the time the contest begins, the circulating blood should be freed from that task and should be available instead to carry oxygen and fuel to the muscles. Liquid nutritional products can be eaten closer to the event (one to two hours) because they are emptied relatively rapidly from the stomach. In addition, they supply an effective way to assure hydration. These products yield low stool residues, an important consideration for wrestlers and other athletes in limited-weight sports.[38]

A person who eats a snack closer to competition time should choose a food that is mostly carbohydrate because it is quickly digested. Better yet, just fill your fluid banks with beverages lacking sugar, such as water. To repeat, sugar eaten immediately before the game can impair performance; fluids will enhance it. Table 9–6 gives guidelines for choosing pregame snacks.

Table 9–6

Guidelines for Pregame Snacks

These foods, to be eaten three to four hours before competition, do *not* have many vitamins or minerals for the most part and should not be overemphasized in the daily diet. The hours before competition are too late for vitamins and minerals, but the special needs for energy and fluid can be met by eating the following snacks.

Food	Serving Size	Calories	Energy Donated by Carbohydrate (% of calories)
Sample Snack #1			
White bread	2 slices	140	74
Jam or jelly	2 tbsp	130	100
Gelatin dessert	1 c	70	97
Grape juice	1 c	165	100
Total		505	94
Sample Snack #2			
Spaghetti and tomato sauce (canned, plain)	1 c	190	80
Roll (white flour)	1	85	71
Popsicle (3 oz)	2	140	100
Limeade	1 c	100	100
Total		515	90
Sample Snack #3			
Banana	1	100	100
Sweetened dry cereal	¾ c	115	90
Nonfat milk	½ c	45	53
Cranberry juice cocktail	⅔ c	109	100
Gumdrops	1 oz	100	100
Total		469	95

Note: Substitutions can be made for cereal (1 c), or bread (2 slices):
- 1 c white or flavored rice.
- 1 3-inch-diameter muffin (plain).
- 1 piece angel food cake.
- 3 small pancakes and syrup.

To substitute liquids (gelatin, juices, limeade), use 1 c any sugar-sweetened beverage.

On Pill Popping to Win and Other Fitness Follies

Competitors in the ancient Greek Olympiad reportedly used mushrooms and herbs.[39] Since then, virtually every food has at one time or another been touted as the "magic bullet" that will enhance performance. Athletes have been known to swallow everything from bee pollen to brewer's yeast to kelp to wheat germ in their quest to gain the competitive edge.

Seductive as the idea of using pills and potions to achieve peak performance may be, the scientific evidence to support claims that special supplements will make an athlete run farther or jump higher is sorely lacking. Most so-called **ergogenic aids**, that is, substances that increase the ability to exercise harder, are costly versions of vitamins, minerals, sugar, and other nutrients provided easily by a balanced diet.[40]

Ergogenic aids anything that helps increase the capacity to work or exercise (*ergo* means "work"; *genic* means "give rise to").

Take bee pollen, a mixture of protein, carbohydrate, a bit of fat, and a few vitamins and minerals.[41] Though touted by one manufacturer as a "natural and balanced source of extra energy" appreciated by "athletes worldwide," it has been tested at Louisiana State University among both runners and swimmers and found to confer no benefit whatsoever on an athlete's training or performance abilities.[42] The same goes for pangamic acid, also known as vitamin B_{15}. While the substance purportedly helps keep muscles working at peak capacity during exercise, the evidence used to support the claim comes from studies conducted in Russia using questionable research methods. Yet a carefully controlled investigation into the matter did not come to the same conclusion.

Surveys of athletes have found that between 53 percent and 80 percent use a vitamin or mineral supplement, although no evidence exists that it improves performance.[43] More than 40 years of research has provided no strong evidence that popping vitamins and minerals increases energy or athletic prowess of adequately nourished people.[44] Except for iron, vitamin and mineral deficiencies are rare among athletes. Since most athletes eat more food than nonathletes eat to meet their increased energy demands, they usually get the additional vitamins and minerals they need, provided they eat a well-balanced diet.

An ordinary multivitamin and mineral supplement might be prudent in one instance: when an athlete's need for energy outstrips the ability to eat the quantity of food required to supply it. Then, many athletes must turn to

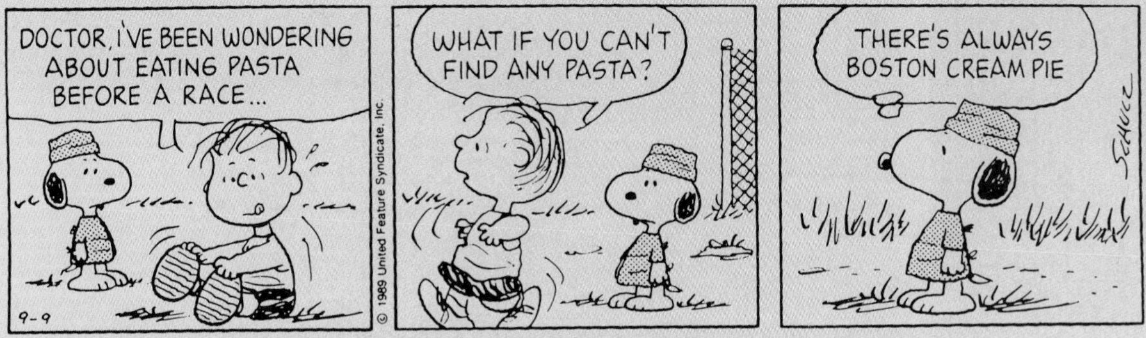
DOCTOR, I'VE BEEN WONDERING ABOUT EATING PASTA BEFORE A RACE...
© 1989 United Feature Syndicate, Inc.
WHAT IF YOU CAN'T FIND ANY PASTA?
THERE'S ALWAYS BOSTON CREAM PIE

concentrated energy sources, such as sugars and fats. While such foods supply abundant energy, they are practically devoid of vitamins and minerals—thus the name "empty calories." The energy they supply, though, requires processing by vitamin- and mineral-containing enzymes. For a short time, say, during the heaviest training, a supplement may be appropriate. It's best to choose one based on the information in the Spotlight feature in Chapter 6. Don't be led astray by the word *athlete* or *fitness* on a label.

Of course, when athletes firmly hold that one or another ergogenic aid does indeed improve performance, convincing them otherwise can be extremely difficult. One reason is that the profound belief that a substance will help can actually produce a psychological benefit known as the **placebo effect.**

Psychological impact aside, pill popping may be harmful in some cases. Taking large doses of vitamin A or D, for example, can cause liver damage over time. Swallowing supplements known as **anabolic steroids**—synthetic hormones that appear to help build muscle—can be even more dangerous.

A particularly popular practice among weightlifters and bodybuilders, steroid abuse often begins at a young age. According to one survey, the drugs are used by some 7 percent of male high school athletes. But while steroids may help increase muscular size and strength in some people, they can bring about numerous side effects, including acne, liver abnormalities, temporary infertility, and offensive outbursts, often referred to as roid rages. Among adults, many effects of steroid use are reversible. Unfortunately, adolescents aren't so lucky. Several studies show that adolescent steroid users may suffer serious consequences of premature skeletal maturation, decreased spermatogenesis, and elevated risk of injury.[45] Along with being unhealthful, steroid use is considered unethical by domestic and international sports organizations such as the American College of Sports Medicine and the International Olympic Committee. As a case in point, track star Ben Johnson lost his Olympic gold medal for the 100-meter sprint in 1988 after officials discovered he had been using steroids.[46]

Many athletes also swallow amino acid supplements in hopes of building larger muscles. These supplements are advertised as "predigested protein" and so supposedly are easily absorbed and readily available to encourage muscle growth brought on by training. Let's look at the facts.

Your intestinal tract is better prepared to handle protein in its complex form of di- and tripeptides (refer to Chapter 5). You absorb 85 percent to 99

Placebo effect an improvement in a person's sense of well-being or physical health in response to the use of a placebo (a substance having no medicinal properties or medicinal effects).

Anabolic steroids synthetic male hormones with a chemical structure similar to that of cholesterol; such hormones have wide-ranging effects on body functioning.

Losing with Steroids[47]

Side effects include:
acne
cancer
heart disease
irreversible baldness in women
jaundice
liver disease
male pattern baldness
oily skin (females only)
shrunken testicles
sterility (reversible)
stunted growth
swelling of feet or lower legs
yellowing of the eyes or skin

percent of the animal protein you eat and 90 percent of protein from vegetable sources. Amino acid solutions, on the other hand, will draw water into your intestinal tract, and their digestion can cause cramping and diarrhea.

In addition, your body can't store extra amino acids, whether they come from food you eat or from supplements. Your body converts the excess into fat. This conversion of amino acids to fat generates urea, which increases your body's need for water. Both diarrhea and increased urination of urea can lead to dehydration, impeding training and performance.

There is no benefit to rapid absorption of amino acids. It takes your body hours, not minutes, to rebuild muscle protein damaged by exercise. Protein from food also supplies iron, vitamin B_{12}, vitamin B_6, and riboflavin. Taking amino acid supplements instead of eating protein-rich foods can deprive your body of these necessary nutrients. To date, there are no known benefits of taking amino acid supplements. And as mentioned before, most athletes already eat more protein than they need.

In addition to pill popping, some athletes look to other dietary means to promote athletic prowess. For instance, many exercisers drink caffeine-containing beverages such as coffee, tea, or cola to enhance performance and endurance. Caffeine apparently stimulates the release of fats into the blood which the body can then use instead of glycogen as a source of energy. Thus, the glycogen is "spared," or saved, for later use, and the amount of time an exerciser can endure physical activity before running out of fuel is prolonged.

The glycogen-sparing effect of caffeine, however, is beneficial only for athletes who exercise for more than one and a half to two hours at a time. The reason is that the muscles generally store enough glycogen to fuel as many as 90 minutes of activity. Moreover, even endurance athletes can experience certain downsides to consuming caffeine. A diuretic, the drug promotes frequent urination and fluid loss that can lead to dehydration. In addition, caffeine can induce rapid heart rate and jitters, which can interfere with performance. Athletes would also do well to remember that caffeine is a drug that neither the American College of Sports Medicine nor the International Olympic Committee condones for use among athletes.

Along with caffeinated beverages, alcoholic drinks are often touted as choice fluids for athletes. Beer, for example, is sometimes portrayed as the perfect carbohydrate-containing complement to both before- and after-competition meals. Despite such images, alcoholic drinks rank as poor sources of fluid and energy for several reasons. For one, alcohol is a diuretic that can bring about fluid loss and dehydration. More importantly, the amount of alcohol in just one beer or glass of wine depresses the nervous system, thereby slowing an athlete's reaction time and interfering with reflexes and coordination. Also, one can of beer provides only 50 carbohydrate calories. The rest of the calories come from alcohol, which must be metabolized by your liver, not your muscles. The American College of Sports Medicine and the American Dietetic Association both conclude that use of alcohol hurts performance. (See the Spotlight feature in Chapter 10 for a detailed explanation of how alcohol affects the body.)

The special supplements and drinks mentioned here are just a sampling of the many "magic" pills and potions promoted to athletes. If you're in doubt about a particular product you see boasted as an ergogenic aid, use the Fitness Quackery Scorecard to separate legitimate claims from bogus ones.

Fitness Quackery Scorecard

Here are a few questions to ask yourself about any health gimmick, product, or device that you see advertised or that someone tries to sell you. Every "yes" answer gets one point:

1. Is the promised action of the product based on magical thinking? ("Eat all you want and lose weight." "Develop a trim body with no exercise.")
2. Does the promotion claim that "doctors agree" or "research has determined," without clarification? (Which doctors? What research?)
3. Does the promotion state that hormones, drugs, or nutrient doses useful in correcting an abnormal condition are needed to make the normal, healthy person more fit?
4. Does the promoter use scare tactics to pressure you into buying the product? ("It's the only one available without poisons.")
5. Is the product being sold or promoted by a crusading organization, a faith-healing group, or a self-styled health adviser who has no acceptable credentials?
6. Is the product advertised as having a multitude of different beneficial effects? ("Makes bigger muscles; gives that 'pumped-up feeling'; improves digestion, coordination, and breathing.")
7. Does the sponsor claim persecution by the medical community and the government because they do not accept this wonderful discovery?
8. Is the product available only from the sponsor by mail order and with payment in advance?
9. Does the promoter use many case histories or testimonials from grateful users?
10. Is the product a special or "secret" formula not available from any other source?

Scoring: Even 1 point is a point against the claimant: it's your warning signal that you are dealing with misinformation. Three or more points is a sure sign of quackery.

Consumer Tips

Advice on Brown Bagging It

Whether you carry your lunch to work or school to save time and money, the following tips can help you pack nutritious meals and add variety to your noontime routine. Even if you don't carry your lunch regularly, you can use this advice when you take food on hikes, day trips, or picnics.

- Choose breads made with whole wheat, bran, or oatmeal to add fiber to your lunch.
- Get out of the peanut butter and jelly rut by filling sandwiches with water-packed tuna mixed with mandarin oranges, bean sprouts, and a bit of plain low-fat yogurt; chopped, cooked, skinless chicken combined with raw sliced vegetables and a little French dressing; cooked, mashed dried beans seasoned with chopped onion, garlic powder, rosemary, thyme, and pepper; or low-fat cottage cheese flavored with drained, chopped pineapple and a dash of cinnamon.
- Bring a thermos bottle filled with chili, vegetable soup, or a milk-based soup, such as cream of tomato, prepared with nonfat milk instead of a sandwich. Try cold lunches such as low-fat or nonfat yogurt and fruit; brown rice with cubes of skinless poultry or lean meat; or cooked pasta tossed with raw vegetables, low-fat cheese, and a bit of Italian dressing.
- Pack fresh fruit such as an apple, a banana, or grapes along with your sandwich or main dish.
- Substitute unsalted pretzels or air-popped popcorn for potato, corn, or tortilla chips.
- Replace Oreos and candy bars with lower fat treats, including fig bars, graham crackers, gingersnaps, or vanilla wafers.
- Drink low-fat or nonfat milk or fruit juice with your lunch instead of soda pop. Freeze small cans or cartons of juice to take along, for instance. Put them in plastic wrap (they "sweat" as they defrost) and pack them into your lunch to help keep the other foods chilled. By lunchtime, the beverage will be thawed and ready to drink.
- Take along fresh cauliflower or broccoli florets, green pepper strips, cucumber or zucchini slices, or cherry tomatoes to munch on.

If you like the idea of packing a lunch every day but often feel too rushed in the morning to do so:

- Pack your lunch the night before and store it in the refrigerator; the food will be thoroughly chilled the following morning and remain fresher longer.
- Make several sandwiches at one time and store them in the freezer. Pull one out to take with you in the morning, and it will be thawed by noon. Although sliced meats, sliced cheese, and mustard freeze well, egg salad, lettuce, tomatoes, jelly, and mayonnaise do not, and they will make a sandwich soggy.

Source: Adapted from the U.S. Department of Agriculture, Human Nutrition Information Service, *Making Bag Lunches, Snacks & Desserts Using the Dietary Guidelines* (Home and Garden Bulletin No. 232-9), pp. 9–22.

Spotlight Nutrition and Stress

Are you one of those people who get the "munchies" when they are stressed out? Or does stress take away your appetite, making it just about impossible for you to eat or drink? Whatever your reaction may be, it is virtually certain that your eating behavior is one of the many things stress affects. Because stress can literally "take a lot out of you," as people so often remark, it is important to know what happens to your body during periods of stress and what you can do before, during, and after to protect yourself from the most severe effects.

● How would you define stress?

Stress can be loosely described as anything that pushes your body out of balance. For example, if you walk outside in the cold air, your body shivers trying to warm up. If you eat a candy bar, your blood sugar rises, so your pancreas secretes insulin in an attempt to restore normal blood sugar levels. Your body likes to maintain status quo and works hard at it. But both physical and psychological stresses intrude daily on your steady state, triggering your body's **stress response.**

Major physical stresses include pain, illness of any kind, surgery, wounds, burns, infections, a very hot or humid climate, toxic compounds, radiation, and pollution. Life's events—even happy ones such as getting married—can also stress us out. These differ for every person. One person may not be affected at all by a situation because he or she previously handled a similar scenario successfully. For a person experiencing a situation for the first time, however, the event can be pressure packed!

One criterion for judging an event as stressful is the amount of change in daily activities the event demands and how many coping behaviors are necessary to deal with the event. Look at the life events listed in Table 9–7. The Holmes scale rates life events from the most to the least stressful. See how you rate.

● How does the body react during times of stress?

While many of the stresses we experience today are psychological, the stress response readies our body for vigorous muscular action—called the fight or flight reaction. Your body mobilizes its defenses to either fight the enemy (stress) or run away. The stress response begins when your equilibrium is threatened. The sight of a car hurtling toward you, the terror that an intruder is present, the excitement of planning for a party, a move, or a wedding, the feeling of pain, the anxiety of a mid-term exam, or any other event that threatens your body or mind signals your stress alarm to go off. A chain of events ensues through both nerves and hormones to prepare your body for battle.

The pupils of your eyes widen to allow more light to enter; your muscles tense up so that you can jump, run, or struggle with maximum strength; your breathing quickens to bring more oxygen into your lungs; and your heart races to rush this oxygen to your muscles so they can burn the fuel they need for energy. The liver pours forth the needed fuels—glucose and ketone bodies—from its stored supply, and the fat cells release fatty acids as alternative fuels. Body protein tissues break down to supply amino acids to back up the glucose supply and to be ready to heal wounds, if necessary. The muscles' blood vessels expand to feed the muscles better, while those of the digestive tract constrict (digestion becomes a low-priority process in time of danger). Less blood flows to the kidneys so that fluid is conserved, and less blood flows to the skin so that blood loss will be minimized at any wound site. More clotting factors form to allow the blood to clot faster, if need be. Hearing sharpens, and the brain produces local opiumlike substances that dull its sensation of pain, which during an emergency might distract you from taking the needed action. And your hair stands on end—a reminder that there was a time when your ancestors had enough hair to bristle, look bigger, and frighten off their enemies.

This tightly synchronized, adaptive reaction to threat provides superb support for emergency physical action. You probably remember having had to take such action. You may have performed an amazing feat of strength or speed for a few minutes, and only after it was over did you notice that your heart was pounding, your breathing was fast, your fingers were cold, your skin was tingling, your mouth was dry, and the sensation of pain or exhaustion was just beginning to come through as the adrenaline drained away.

● Is the stress response harmful to the body?

Fortunately, many of the stresses that you deal with every day don't require you to engage in a fistfight or to run away. Navigating traffic jams, studying for final exams, and searching for employment all require calm, rational thought. Nevertheless, your body prepares for heavy physical activity. This response literally needs to be worked off. Keeping the stress bottled up inside of you may cause you harm. The fat, for example, that was released for energy stays in circulation and has more opportunity to enter the artery walls and form plaque (refer to Chapter 4). When you are under stress, go dance, run, jump rope, climb trees, swim, walk, run up and down a flight of steps, or engage in any type of physical activity until you are exhausted. Avoid the use of drugs (including alcohol and tranquilizers) that would discourage activity and exercise.

Table 9–7 Events People Perceive as Stressful

People ranked these events, according to how stressful they perceived them to be, on a scale from 1 to 100. Note that some "happy" events are included here. Individual people may score these events higher or lower than they are here. We have added in parentheses events that might be comparable to these in the lives of students.

LIFE EVENT	STRESS POINTS	LIFE EVENT	STRESS POINTS
Death of spouse	100	Change in responsibilities at work (change in course demands)	29
Divorce	73	Son or daughter leaving home	29
Marital separation (breakup with boyfriend/girlfriend)	65	Trouble with in-laws (trouble with parents)	29
Jail term	63	Outstanding personal achievement	28
Death of close family member (except spouse)	63	Spouse beginning or stopping work	26
Major personal injury or illness	53	School beginning or ending (final exams)	26
Marriage	50	Change in living conditions	25
Being fired from a job (expulsion from school)	47	Revision of personal habits (self or family)	24
Marital reconciliation	45	Trouble with boss (trouble with professor)	23
Retirement	45	Change in work (or school) hours or conditions	20
Change in health of a family member (not self)	44	Change in residence (moving to school, moving home)	20
Pregnancy	40	Change in schools	20
Sex difficulties	39	Change in recreation	19
Gain of new family member (change of roommate)	39	Change in church activities	19
Business readjustment	39	Change in social activities (joining a new group)	18
Change in financial state	38	Taking on a small mortgage or loan	17
Death of a close friend	37	Change in sleeping habits	16
Change to different line of work (change of major)	36	Change in number of family get-togethers	15
Change in number of arguments with spouse	35	Change in eating habits	13
Taking on a large mortgage (taking on financial aid)	31	Vacation	13
Foreclosure of a mortgage or loan	30	Christmas	12
		Minor violations of the law	11

Check the list and identify the events that have happened to you in the past year or that you expect within the next year. Use the number system to determine how many stress points you are experiencing in this period of your life. Then score yourself as follows: over 200—urgent need of intelligent stress management; 150 to 199—careful stress management indicated; 100 to 149—stressful life, keep tabs on your mental health; under 100—no present cause for concern about stress.

Source: Adapted from Lifescore: Holmes scale, *Family Health,* January 1979, p. 32.

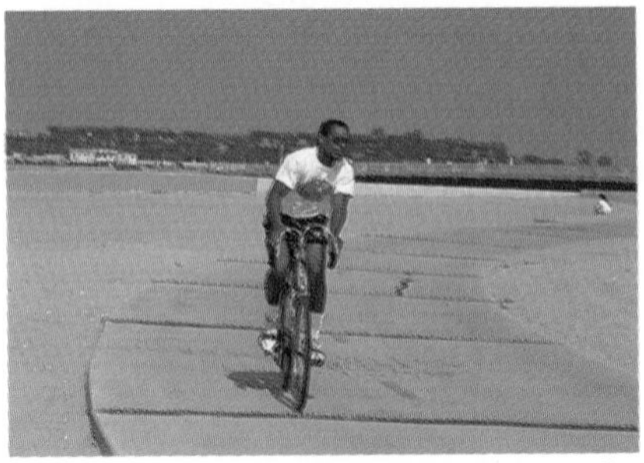

The stress response needs to be worked off physically.

Anyone can respond in this magnificent fashion to sudden physical stress for a short time. But if stress is prolonged—and especially if physical activity is avoided—the stress can drain the body of its reserves. Many of the biochemical pathways used during the stress response rely on nutrients to run. If nutrients are not replaced as they are used up, deficiencies can develop, leaving the body weakened and susceptible to illness. Water, protein, carbohydrate, fat, calcium, and potassium are some of the key players in the stress response.

Which body reserves are most drawn upon during stress?

In preparation for potential blood loss that might occur with a physical injury, your body conserves water during stress. It does so by retaining sodium, because water clings to this mineral in your body. But to retain sodium, your kidneys must expel potassium. Thus, you need ample stores of potassium to be able to afford losses of this mineral.

All three energy-yielding nutrients—carbohydrate, fat, and

protein—are drawn upon in increased quantities if the stress requires vigorous physical action or if there is injury. While the body is busy responding and not eating, the fuels must be drawn from internal sources. Carbohydrate is your body's preferred source of fuel. Initially, carbohydrate is taken from the liver's stores, but that supply lasts only about a day. Thereafter, your muscles and some of your organs—heart, liver, and lungs—are broken down to supply protein that your body converts into carbohydrate for fuel. The breakdown of muscles also provides your body with available protein that the body can use to make scar tissue to heal wounds.

Some tissues can burn fat for fuel. In a normally nourished person, fat stores are adequate to meet energy needs for many days. Chapter 8 described these processes as they occur during the stress of fasting. For now, what is important to notice is that the body uses not only dispensable supplies (those that are stored for time of need, like body fat) but also vital tissue—like muscle tissue—that your body can ill afford to lose.

Another nutrient lost from the body during stress is calcium from the bones. The evidence is not completely clear on this, but it has been observed that people lose widely varying amounts of this important bone mineral, depending partly on their hormonal state.[48]

The best nutritional preparation for stress is a balanced and varied diet as part of a lifestyle in which exercise plays a constant part. Notice that nothing is said here about supplements or gimmicks. Just eat well to obtain the nutrients and exercise regularly to promote the nutrients' storage and your body will be as well prepared as it can be to withstand the impacts of periods of unavoidable stress.

• Is it best not to eat during times of stress?

How much you should eat and what you should eat during a stressful time depends in part on what your stomach can tolerate. During severe stress, the appetite is suppressed. This is an adaptive reaction to a physical threat. Energy at such a time is needed to fight off the threat. It would be wasteful and risky to spend energy looking for or eating food. The blood supply has been diverted to the muscles to maximize strength and speed, so even if you swallow food, you may not be able to digest or absorb it efficiently. (In a severe upset, the stomach and intestines will even reject solid food. Vomiting and diarrhea are their way of disposing of a burden they can't handle.) All of this means that it is poor advice to tell someone under severe stress to eat. He or she can't. And if the person forces him or herself to eat, the person cannot assimilate what he or she has eaten.

On the other hand, fasting is itself a stress on the body, and the longer a person goes without eating, the harder it can be to get started again. Thus, fasting can be a no-win situation. People often get into a downward spiral once they have let stress affect them to the point where they cannot eat, and not eating makes it harder for them to handle the stress. It is therefore desirable not to let stress become so overwhelming that eating becomes impossible. Managing stress so that it does not overwhelm one is a psychological task, and it may require the help of a counselor.

If you can eat, do so, of course. Take only a little, if that is all you can handle, and eat more often to keep meeting your energy and nutrient needs. Choose a variety of foods. Drink fluids, too, but not too much with meals. Drinking too much water with your meals can make you feel full faster and cause you to cut back on the amount of food you eat. Try to drink water and other fluids between meals. Although your body conserves fluids during stress, it will excrete what it does not need, and by taking in water, you enable your kidneys to excrete the sodium they might otherwise have to retain.

• What if I choose not to eat during stressful times?

If you choose not to eat at all while under stress, you will deplete your body of vital nutrients. Aside from the protein, calcium, and potassium already mentioned, the nutrients most susceptible to this depletion are the vitamins and minerals that are not stored in substantial quantities. You may already be aware that the water-soluble vitamins (B vitamins and vitamir C) fall into this category. But do you know that about two dozen minerals also fall into this category? When the question arises whether you should take vitamin supplements during periods of stress, the answer should probably be yes if you can't eat—but not just vitamin supplements. Take a vitamin-mineral preparation that supplies a balanced assortment of all the nutrients that you might need, not in megadoses, but in amounts comparable to the RDA. Refer to the Nutrition Action feature in Chapter 6 for information on selecting a well-balanced vitamin and mineral supplement.

• What causes some people to overeat during times of stress?

While some people can't eat under stress, others get the munchies. One possible explanation is that as carbohydrate is drawn from body stores and the body fails to use it up by exercising, it becomes stored as body fat. The net effect is that body carbohydrate stores are used up. When your circulating blood carbohydrate levels (known as blood sugar) fall, you get hungry. If stress empties your body stores of carbohydrate and your blood glucose levels fall, you will get hungrier sooner than you should.

Another possibility is that the behavior of eating helps to relieve stress by occupying the nervous system with a familiar activity that discharges its nerves without doing them harm, as fighting might do.[49] It may be that eating—or the food eaten—leads to the release of substances in the brain that are experienced as soothing. Much remains to be learned about stress-induced eating. The person who is caught up in this behavior and who is prone to obesity because of it would be well advised to find an alternative

Miniglossary

Stress any threat to a person's well-being. The threat may be physical or psychological, desired or feared, but the reaction is always the same.

Stress response the body's response to stress, mediated by both nerves and hormones initially; begins with an alarm reaction, proceeds through a stage of resistance, and then leads to recovery or, if prolonged, to exhaustion.

behavior with which to respond to stress—exercising, strolling, window shopping, gardening, listening to music, talking with others, or other relaxing, non-food-related activities.

● Any advice on the psychological part of handling stress?

Although this is outside our province, perhaps a word or two would not be amiss. A clue to the management of stress comes from the fact that it is not the stressful event itself, but your reaction to the event that determines how much stress the event will cause. Remember, stress is defined as anything you *perceive* as a threat to your status quo. Psychological counselors urge that you learn stress management techniques to help get you through the disruptive changes in your life. They suggest that you:

- *Change how you perceive the event.* View the event as one you can handle and as an opportunity to learn from instead of a disaster that you can't cope with.
- *Express yourself.* Air your feelings so that you will be less tense.
- *Take time out.* Meet your need for relief from pain, sadness, anxiety, or anger by exercising or using relaxation techniques.
- *Expand your social support system.* Much that is exhausting and painful to handle alone is easier to manage when you have understanding from a circle of supportive friends and helpers.

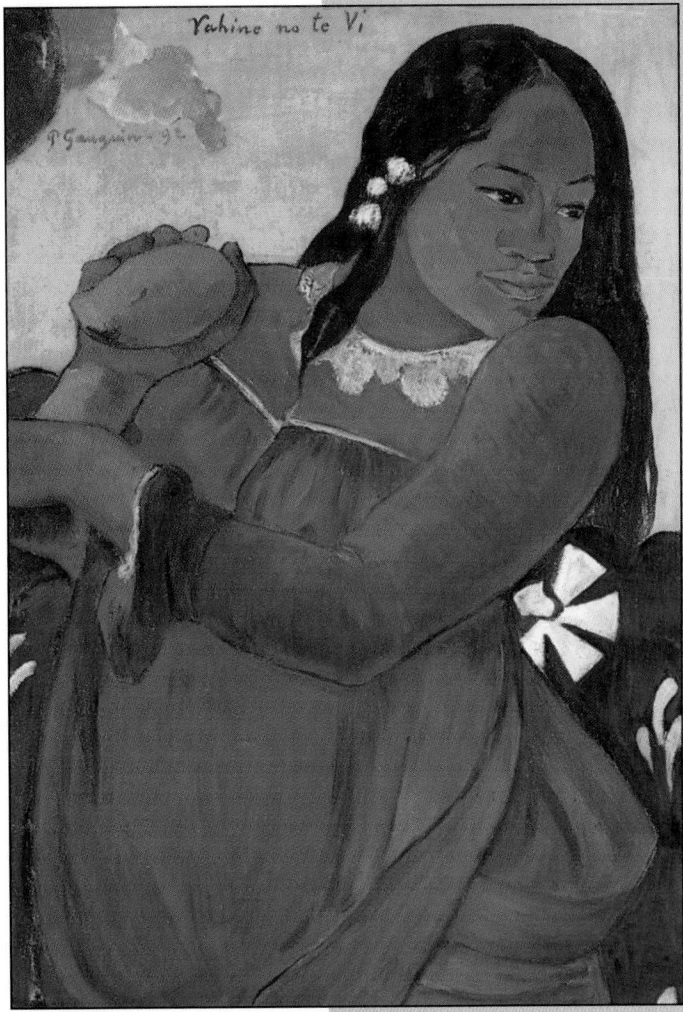

> *Nutrition undergirds the quality of life throughout the human life cycle: it supports the right to be well born; it ensures optimum growth and development; it maintains productive adulthood; it cushions and enriches old age.*
>
> *—S. R. Williams*

Vahine No Te Vi *(Woman of the Mango) by Paul Gauguin, The Baltimore Museum of Art: The Cone Collection, formed by Dr. Claribel Cone and Miss Etta Cone of Baltimore, Maryland. BMA 1950-213.*

CHAPTER 10
The Life Cycle: Conception Through Adulthood

Contents

Ask Yourself . . . ?

Which of these statements about nutrition are true, and which are false? For the false statements, what *is* true?

1. The poor nutrition of a woman during her pregnancy can impair the health of her grandchild, even after that child has grown up.
2. A woman needs twice as many calories per day in late pregnancy as she did before she was pregnant.
3. Even one alcoholic beverage, if taken at the wrong time during pregnancy, can damage the development of the nervous system in the unborn infant.
4. If a woman craves a food during pregnancy, it is probably because she instinctively knows that she needs the nutrients in that food.
5. Substances in a mother's milk can protect the breastfeeding infant against diseases to which the mother has been exposed.
6. If a child loses his or her appetite, the caretaker must insist that the child eat his or her meals anyway, because it is bad for a growing child to go without food.
7. School lunch is designed to provide all of the nutrients schoolchildren need in a day.
8. For older adults, the most important nutrient is water.
9. Caffeine is fine for young adults, but older people may suffer anxiety attacks if they ingest too much caffeine.
10. When you drink alcohol, your body loses water.

Answers: 1. True. 2. False. A woman needs only 15 percent more calories per day during pregnancy than she did before. 3. True. 4. False. Women's cravings during pregnancy do not seem to reflect real physiological needs. 5. True. 6. False. A child's appetite regulates food intake to meet need; caretakers should not force food on children, because this will only create conflict. 7. False. School lunch is designed to provide one-third of the nutrients schoolchildren need in a day. 8. True. 9. False. Too much caffeine can cause anxiety attacks in individuals of any age, even children. 10. True.

By the time you are 65 years old, you will have eaten about 100,000 pounds of food. Each bite may or may not have brought with it the nutrients you needed. The impact of the food you have eaten, together with your lifestyle habits, accumulates over a lifetime, and people who have lived and eaten differently all their lives are in widely different states of health by the time they reach 65.

Nutrition shares with other lifestyle factors the responsibility for maintaining good health. The complete prescription for good health presented in Chapter 1 reads as follows: get regular sleep; eat regular meals; maintain desirable weight; don't smoke; drink alcohol moderately or not at all; and get regular exercise. Nutrition is represented by three of the six items in this list—one-half of the total. A person who abides by all six practices can expect by later midlife to be physiologically 30 years younger than a person who abides by few or none of them.[1] If you subscribe to the view that your job is to accept the things you can't control and control the things you can, your nutritional health falls in the second category and deserves your conscientious attention.

The effects of nutrition extend from one generation to the next, and this is particularly evident during pregnancy. Research has demonstrated that the poor nutrition of a woman during her early pregnancy can impair the health of her *grandchild,* even after that child has become an adult.[2] A woman should attend to her nutrition even before she becomes pregnant: if she needs supplementation, she should be taking a supplement; if she is underweight or overweight, she should try to gain or lose weight before she becomes pregnant to maximize her chances of having a healthy baby.

Similarly—to give but two of dozens of possible examples—the nutrition of a girl in her teens will help determine the soundness of her skeleton when she is 80 years old, and the nutrition of a boy in his teens will affect his chances of contracting heart disease decades later. This chapter follows people through the life cycle and attends to their special nutritional needs at each stage.

Pregnancy: Nutrition for the Future

The only way nutrients can reach the developing fetus in the uterus is through the **placenta**, the special organ that grows inside the uterus to support the new life (see Figure 10–1). If the mother's nutrient stores are inadequate early in pregnancy when the placenta is developing, the fetus will develop poorly, no matter how well the mother eats later. After getting such a poor start on life, a girl child may grow up poorly equipped to support a normal pregnancy, and she, too, may bear a poorly developed infant.

Infants born of malnourished mothers are more likely than healthy women's infants to become ill, to have birth defects, and to suffer retarded mental or physical development. This remains true even if they later receive abundant, nourishing food. Among the many growth-retarded Korean orphans adopted by U.S. families after the Korean War, for example, several years of catch-up growth occurred but did not completely remedy the growth deficits caused by early malnutrition.[3] Malnutrition in the **prenatal** and early **postnatal** periods also affects learning ability and behavior. Clearly, it is critical to provide the best nutrition at the early stages of life.

Placenta (pla-SEN-tuh) the organ inside the uterus in which the mother's and fetus's circulatory systems intertwine and in which exchange of materials between maternal and fetal blood takes place. The fetus receives nutrients and oxygen across the placenta; the mother's blood picks up carbon dioxide and other waste materials to be excreted via her lungs and kidneys.

Prenatal prior to birth.

Postnatal after birth.

Most severe risk factors for malnutrition in pregnancy:

Age 15 or under.
Unwanted pregnancy.
Many pregnancies close together.
History of poor outcome.
Poverty.
Food faddism.
Heavy smoking.
Drug addiction.
Alcohol abuse.
Chronic disease requiring special diet.
More than 15% underweight.
More than 15% overweight.

These factors at the start of pregnancy indicate that poor nutrition is very likely to be present and to affect the pregnancy adversely.

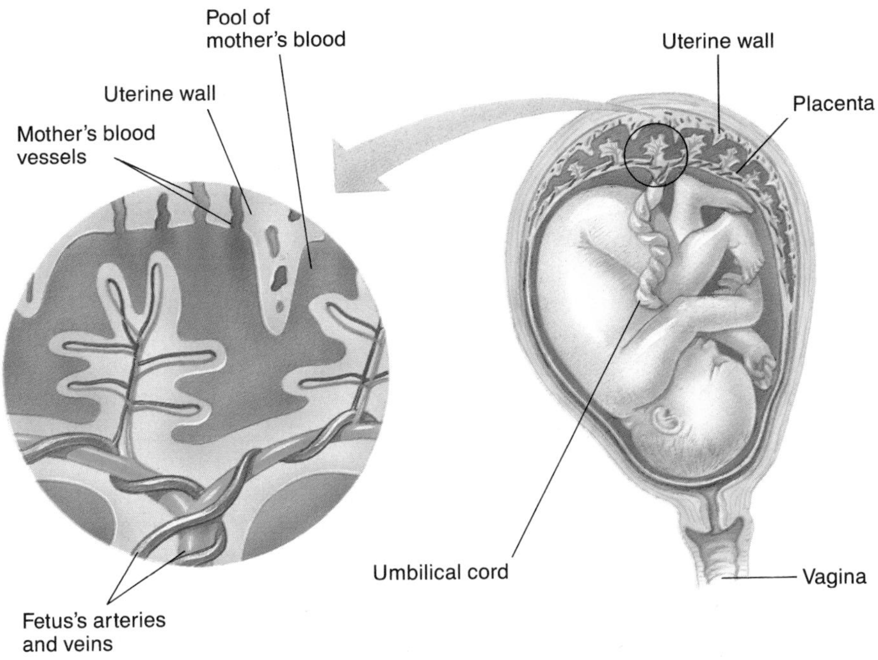

Figure 10–1

The Placenta

The placenta is a sort of pillow of tissue in which maternal blood vessels lie side by side with fetal blood vessels entering it through the umbilical cord. This close association between the two circulatory systems permits the mother's bloodstream to deliver nutrients and oxygen to the fetus and to carry away fetal waste products.

Pregnancy Readiness Scorecard

Are you nutritionally ready for pregnancy? Score each question as shown. A score of 15 is perfect; scores below 3 per question identify areas that need improvement.

1. My body weight is desirable for my height, according to the standards given in this book.
   a. Right on target — 3 points
   b. Within 10% — 2 points
   c. 10% to 20% above — 1 point
   d. More than 20% above or 20% below — 0 points

2. I drink milk and use milk products every day.
   a. Equivalent of 3 c or more a day — 3 points
   b. About 2 c a day — 2 points
   c. About 1 c a day — 1 point
   d. No milk or milk products — 0 points

3. I eat vegetables and fruits daily.
   a. Four servings a day — 3 points
   b. Three servings a day — 2 points
   c. Two servings a day — 1 point
   d. One or fewer servings a day — 0 points

4. I eat iron-rich foods, such as meats or legumes, daily.
   a. Two servings, or enough to meet the RDA — 3 points
   b. One serving, or enough to meet about half the RDA — 1 point
   c. Less than one serving, or less than half the RDA — 0 points

5. I am physically fit, because I have a well-established habit of exercising daily or every other day, and I will be able to continue exercising during pregnancy.
   a. I am as fit as I can be. — 3 points
   b. I am fairly fit. — 2 points
   c. I am not fit. — 0 points

Ideally, a woman will start pregnancy at a healthful weight and with the firmly established habit of eating a balanced and varied diet. The Pregnancy Readiness Scorecard permits women to evaluate their nutritional readiness for pregnancy and to identify the eating habits that might need improvement.

Weight Gain

The average pregnant woman needs to gain between 25 and 35 pounds during her pregnancy. Her infant at birth will weigh only about 6 to 8 pounds, but the body tissues the mother builds (blood, blood vessels, muscle, fat stores, and others) to provide a healthful environment for the infant's development weigh more than 16 pounds (see Table 10–1). If the woman is a growing teenager or is overly thin to begin with, she needs to gain more; if she is obese at the start of pregnancy, she still should gain at least 16 to 24 pounds, for less would jeopardize the development process. Weight gain should be at its lowest during the first **trimester** and should steadily increase, with the most weight gained in the third trimester, when the fetus and placenta are growing the most. If a woman gains more than the expected amount of weight early in pregnancy, she should not try to diet in the last weeks. (Dieting during pregnancy is not recommended.) Women have been known to gain up to 60 pounds in pregnancy without negative effects. (A *sudden* large weight gain, however, is a danger signal that may indicate the onset of **pregnancy-induced hypertension (PIH)**; a woman experiencing this type of weight gain should see her health care provider.)

Most of the weight a woman gains in pregnancy is lost at delivery. For the woman who has gained the recommended 25 to 35 pounds, the remainder is generally lost within a few months as her blood volume returns to normal and she loses the fluids she has accumulated.

Trimester a normal pregnancy (38 to 42 weeks) is divided into 3 periods of 13 to 14 weeks, called trimesters.

Pregnancy-induced hypertension (PIH), formerly known as **toxemia (tox-EEM-ee-uh)** a cluster of symptoms seen in pregnancy, including edema, hypertension, and kidney complications. A variety of terms are associated with PIH. Most common is **eclampsia;** its symptoms include convulsions and coma, associated with high blood pressure, edema, and protein in the urine. Eclampsia may be preceded by **pre-eclampsia,** from mild to severe.

Nutrient Needs

A woman's nutrient needs during pregnancy are much higher than usual, but her energy needs are not. An increase of only 15 percent of maintenance calories is recommended—just enough to spare the protein she eats for its all-important tissue-building work. However, protein, vitamin, and mineral needs increase twofold or more. Most women are already eating enough protein to cover the increased demand of pregnancy—from about 45 grams in a nonpregnant woman to about 60 grams per day for a pregnant woman—but their carbohydrate, vitamin, and mineral intakes might not be ample.

Carbohydrate should provide about 50 percent to 60 percent of total food energy. Think for a moment what that means: in a 2,000 calorie-per-day intake, this would represent at least 1,000 calories from carbohydrate, or about 250 grams. Four cups of milk a day would contribute about 50 grams of carbohydrate, an apple provides 15 grams of carbohydrate, and a slice of bread provides 15 grams. This recommendation implies many servings of fruits, vegetables, legumes, and breads.

The pregnant woman's recommended folate intake is more than twice that of the nonpregnant woman due to the large increase in her blood volume and the rapid growth of the fetus.* Folate needs can be met by a well-selected diet. Therefore, the routine use of a folate supplement is not recommended, unless the physician has reason to believe the pregnant woman's folate intake is low.

Among the minerals, those involved in building the fetus's skeleton—calcium, phosphorus, and magnesium—are in great demand during pregnancy, and increases of about 50 percent over pre-pregnancy needs are recommended. Intestinal absorption of calcium doubles early in pregnancy, and the mineral is stored in the mother's bones. Later, the mother's bone stores give up their calcium as the fetal bones begin to calcify. The mother whose calcium intake is less than 1,200 milligrams per day will lose more calcium from her bones than she has stored to support fetal bone growth.[4]

Calcification of the baby's teeth begins in the fifth month after conception; 32 teeth are well along in development before birth. Children whose mothers have received adequate fluoride during pregnancy have teeth that are more decay free at 5 to 9 years of age than other children have.[5] If the drinking water is not fluoridated, a physician-prescribed supplement may be desirable.

The body conserves iron even more than usual during pregnancy: menstruation ceases, and absorption of iron increases up to threefold. However, the developing fetus draws on its mother's iron stores to create stores of its own to carry it through the first three to six months of life. Additional iron is needed due to the increase in maternal blood volume by as much as 50 percent. This drain on the mother's supply may precipitate a deficiency; furthermore, the mother loses blood when she gives birth. Since few women enter pregnancy with adequate iron stores to meet these demands, an iron supplement throughout pregnancy may be beneficial.[6]

Because energy needs increase less than nutrient needs, the pregnant woman must select foods of high nutrient density. A woman who already eats

*In certain studies folate has been shown to be important in preventing neural tube defects, such as spina bifida.

Table 10–1

An Example of the Pregnant Woman's Weight Gain

DEVELOPMENT	WEIGHT GAIN (lb)
Infant at birth	7½
Placenta	1
Increase in mother's blood volume to supply placenta	4
Increase in size of mother's uterus and the muscles to support it	2½
Increase in size of mother's breasts	3
Fluid to surround infant in amniotic sac	2
Mother's fat stores	5 to 10
Total	25 to 30

Note: The pattern of gain should be about a pound a month for the first three months and a pound a week thereafter. Different patterns of weight gain are suggested for underweight, normal-weight, and overweight women, described by E. McCarthy, Report of a Montreal Diet Dispensary experience, *Journal of the Canadian Dietetic Association* 44 (1983): 71–75.

Foods containing folate:
green, leafy vegetables
legumes (dried beans, peas, and lima beans)
orange juice and cantaloupe
other vegetables
whole-wheat products

Foods containing calcium:
Four cups of milk a day will supply 1,200 mg of calcium. (For other food sources, see Chapter 7.) The milk should be fortified with vitamin D; if it is not, a vitamin D supplement may be needed.

Food sources of iron:
red meat, fish, and other meat
dried fruits
legumes
dark green vegetables

Iron supplementation in the form of thirty milligrams of ferrous iron is recommended for pregnant women. This iron supplement should be taken daily between meals or at bedtime on an empty stomach during the second and third trimesters.

For high-risk pregnant women—that is, those who are carrying twins, who smoke cigarettes, or who abuse drugs—a generally low-dose vitamin-mineral supplement may be appropriate. A multivitamin-mineral supplement may benefit pregnant women who do not consume an adequate diet, despite dietary counseling.

Low birthweight (LBW) a birthweight of 5 1/2 lb (2,500 g) or less, used as a predictor of poor health in the newborn and as a probable indicator of poor nutrition status of the mother during and/or before pregnancy. Normal birthweight is 6 1/2 lb or more. Low-birthweight infants are of two different types. Some are **premature;** they are born early (prior to 38 weeks of gestation) and are the right size for their gestational age. Others have suffered growth failure in the uterus; they may or may not be born early, but they are **small for gestational age (small for date).**

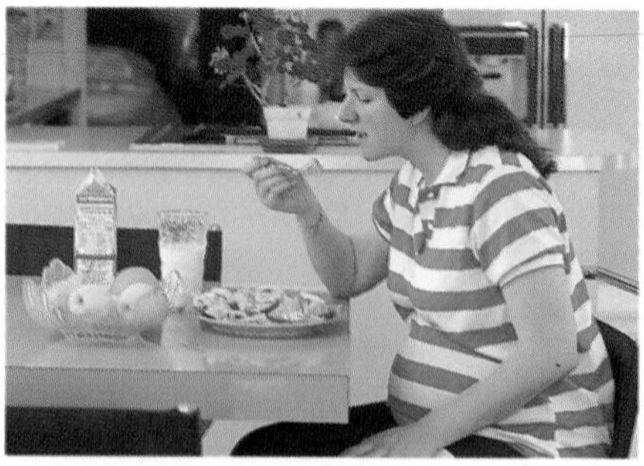

Adequate nutrition prior to conception and during pregnancy helps ensure the health of both the mother and the fetus.

well can simply increase her servings of nutritious foods to meet her increasing nutrient needs. For most women, appropriate choices include foods like nonfat milk, cottage cheese, lean meats, legumes, eggs, dark green vegetables, whole-grain breads and cereals, and generous quantities of vitamin C-rich foods. A suggested food pattern is shown in Table 10–2.

If the mother does not receive adequate nourishment and does not gain the full recommended amount of weight, she may give birth to a baby of **low birthweight (LBW).** Not all small babies are unhealthy, but birthweight and length of gestation are the primary indicators of an infant's future health status. Nutritional deficiency, coupled with low birthweight, is the underlying or associated cause of more than half of all the deaths, worldwide, of children under five years old.

Practices to Avoid

Some nutritional practices should be avoided during pregnancy, but some have an undeserved bad reputation. One or two cups of coffee or tea a day or the equivalent is probably within safe limits (see the Nutrition Action feature regarding caffeine later in the chapter). A general guideline can be offered: eat a varied, balanced diet that meets the Dietary Guidelines and practice moderation. Some practices are truly harmful, and their potential impact is too great to risk.

One such harmful practice is smoking. Smoking restricts the blood supply to the growing fetus and so limits the delivery of nutrients and removal of wastes. It stunts growth, thus increasing the risk of retarded development and complications at birth.

Dieting, even for short periods, is also hazardous. Low-carbohydrate diets or fasts that cause ketosis deprive the fetus's growing brain of needed glucose and cause congenital deformity. Most serious may be the invisible effects. For example, carbohydrate metabolism may be rendered permanently defective, or the infant's brain may be permanently damaged. Protein deprivation can

Table 10–2

Food Guides for Pregnant and Lactating Women

	NUMBER OF SERVINGS		
FOOD[a]	Nonpregnant Woman	Pregnant Woman[b]	Lactating Woman
Protein foods	2	2 (2 +)	2
Milk and milk products	2	4 (4 +)	4
Enriched or whole-grain breads and cereals	4	4 (5 to 6)	4
Vitamin C-rich fruits and vegetables	1	1 (1 +)	1
Dark green vegetables	1	1	1
Other fruits and vegetables	2	2 (2 +)	2

[a]See Table 2–6 in Chapter 2 for details on serving sizes and food sources.
[b]Numbers in parentheses indicate numbers of servings recommended for the pregnant teenager.

cause children's height and head circumference to diminish markedly and irreversibly. Iron deficiency during pregnancy in animals has been seen to alter their brains permanently.

Most important, drinking alcohol during pregnancy—even as few as 1 or 2 drinks a day—can cause irreversible brain damage and mental and physical retardation in the fetus (**fetal alcohol syndrome**, or **FAS**). The most severe impact of maternal drinking is likely to be in the first month, before the woman even is sure she is pregnant. About 1 in every 750 children born in the United States is a victim of this preventable damage, the leading known cause of mental retardation in the United States.[7]

Fetal alcohol syndrome (FAS) the cluster of symptoms seen in an infant or child whose mother consumed excess alcohol during her pregnancy; includes mental and physical retardation with facial and other body deformities.

Oxygen is indispensable on a minute-to-minute basis to the development of the fetus's central nervous system, and a sudden dose of alcohol can halt the delivery of oxygen through the umbilical cord. During the first month of pregnancy, the fetal brain is growing at the rate of 100,000 new brain cells a minute, so even a few minutes of such deprivation can have a major effect. Birth defects, low birthweight, and spontaneous abortions occur more often in pregnancies of women who drink even as little as 2 ounces of alcohol daily during pregnancy. Accumulating evidence that even one drink may be too much has led the *Journal of the American Medical Association* to take the position that women should stop drinking as soon as they *plan* to become pregnant.[8] Experiments using animals have even shown that alcohol in the female *before fertilization* may damage the outcome of pregnancy.[9]

As a result of findings like these, the following position seems justified:

- The pregnant woman who drinks is more likely to give birth to a baby with FAS defects.
- The woman who is pregnant should not drink.
- The woman who is addicted to alcohol should be advised to avoid pregnancy at all costs.[10]

We might add that it is important for a woman who drinks heavily during the first two-thirds of her pregnancy to know that she can still prevent some damage by stopping heavy drinking during the third trimester.[11]

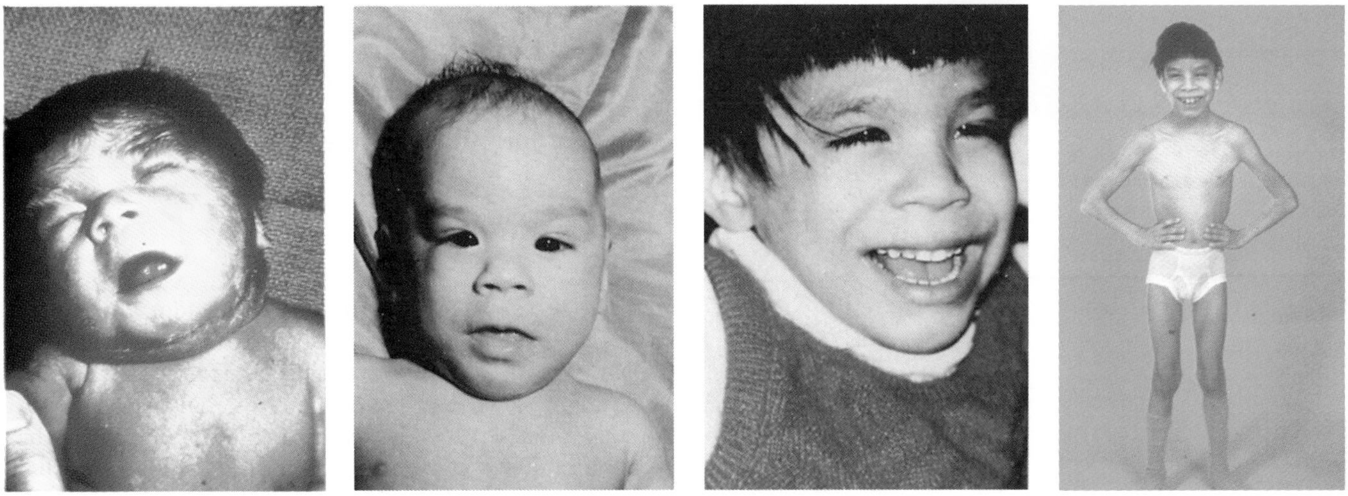

These facial traits reflect fetal alcohol syndrome, caused by maternal drinking. Irreversible abnormalities of the brain and internal organs accompany these surface features.

Drugs other than alcohol, taken during pregnancy, can also cause birth defects. A particularly dramatic example is the acne medication Accutane (isotretinoin), which causes major deformities during fetal development. Pregnant women should avoid taking all drugs except on the advice of their physicians.

Common Problems of Pregnancy

Common physical problems in pregnancy include "morning" (actually, any time) sickness and, later, constipation. The nausea of morning sickness seems unavoidable because it arises from the hormonal changes taking place early in pregnancy, but it can sometimes be alleviated. A strategy some expectant mothers have found effective in quelling nausea is to start the day with a few sips of water and a few nibbles of a soda cracker or other bland carbohydrate food to get something in their stomachs before getting out of bed. Carbonated beverages also may help between meals.

Later, as the hormones of pregnancy alter her muscle tone and the thriving infant crowds her intestinal organs, an expectant mother may complain of constipation. A high-fiber diet, plentiful water intake, and moderate exercise will help to relieve this condition. Laxatives should be used only if the physician orders them.

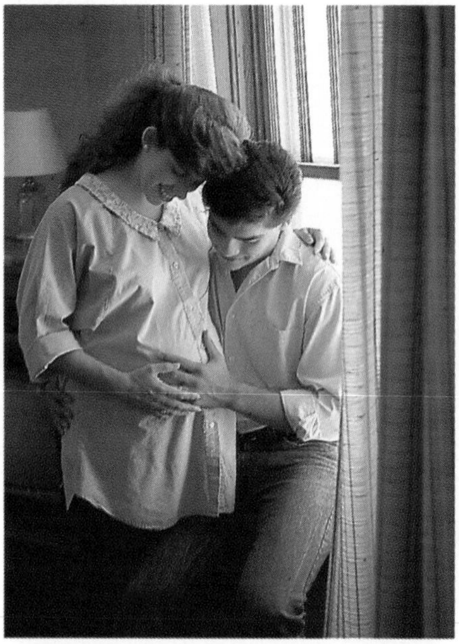

The pregnant woman, like all people, thrives on support, understanding, and love.

Pregnancy for many women is a time of adjustment to major changes. The woman who is expecting a baby is a growing person in more ways than one. Not only her physical needs but also her emotional needs are changing. If it is her first baby, she senses that her lifestyle will change as she takes on the new responsibility of caring for a child. Ideally, she will be encouraged to develop this sense of responsibility by caring for herself during pregnancy. The expectant mother needs support in thinking of herself as a thoroughly worthwhile and important person with a new and challenging task that she can and will perform well. Oftentimes, as a young adult, she is still working out her relationship with her partner; and they both know that the coming of a first baby will affect that relationship profoundly. There is a need for sensitive communication and understanding on both parts in this time of transition.

Women's cravings during pregnancy do not seem to reflect real physiological needs. People should not laugh at women going through this major experience and should recognize the validity of these women's feelings. If a woman craves pickles and chocolate sauce at 2 o'clock in the morning for example, it is probably not because she lacks a combination of nutrients uniquely supplied by these foods. She is, however, expressing a need as real and as important as her need for nutrients—the need for support, understanding, and love.

Milk for the Infant

Toward the end of her pregnancy, a woman needs to decide whether to breastfeed her baby or not. If she plans to breastfeed, she should begin to prepare so that she can get started smoothly. It is wise ahead of time to read a handbook on breastfeeding, talk with other women who have successfully breastfed their babies, and seek family and medical support. Ideally, the mother and a partner can attend classes together before the baby is born that will provide basic information regarding breastfeeding.

Breastfeeding

Breastfeeding has both emotional and physical advantages. Emotional **bonding** is facilitated by many events and behaviors of mother and infant during the early months and years; one of the first can be breastfeeding, beginning right after birth. Since a critical event in bonding, thought to be mediated by chemical messengers in breast milk, may occur in the first 45 minutes after birth, this may be an especially important feeding time.[12]

During the first two or three days of lactation, the breasts produce **colostrum**, a premilk substance containing antibodies and white cells from the mother's blood. Colostrum is sterile as it leaves the breast, and the baby cannot contract a bacterial infection from it even if the mother has one. Because it contains immunity factors, colostrum helps protect the newborn infant from those infections against which the mother has developed immunity—precisely those in the environment against which the infant needs protection. Entering the infant's body with the milk, these antibodies inactivate bacteria within the digestive tract, where they could otherwise cause intestinal infections.

Breast milk also contains antibodies, although not as much as colostrum. Colostrum and breast milk also contain a factor (the **bifidus factor**) that favors the growth of the "friendly" bacteria *Lactobacillus bifidus* in the infant's digestive tract so that other, harmful bacteria cannot grow there.

Breast milk is also tailor-made to meet the nutrient needs of the human infant. It offers its carbohydrate in the easy-to-assimilate form of lactose; its fat contains a generous proportion of the essential fatty acid linoleic acid; and its protein in a form the human infant can easily digest. Its vitamin contents are ample. Even vitamin C, for which cow's milk is not a good source, is supplied generously by breast milk.

As for minerals, calcium, phosphorus, and magnesium are present in amounts appropriate for the rate of growth expected in a human infant, and breast milk is low in sodium. Breast milk contains special factors that favor absorption of the iron and zinc it contains.

Powerful agents against bacterial infection also occur in breast milk. Among them is **lactoferrin**, an iron-grabbing compound that keeps bacteria from getting the iron they need to grow on, helps absorb iron into the infant's bloodstream, and works directly to kill some bacteria.

Other factors in breast milk include several enzymes, several hormones, lipids that protect the infant against infection, and a morphinelike compound for which there are corresponding receptors in the infant's brain.[13] Much remains to be learned about the composition and characteristics of human milk, but clearly it is a very special substance.

Breastfeeding provides other benefits. It protects against allergy development during the vulnerable first few weeks; the act of suckling favors normal tooth and jaw alignment; and breastfed babies are less likely to be obese because they are less likely to be overfed. Some studies suggest that mothers who breastfeed are less likely to develop breast cancer and to form unwanted clots in the bloodstream after delivery. A woman who wants to breastfeed can derive justification and satisfaction from all these advantages.

Under most circumstances, a woman can freely choose to feed breast milk or formula, knowing that the two modes of feeding are equally beneficial to the infant. However, if the infant is premature, or if other factors act to the

Bonding the formation of an emotional and physical tie between parent and infant.

Colostrum (co-LAHS-trum) a milklike secretion from the breast, rich in protective factors, present during the first day or so after delivery and before milk appears.

Bifidus factor (BIFF-id-us) a factor in colostrum and breast milk that favors the growth in the infant's intestinal tract of the "friendly" bacteria *Lactobacillus* (lack-toh-ba-SILL-us) *bifidus* so that other, less-desirable intestinal inhabitants will not flourish.

Lactoferrin (lak-toe-FERR-in) a factor in breast milk that binds iron and keeps it from supporting the growth of the infant's intestinal bacteria.

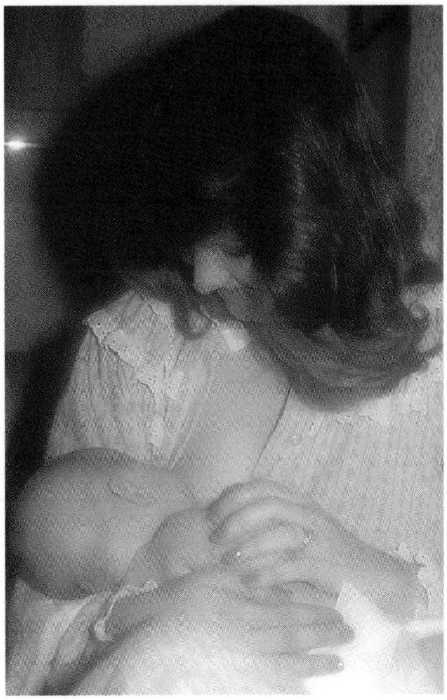

Breast milk is a very special substance.

baby's disadvantage, breastfeeding becomes the preferred choice. Even when separation prevents the mother from breastfeeding, she can express her milk to be given to the infant; the composition of the milk from a premature infant's mother is ideal for the premature infant. Breastfeeding manuals show how to use manual massage or breast pumps to obtain milk. If the mother chooses not to breastfeed, a premature baby can, however, be successfully nourished on special formula for premature infants.

If a woman has a communicable disease such as AIDS, tuberculosis, or hepatitis, or if she must take medication that is secreted in breast milk and is known to affect the infant, she must not breastfeed. Drug addicts—including alcohol abusers—are capable of ingesting such high doses that their infants can become addicts by way of breast milk. In such cases, breastfeeding is also contraindicated.

Most prescription drugs do not reach nursing infants in sufficiently large quantities to affect them adversely. As a precaution, a nursing mother should consult with the prescribing physician prior to taking any drug. Minimal use of alcohol is compatible with breastfeeding. Smoking between feedings is permissible, although it is desirable not to expose an infant to secondhand smoke in the air. Coffee drinking is fine in moderation (2 to 3 cups of coffee a day), as is the eating of foods such as garlic and spices. A particular food may affect the baby's liking for the mother's milk; this is a matter that requires individual detective work. (Examples are chocolate for some babies, excess caffeine for others, and foods that cause gas in the mother for still others.) If a woman has an ordinary cold, she can go on nursing without worry. The infant may well catch it from her anyway but may actually be less susceptible than a bottle-fed baby would be, thanks to the immunologic protection offered by breast milk.

A woman sometimes hesitates to breastfeed because she has heard that environmental contaminants may enter her milk and harm her baby. The decision whether to breastfeed on this basis might best be made after consulting with a physician or dietitian familiar with the local environment or with the state health department.

Feeding Formula

The substitution of formula feeding for breastfeeding involves copying nature as closely as possible. The milk of humans and that of cows differ: cow's milk is significantly higher in protein, calcium, and phosphorus, for example, to support the calf's faster growth rate. But a formula for human babies can be prepared from cow's milk that does not differ significantly from human milk in these respects. The formula makers first dilute the milk and then add carbohydrate and nutrients to make the formula nutritionally comparable to human milk.

The antibodies in cow's milk do not protect the human baby from disease (they protect the calf from cattle diseases), but the high level of preventive medical care (vaccinations) and public health measures achieved in developed countries, especially the United States and Canada, make this consideration less important than it was in the past. Safety and sanitation can be achieved with either mode of feeding by the educated mother whose drinking water supply is reliable.

Like the breastfeeding mother, the woman who offers formula to her baby has reasons for making her choice, and her feelings should be honored.

Bearing and nurturing a baby involves much more than merely nursing it. The mother and her baby can benefit in many ways from the supportive approval of those around them.

One of the major advantages of formula feeding is that gained by the mother whose attempts at breastfeeding have met with frustration. Formula provides adequate nourishment for the infant, and a mother can choose this alternative with confidence. Other advantages:

- The parents can see that the baby is getting enough milk during feedings.
- The mother can offer similar closeness, warmth, and stimulation during feedings as the breastfeeding mother does.
- Other family members can get close to the baby and develop a warm relationship in feeding sessions.

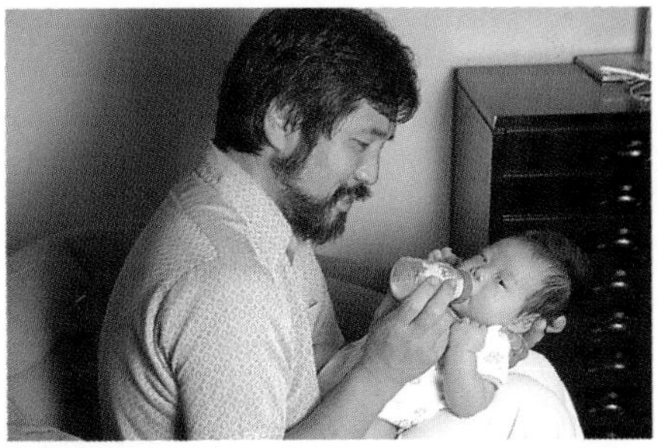
Formula feeding allows other family members to enjoy feeding the infant.

Many mothers breastfeed at first and then wean within the first one to six months. A few weeks of breastfeeding significantly reduce the likelihood of the baby's developing an allergy to cow's milk and confer on the baby the immunologic protection of breastfeeding during the earliest, critical first few weeks.

When a mother chooses to wean her infant during the first six months of life, it is imperative that she shift to *formula,* not to plain milk of any kind—whole, low-fat, or nonfat. Only formula contains enough iron (to name but one of many, many factors) to support normal development in the baby's first months of life. National and international standards have been set for the nutrient content of infant formulas. The Infant Formula Act of 1980 requires that formulas meet nutrient standards based on the American Academy of Pediatrics (AAP) recommendations; and in 1982, the FDA adopted quality control procedures to be sure that infant formulas do. Formulas that meet the standards are nutritionally similar; small differences in nutrient content are sometimes confusing but not usually important.

For infants with special problems, formulas can be adapted to make them closer in composition to human milk (adjusted protein ratio, lower linoleic acid, lower sodium and other minerals). For premature babies, special premature formulas are available. Special formulas based on soy protein are available for infants allergic to milk protein, and formulas with the lactose replaced can be used for infants with lactose intolerance. For infants with other special needs, many other variations are available.

Once the baby is obtaining at least a third of the total daily food energy from a balanced mixture of cereal, vegetables, fruits, and other foods (usually after six months of age), whole cow's milk fortified with vitamins A and D is acceptable as an accompanying beverage.[14] The AAP recommends introducing cow's milk at six months, but many pediatricians advise continued use of formula throughout the first year because of the iron it provides. In any case, do not offer plain, unmodified cow's milk before six months, because an infant's digestive tract may be sensitive to its protein and, if so, may bleed.

Nutrition of the Breastfeeding Mother

Adequate nutrition of the mother makes a highly significant contribution to successful lactation; without it, lactation is likely to falter or fail. The mother should continue to eat high-quality foods to the end of her pregnancy, not attempt to restrict her weight gain unduly, and plan to enjoy ample food and fluid at frequent intervals.

A nursing mother produces 30 ounces of milk a day on the average, with wide variations possible. The RDA table suggests that 500 calories to support this milk production come from added food and that the rest come from the stores of fat the mother's body has accumulated during pregnancy for this purpose. Table 10–2 showed a food pattern that would meet the lactating woman's nutrient needs.

The period of lactation is the natural time for a woman to lose the extra body fat she accumulated during pregnancy. Once lactation has been established, if her choice of foods is judicious, she can tolerate an energy deficit and a gradual loss of weight (1 pound per week) without any effect on her milk output. Fat can only be mobilized slowly, however, and too large an energy deficit will inhibit lactation. On the other hand, if a mother does not breastfeed, she may not as easily lose the fat she gained during pregnancy.

Supplements for the Infant

Breast milk or formula and the infant's own internal stores will meet most nutrient needs for the first four to six months. Thereafter, the introduction of intelligently chosen juices and foods will normally keep up with the infant's changing requirements. But if the time during which an infant is receiving only milk (either breast milk or formula) is prolonged beyond six months, some supplementation may be appropriate.

Breast milk does not provide enough vitamin D for the infant who has little exposure to sunlight. This is not a problem in the South, but in northern, smoggy, or fogbound cities, vitamin D deficiency in breastfed babies—especially dark-skinned ones—can cause rickets. A light-skinned baby wearing just a diaper in strong summer sun and clear air might make enough vitamin D in 15 to 30 minutes to meet his or her daily need. A dark-skinned baby wrapped up for cold weather in a smoggy city might not make enough even if he or she was outside for several hours. For most babies in most circumstances, some daily exposure of a small amount of skin to the sun will provide a protective dose of vitamin D.

Supplemental fluoride may also be needed if the baby's only source of fluoride is breast milk. The pediatrician should prescribe it if appropriate. Fluoride does not appear to be secreted into breast milk even if the mother's fluoride supply is ample. As for iron, breast milk makes it easily absorbable. When breast milk ceases to be the infant's main food, iron-fortified cereals become important.

For the formula-fed infant, the makeup of the formula determines what further supplementation may be necessary. The pediatrician is the expert to consult on individual needs. In a baby's first six months, the choice of formula is important because whatever is chosen must supply the nutrients of human milk in similar forms and proportions.

Food for the Infant

The growth of infants and children directly reflects their nutritional well-being and is the major indicator of their nutritional status. A baby grows faster during the first year than ever again, tripling its birthweight. Clearly, from the point of view of nutrition, the first year is the most important year

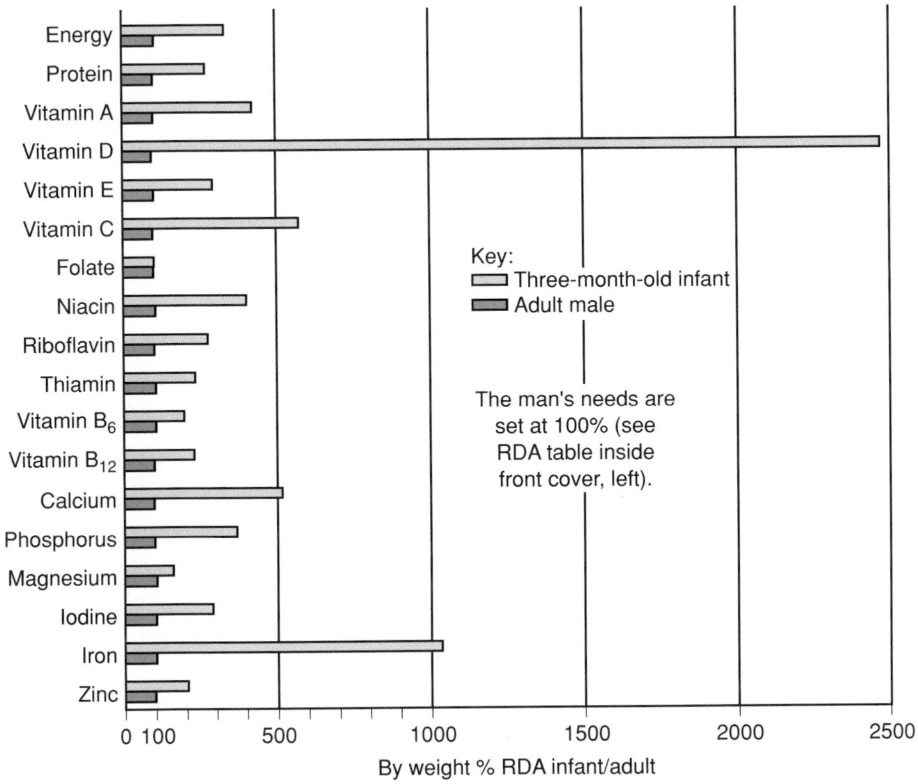

Figure 10–2

Nutrient Recommendations for a Three-Month-Old Infant and an Adult Male, Per Unit of Body Weight

of a person's life. Figure 10–2 compares a three-month-old baby's needs with those of an adult man; as you can see, some of the differences are extraordinary. After six months, energy needs increase less rapidly as the growth rate begins to slow down, but some of the energy saved by slower growth is spent in increased activity.

The most important nutrient of all—for infants as for everyone—is the one easiest to forget: water. The younger a child, the greater the percentage of the body weight is water and the more rapid the turnover. Since proportionately more of the infant's body water than the adult's is between the cells and in the vascular spaces, this water is easy to lose. Conditions that cause fluid loss, such as vomiting, diarrhea, sweating, or normal urinary loss without replacement, can rapidly propel an infant into life-threatening dehydration. Fluid and electrolyte imbalances caused by infection kill more of the world's children than any disease or disaster. Because infants can only cry and cannot tell you what they are crying for, it is important to remember that they may need fluid and to let them drink it until their thirst is quenched.

Iron is the nutrient hardest to provide for infants after weaning from breast milk or formula because its concentration in milk, the infant's major food, is low. By the end of the first year, half or more of all infants are receiving less than the RDA for iron, and one-fourth are receiving less than two-thirds of the RDA. Iron may be the nutrient most needing attention in infant nutrition.

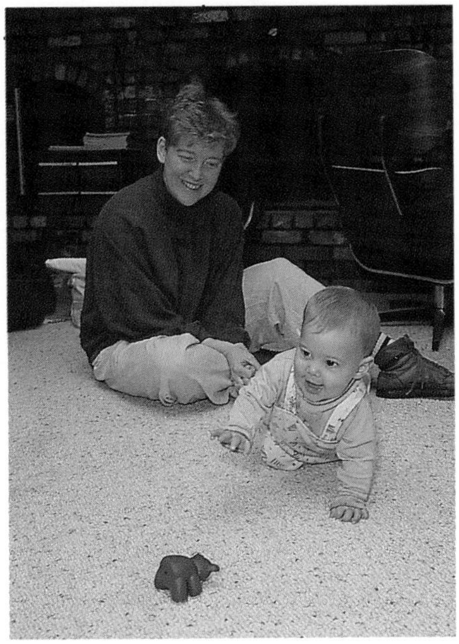

Energy saved by slower growth is spent in increased activity.

The addition of solid foods to a breastfed baby's diet should normally take place between six months and a year. A baby who is formula fed might be started on solid foods gradually beginning at three to four months, depending on readiness. Indications of readiness are:

- When the infant's birthweight has doubled.
- When the infant can consume 8 ounces of formula and still be hungry in less than four hours.
- When the infant is consuming 32 ounces (about 1 liter) of formula a day and wants more.
- When the infant is six months old.

Solids should not be introduced too early, because infants are more likely to develop allergies to them in the early months. But all babies are different, and the program of additions should depend on the individual baby, not on any rigid schedule. Table 10–3 presents a suggested sequence.

The addition of foods to a baby's diet should be governed by three considerations: the baby's nutrient needs, the baby's physical readiness to handle different forms of foods, and the need to detect and control allergic reactions. Nutrients needed early are iron and vitamin C. Juices and fruits that contain vitamin C are usually among the first foods introduced. Since a baby's stored iron supply from before birth runs out after the birthweight doubles, formula with iron, iron-fortified cereals, and, later, meat or meat alternates such as legumes, are recommended.

It has been suggested that the early introduction of sweet fruits to babies' diets might favor their developing a preference for sweets and lessen their liking for vegetables introduced later. To prevent this, the order should perhaps be vegetables first, fruits later. This practice now has a wide following. As for sweets of any other kind, they have no place in a baby's diet. The added food energy they contribute can promote obesity and perhaps the irreversible multiplication of fat cells, but they convey no nutrients to support growth.

Table 10–3

First Foods for the Infant

AGE (months)	ADDITION
4–6	Iron-fortified rice cereal, followed by other cereals (for iron; the baby can swallow and can digest starch now)[a]
5–7	Strained vegetables and/or fruits and their juices,[b] one by one (perhaps vegetables before fruits so the baby will learn to like vegetables' less-sweet flavors)
6–8	Protein foods (cheese, yogurt, tofu, cooked beans, meat, fish, chicken, egg yolk)
9	Finely chopped meat (the baby can chew now), toast, teething crackers (for emerging teeth)
10–12	Whole egg (allergies are less likely now), whole milk

[a]Later you can change cereals, but don't forget to keep on using the iron-fortified varieties.
[b]All baby juices are fortified with vitamin C. Orange juice causes allergies in some babies; apple juice is often recommended as the first juice to feed. Juices should be offered in a cup, not a bottle, to prevent nursing bottle syndrome (a form of tooth decay). (Prolonged sucking on a bottle of milk or juice bathes the upper teeth in a carbohydrate-rich fluid that favors the growth of decay-producing bacteria.)

Physical readiness to handle foods develops in many small steps. For example, the ability to swallow solid food develops at around four to six months, and experience with solid food at that time helps to develop swallowing ability by desensitizing the gag reflex. Later still, when a baby can sit up, can handle finger foods, and is teething, hard crackers and other hard finger foods may be introduced. Such foods promote the development of manual dexterity and control of the jaw muscles. (An infant can choke on these foods, however, so an adult should keep a watchful eye on the learning process.)

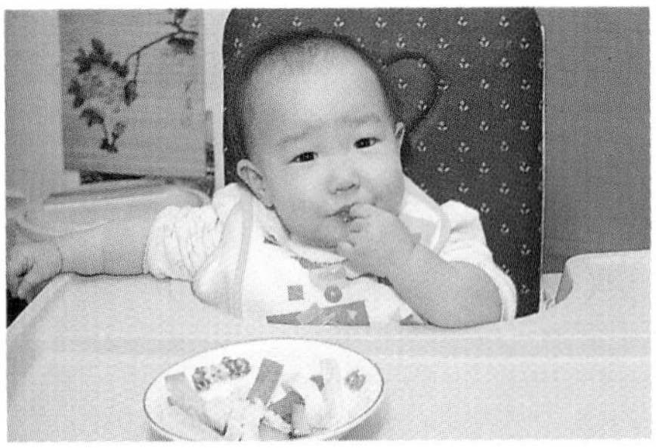

Let infants handle food as they become ready.

Some parents want to feed solids at an earlier age on the theory that "stuffing the baby" at bedtime promotes sleeping through the night. There is no proof for this theory. On the average, babies start to sleep through the night at about the same age regardless of when solid foods are introduced. By three months, 75 percent are sleeping through the night whether or not they are receiving any solid foods.[15]

New foods should be introduced singly to facilitate prompt detection of allergies. For example, when cereals are introduced, try rice cereal first for several days; it causes allergy least often. Try wheat cereal last; it is the most common offender. If a cereal causes irritability due to skin rash, digestive upset, or respiratory discomfort, discontinue its use before going on to the next food. About nine times out of ten, the allergy won't be evident immediately but will manifest itself in vague symptoms occurring up to five days after the offending food is eaten, so it isn't easy to detect. If parents detect allergies in their infant's early life, they can spare the whole family much grief.

As for the choice of foods, baby foods commercially prepared in the United States and Canada are generally safe, nutritious, and of high quality. In response to consumer demand, baby food companies have removed much of the added salt and sugar their products contained in the past, and baby foods also contain few or no additives. They generally have high nutrient density, except for mixed dinners (which contain little meat) and desserts (which are heavily sweetened). An alternative for the parent who wants the baby to have family foods is to "blenderize" a small portion of the table food at each meal. This necessitates cooking without salt, though. Foods adults prepare for themselves often contain much more salt than commercial baby foods. The adults can salt their own food after the baby's portion has been taken. Babies should never be fed canned vegetables; not only is the sodium content too high, but some nutrient value is lost in the canning process. It is also important to take precautions against food poisoning and to avoid the use of vegetables in which nitrites are likely to form—notably, home-prepared carrots, beets, and spinach. Honey should never be fed to infants because of the risk of botulism. Babies and even young children have difficulty swallowing certain foods—popcorn, grapes, bite-size hot dogs, and nuts, for instance. Small round pieces of food should be avoided. An infant can easily choke on these foods; it is not worth the risk to give such foods to infants.

At a year of age, the obvious food to supply most of the nutrients the baby needs is still milk; 2 to 3 1/2 cups a day are now sufficient. More milk than this would displace foods necessary to provide iron and would cause the iron-deficiency anemia known as **milk anemia.** Infants under a year old should not drink low-fat or nonfat milk; they need the fat and vitamins A and D of fortified whole milk until two years of age. The other foods—meat,

Milk anemia iron-deficiency anemia caused by drinking so much milk that iron-rich foods are displaced from the diet.

Table 10–4

Meal Plan for a One-Year-Old

BREAKFAST	SNACK
1 c milk 3 tbsp cereal 2–3 tbsp strained fruit Teething crackers	½ c milk Teething crackers 1 tbsp peanut butter
LUNCH	**SUPPER**
1 c milk 2–3 tbsp vegetables 2 tbsp chopped meat or well-cooked, mashed legumes	1 c milk 1 egg 2 tbsp cereal or potato 2 to 3 tbsp vegetables 2–3 tbsp fruit Teething crackers

Figure 10–3

One-Year-Old and Two-Year-Old

The two-year-old has lost much of the baby fat; the muscles (especially in the back, buttocks, and legs) have firmed and strengthened, and the leg bones have lengthened and increased in density.

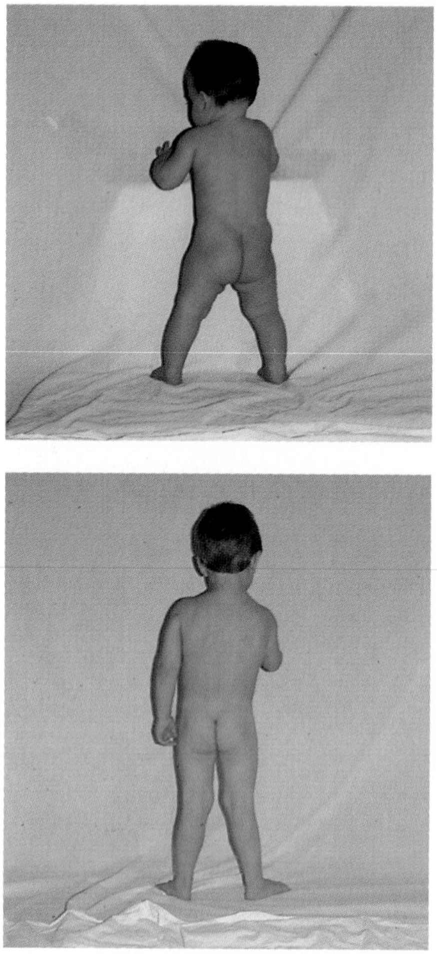

iron-fortified cereal, enriched or whole-grain bread, fruit, and vegetables—should be supplied in variety and in amounts sufficient to round out total energy needs. Ideally, the one-year-old is sitting at the table and eating many of the same foods everyone else eats. A meal plan that meets the requirements for the one-year-old is shown in Table 10–4.

The wise parent of a one-year-old offers nutrition and love together. Both promote growth. It is literally true that "feeding with love" produces better growth in both weight and height of children than feeding the same food in an emotionally negative climate.[16] It also promotes better brain development. The formation of nerve-to-nerve connections in the brain depends both on nutrients and on environmental stimulation.[17]

The person feeding a one-year-old should keep in mind that the baby is also developing eating habits that will persist throughout life. Mealtimes should be relaxed and leisurely. Children should learn to eat slowly, pause and enjoy their table companions, and stop eating when they are full. The "clean your plate" dictum should be stamped out for all time, and in its place, parents who wish to avoid waste should learn to serve smaller portions or teach their children to serve themselves as much as they truly want to eat. Physical activity should be encouraged on a daily basis to promote strong skeletal and muscular development and to establish habits that will undergird good health throughout life.

Early and Middle Childhood

After the age of one, a child's growth rate slows, but the body continues to change dramatically. At one, most babies have just learned to stand and toddle; by two, they can take long strides with solid confidence and are learning to run, jump, and climb. The internal change that makes these new accomplishments possible is the accumulation of a larger mass and greater density of bone and muscle tissue. The changes are obvious in Figure 10–3.

Growth and Nutrient Needs of Children

A one-year-old child needs perhaps 1,000 calories a day; a three-year-old needs only 300 to 500 calories more. Appetite decreases markedly around the age of one year in line with the great reduction in growth rate. Thereafter, the appetite fluctuates; a child will need and demand much more food during periods of rapid growth than during slow periods.

The gradually increasing needs for all nutrients during the growing years are evident from the RDA table and the RNI for Canadians, which list separate averages for each span of three years. To provide these nutrients, the Four Food Group Plan recommends a balance among milk and milk products; eggs, meats, and meat alternates; fruits and vegetables; and breads and cereals (see Table 10–5). Because the serving sizes adjust as the child grows older, these recommendations are good from age two to the teen years.

Table 10–5

Children's Daily Food Pattern for Good Nutrition

FOOD GROUP	SERVINGS PER DAY	AVERAGE SIZE OF SERVING: 1 to 3 Years	4 to 5 Years	6 to 12 Years
Milk and cheese (1 oz cheese = 1 c milk)	4	½–¾ c	¾ c	¾–1 c
Protein foods	2 or more			
Eggs		1	1	1
Lean meat, fish, poultry, legumes		2 tbsp	4 tbsp	2–4 oz
Peanut butter		0–1 tbsp	2 tbsp	2–3 tbsp
Fruits and vegetables	4 (more recommended)			
Vitamin C source (citrus fruits, berries, tomatoes, cabbage, cantaloupe)	1 or more	⅓–½ c	½ c	1 medium orange
Vitamin A source (green or orange fruits/vegetables)	1 or more	2–3 tbsp	4 tbsp (¼ c)	¼–⅓ c
Other vegetables (including potatoes)	2	2–3 tbsp	4 tbsp (¼ c)	⅓–½ c
Other fruits		¼–⅓ c	½ c	1 medium
Cereals (whole grain or enriched)	4 (more recommended)			
Bread, buns, pizza		½–1 slice	1½ slices	1 to 2 slices
Ready-to-eat cereals		½–¾ oz	1 oz	1 oz
Cooked grains (cereals, macaroni, grits, rice)		¼–⅓ c	½ c	½–¾ c
OPTIONAL				
Fats and sugars	These foods can be used to meet energy needs when the required servings of nutritious foods do not. Serving sizes listed here are maximum.			
Butter, margarine, mayonnaise, oils	1	1 tbsp	1 tbsp	2 tbsp
Desserts and sweets (100-cal portions)[a]	1	1–1½ portions	1½ portions	3 portions

[a] ⅓ c pudding or ice cream; 2 to 3 cookies; 1 oz cake; 1⅓ oz pie; or 2 tbsp jelly, jam, honey, or sugar.

Source: Adapted from B. B. Alford and M. L. Bogle, *Nutrition during the Life Cycle* (Englewood Cliffs, N.J.: Prentice-Hall, 1982), pp. 60–61.

After the crucial first year, there is still much a parent can do to foster the development of healthful eating habits. The goal is to teach children to like nutritious foods in all four food categories.

Experimentation with children's food patterns shows that candy, cola, and other concentrated sweets must be limited in a child's diet if the needed nutrients are to be supplied. If such foods are permitted in large quantities, there are only three possible outcomes: nutrient deficiencies, obesity, or both. A child can't be trusted to choose nutritious foods on the basis of taste alone; the preference for sweets is innate. On the other hand, an active child can enjoy the higher-calorie nutritious foods in each category: ice cream or pudding in the milk group and whole-grain cookies in the bread group. These foods, made from milk and grain, carry valuable nutrients and encourage a child to learn, appropriately, that eating is fun.

Children sometimes seem to lose their appetites for a while; this is nothing to worry about. The perfection of appetite regulation in children of normal weight guarantees that such children's energy intakes will be right for each stage of growth. As long as the food energy they do consume is from nutritious foods, they are well provided for. An overzealous parent, however, unaware that a one-year-old is supposed to slow down, may begin a lifelong conflict over food by trying to force more food on the child than the child feels like eating.

Other Factors that Influence Childhood Nutrition

While parents are doing what they can to establish favorable eating behaviors during the transition from infancy to childhood, children in preschool or grade school are encountering foods prepared and served by outsiders. The U.S. government funds several programs to provide nutritious, high-quality meals for children at school. School lunches are designed to meet certain requirements. They must include specified servings of milk, protein-rich foods (meat, cheese, eggs, legumes, or peanut butter), vegetables, fruits, bread or other grain foods, and butter or margarine. They are intended to provide at least a third of the RDA for each of the nutrients, and they are split into several patterns to provide for the nutritional needs of different ages. Coincident with the school lunch program is a program of nutrition education and training (NET program) in all the public schools.[18] Children growing up today need not only to be fed well in the interest of their growth and development but also to learn enough about nutrition to become able to make adaptive food choices when the choices become theirs to make.

Children hear a great deal about foods from the television set. Many authorities are concerned that television commercials may have a less than desirable impact on children. It is estimated that the average child sees more than 21,000 commercials a year, of which approximately half are for sugary foods. Hundreds of millions of dollars are spent in the effort to sell these foods to children.

Most of the concern centers on the issue of sugar. You may recall that not all the public disapproval of sugar is based on scientific findings. There is widespread agreement on one point: sticky, sugary foods left on the teeth provide an ideal environment for the growth of mouth bacteria and the formation of cavities, as the Nutrition Action feature later in the chapter points out. No regulations to prevent the promotion of sticky, sugary foods are in force, however. Parents and health professionals (especially dentists) need to compensate for the misinformation provided by advertisements. To promote dental health, they need to teach children to:

- Brush their teeth, or at least rinse their mouths with water, after meals or snacks.
- Eat foods rich in calcium and phosphorus.
- Eat a variety of firm, fibrous foods to brush over the teeth and stimulate the rinsing action of the salivary glands.
- Brush and floss daily.

Another environmental force affecting children's food choices is the vending machine, especially in schools. The American Dental Association (ADA) would like to eliminate the sale of confections as snacks in schools, but so far it has met with little success. Most progress has been made by way of individual, voluntary initiatives. Experiments have shown that children choose more nutritious snacks if such snacks are offered side by side with sugary foods. When apples are made available in vending machines, children choose chocolate bars less often. When milk is made available, soft drink use drops considerably. As long as such undeniably attractive temptations as cola beverages and candy bars surround children, barriers against their abuse have to be provided by parents and other concerned adults and by teaching the children themselves.

Of all nutritional disorders other than obesity found in U.S. children, the most common is iron-deficiency anemia. It is most prevalent in low-birthweight infants, babies from six months to two years of age, and children and adolescents from low-income families. To ensure adequate iron nutrition, parents should offer an abundance of such iron-rich foods as lean meats, fish, poultry, eggs, and legumes. Grain products should be whole-grain or enriched only, and children should learn to avoid candies, soft drinks, and bakery goods unfortified with iron. Even milk, beneficial as it is, should be limited, because it is a poor iron source; dairy products should be consumed only in the amounts needed to ensure adequate calcium and riboflavin intakes.

It is desirable for children to learn to like nutritious foods in all of the food groups. With one exception, this liking usually develops naturally. The exception is vegetables, which young children frequently dislike and refuse. Even a tiny serving of spinach, cooked carrots, or squash may elicit an expression of disgust. Since most youngsters need to eat more vegetables, parents need to know how to make them appealing to children. Children prefer vegetables that are slightly undercooked and crunchy, attractive in color and shape, and easy to eat. Vegetables should be warm, not hot, because a child's mouth is much more sensitive than an adult's. The flavor should be mild (a child has more taste buds), and smooth foods like mashed potatoes or pea soup should have no lumps in them (a child wonders, with some disgust, what the lumps might be). Irrational as the child's fear of strangeness may seem, the parent must realize that it is practically universal among children and may even have a built-in biological basis.

Little children like to eat at little tables and to be served small portions of food. They also love to eat with other children and have been observed to stay at the table longer and eat much more when in the company of their peers. A bright, unhurried atmosphere free of conflict is also conducive to good appetite. Parents who serve the food in a relaxed and casual manner and without anxiety provide the emotional climate in which a child's negative emotions will be minimized.

Ideally, each meal is preceded, not followed, by the activity the child looks forward to the most. In a number of schools, it has been discovered that children eat a much better lunch if recess occurs before rather than after the meal. With recess after, they are likely to hurry out to play, leaving food on their plates that they were hungry for and would otherwise have eaten. Before sitting down to eat, small children should be helped to wash their hands and faces to decrease the likelihood of contaminating the food with bacteria.

Many little children—both boys and girls—enjoy helping in the kitchen. Their participation provides many opportunities to encourage good food habits. Vegetables are pretty, especially when fresh, and provide opportunities to learn about color, about growing things and their seeds, about shapes and textures—all of which are fascinating to young children. Measuring, stirring, decorating, cutting, and arranging vegetables are skills even a very small child can practice with enjoyment and pride.

When introducing new foods at the table, parents are advised to offer them one at a time—and only a small amount at first. Whenever possible, the new food should be presented at the beginning of the meal, when the child is hungry. If the child is cross, irritable, or feeling sick, don't insist, but withdraw the new food and try it again a few days later. Remember, parents have inclinations and dislikes to which they feel entitled; children should be accorded the same privilege. Never make an issue of food acceptance; a power struggle almost invariably results in a permanently closed mind on the child's part. Rather, let children participate in the planning and preparation of meals. If the beginnings are right, children will grow up with positive feelings toward themselves and the ways they relate to food. Remember too, that parents can act as good role models—enjoying healthful meals and keeping in good physical shape themselves.

The Importance of Teen Nutrition

When children become teenagers, they often assume responsibility for their own food intakes. At the same time, they are intensely involved in day-to-day life with their peers and preparation for their future lives as adults. Few become interested in foods and nutrition except as part of the effort to define themselves such as by way of vegetarianism or crash dieting. Yet the changes that are taking place in their bodies impose tremendous nutrient demands on them. An added need for iron is caused by the onset of menstruation in girls and by the great increase in lean body mass in boys. A rapidly growing, active boy of 15 may need 4,000 calories or more a day just to maintain his weight. At the same time, an inactive girl of the same age, whose growth is nearly at a standstill, may need fewer than 2,000 calories if she is to avoid becoming obese. Thus, there is tremendous variation in the nutrient needs of adolescents.

There is also tremendous variation in the rates and patterns of adolescents' growth. Growth charts used for children can no longer be used when the signs of puberty begin to appear. The only way to be sure teenagers are growing normally is to compare their heights and weights with their own previous measures taken at intervals and note whether reasonably smooth progress is being made.

Keeping Out from under the Dental Drill

For years conventional wisdom has held that staying away from candy, cookies, sugary soda pop, and the like is the most important line of dietary defense against cavities. Even Aristotle asked in about 350 B.C., "Why do figs when they are sweet, produce damage to the teeth?"[19]

These days dentists advise that cutting down on the amount of sugar eaten is not the only way to prevent **dental caries.** Every bit as—if not more—important to consider is whether a food clings to the teeth and lingers in the mouth as well as when and how often it's eaten. It has to do with the mouth's level of acid. Each time you bite into a food, the bacteria that live in your mouth feed on the sugar in it and release an acid that eats away at tooth enamel. When a large number of bacteria living in a film referred to as **dental plaque** produce enough acid to dissolve a "hole" in the enamel over a period of time, the result is a cavity.

While consuming sugary items such as soda pop boosts acid production in the mouth, so does munching on starchy foods such as crackers or pretzels. That's because enzymes in the saliva can break the carbohydrate in the cracker or pretzel into the simple sugars that bacteria feast on. If a crumb or two from starchy foods gets caught between the teeth, it may provide enough carbohydrate for bacteria to feed on for hours, thereby prolonging the teeth's exposure to acid. In fact, after comparing the acid levels in the mouth produced by eating sugary chocolate nougats, caramels, and fruit chews with acid levels prompted by chewing potato chips, cornflakes, croissants, and breadsticks, a group of dentists in Rochester, New York, found that the sugary foods caused short-lived rises in the mouth's acid level. The starchy foods, on the other hand, brought about increases in acid levels for relatively long periods of time. In other words, starchy foods that linger in the mouth can cause more prolonged acid attacks than sugary items that don't stick to the teeth.[20]

Regardless of starch or sugar content, foods tend to be less harmful to the teeth when eaten with a meal than when consumed alone. One reason may be that the mouth makes more saliva during a full meal. That's crucial, because even though saliva helps make sugar for bacteria, it also clears food particles from the mouth and neutralizes destructive acids before they dissolve the teeth. Consider that one study at the University of Iowa's College of Dentistry found that after people nibbled on foods with a strong tendency to produce acid, such as raisins and chocolate bars, and then chewed sugarless gum, within ten minutes the gum helped stimulate the release of enough saliva to neutralize the acid flow that the sweets had caused.[21]

Dental caries decay of the teeth, or cavities (*caries* = rottenness).

Dental plaque a colorless film consisting of bacteria and their by-products that is constantly forming on the teeth.

For optimal dental health, the American Dental Association recommends that you:[22]

- Eat a balanced diet.
- Keep snacking to a minimum, if possible. The ADA recognizes that some people, such as diabetics, may require snacks. For others, however, the Association suggests limiting the number of snacks if brushing the teeth is not possible shortly after eating them.
- Eat sweets with meals rather than between them.
- Brush and floss thoroughly each day to remove dental plaque.
- Use an ADA-accepted fluoride toothpaste and mouth rinse and talk to your dentist about the need for supplemental fluoride.
- Visit a dentist regularly.
- Do not allow infants to sleep with bottles containing sweetened liquids, fruit juices, milk, or formula.

Of course, while saliva helps fight cavities, the best way to ensure good dental health is to brush your teeth as soon as possible after eating, or at least swish the mouth with water or milk after a meal to help rinse the teeth and dislodge stuck particles. Flossing daily is important as well, because flossing rids the mouth of not only food but also plaque before it becomes so widespread that it produces tooth-threatening levels of acid. Regular visits to the dentist also play a role in keeping dental health up to snuff. In addition, drinking water containing fluoride, a mineral that helps strengthen tooth enamel, prevents cavities. People whose water supplies may not supply fluoride should check with a dentist about the need for fluoride supplements.

Along with practicing good dental hygiene, eating a balanced diet helps keep the mouth healthy. One reason is that if the diet lacks essential nutrients, mouth tissues can become compromised, leaving them particularly vulnerable to infection. In fact, some experts believe that **periodontal disease** is especially severe among people who have poor diets. Another reason to eat an adequate diet, particularly for children, is that it helps to ensure proper development of the teeth. Similarly, eating well should rank as a high priority for a pregnant woman, whose unborn baby's teeth, among other things, start forming after just six weeks and begin to harden between the first and second trimester of pregnancy.[23]

Periodontal disease inflammation or degeneration of the tissues that surround and support the teeth.

Nursing bottle syndrome (also called baby bottle tooth decay) decay of all the upper and sometimes the back lower teeth that occurs in infants given carbohydrate-containing liquids when they sleep. The syndrome can also develop in babies given bottles of liquid to carry around and sip all day.

Incidentally, parents should never allow an infant to sleep with a bottle filled with sweetened liquids, fruit juices, milk, or formula. Little ones allowed to do so often develop what is known as **nursing bottle syndrome.** As a baby sucks on a bottle, the tongue pushes outward slightly and covers the lower teeth. If the infant falls asleep with the bottle in the mouth, the liquid bathes the teeth, particularly the upper teeth not protected by the tongue, thereby literally soaking them in potentially cavity-causing carbohydrates for hours at a time.[24]

Teenagers who want to know what they should weigh should be reassured that any of a wide range of weights is considered normal at this time in life. A rule of thumb regarding weight can be applied to teenage girls (see margin); the result can be considered a weight to aim at, but weights well in excess of these are normal, too. Teenage boys can be told that when they have finished growing, they should expect to weigh what the adult charts show, but that while they are growing, it is not unusual for their weights to be quite different from the adult standards.

Rule of thumb for teenage girls:

For 5 ft, consider 100 lb a reasonable weight. For each inch over 5 ft, add 5 lb.

For each year under 25 (down to 18), subtract 1 lb.

For teen boys, see the inside back cover.

Teenagers as a group do have nutritional problems. Nearly every nutrient can be found lacking in one or another group of teenagers. In sedentary teenagers, obesity often sets in. Serious nutrient deficiencies often arise in pregnant teenage girls.

On the average, about a third of teenagers' total daily energy intake and a fifth of their vitamin and mineral consumption comes from snacks. Snacks can offer substantial amounts of many nutrients—for example, calcium, if dairy products are chosen. (See the Nutrition Action feature in Chapter 2 for more information about snacks.)

Teenage pregnancy presents special nutrient needs. About one out of every five babies is born to a teenager, and more than a tenth of these mothers are 15 or younger. Emphasis on preparing young girls for future pregnancy is needed in public schools and public health programs. A model program for giving nutritional help to teenage mothers, among others, is the WIC (Women's, Infants' and Children's) program, a federally funded program that provides nutrition information and low-cost nutritious foods to low-income pregnant women and their children.

Nutrition in Later Life

It is easy to get the impression from mortality statistics that people are living longer and longer lives, but this is not true. The *average* age at death (life expectancy) is greater than it used to be. Most men die at a little past 70, and most women die at a little past 75 years of age. On the other hand, the *maximum* age at which people die—that is, the *maximum life span*— has changed very little. It seems that aging—whatever that is—cuts off life at a rather fixed point in time.

Why we age as we do and why we die, no one knows, although many researchers are trying to find out. Among the questions they are asking are:

- To what extent is aging inevitable? Can we retard it through changes in our lifestyle and environment?
- What roles does nutrition play in aging, and what roles can it play in retarding aging?

With respect to the first question, it seems that aging is an inevitable, natural process programmed into our genes at conception but that we can adopt lifestyle habits, such as exercising and paying attention to our work and recreational environments, that will slow the process within the natural limits set by heredity. With respect to the second question, clearly, good nutrition can retard and ease the aging process in many significant ways. However, no potions, foods, or pills will prolong your youth, despite the efforts of quacks to persuade you otherwise. People who claim to have found the fountain of youth have been selling its waters for centuries, but products advertised to prevent aging profit only the sellers, not the buyers.

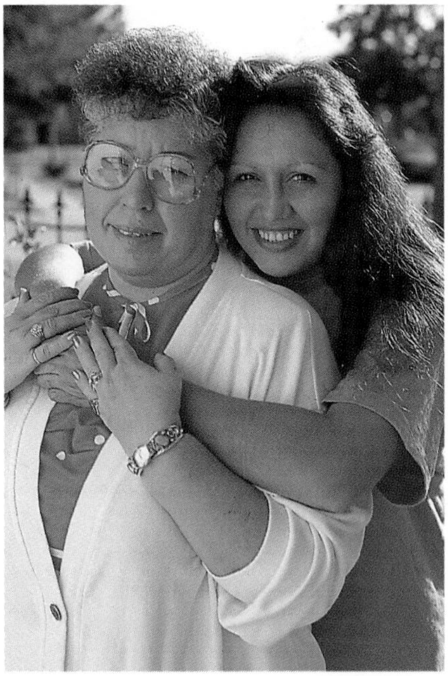

If age is venerated, people will claim to be old.

An approach to the prevention of aging has been to study other cultures in the hope of finding an extremely long-lived race of people and then learning from them their secrets of long life. One scientist traveled far and wide in search of such people and for a while thought that he had found them in two different geographical areas because many people in the areas claimed to have lived for over 100 years. Further study revealed, however, that the old-age range in these populations was unremarkable—about 70 to 80, as elsewhere. These people only claimed to be 100 or older, because in their societies age was venerated. The oldsters were remarkably healthy and justifiably proud of it, but not because they ate according to any particular formula. One group ate a lot of meats and sweets; another used large amounts of alcohol and sugar. The secret—the one thing they all seemed to have in common—was that they lived physically active lives. The lesson of this story seems to be that people will always lie about their age, but not always in the same direction.

Another approach to preventing aging has been drastic manipulation of the diet in animals, which has given rise to some interesting and suggestive findings. Rats live longer when their food intake is restricted in the early weeks of their lives, or even when it is restricted during adulthood. The restriction has to be severe, though: 60 percent of the normal energy intake, or even less. These experiments have inspired articles in the popular press with titles like "Eat Less—Live Longer," but in reality, they did not suggest any direct applications to human nutrition. Half of the animals given restricted feedings died *very* early (before 300 days). The average length of life was long because the few survivors lived a very long time. Also, the restriction was severe: "even the shortest period of food restriction in this study was comparable to restriction of the food intake of a human infant kept in an isolated environment for 20 to 25 years to an amount that would permit the infant to grow during that time to about the size of a one-year-old child."[25] Furthermore, the restricted animals that survived were retarded and malformed in a number of ways.

Old people, then, need not conclude on the basis of this evidence that their parents should have starved them when they were younger. Moderation in energy intake is desirable, of course, but extreme starvation, like any extreme, is hardly worth the price.

The food restriction experiments have stimulated much discussion. The views of the experts can best be summed up by saying that disease can *shorten* people's lives and that poor nutrition practices make diseases more likely to occur. Optimal nutrition, then, by postponing and slowing disease processes, can help to relengthen life back to the maximum life span—but can't extend it further.[26] This brings us to a consideration of the many diseases that seem to come with age and the relevance of nutrition to them, but first, test your own knowledge of the aging process with the Aging Scorecard found on page 301.

Nutrition and Disease

Among the diseases that befall some people in later life are heart disease, cancer, diverticulosis, bone disease, brain disease, diabetes, and gum disease. To what extent can nutrition prevent or retard the development of these diseases? Table 10–6 on page 302 sums up the answers to this question. Clearly, an adequate intake throughout life of nutrients and fiber from a variety of foods, together with moderate intakes of food energy and fat, helps immensely to promote good health in the later years.

Lest Table 10–6 should seem to overstate the case in favor of nutrition, Figure 10–4 on page 303 puts nutrition (a factor you can control) in perspective with respect to heredity (a factor you can't control). It illustrates the point that some diseases are much more responsive to nutrition than others and that some are not responsive at all. At one extreme are diseases that can be completely cured by supplying missing nutrients, and at the other extreme are certain genetic, or inherited, diseases that are completely unaltered by nutrition. Most fall in between, being influenced by inherited susceptibility but responsive to dietary manipulations that help to normalize metabolism and counteract the disease process. Thus, diabetes may be controlled by means of a diet low in sugar and fat and high in complex carbohydrate; arthritis may be somewhat relieved by weight reduction; and cardiovascular disease may respond favorably to a diet low in fat and cholesterol.

These scientific approaches differ markedly from nutrition quackery aimed at the aging population. Nutrition quackery is largely based on the notion that certain foods and nutrients have almost miraculous powers to

Aging Scorecard

True	False	
☐	☐	1. Everyone becomes "senile" sooner or later, if he or she lives long enough.
☐	☐	2. American families have by and large abandoned their older members.
☐	☐	3. Depression is a serious problem for older people.
☐	☐	4. The numbers of older people are growing.
☐	☐	5. The vast majority of older people are self-sufficient.
☐	☐	6. Mental confusion is an inevitable, incurable consequence of old age.
☐	☐	7. Intelligence declines with age.
☐	☐	8. Sexual urges and activity normally cease around age 55–60.
☐	☐	9. If a person has been smoking for 30 or 40 years, it does no good to quit.
☐	☐	10. Older people should stop exercising and rest.
☐	☐	11. As you grow older, you need more vitamins and minerals to stay healthy.
☐	☐	12. Only children need to be concerned about calcium for strong bones and teeth.
☐	☐	13. Extremes of heat and cold can be particularly dangerous to older people.
☐	☐	14. Many older people are hurt in accidents that could have been prevented.
☐	☐	15. More men than women survive to old age.
☐	☐	16. Deaths from stroke and heart disease are declining.
☐	☐	17. Older people on the average take more medications than younger people.
☐	☐	18. Snake oil salesmen are as common today as they were on the frontier.
☐	☐	19. Personality changes with age, just like hair color and skin texture.
☐	☐	20. Sight declines with age.

Answers

1. False. Even among those who live to be 80 or older, only 20-25 percent develop Alzheimer's disease or some other incurable form of brain disease. "Senility" is a meaningless term which should be discarded.
2. False. The American family is still the number one caretaker of older Americans. Most older people live close to their children and see them often; many live with their spouses. In all, 8 out of 10 men and 6 out of 10 women live in family settings.
3. True. Depression, loss of self-esteem, loneliness, and anxiety can become more common as older people face retirement, the deaths of relatives and friends, and other such crises—often at the same time. Fortunately, depression is treatable.
4. True. Today, 12 percent of the U.S. population are 65 or older. By the year 2030, one in five people will be over 65 years of age.
5. True. Only 5 percent of the older population live in nursing homes; the rest are basically healthy and self-sufficient.
6. False. Mental confusion and serious forgetfulness in old age can be caused by Alzheimer's disease or other conditions which cause incurable damage to the brain, but some 100 other problems can cause the same symptoms. A minor head injury, a high fever, poor nutrition, adverse drug reactions, and depression can all be treated and the confusion will be cured.
7. False. Intelligence per se does not decline without reason. Most people maintain their intellect or improve as they grow older.
8. False. Most older people can lead an active, satisfying sex life.
9. False. Stopping smoking at any age not only reduces the risk of cancer and heart disease, it also leads to healthier lungs.
10. False. Many older people enjoy—and benefit from—exercises such as walking, swimming, and bicycle riding. Exercise at any age can help strengthen the heart and lungs, and lower blood pressure. See your physician before beginning a new exercise program.
11. False. Older people need the same amounts of most vitamins and minerals as younger people.
12. False. Older people require fewer calories, but adequate intake of calcium for strong bones can become more important as you grow older. This is particularly true for women, whose risk of osteoporosis increases after menopause.
13. True. The body's thermostat tends to function less efficiently with age and the older person's body may be less able to adapt to heat or cold.
14. True. Falls are the most common cause of injuries among the elderly. Good safety habits, including proper lighting, nonskid carpets, and keeping living areas free of obstacles, can help prevent serious accidents.
15. False. Women tend to outlive men by an average of 8 years. There are 150 women for every 100 men over age 65, and nearly 250 women for every 100 men over 85.
16. True. Fewer men and women are dying of stroke or heart disease. This has been a major factor in the increase in life expectancy.
17. True. The elderly consume 25 percent of all medications and, as a result, have many more problems with adverse drug reactions.
18. True. Medical quackery is a $10 billion business in the United States. People of all ages are commonly duped into "quick cures" for aging, arthritis, and cancer.
19. False. Personality doesn't change with age. Therefore, all old people can't be described as rigid and cantankerous. You are what you are for as long as you live.
20. False. Although changes in vision become more common with age, any change in vision, regardless of age, is related to a specific disease. If you are having problems with your vision, see your doctor.

Source: Adapted from What is your Aging I.Q.? U.S. Department of Health and Human Services, Public Health Service, National Institutes of Health (Washington, D.C.: U.S. Government Printing Office), November 1986.

promote health. People with cancer, particularly those who feel they can't be helped by therapy, are easy targets for peddlers of nutrition "cures." They may take massive doses of vitamins and/or minerals, some of which may be toxic. Table 10–6 displays an impressive list of health-promoting effects of good

Table 10–6

Examples of Preventive Effects of Good Nutrition

Adequate intake of protein, food energy, or essential nutrients helps prevent:
- In pregnancy:
  - Some birth defects
  - Some forms of mental/physical retardation
  - Low birthweight
  - Poor resistance to disease
- In infancy and childhood:
  - Growth deficits
  - Poor resistance to disease
- In adulthood and old age:
  - Malnutrition
  - Poor resistance to infectious and degenerative diseases

Moderation in food energy intake helps prevent:
- Obesity and related diseases, such as diabetes and hypertension

Adequate intake of any essential nutrient prevents:
- Deficiency diseases, such as cretinism, scurvy, and folate-deficiency anemia

Adequate calcium intake helps prevent:
- Adult bone loss

Adequate iron intake helps prevent:
- Anemia

Adequate fluoride intake helps prevent:
- Dental caries

Moderation in sodium intake helps prevent:
- Hypertension and related diseases of the heart and kidney

Adequate fiber intake helps prevent:
- Digestive malfunctions, such as constipation and diverticulosis, and possibly colon or other cancers

Adequate vitamin A intake helps prevent:
- Susceptibility to certain cancers

Moderation in fat intake helps prevent:
- Susceptibility to some cancers and atherosclerosis

Moderation in sugar intake helps prevent:
- Dental caries

Moderation in alcohol intake helps prevent:
- Liver disease
- Malnutrition

Moderation in intake of essential nutrients prevents:
- Toxicity states

Not effective against arthritis:

alfalfa tea
aloe vera liquid
burdock root
calcium
celery juice
fasting
fish liver oil
fresh fruit
honey
kelp
lecithin
megadoses of vitamins
raw liver
superoxide dismutase (SOD)
vitamin D
watercress
yeast
100 others

nutrition, but there is a difference. It does not advocate the use of specific foods—and certainly not of nutrient supplements—nor does it imply that even the most scrupulous attention to nutrition will guarantee freedom from disease. Taken together, the recommendations of the table simply add up to an adequate, balanced, and varied diet composed of nutritious foods—a quiet, sensible prescription for good nutritional health.

Similarly, many bizarre diets advertise themselves as arthritis cures, but no known diet prevents, relieves, or cures arthritis.[27] Research does, however, support the notion that arthritis prevention is helped by adequate, balanced diets.[28] This is an undramatic conclusion, perhaps, but it is honest, good advice.

Weight loss is important for overweight persons with arthritis because the joints affected are often weight-bearing joints that are stressed and irritated by having to carry excess poundage. Weight loss alone often relieves the worst of

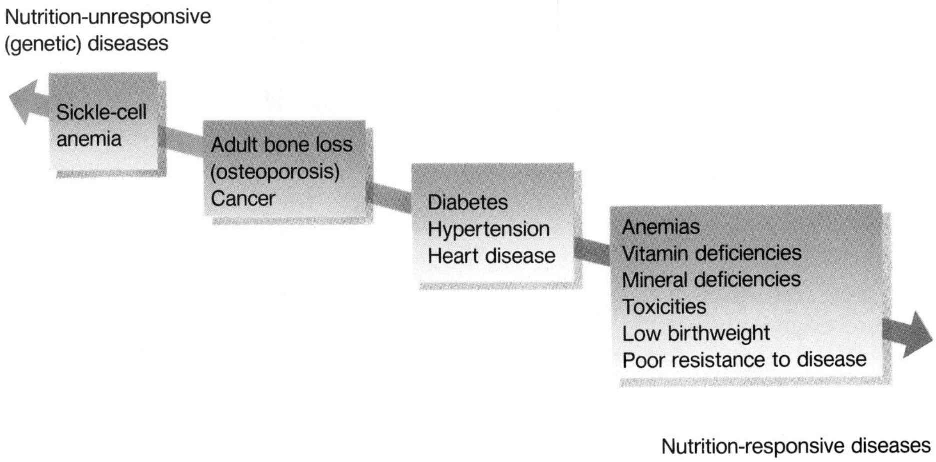

Figure 10–4

Nutrition and Disease

Not all diseases are equally influenced by diet. Some are purely hereditary, like sickle-cell anemia. Some may be inherited (or the tendency to develop them may be inherited) but may be influenced by diet, like some forms of diabetes. Some are purely dietary, like the vitamin and mineral deficiency diseases. Some authorities are concerned that the offering of dietary advice to the public may seem to exaggerate the power of nutrition in preventing disease. Nutrition alone is certainly not enough to prevent many diseases, but it helps.

the pain in arthritis victims. Weight loss may confer a benefit even on arthritis in the hands, though for reasons unknown. Perhaps the drastic reduction in fat intake that accompanies the adoption of a calorie-restricted diet is in some way beneficial to arthritis sufferers.[29]

Aging affects every body tissue and organ: the brain, the heart, the digestive tract, the bones. Many of the changes are inevitable, but a nutrition lifestyle that combines moderation with adequate intakes of all essential nutrients can forestall degeneration and improve the quality of life into the later years.

Nutrient Needs in Later Life

Many of the nutrient needs of the elderly are the same as for younger persons, but some special considerations deserve emphasis. Table 10–7 shows eating patterns that would supply the amounts of food energy recommended by the RDA tables. Because overweight is well recognized as a shortener of the life span, these seem to be life-sustaining recommendations.

Food energy intake should be adequate, however. Deficiency can cause protein-energy malnutrition (PEM), which is common in older people and often goes unnoticed (see Chapter 5). An observer, seeing the wasted muscle, weakness, and sometimes swelling of protein deficiency, may think, "That person looks old," when in fact the observer should recognize the symptoms of PEM. Older people who have been trying to lose weight or have been eating monotonous or bizarre diets are most likely to be affected.[30]

On one side of the energy budget, energy is taken in; on the other side, it is spent. If you are motivated to maintain your good health into the later years, you should plan regular exercise into your days. People responsible for the care of older adults should encourage more activity of all kinds and shorter recuperation periods in bed following illnesses.

Ideally, the exercise should be intense enough to increase the heartbeat and respiration rate and to prevent the atrophy of all muscles (not only the heart) that otherwise takes place. Many older people believe that they can't participate in strenuous exercise, but studies have shown that they can do more than they think they can. Any exercise—even a ten-minute walk a day—is better than none, and with persistence, great improvement can be achieved. Modest endurance training can improve cardiovascular and respi-

Table 10–7

Eating Patterns for Older People

EXCHANGE LIST	NUMBER OF EXCHANGES: Woman (1,500 cal)	NUMBER OF EXCHANGES: Man (2,000 cal)
Milk (nonfat)	4	4
Vegetable	2	3
Fruit	4	6
Bread	5	9
Meat (lean)	6	7
Fat	6	8

Note: These patterns supply the food energy amounts recommended by the RDA for people over 50.

ratory function and promote good muscle tone while controlling the accumulation of body fat.

The older person who has never worked out hard before may be encouraged to learn that the trainability of older people does not depend on their physical prowess in their youth. Improvement during training is due not only to improvement in muscles but also to the increased blood flow to the brain engendered by the exercise. A major benefit is that with an increased energy output, a person can afford to eat more food and so obtain more nutrients.

Perhaps the most important nutrient of all is *water.* The elderly need to be reminded to take in fluids because they are likely to be somewhat insensitive to their own thirst signals. They should take in six to eight glasses of fluid a day—enough to bring their urine output to about 6 cups per day. A large percentage of nursing home operators note that one of the biggest problems with their elderly clients is getting them to drink more water and fruit juices.

You can tell from the color of your urine if you're getting enough water. Bright yellow or dark yellow urine is too concentrated; you need more water. Pale yellow, almost colorless urine is dilute enough; your water intake is ample.

The recommended intakes of many of the vitamins and minerals are thought by some nutritionists to be too low for the over-65 group. They recommend supplements, particularly for the water-soluble vitamins, because large amounts pose no great threat of toxicity. However, other nutritionists feel that recommending vitamin supplements is a cop-out, laying the elderly open to exploitation by quacks. Money is better spent, they say, on food of higher quality.

Surveys designed to find out what kinds of nutrient supplements older people are using tend to support the view that in many cases, older people are wasting their money. A study in a Southern California retirement community showed that 72 percent of the subjects were taking nutrient supplements—mostly of vitamins C and E—but that these choices were not related to the users' dietary intakes; that is, they were not appropriate.[31] Another study, in upper New York State, showed that 10 percent of an elderly population who needed vitamin and mineral supplements either were not taking any or were taking the wrong ones and, in fact, that their doctors had prescribed the wrong ones.[32] Advertising of supplements to the elderly muddies the waters further. Tonics that promise rejuvenation and renewed youth and vigor either hold out false hopes, are incomplete, or are laced with so much alcohol that the lift they seem to provide may in fact be an illusion with a negative effect, if any, on nutrition status.

The older person would probably be wise to follow the rule of thumb that if the food energy intake is below about 1,500 calories, a vitamin-mineral supplement is recommended—not a megavitamin, but just a once-daily type of supplement.

How to choose a vitamin-mineral supplement: see Chapter 6.

Sources of Nutritional Assistance

Two programs are helpful to older people with nutrition problems, although they are not designed specifically for older people but rather for low-income people of all ages. The Food Stamp program enables people who qualify to obtain stamps with which to buy food. The Supplemental Security Income (SSI) program is aimed at directly improving the financial plight of the very poor by increasing a person's or family's income to the defined poverty level. This sometimes helps older people retain their independence.

Consumer Tips

Meals for One

Planning nourishing meals for one that offer variety and optimal nutrition can be particularly challenging. The following tips help solve some of the problems that singles of any age face concerning buying and preparing foods.

- Buy only what you will use: the individual-sized containers may be expensive, but it is also expensive to let the unused portion of a large-sized container spoil before you are ready to use it. Don't be timid about asking the grocer to break up a package of meat, eggs, fresh fruits, or vegetables and wrap a smaller quantity for you.
- Buy a loaf of bread and store half in the freezer. The freezer keeps it fresher than the refrigerator.
- Think up a variety of ways to use a vegetable when you buy it in a large quantity. For example, you can divide a head of broccoli into thirds. Cook one-third and eat it as a hot vegetable. Put one-third into a soup, and use one-third as an appetizer or in a salad. Buy large quantities of frozen vegetables if you have sufficient freezer space. You can take out the exact amount you need at mealtime.
- Buy large packages of meat such as pork chops, ground meat, or chicken when they are on special sale. Divide the package into individual servings, and freeze them separately.
- Get the maximum nutritive value out of what you cook. Steam vegetables over water rather than boiling them. Broil meats rather than frying them. Experiment with stir-fried foods. A variety of vegetables and meats can be enjoyed this way; inexpensive vegetables such as cabbage and celery are delicious when crisp-cooked in a little oil with soy sauce and lemon or ginger added. Cooked, leftover vegetables can be dropped in at the last minute.
- Get the maximum value out of the time you spend cooking. Cook for several meals at a time. For example, boil three potatoes with skins. Eat one hot, with butter or margarine and herbs. When the others have cooled, use one to make a potato-cheese casserole ready to be put into the oven for the next evening's meal. Slice the third one and pour your favorite salad dressing over it. The potato will keep several days in the refrigerator and can be used in a salad.
- Make twice as much as you need of a recipe that takes time to prepare: spaghetti sauce, a casserole, vegetable pie, chili, or meat loaf. Label and store the extra servings in the freezer. Be sure to date these so you will use the oldest first.
- Make mixtures of leftovers you have on hand: a thick stew prepared from leftover green beans, carrots, cauliflower, broccoli, and any beans or meat, with some added fresh herbs, onion, pepper, celery, and potatoes, makes a complete and balanced meal—except for milk.
- Set aside a place in your kitchen for rows of shelf staple items that you can't buy in single-serving quantities—rice, tapioca, lentils or other dried beans, flour, cornmeal, dry nonfat milk, pasta, or cereal, to name only a few possibilities. Place each jar, tightly sealed, in the freezer for a few days to kill any eggs or organisms before storing it on the shelf. The jars make an attractive display and will remind you of possibilities for variety in your menus. Include the directions-for-use labels from the packages in the jars.
- Cook for yourself with the idea that you are cooking for special guests. Invite guests when you can and make enough food so that you will have enough for a later meal.

In several areas, a self-help effort aimed at enabling older people on limited incomes to buy good food for less money is the establishment of food banks. A food bank project buys industry's "irregulars"—products that have been mislabeled, underweighted, redesigned, or mispackaged and therefore would ordinarily be thrown away. Nothing is wrong with this food; the industry can credit it as a donation, and the buyer (often a food-preparing site) can buy the food for a small handling fee and make it available at a greatly reduced price.

The federal Nutrition Program for the Elderly (Title IIIC) is intended to improve older people's nutrition status and enable older people to avoid medical problems, continue living in communities of their own choice, and stay out of institutions. The program's specific goals are to provide:

- Low-cost, nutritious meals.
- An opportunity for social interaction.

- Auxiliary nutrition, homemaker education, and shopping assistance.
- Counseling and referral to other social and rehabilitation services.
- Transportation services.

Sites chosen for congregate meals under this program must be accessible to most of the target population. Volunteers deliver meals to those who are either permanently or temporarily homebound. Every effort is made to persuade the elderly person to come to the congregate meal site, as the social atmosphere there is as valuable as the nutrition.

Sometimes assistance programs are not enough to meet the needs of older people. Some people require institutional care. A variety of options exist; a familiar alternative is the nursing home. A nursing home is a medical solution to what, in many cases, is a social problem, but it may be necessary for people who need constant medical care.

The relative inquiring into nursing homes should ask the director or dietitian some questions about the food service. Is a choice given the resident in the selection of food? How often are the menus repeated (is the cycle monotonous)? How often are fresh fruits and vegetables served? Is the food fresh and tasty when served? Is a plate check conducted regularly, at least once a week, to discover what the resident is consuming? Does the staff keep track of each person's weight? Is there good communication between the nursing staff and the dietitian so that the dietitian will know if someone is not eating? Is the resident encouraged and helped to go to the dining room to eat so that some socializing will occur? Is the dining room attractive? Does someone help those who can't manage feeding themselves? Are minced meats offered to those who have problems with their teeth or dentures? Are religious dietary restrictions honored? How high a proportion of the food is prepackaged? (No guide can be given for what proportion is desirable, but it should be remembered that processed foods are often low in vitamin content and high in salt.) Other questions that the investigator will want to ask have to do with the general atmosphere of the nursing home, in recognition of the effect of social climate on a person's appetite. A nursing home that views residents as people, not as patients, gets a mark in its favor.

In the nursing home, the dietitian, nutritionist, or nurse responsible for the residents' care should keep in mind the special needs associated with the residents' time in life. The average age of a nursing home resident is 81, and many have problems or habits that can affect their nutrition status:

- At least one chronic disease.
- Constipation or incontinence.
- Confusion due to the change in environment.
- Poor eyesight or hearing.
- Ill-fitting or missing dentures.
- Inability to feed themselves because of arthritis or stroke.
- Psychological problems, especially depression.
- Anorexia and loss of interest in eating.
- Lack of opportunity to socialize at mealtimes.
- Long-established food preferences.
- Slowed reactions (seeing, holding utensils, chewing, swallowing).[33]

On admission to the nursing home, a resident's nutrition status should be assessed immediately, and the person responsible for the resident's nutritional care should make every effort to rectify any problems promptly. Thereafter the resident should be reassessed at regular, frequent intervals, and adjustments should be made as needed.

Opinions differ on the philosophy to adopt for nursing home menus. A multitude of different special diets is difficult and expensive to manage, and one authority recommends for most residents a "liberalized geriatric diet" rather than modified diets. Based on the assumption that older people "should have the right to choose the food they eat," this approach provides in one package the key characteristics of several special diets:

- 1,500 to 2,000 calories per day, mostly from nutrient-dense foods, with simple desserts not too high in food energy.
- Minimal salt used in preparation.
- 65 to 70 grams of protein per day from 2 cups of milk and 4 to 6 ounces of meat or meat alternates.
- At least 6 milligrams of iron per day (the RDA for older people is 10 milligrams per day).
- Generous amounts of natural fiber and 64 ounces of fluid per day.[34]

Further modifications can be made available for people with severe diseases.

The very best help we could give our elderly citizens would be a changed attitude toward them. As a nation, we value the future more than the present, putting off enjoying today so that tomorrow we will have money or prestige or time to have fun. The elderly feel this loss of future. The present is their time for leisure and enjoyment, but they have no experience in the use of leisure time.

It would take a near miracle to change the attitude of a nation, but there is a change in attitude that individual persons can make toward themselves as they age. Preparation for this period should, of course, include financial planning, but other lifelong habits should be developed as well. Each adult needs to learn to reach out to others to forestall the loneliness that will otherwise ensue. Adults need to learn some skills or activities that they can continue into their later years—volunteer work with organizations, reading, games, hobbies, or intellectual pursuits—and that will give meaning to their lives. Each adult needs to develop the habit of adjusting to change, especially when it comes without consent, so that it will not be seen as a loss of control over one's life. The goal is to arrive at maturity with as healthy a mind and body as possible; this means cultivating good nutrition status and maintaining a program of daily exercise.

Preparation for the later years begins early in life, both psychologically and nutritionally. Everyone knows older people who have gathered around themselves many contacts—through relatives, church, synagogue, or fraternal orders—and have not allowed themselves to drift into isolation. Upon analysis, you will see that their favorable environment came through a lifetime of effort. These people spent their entire lives reaching out to others and practicing the art of weaving others into their own lives. Likewise, a lifetime of effort is required for good nutrition status in the later years. A person who has eaten a wide variety of foods, has stayed trim, and has remained physically active will be most able to withstand the assaults of change.

Not for Coffee Drinkers Only

In 1657 when merchants first introduced Londoners to a Middle Eastern brew known as coffee, they boasted it to be a "wholesome and physical drink," an elixir of health suitable for treating colds, coughs, gout, and many other ills.[35] Modern-day coffee drinkers have heard otherwise. During the past decade, the "coffee generation" has been subject to a barrage of reports linking coffee and other **caffeine**-containing products such as colas and tea with more than 100 diseases. Fingers have repeatedly pointed at caffeine as the culprit behind breast disease, cancer, heart disease, birth defects, and high blood pressure, to name just a few.[36]

Caffeine a type of compound, called a methylxanthine, found in coffee beans, cola nuts, cocoa beans, and tea leaves. A central nervous system stimulant, caffeine's effects include increasing the heart rate, boosting urine production, and raising the metabolic rate.

Despite the brouhaha over the substance, the jury is still out as to whether caffeine is truly to blame. Scientists have yet to confirm long-standing suspicions that caffeine contributes to any health problems other than jitteriness. One reason for all the controversy is that much of the evidence linking the substance with different diseases has been clouded by a number of issues. Some studies do not measure sources of caffeine other than coffee and tea, such as soft drinks, chocolate, and certain medications. In addition, the amount of caffeine and other substances in coffee or tea can vary considerably depending on how the beverage is brewed, a fact most studies fail to take into account.

At least 8 out of 10 Americans consume caffeine, the most widely used behaviorally active drug in the world.[37]

Consider the widely debated question of whether drinking coffee raises blood cholesterol. Granted, a great deal of strong evidence suggests that the beverage does contribute to high blood cholesterol and, therefore, to heart disease. The hitch is that most of the evidence comes from Scandinavia, where coffee is boiled rather than brewed in automatic drip coffee makers or electric percolators. Subsequent research has found that whereas boiled coffee appears to boost blood cholesterol levels, filtered coffee does not. In other words, some substance other than caffeine found in boiled coffee may be the cholesterol-raising culprit.[38]

Contrary to popular belief, black coffee will not sober up a person who has had too many beers or other alcoholic drinks.

Another issue that most research has not filtered out is that while coffee drinking may not contribute to ill health in and of itself, it seems to be part of a lifestyle that does. After questioning some 2,300 men and women about their habits, researchers at the University of California in San Diego found that coffee drinkers were more likely to smoke, drink alcohol, and eat high-fat diets than abstainers. Thus, it may not be the coffee but rather the donut or cigarette that goes along with it that contributes to health problems.[39]

None of this is to say that caffeine is necessarily good for people. As anyone who can't get going in the morning without a cup of coffee or can of caffeinated soda pop is well aware, consuming caffeine day in and day out can be habit forming. People with certain medical conditions would do well to

Table 10–8

Caffeine Sources

DRINKS AND FOODS	AVERAGE (mg)	RANGE (mg)
Coffee (5-oz cup)		
Brewed, drip method	130	110–150
Brewed, percolator	94	64–124
Instant	74	40–108
Decaffeinated, brewed or instant	3	1–5
Tea (5-oz cup)		
Brewed, major U.S. brands	40	20–90
Brewed, imported brands	60	25–110
Instant	30	25–50
Iced (12-oz glass)	70	67–76
Soft drinks (12-oz can)		
Dr. Pepper		40
Colas and cherry colas:		
Regular		30–46
Diet		2–58
Caffeine free		0–trace
Jolt		72
Mountain Dew, Mello Yello		52
Big Red		38
Fresca, Hires root beer, 7-Up, Sprite, Squirt, Sunkist Orange		0
Cocoa beverage (5-oz cup)	4	2–20
Chocolate milk beverage (8 oz)	5	2–7
Milk chocolate candy (1 oz)	6	1–15
Dark chocolate, semisweet (1 oz)	20	5–35
Baker's chocolate (1 oz)	26	26
Chocolate-flavored syrup (1 oz)	4	4
DRUGS[a]		
Cold remedies (standard dose)		
Dristan		0
Coryban-D, Triaminicin		30
Diuretics (standard dose)		
Aqua-ban, Permathene H_2Off		200
Pre-Mens Forte		100
Pain relievers (standard dose)		
Excedrin		130
Midol, Anacin		65
Aspirin, plain (any brand)		0
Stimulants		
Caffedrin, NoDoz, Vivarin		200
Weight-control aids (daily dose)		
Prolamine		280
Dexatrim, Dietac		200

[a]Because products change, contact the manufacturer for an update on products you use regularly.

Source: Data from C. Lecos, The latest caffeine scoreboard, *FDA Consumer,* March 1984, p. 14; Measuring your life with coffee spoons, *Tufts University Diet and Nutrition Letter,* April 1984, pp. 3–6; Institute of Food Technologists, Expert Panel on Food Safety and Nutrition, *Evaluation of Caffeine Safety,* a publication (1986) available from the Institute of Food Technologists, 221 N. LaSalle St., Chicago, IL 60601.

consume caffeine in moderation or avoid it completely. Pregnant women, for example, should limit the amount of caffeine they take in. While the substance has never been proved to cause birth defects, it does cross the placenta and enter the fetus, where large amounts can affect the unborn baby's heart rate and breathing.[40] Some people with heart rhythm disorders also need to stay away from caffeine because it may promote dangerous irregularities in the heartbeat. Finally, those with ulcers should steer clear of caffeinated *and* decaffeinated coffee, both of which stimulate the secretion of acid, which can irritate the stomach's lining.

For a healthy person, drinking a few (2 to 3) cups of coffee, tea, or cola a day does not seem to pose any hazard. Only those who are particularly sensitive to caffeine and suffer symptoms such as headaches, nervousness, and insomnia after consuming it really need to consider avoiding—or at least cutting back on—it. (See Table 10–8 to figure out how much caffeine you're taking in each day.)

If you drink coffee or a can or two of cola every day and decide to quit, make sure you do it gradually. Even moderate caffeine users who try to stop cold turkey often suffer from withdrawal symptoms, such as splitting headaches, fatigue, moodiness, and nausea. Try instead to cut back gradually by, say, no more than a cup or so every couple of days. You can do that by substituting decaffeinated coffee for some of the regular roast in your morning brew and gradually using more and more decaf and less regular coffee. Likewise, you can drink a glass of decaffeinated instead of caffeinated soda pop here and there until you've weaned yourself off the caffeinated version over time.

Smokers, incidentally, metabolize the caffeine in their bloodstreams more quickly than nonsmokers, thereby needing more of the substance to obtain its stimulating effect. When smokers try to give up cigarettes, however, the caffeine stays in the bloodstream longer, giving them a stronger than usual dose and possibly causing jitteriness and irritability on top of the jitters already occurring as a result of giving up nicotine. Thus, smokers who kick the cigarette habit may want to try to cut back on caffeine at the same time to avoid that problem.[41]

See Chapter 9 for a discussion of caffeine's effect on physical performance.

Spotlight

Alcohol and Nutrition

One of the many drugs—and usually the most common one—that enters people's lives as they arrive at their teen and adult years is alcohol. The National Institute on Alcohol Abuse and Alcoholism has estimated that about two-thirds of all adults in the United States drink alcohol. Of these, 33 percent are classified as light drinkers, about 24 percent are moderate drinkers, and 9 percent are heavy drinkers. A heavy drinker is defined as one whose alcohol intake exceeds 0.8 grams per kilogram of body weight per day (this represents 80 grams of alcohol) or an average of 0.7 grams per kilogram of body weight in a three-day period.

Even though people in the 20- to 40-year-old age group have the greatest alcohol consumption, many teenagers are regular alcohol users. A 1985 survey showed that two-thirds of the high school seniors interviewed reported that they had consumed alcohol within the past month and 5 percent indicated that they drank alcohol every day. In addition, men are more likely to consume alcohol and to drink more heavily than women.

Alcohol abuse and alcoholism are recognized as major public health problems in the United States today. Whether an individual is a "social drinker," an alcohol abuser, or an alcoholic, the common element is managing the physiological, psychological, and social consequences of alcohol consumption. (The difference between the alcohol abuser and the alcoholic is generally one of degree, with the alcoholic experiencing more difficulties in terms of illness, dependence on alcohol, loss-of-control symptoms, and disruption of family and work life than the alcohol abuser.) As we will see, alcohol has a profound effect on all aspects of metabolism and health.[42]

• Why doesn't everyone who drinks alcohol become an alcoholic?

As the concept grew that alcoholism is a disease and not a mental illness or a lack of self-discipline, it also became apparent that alcoholism tends to run in families. Studies have shown that the natural sons of alcoholics are three to four times more likely to be alcoholic themselves than are the biological sons of nonalcoholic parents. This observation tends to hold true whether the child was raised by its natural parent or by an adoptive parent.[43] Research is under way to understand this process in greater detail and develop biochemical markers that will identify individuals who are at risk of becoming alcoholic.

• How does alcohol affect the body?

Alcohol (specifically, ethanol, the form found in alcoholic beverages) affects every organ, but the most dramatic evidence of its disruptive behavior appears in the liver. This is the only organ whose cells can oxidize alcohol for fuel to any great extent. All other cells are affected by the presence of alcohol but can do practically nothing about getting rid of it. Ethanol, like the other alcohols, is toxic—but less so than some. Sufficiently diluted and taken in small enough doses, it produces **euphoria**—an effect that people seek—not with zero risk but with a low enough risk (if the doses are low enough) to be tolerable. Used to achieve these effects, alcohol is a **drug**—that is, a substance that can modify one or more of the body's functions. Like all drugs, alcohol offers some benefits; it also has tremendous abuse potential.

• What are the benefits offered by alcohol?

The beneficial effects of alcohol have long been appreciated and praised. Wine, beer, and other fermented beverages have given pleasure and relaxation to people for more than 5,000 years. Only recently have we begun to learn exactly how the little ethanol molecule acts in our bodies, but people have always known that it affects their mood, sensations, and behavior. Because it alters mood, alcohol has many uses. Taken in moderation, alcohol relaxes people, reduces their inhibitions, and encourages desirable social interactions. The regular and moderate consumption of alcohol, especially wine, by elderly people results in better sleep patterns, improved mood, a lower heart rate, and reduced anxiety levels.[44]

Alcohol may even lower an individual's susceptibility to heart disease, possibly by increasing the blood HDL level. Among middle-aged women, *moderate* alcohol consumption has been shown to decrease the risk of both stroke and heart disease (although it may increase the risk of brain hemorrhage).[45]

• What do you mean by *moderation*?

We can't name an exact amount of alcohol per day that would be appropriate for everyone, because people differ in their tolerance levels. In fact, it is even hard to define what is meant by a **drink.** Still, authorities have attempted to set a limit that is appropriate for most healthy people: not more than 1 ounce of pure alcohol in a single day for men and not more than one-half ounce for women. For men, this is the equivalent of two cans of beer (12 ounces for women), two small glasses of wine (5 ounces for women), or two average cocktails (one for women). This amount is supposed to be enough to produce euphoria without incurring any long-term harm to health. Doubtless some people could consume slightly more; others could definitely not handle nearly so much without significant risk.

How does the body handle alcohol?

From the moment alcohol enters the body in a beverage, it is treated as if it has special privileges. Foods sit around in the stomach for a while, but not alcohol. The tiny alcohol molecules need no digestion; they can diffuse as soon as they arrive, right through the walls of the stomach, and they reach the brain within a minute.

A small amount of alcohol can be metabolized by the enzyme **alcohol dehydrogenase** housed within the cells lining the stomach. The extent to which the stomach cells metabolize this "first-pass" alcohol differs between women and men. The observation that "women can't seem to hold their liquor" compared with men is explained in part by a woman's lower alcohol dehydrogenase activity in the stomach. Women's inability to handle this first-pass alcohol holds true even when adjustments are made for the differences in body size between women and men.[46]

Regardless of your gender, you can feel euphoric right away when you drink, especially if your stomach is empty. When your stomach is full of food, the molecules of alcohol have less chance of touching the walls and diffusing through, so you don't feel the effects of alcohol as quickly. If you don't want to become intoxicated at parties, eat the snacks provided by the host. Carbohydrate snacks are best suited for slowing alcohol absorption. High-fat snacks help, too, because they slow peristalsis (see Appendix B).[47] But when the stomach contents are emptied into the duodenum, it doesn't matter that plenty of food is mixed with the alcohol. The alcohol is absorbed rapidly anyway and transported to the liver "as if it were a V.I.P. (Very Important Person)."[48]

What does the alcohol do once it arrives at the liver?

Although a small amount of alcohol can be metabolized by stomach cells, liver cells are the only cells in the body that can make enough alcohol dehydrogenase to oxidize alcohol at an appreciable rate. However, there is a limit to the amount of alcohol anyone can process in a given time. This limit is set by the number of molecules of the alcohol-processing enzymes in the liver. If more molecules of alcohol arrive at the liver cells than the enzymes can handle, the extra alcohol must wait. It enters the general circulation and moves on past the liver. From the liver, it is carried to all parts of the body, circulating again and again through the liver until enzymes are available to convert it to **acetaldehyde.** The rate at which the liver enzymes can work limits the rate of the body's handling of alcohol.

How fast do the liver enzymes work?

That depends on many individual factors. For example, the amount of enzymes present depends on when you last ate a good meal. Fasting for as little as a day causes degradation of the enzyme (protein) within the cells, and it can reduce the rate of alcohol metabolism by half. Drinking on an empty stomach thus not only lets the drinker feel the effects more promptly but also brings about higher blood alcohol levels for longer periods of time and increases the effect of alcohol in anesthetizing the brain.

What if you drink too fast?

If you drink so fast that your liver enzymes can't keep up with the load, metabolic products of alcohol's metabolism accumulate in the blood and body organs. One is acid—dangerous for all body processes. Another is acetaldehyde, already mentioned, which is toxic to the brain and other organs. Another is fat, which accumulates in the liver itself and can't be moved out until the body is free of alcohol.

Alcohol also causes loss of body water by excretion, and that leads to thirst. Many people have observed the increase in urination that accompanies drinking, but they may not realize that they can easily get into a vicious cycle as a result. Loss of body water leads to thirst. Thirst leads to more drinking—but drinking of what? The only fluid that will relieve dehydration is water, but the thirsty person welcomes any cold fluid—even concentrated alcohol—that relieves the dry mouth associated with thirst. If a person tries to quench thirst with concentrated alcoholic beverages, the thirst only becomes worse. The smart drinker, then, either drinks beer (which contains plenty of water) or drinks wine or hard liquor with mixers or chasers. Better still, the drinker limits the total amount consumed.

What are the nutritional consequences of drinking alcohol regularly?

If you are a light drinker in good health and otherwise well nourished, the occasional consumption of alcohol will probably have little effect on your nutritional status. The biggest risk to you will come most likely from the additional calories provided by alcohol; these extra calories may contribute to unwanted weight gain. This is not to say that alcohol has *no effect* on your nutritional status, for it does. Alcohol causes fundamental changes in metabolism which occur whenever you consume alcohol. The extent to which alcohol affects your nutritional status depends on how much alcohol you consume and your current nutritional and health status.

If you drink excessively on a regular basis, your nutritional status will become compromised. Protein deficiency can develop, both from the depression of protein synthesis in the cells and, in the drinker who substitutes alcohol for food, from poor diet. Eating well does not protect the drinker from protein depletion. One has to stop drinking alcohol for complete protection.

Alcohol affects every tissue's metabolism of nutrients in other ways as well. Stomach cells become inflamed and vulnerable to ulcer formation. Intestinal cells fail to absorb thiamin, folate, and vitamin B_{12}. Liver cells lose efficiency in activating vitamin D, and they alter their production and excretion of bile. Rod cells in the retina, which normally process vitamin A alcohol (retinol) to the form needed in vision (retinal), find themselves processing drinking alcohol instead. The kidney excretes increased quantities of magnesium, calcium, potassium, and zinc.

Acetaldehyde interferes with metabolism, too. It dislodges vitamin B_6 from its protective binding protein so that it is destroyed, causing a vitamin B_6 deficiency and, thereby, lowered production of red blood cells.

• Do alcoholics have special nutritional problems?

Definitely. Some alcoholics tend to substitute alcohol for food and can consume more than 50 percent of their calories from alcohol. Because of the metabolic derangements that occur with alcohol consumption, the chronic alcoholic tends to develop hyperlipidemia (a high blood triglyceride level), a **fatty liver** which ultimately leads to **cirrhosis** of the liver, and impaired kidney function. Over time, a high level of alcohol intake may also damage the lining of the stomach, produce low blood sugar and high blood concentrations of uric acid, and cause metabolic bone disease. Even fairly young men in their 30s and 40s can develop osteoporosis from consuming excessive alcohol over the course of 10 to 15 years.[49] In addition, alcoholics have an increased risk of hypertension, stroke, and a variety of cancers, particularly cancers of the tongue, mouth, pharynx, esophagus, larynx, and liver, the latter occurring because of cirrhosis.

• I've heard that alcohol and other drugs interact in a dangerous way. Is this true?

Yes, they do. The liver's V.I.P. treatment of alcohol is reflected in its altered handling of **drugs** as well as nutrients. The liver possesses an enzyme system in addition to the enzyme alcohol dehydrogenase that metabolizes *both* alcohol *and* drugs—any compounds that have certain chemical features in common. Called the **MEOS (microsomal ethanol-oxidizing system),** this system handles only about one-fifth of the total alcohol a person consumes, but the MEOS enlarges if repeatedly exposed to alcohol. This may not make the drinker able to handle much more alcohol at a time than before, because the total alcohol-metabolizing ability of the MEOS is small, but the effect on the ability to metabolize other drugs is considerable.

When the MEOS enlarges, it makes the body able to metabolize other drugs much faster than before. This can make it confusing and tricky to work out the correct doses of medications. The physician who prescribes sedatives to be taken every four hours, for example, assumes that the MEOS will dispose of the drug at a certain predicted rate. Well and good; but in a client who is a heavy drinker, the MEOS is adapted to metabolizing large quantities of alcohol. It therefore metabolizes the drug extra fast. The drug's effects wear off unexpectedly fast, leaving the client undersedated. Imagine a surgeon's alarm if a client wakes up on the table during an operation! A skilled anesthesiologist always asks clients about their drinking patterns before putting them to sleep.

An enlarged MEOS will oxidize drugs *faster* than expected, but only as long as there is no alcohol in the system. If the person drinks and uses the drug at the same time, the drug will be metabolized more *slowly* and so will be much more potent. Since the MEOS is busy disposing of alcohol, the drug can't be handled until later, and the dose may build up to where it greatly oversedates, or even kills, the user.

• What does alcohol do to the brain?

Alcohol is a **narcotic.** It was used for centuries as an anesthetic because of its ability to deaden pain. But it wasn't a very good anesthetic, because one could never be sure how much a person would need and how much would be a lethal dose. As new, more predictable anesthetics were discovered, they quickly replaced alcohol. However, alcohol continues to be used today as a kind of anesthetic on social occasions, to help people relax or to relieve anxiety. People think that alcohol is a stimulant, because it seems to make them lively and uninhibited at first. Actually, though, the way it does this is by sedating *inhibitory* nerves, which are more numerous than excitatory nerves. Ultimately, alcohol acts as a depressant because it affects all the nerve cells.

When alcohol flows to the brain, it first sedates the frontal lobe, the reasoning part. As the alcohol molecules diffuse into the cells of this lobe, they interfere with reasoning and judgment. If the drinker drinks faster than the rate at which the liver can oxidize the alcohol, the speech center of the brain becomes narcotized, and the area that governs reasoning becomes more incapacitated. Later, the cells of the brain responsible for large-muscle control are affected; at this point, people "under the influence" stagger or weave when they try to walk. Finally, the conscious brain is completely subdued, and the person passes out. Now, luckily, the person can drink no more. This is lucky because a higher dose's anesthetic effect could reach the deepest brain centers that control breathing and heartbeat, and the person could die. Table 10–9 shows the blood alcohol

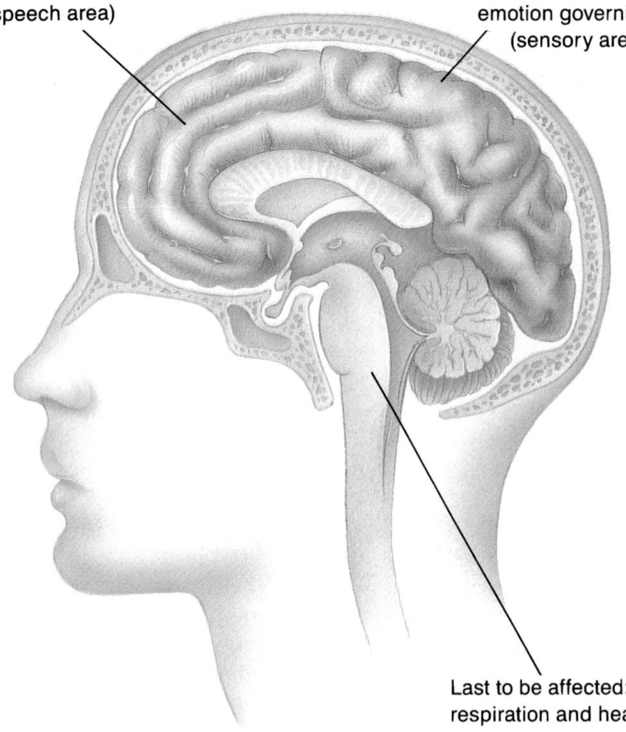

Alcohol is rightly termed an anesthetic because it puts brain centers to sleep in order: first the cortex; then the emotion-governing centers; then the centers that govern muscular control; and, finally, the deep centers that control respiration and heartbeat.

levels that correspond with progressively greater intoxication.

• Why, then, don't people die from drinking alcohol?

Luckily, the brain centers respond to alcohol in the order just described, so people pass out before they can drink enough to kill them. It is possible, though, to drink fast enough that the effects of alcohol continue to accelerate after one has gone to sleep. The occasional death that takes place during a drinking contest is attributed to this effect. The drinker drinks fast enough, before passing out, to receive a lethal dose.

The lack of glucose for the brain's function (once again, because of the body's V.I.P. treatment of alcohol) and the length of time needed to clear the blood of alcohol account for some diverse consequences of drinking. Responsible aircraft pilots know that they must allow 24 hours for their bodies to clear alcohol completely, and they refuse to fly any sooner. Major airlines enforce this rule. Women who may become pregnant are warned to abstain from the use of alcohol, as mentioned earlier in the chapter. One of the effects of an acute dose in experimental animals is to collapse the umbilical cord temporarily, depriving the developing fetus of oxygen.[50] Remember, this can occur even before a woman knows that she is pregnant.

• Does alcohol cause brain damage?

Yes, and the damage is permanent in both the drinker and the child born to a pregnant woman who drinks. When liver cells have died, other cells may later multiply to replace them, but there is no regeneration of brain cells.

• Suppose I want to drink but not get drunk. How can I go about drinking in moderation?

If you want to drink socially, you should drink slowly, and you should sip, not gulp, your drinks. You should eat available snacks or a light meal along with the alcoholic beverages. With this strategy, the alcohol molecules should dribble slowly enough into the liver cells, allowing the enzymes to handle the load. Spacing of drinks is important, too. It takes about an hour and a half to metabolize one drink, depending on your body size, on previous drinking experience, on how

Table 10–9 Alcohol Doses and Brain Responses

Number of Drinks[a]	Blood Alcohol Level (%)	Brain Response
2	0.05	Judgment impaired
4	0.10	Emotional control impaired
6	0.15	Muscle coordination and reflexes impaired
8	0.20	Vision impaired
12	0.30	Drunk, totally out of control
14	0.35	Stupor
More than 14	0.50–0.60	Total loss of consciousness; finally, death

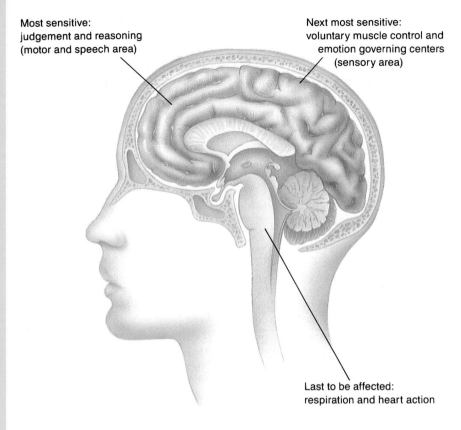

[a]Taken within an hour or so.

recently you have eaten, and on how you are feeling at the time.

Finally, you might elect to dilute your alcoholic beverages over the course of the "happy hour." For example, after you've drunk half a glass of wine, fill up the glass with a non-cola soft drink to make a wine spritzer. If you choose a low-calorie carbonated drink, you eliminate extra calories and alcohol. Or choose a low-alcohol beer or wine cooler.

• What can I do to help a friend who has drunk too much? Does it help to walk my friend around?

No, don't wear yourself out walking your friend around the block. The muscles have to work harder, but since they can't metabolize alcohol, they can't help clear it from the blood. Time is the only thing that will do the job; each person has a particular level of the enzyme alcohol dehydrogenase, and it clears the blood at a steady rate. This is not true for most nutrients. If you bring in more of a nutrient, generally the body can promptly step up the rate at which it metabolizes that nutrient. But not with alcohol.

Nor will it help to give your friend a cup of coffee. Caffeine is a stimulant, but it won't speed up the metabolism of alcohol. The police say ruefully, "If you give a cup of coffee to a drunk, you'll just have a wide-awake drunk on your hands."

You may have heard the story of the country woman who kept saying "Amen!" as the preacher ranted about one sin after another; but when he got to her favorite sin, she whispered to her husband that the preacher had "quit preachin' and gone to meddlin'." We've tried to stick to scientific facts, so the only "meddlin'" that we'll do is to urge you to look again at the accompanying drawing of the brain and note that judgment is affected first when someone drinks. A man's judgment may tell him that he should limit himself to two drinks at a party, but the first drink may take his judgment away, so he has many more. The failure to stop drinking as planned, on repeated occasions, is a danger sign that indicates that the person should not drink at all.

Alcohol interferes with a multitude of chemical and hormonal reactions in the body—many more than have been enumerated here. The point of this discussion, however, was not to summarize every effect of alcohol; the point was to offer a reward to the reader for learning the basics of nutrition. The understandings gained permit a profound appreciation of processes like those described here.

Miniglossary

Acetaldehyde (ass-et-AL-duh-hide) a substance to which drinking alcohol is metabolized.

Alcohol dehydrogenase a liver enzyme that converts ethanol to acetaldehyde. The MEOS also oxidizes alcohol.

Cirrhosis (seer-OH-sis) advanced liver disease, often associated with alcoholism, in which liver cells have died and hardened and have permanently lost their function.

Drink a dose of any alcoholic beverage that delivers ½ ounce of pure ethanol:
- 3 to 4 ounces of wine
- 8 to 12 ounces of beer
- 1 ounce of hard liquor (whiskey, scotch, rum, or vodka)

Drugs substances that can modify one or more of the body's functions.

Euphoria (you-FORE-ee-uh) a feeling of great well-being which people often seek through the use of drugs such as alcohol.
- *eu* = good
- *phoria* = bearing

Fatty liver an early stage of liver disease seen in several conditions (kwashiorkor, alcoholic liver disease), characterized by accumulation of fat in the liver cells.

MEOS (microsomal ethanol-oxidizing system) a system of enzymes in the liver that oxidize not only alcohol but also several classes of drugs. (The **microsomes** are tiny particles of membranes with associated enzymes that can be collected from broken-up cells.)
- *micro* = tiny
- *soma* = body

Narcotic (nar-KOT-ic) any drug that dulls the senses, induces sleep, and becomes addictive with prolonged use.

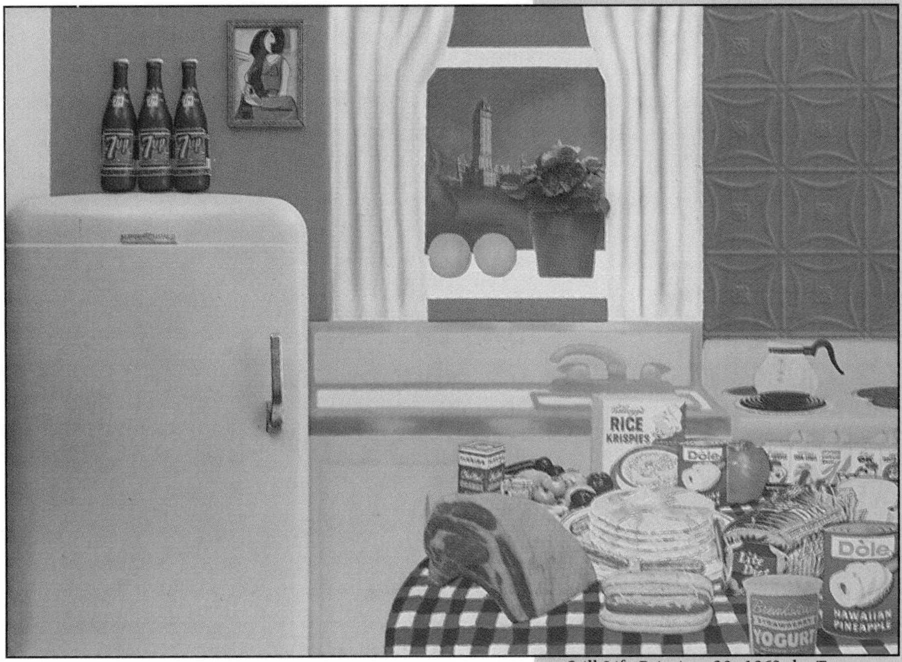

Still Life Painting, 30, *1963, by Tom Wesselmann. Assemblage, oil, enamel, and synthetic polymer paint on composition with collage of printed advertisements, plastic artificial flowers, etc., 48½ × 66 × 4″. Collection, the Museum of Modern Art, New York. Gift of Philip Johnson.*

> *Nutrition is one of those rare comprehensive arts and sciences whose many disciplines, ranging from food technology and cultural anthropology to biochemistry and medical epidemiology, fit together into a beautiful mosaic. Food, because it is one of the major determinants of human ecology, can act as a potent and effective vehicle for health . . . the reason is simple; everyone eats.*
>
> *G. Christakis*

CHAPTER 11

Food Safety and Nutrition: Today and Tomorrow

Contents

Ask Yourself . . . ?

Which of these statements about nutrition are true, and which are false? For the false statements, what *is* true?

1. The greatest hazard present in the U.S. food supply today is inadequately tested, irresponsibly used food additives.
2. Honey and mayonnaise are likely carriers of food poisoning.
3. If a food contains toxic substances, a person who consumes it will become ill.
4. Legal pesticides are poisonous only to pests, not to human beings.
5. Imported foods may contain residues of pesticides that are illegal in the United States because they are not tested for them.
6. Now that the law requires U.S. drivers to use unleaded gasoline in their cars, lead contamination of food is becoming a negligible problem.
7. The most frequent cause of foodborne illness in homes and restaurants is the inadequate cooling of foods.
8. The safety of a GRAS substance is guaranteed by the Food and Drug Administration.
9. Most outbreaks of foodborne disease can be prevented by handling food properly.
10. Hunger in the United States is found almost exclusively among the unemployed homeless.

Answers: 1. False. The greatest hazard present in the U.S. food supply today is not food additives but microbial food poisoning. 2. False. Honey is a likely carrier of food poisoning, but mayonnaise is not. 3. False. If a food contains toxic substances, a person who consumes it *may* become ill, but may not; it depends on the amounts present. 4. False. Legal pesticides are poisonous both to pests and to human beings. 5. True. 6. False. Lead contamination of food is a serious problem, with a magnitude greater than has been previously thought. 7. True. 8. False. The Food and Drug Administration continually reviews the safety of all GRAS substances; if new data suggest a GRAS substance is unsafe, it is removed from the GRAS list. 9. True. 10. False. Hunger in the United States appears not only among the unemployed homeless, but also among home owners and the working poor.

So far, this book has dealt primarily with the nutrients and how your body handles them. Along the way, it has offered some practical pointers about foods. Chapter 2 showed how to plan balanced and varied diets using food grouping systems. Chapter 5 dealt with diet planning for the vegetarian. Chapters 6 and 7 contained tables showing the vitamin and mineral contents of foods. Chapter 8 showed how to plan weight-loss and weight-gain diets, but no chapter has focused on foods themselves. What are foods made of besides nutrients? What sorts of additives do foods contain, and what are the effects of those additives? Are foods ever contaminated? If so, with what, and how seriously? How can the consumer prepare foods both nutritiously and safely? This chapter deals with these and other questions.

Today's Food Supply

An abundant, safe, and diverse food supply is surely the goal of all nations. Achieving this goal requires careful and thorough monitoring of the entire food supply, from food production on farms—whether they be owned by a single farmer or a large agribusiness—to the distribution of foodstuffs to food processors and wholesalers and the eventual sale of wholesome food to consumers in the marketplace.

Here in the United States, we have the safest, most plentiful food supply in the entire world.[1] This is due to the concerted efforts of food suppliers, food processors, and federal, state, and local governments, all of whom are concerned with food safety.

We also have the most diverse food supply in the world and enjoy an incredible array of fresh and processed foods. Consider, for example, the growth in recent years of the international food market. Most U.S. supermarkets today have set aside shelf space for a variety of foods from other countries—cookies and crackers from Denmark and the United Kingdom, Belgian chocolates, Italian cheeses, beef and veal products from New Zealand and Australia, goose liver paté from France, and specialty foods such as pasta, egg rolls, and noodle soups from Japan, Mexico, and even China. Our international bent can be seen in the produce section as well, where exotic star fruit, papaya, and mango from overseas markets are widely available.[2] The diversity of the U.S. food supply is due partly to innovations of the food industry. Food companies, through their research and development programs, have brought new food products and ingredients such as artificial sweeteners and fat substitutes to the marketplace.[3]

You might ask at this point, Do consumers have an effect on the food supply? The answer is a resounding yes. The expectations consumers have about foods drive the marketplace in many respects, and consumers' opinions and purchasing practices influence product development. Surveys have shown that consumers expect foods to be fresh, safe to eat, and of high quality. Consumers also want convenience foods, a reflection perhaps of their on-the-go lifestyles. Their growing interest in diet and health, sparked in part by evidence linking a high-fat diet to heart disease and other chronic diseases, has led to the marketing of low-fat, "heart healthy" food products. U.S. consumers also still expect value for their food dollar and demand high-quality foods at reasonable prices. Altogether, these expectations help the food industry focus on new technologies and ingredients designed to bring the freshest and safest food products to the marketplace.[4]

Food Safety in the Twentieth-century Marketplace

The diverse mix of fresh and processed foods available to consumers in North America from local, national, and international markets underscores the need for careful monitoring of the food supply. How is this accomplished so that foods don't deteriorate during transit and storage or become contaminated with microorganisms or other environmental agents before they reach the consumer's dinner table? This section describes the agents that cause foodborne disease, the laws and regulations that ensure a safe and adequate food supply, the substances found in human food, and the agencies responsible for safeguarding the food supply.

Foodborne Diseases

Foodborne illness is one of the greatest concerns of the regulatory agencies and the food industry with respect to food. It is estimated to cause between 24 million and 81 million cases of illness each year in the United States and to cost between $5 billion and $17 billion in medical care and lost productivity.[5] Incredible as these figures are, they probably represent only about 75 percent of the whole picture. The overwhelming majority of mild cases are never reported, because the victims pass them off as flu. (Some viruses do cause intestinal distress, and those that do are usually transmitted via food; true influenza viruses cause symptoms primarily in the upper respiratory tract.) If you experience diarrhea, nausea, abdominal pain, or vomiting as the major or only symptoms of your next bout of flu, chances are excellent that what you really have is food poisoning. If you take the proper precautions, you may never have it again.

Food supports the growth of contaminating microorganisms. This isn't surprising, when you consider that food is biological in nature and contains nutrients important in animal and human—and microbial—nutrition. Since disease-producing microorganisms are widespread in our environment, the potential for food-related illness is enormous. Foods can pick up microbes during production, processing, packaging, transport, storage, or preparation. Raw food contains microbes, as do all things.

The food industry uses different types of control measures to limit the risk of foodborne disease to consumers. Destruction or inactivation of bacteria or their spores can be accomplished through the use of heat treatments such as pasteurization and canning. Freezing, dehydrating, and refrigerating food halts or slows down bacterial growth. Special packaging techniques—for example, aseptic packaging, a process used in manufacturing the so-called paper bottle—and the use of approved antimicrobial preservatives also help control food-related pathogens.

Given the quantity of food processed by industry, you might think that food processors are responsible for most cases of foodborne illness. In fact, food processing plants account for only about 3 percent of outbreaks of foodborne disease.

Consider the safety record of the dairy industry. In 1938, illness due to contaminated milk and fluid milk products accounted for 25 percent of all reported foodborne disease; today these foods account for less than 1 percent of all such disease outbreaks. (Over the past 25 to 30 years, about 95 percent of all outbreaks associated with dairy products were due to the consumption of raw, unpasteurized milk.)[6]

According to figures from the Centers for Disease Control in Atlanta, Georgia, food service establishments—that is, cafeterias and restaurants (both traditional and fast-food)—account for about 77 percent and food preparation practices in homes, for about 20 percent of reported cases. Clearly, most cases of foodborne disease are caused by faulty handling, cooking, and storing of food in food service operations or in the home. Many of the food safety principles outlined in the Safe Food Preparation section apply to food-handling procedures in the home and in food service establishments.

Table 11–1 lists the leading causes of foodborne disease. Note that inadequate cooling of foods is the most common cause.[7] Inadequate cooling refers to leaving foods at room temperature for a long period of time, storing leftovers in large quantities in large containers (small containers cool down rapidly and slow the growth of microorganisms faster than large containers), not transporting perishable foods in a refrigerated container, and holding foods in ovens before serving them.

Foodborne disease, food poisoning illness transmitted by ingesting poisonous plants or animals or food contaminated with infectious microorganisms or toxic substances.

Agents That Cause Foodborne Disease

When we speak of **foodborne disease** or **food poisoning**, we are referring to the ingestion of food contaminated with infectious microorganisms or toxic substances—the most common types of foodborne disease in the United

Table 11–1

Most Important Factors Contributing to Outbreaks of Foodborne Disease in Homes and Restaurants

FACTOR	% OF OUTBREAKS
Inadequate cooling	46
Lapse of a day or more between preparation and service	21
Infected person touching cooked foods	20
Inadequate heat processing, canning, or cooking	16
Inadequate hot storage	16
Inadequate reheating	12
Contaminated raw food	11
Cross-contamination	7
Inadequate cleaning of equipment	7
Use of leftovers	4

Source: Adapted from N. H. Mermelstein (Ed.), New bacteria in the news—A special symposium, *Food Technology* 40 (1986): 16–26.

States—or the consumption of poisonous plants or animals. For the purpose of tracking and controlling outbreaks of food-related illness, experts classify foodborne diseases into two types: intoxications and infections.

An example of **foodborne bacterial intoxication** is the vomiting, nausea, abdominal cramping, sweating, chills, and subnormal body temperature that result from eating food contaminated with the pathogen, *Staphylococcus aureus.* This bacterium produces a toxin (specifically, an **enterotoxin**) that causes a severe inflammation of the lining of the gastrointestinal tract. Foodborne intoxication can also be caused by eating food that has been chemically contaminated, as with heavy metal poisoning. Salmonellosis, an illness caused by the bacterium *Salmonella,* is an example of **foodborne infection.**

Foodborne bacterial intoxication illness caused by eating food which contains a bacterial toxin resulting from bacterial growth in food.

Enterotoxin a toxic compound produced by microorganisms that distresses the gastrointestinal tract.

Foodborne infection illness caused by eating food that contains bacteria which grow and thrive in the host's tissues.

An important question to ask at this point is, How much contaminated food do I have to eat to come down with food poisoning? The answer isn't exactly straightforward. The mere presence of a pathogenic microorganism in or on foods is not usually enough to cause illness. Instead, the offending microorganism, toxin, or even toxic chemical must be present in food in a large enough quantity to produce illness. Bacteria that cause food poisoning must multiply to large numbers to cause the familiar symptoms of nausea, abdominal cramps, and diarrhea. To reach the critical mass that could produce such unpleasant symptoms, the bacteria require nutrients, moisture, a neutral or slightly acidic environment, and warmth—growth-enhancing factors all conveniently found in foods.

As indicated previously, not all foodborne illness is the result of bacterial contamination. Some outbreaks of food poisoning are caused by naturally occurring toxins in plants and animals or by heavy metals. These are discussed below, together with a brief review of the major types of bacterial agents that cause foodborne disease.

Microbial Agents When we scan a restaurant menu or reach for a food from the refrigerator at home, we aren't usually thinking about microorganisms, their possible presence in the foods we eat, or their potential to cause illness. We tend to assume that the foods and beverages we consume are safe to eat or drink. Most of the time we don't need to worry. But when proper food-

Table 11–2 Common Microbial Agents That Cause Foodborne Illness

ORGANISM & FOODS	ONSET	TOXIN	SYMPTOMS
Food infections			
Salmonella Raw meats, poultry, cracked eggs, milk and dairy products, shrimp, pasta, chocolate, and coconut	12–36 hrs	No	Vomiting, diarrhea, headache, malaise, anorexia, fever
Shigella Chocolate pudding, tossed salad, turkey salad, and spaghetti	1–7 days	No	Abdominal pains, fever, diarrhea, dehydration
Listeria monocytogenes Coleslaw, soft-style Mexican cheese, and pasteurized milk (contaminated after pasteurization process)	4 days–3 wks	No	Malaise, fever, flu-like symptoms, diarrhea, meningitis
Food intoxications			
Staphylococcus aureus Meats, poultry, egg products, tuna, potato and macaroni salads, puddings, and cream-filled pastries	1–7 hrs	Yes	Nausea, vomiting, abdominal cramping, prostration, weak pulse, shock
Clostridium botulinum Low-acid products such as canned corn, peppers, soups, mushrooms, ripe olives, spinach, tuna, chicken, luncheon meats, ham, sausage, and smoked fish	12–72 hrs	Yes	Nausea, vomiting, dizziness, blurred vision, respiratory failure, muscle paralysis
Bacillus cereus Common on vegetation; found in dairy products, meats, spices, and cereals (especially rice)	8–20 hrs	Yes	Nausea, vomiting, abdominal cramps, diarrhea
Clostridium perfringens Meats and meat products stored at between 120 and 130° F	4–24 hrs	Yes	Abdominal cramps, headache, shivering, diarrhea

handling procedures are not followed carefully, there is the risk of food poisoning. The symptoms of foodborne disease are usually mild, but they can be severe and truly life threatening, especially in the elderly, young children, or people with certain health problems, such as liver disease.

Several microorganisms can cause foodborne disease in humans. Here in North America, among the microorganisms responsible for most food-related disease outbreaks are *Staphylococcus aureus, Salmonella,* and *Clostridium botulinum.*[8] Table 11–2 summarizes the common food sources of these and other microbial agents responsible for outbreaks of foodborne illness.

Of the common disease-producing pathogens, *Staphylococcus aureus* is responsible for 20 percent to 40 percent of reported foodborne illnesses in the United States every year. The bacterium, which is found in the nose and throat and on the skin of most people, isn't responsible directly for the illness. Rather, it produces an enterotoxin that causes the typical symptoms of food poisoning within two to four hours of eating a food contaminated with the staphylococcus enterotoxin. When an individual with an infected wound or boil or one with a respiratory infection handles food improperly, *S. aureus* can be transferred to the food, where it then multiplies. The foods typically implicated in *S. aureus* intoxication include meat and poultry products, cream sauces, salads (chicken, ham, potato, etc.), puddings, and custards. Proper food-handling and sanitation procedures will help prevent food poisoning by this bacterium.

that of remedies taken from plants (or animals) is unreliable and unpredictable. The potential dangers are amplified when a food is mislabeled or misidentified. A root sold as the rare and expensive ginseng root may actually be that of a different plant, indistinguishable to an untrained eye.

As an example of the mistaking of one herb for another, a man confused the foxglove plant (from which a potent heart medication is extracted) with comfrey (a plant popular for making tea). He brewed a tea from the foxglove and drank a little more than a quart of it over several days resulting in digoxin poisoning.[9] Comfrey itself becomes toxic when used regularly, but foxglove is even more so. Such herbal stories are common.

If people are aware of the risks of misusing or overusing herbal teas, they still may not realize that many commonly used plants and plant products also contain naturally occurring toxicants. Mushrooms, already mentioned, are a familiar example, but a number of other common foods have been observed to cause toxic effects. Consider this list:

- Cabbage, mustard, and other plants contain goitrogens; if these plants are consumed as a steady diet, they can enlarge the thyroid gland.
- Spinach and rhubarb contain oxalates, tolerable as usually consumed; but one normal serving of rhubarb contains one-fifth the toxic dose for humans.
- Potatoes contain solanine, a powerful inhibitor of nerve impulses found in the green layer that develops just beneath the skin. Ordinary consumption of potatoes delivers one-tenth the dose of solanine that would be toxic.[10] When potatoes are exposed to light, they develop more solanine. Throw such potatoes away; don't eat them. (Fortunately, most potatoes on the market today are low in solanine, thanks to the efforts of scientists who bred low-solanine varieties of potatoes.)
- Honey can be a host to the botulinum organism and can accumulate enough toxin to kill an infant.[11]

There are 700 other examples of plants that have caused serious illnesses or death in the Western Hemisphere.[12] A well-known environmental scientist has said, "One can predict that if the standards used to test manmade chemicals were applied to 'natural' foods, fully half of the human food supply would have to be banned."[13]

Perhaps the most sensible practical advice to follow in relation to these facts is to avoid using strange and unfamiliar foods except when they are sold by reputable agencies—such as your local grocery store. Especially avoid buying herbal products from sellers that advertise them as having medicinal effects. Should you have questions, ask before you eat.*

Toxic Animals In 1975, one of Japan's most celebrated Kabuki actors, an artist designated "a living national treasure" by the Japanese government, died of convulsions and paralysis several hours after eating fugu liver, the most poisonous part of the globefish (also known as puffer, blowfish, swellfish, and fugu). The actor, Mitsugoro Bando VIII, had a penchant for fugu and had begged the restaurant's chef to prepare fugu liver. Mr. Bando ate four helpings and paid dearly for his passion.

Puffers, long considered a delicacy in Japan, may be the most deadly fish in the sea. They are host to a potent poison—tetrodotoxin—which doesn't

*The FDA's address and telephone number are in Appendix A.

Figure 11–1

How a Food Chain Works

A person whose principal animal protein source is fish may consume about a hundred pounds of fish in a year. These fish will, in turn, have consumed a few tons of plant-eating fish in the course of their lifetimes. The plant eaters, in their lifetimes, will have consumed several tons of photosynthetic producer organisms. If the producer organisms have become contaminated with toxic chemicals, these chemicals become more concentrated in the bodies of the fish that consume them. If none of the chemicals are lost along the way, *one person* ultimately eats the same amount of contaminant as was present in the original *several tons* of producer organisms.

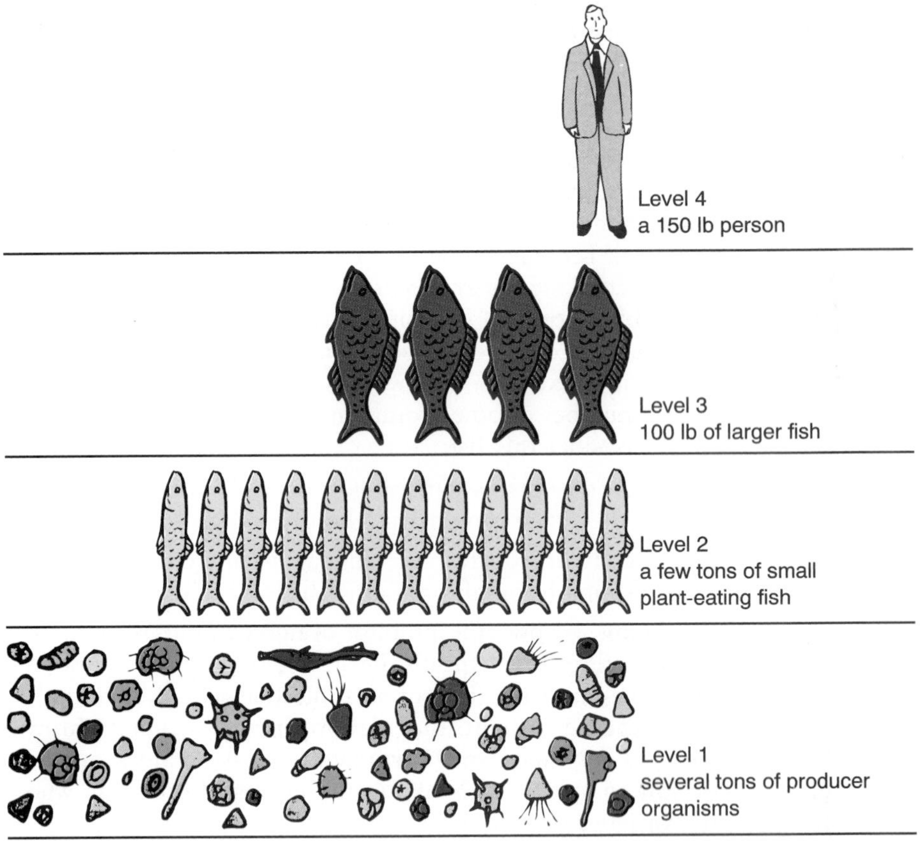

harm them but can be lethal if eaten by humans or other animals. Tetrodotoxin, which is 275 times deadlier than cyanide, works by blocking nerve impulses; over a period of several hours, it will eventually close down a person's entire nervous system.[14]

Puffer poisoning is one example of a foodborne disease traced to eating a toxic animal. Others also exist. Scombroid fish poisoning—which involves the scombroid fish tuna, mackerel, and skipjack—results from ingesting a toxin produced by the action of bacteria on the dark meat in the fish. Fish contaminated with the scombroid toxin have a "honeycombed" look and a sharp, peppery taste. Ciguatera fish poisoning results from eating certain contaminated fish, especially the tropical marine reef fish, grouper and snapper, and brings about symptoms such as nausea, diarrhea, headache, and face pain. These fish are thought to acquire the toxin through the food chain (see Figure 11–1). Finally, there is paralytic shellfish poisoning, which can occur after eating mollusks (clams, mussels, oysters, and scallops) contaminated with marine algae that produce a neurotoxin. The mollusks don't themselves become ill, but people eating these contaminated species do, with symptoms including nausea, vomiting, cramps, and muscle weakness. In each of these cases, the toxin is not destroyed on cooking. Thus, the consumer's best approach to healthful eating is to buy fish from reputable vendors. Additional consumer protection from contaminated fish is provided by the FDA through its new inspection program. The FDA's newly organized Office of Seafood is responsible for inspecting domestic and imported seafood, in addition to developing and implementing shellfish sanitation programs.

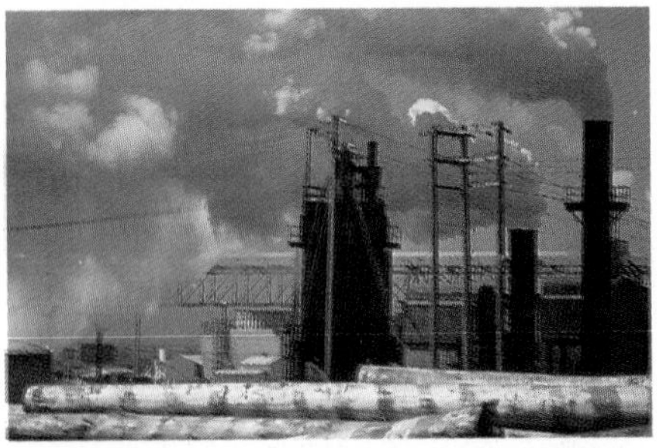

Many of the toxins that contaminate foods are the waste products of industry.

Chemical Agents Despite major efforts by food producers and food processors to maintain a safe food supply, some risk of consuming undesirable substances or **contaminants** is unavoidable. The reliance of our industrial society on chemical processes is such that foods may become contaminated by a variety of chemicals introduced into the environment. Some of the problem chemicals include polychlorinated biphenyl (PCB), polybrominated biphenyl (PBB), and metals such as lead and mercury.

In 1953, a number of people in Minamata, Japan, became ill with a disease no one had seen before. By 1960, 121 cases had been reported, including 23 cases in infants. Mortality was high: 46 died. In the survivors, the symptoms were ugly: "progressive blindness, deafness, incoordination, and intellectual deterioration."[15] The cause was ultimately revealed to be methylmercury contamination of fish from the bay these people lived on. The infants who contracted the disease had not eaten any fish, but their mothers had, and even though the mothers exhibited no symptoms during their pregnancies, the poison had been affecting their unborn babies. Manufacturing plants in the region were discharging mercury into the water of the bay, the mercury was turning into methylmercury upon leaving the factories, and the fish in the bay were accumulating this poison in their bodies. Some of the families who were affected were eating fish from the bay every day.[16]

Another example of the toxicity to humans of an environmentally derived **heavy metal** comes from the work of a physician, Dr. Alice Hamilton. In 1910, Dr. Hamilton began documenting her observations of factory workers intoxicated with lead poisoning. The workers exhibited a wide variety of symptoms, she said, including anemia, constipation, loss of appetite, abnormal kidney function, jaundice due to liver damage, "wrist drop" (loss of muscular control of the hand), irritability, drowsiness, stupor, and coma. Mothers exposed to lead more often had abortions and stillbirths, and their children were more often sick.[17] Lead also finds its way into food, as will be shown below.

In 1973, in Michigan, half a ton of polybrominated biphenyl (PBB), a toxic chemical, was accidentally mixed into some livestock feed that was distributed throughout the state. The chemical found its way into millions of animals and then into humans. The seriousness of the accident began to come to light when dairy farmers reported their cows going dry, aborting their calves, and developing abnormal growths on their hooves. Although more than 30,000 cattle, sheep, and swine and more than a million chickens were destroyed, effects on people were not prevented. By 1982, it was estimated that 97 percent of Michigan's residents had become contaminated with PBB. Nervous system aberrations and alterations in the liver and immune systems were among the effects in exposed farm residents.[18]

Mercury and lead are both heavy metals, and PBB is an **organic halogen.** These two classes of chemicals are among the most toxic and widespread in our environment. The number of contaminants we could discuss here and the amount of information available about them are far beyond our scope. Instead of dealing superficially with many of them, we can illustrate principles that apply to all contaminants by giving details about just a few. A list of some of the chemical contaminants of greatest concern in foods is presented in Table 11–4. Table 11–5 gives more details on a selected few.

On first studying this subject, a reader is likely to want the question answered, How serious is all this—how dangerous is it for *me*? No one who has pursued the subject realistically expects to have that question answered in

Contaminants potentially dangerous substances that can accidentally find their way into foods (lead is an example).

Heavy metal any of a number of mineral ions such as mercury and lead, so called because they are of relatively high atomic weight. Many heavy metals are poisonous.

Organic halogen an organic compound containing one or more atoms of a halogen—fluorine, chlorine, iodine, or bromine.

Table 11–4

Chemical Contaminants of Concern in Foods

Heavy metals
Arsenic
Cadmium
Lead
Mercury
Selenium
Halogenated compounds
Chlorine
Ethylene dichloride
Iodine
Polybrominated biphenyl (PBB)
Polychlorinated biphenyl (PCB)
Trichloroethylene
Vinyl chloride
Others
Acrilonitrile
Antibiotics (in animal feed)
Asbestos
Dioxins
Heat-induced mutagens
Lysinoalanine

Source: E. M. Foster, How safe are our foods? *Nutrition Reviews* (supplement), January 1982, pp. 28–34.

Table 11–5

Examples of Contaminants in Foods

Name and Description	Sources	Toxic Effects	Typical Route to Food Chain
Cadmium (heavy metal)	Used in industrial processes, including electroplating, plastics, batteries, alloys, pigments, smelters, and burning fuels; present in cigarette smoke.	Has immediately detectable symptoms; slowly and irreversibly damages kidneys and liver.	Enters air in smokestack emissions, settles on ground, is absorbed into food plants, is consumed by farm animals, and is eaten in meat and vegetables by people. Sewage sludge and fertilizers leave large amounts in the soil; runoff contaminates shellfish.
Lead (heavy metal)	Added to gasoline; added to paints; sometimes used to seal cans of food; sometimes present in tap water.	Displaces calcium, iron, zinc, and other minerals from their sites of action in the nervous system, bone marrow, kidneys, and liver, causing failure to function; has severe effects in fetuses, infants, and children, who easily absorb and retain lead; causes breakage of red blood cells (anemia) and interferes with the immune response.	Air pollution, gasoline, water pipes, and others.
Mercury (heavy metal)	Widely dispersed in gases from the earth's crust; local high concentrations from industry, electrical equipment, paints, and agriculture.	Methylmercury poisons the nervous system, especially in fetuses.	Inorganic mercury released into waterways by industry and acid rain is converted to methylmercury by bacteria and ingested by food species of fish (tuna, swordfish, and others).
Polychlorinated biphenyl (PCB) (organic compound)	Has no natural source; produced for use in electrical equipment (transformers, capacitors).	Causes long-lasting skin eruptions, eye irritations, growth retardation in children of exposed mothers, anorexia, fatigue, and other effects.	Discarded electrical equipment; accidental industrial leakage, or reuse of PCB containers for food.

any simple way. It may be a negligible problem in your particular area today, but tomorrow it may become a severe one if there is a major spill or other accident. A general answer, then, is that even though the material is toxic, the hazard may be small because most of the time the chemicals are under control. In the event of an accident, though, the hazard can suddenly become very great.

At this point, we should differentiate between **toxicity** (a property of all substances) and **hazard** (the probability of a substance's actually causing harm). "Toxicity—the capacity of a chemical substance to harm living organisms—is a general property of matter; hazard is the capacity of a chemical to produce injury under conditions of use. All substances are potentially toxic, but are hazardous only if consumed in sufficiently large quantities."[19] In other words, the dose makes the poison. For example, eating foods containing preformed vitamin A as part of a nutritionally balanced diet is not hazardous. Eating large portions of polar bear liver, which can contain up to

Toxicity the ability of a substance to harm living organisms. All substances are toxic if high enough concentrations are used.
Hazard state of danger; used to refer to any circumstance in which harm is possible under normal conditions of use.

100,000 IU (international units) of vitamin A per gram of liver tissue, or taking megadoses of vitamin A supplements, can produce acute vitamin A toxicity.*

See Chapter 6 and the inside front cover for recommended intakes of vitamin A.

Table 11–5 shows how pervasively a contaminant can affect the body. The case of lead offers a particularly telling example of something else—how specific nutrients interact with heavy metals in specific ways. Total food intake; fat intake; and calcium, iron, and zinc intakes are also known to alter animals' (and probably humans') susceptibility to lead toxicity:

- A diet low in calcium permits greater amounts of lead to accumulate in the body, probably by permitting more lead to be absorbed.
- Iron deficiency, even mild iron deficiency, permits greater lead intoxication. Iron deficiency in a nursing female increases the lead content of the milk.
- Zinc status affects both tissue accumulation of lead and sensitivity to its effects.[20]
- The absorption of lead is greater when the stomach is empty.[21]

The interaction of nutrients with contaminants like lead raises an important point. When an agency is charged with setting the "maximum permissible level" of an environmental contaminant, it sets about testing animals to see what levels bring about detectable ill effects. Usually these animals are being fed the standard laboratory chow—a very nutritious diet—and the only thing varied is the animals' exposure to the contaminant. Healthy, well-nourished animals are likely to have considerably greater resistance to toxicity than they would if they were sick or malnourished or if they were exposed to other toxins simultaneously. Yet the people to whom the results are applied may be neither healthy nor well-nourished, and all probably encounter numerous toxins every day. These facts must be remembered when the limits are set.

In 1981, 535,000 U.S. children aged six months to five years were screened, and 22,000 were found to have symptoms caused by lead toxicity, reflecting a prevalent national health problem. In the same screening, an almost equal number of children—23,000—were found to need treatment for iron deficiency, a long-familiar, widespread public health problem. Thus, lead toxicity ranks with iron deficiency in prevalence and severity. Today, at least one out of every six children between the ages of 6 months and 5 years, and one out of every nine fetuses are at risk for lead toxicity.[22] Of even greater concern: only one year of exposure can cause irreversible effects on the brain, nervous system, and psychological functioning.[23] Furthermore, recent experiments have shown that the effects occur with *lower* doses than had been thought in the past. Based on these experiments, more than one million children may now be at risk of showing permanent damage caused by lead.[24]

Lead appears in all foods and is also the nation's most significant contaminant in drinking water.[25] (See the Spotlight feature in Chapter 7 for a discussion on lead in drinking water.) Whether some of it is naturally present is not known, but much of it is known to come from industrial pollution. People use lead in gasoline, paint, newspaper ink, shotgun ammunition, batteries, and pesticides and in industrial processes that release lead into the

*Although the vitamin A recommendation is expressed in RE, the amounts of vitamin A in supplements are often expressed in an older unit, IU (international units). To convert, use the factor 3 IU = 1 RE.

air and water. Some domestic pipes are made of lead, which dissolves into water—especially soft, acid water. While food from cans sealed with lead solder used to contain the metal, most canned foods purchased today do not; only about 4 percent of American cans are soldered with lead, and most of these contain dry foods such as coffee, into which lead cannot leach. Many imported cans, however, still have lead-soldered seams. The edges along the joint of such a seam will be folded over and smeared with a silver-gray metal. Seams welded without lead, on the other hand, are flat, with a thick, dark line along the joint.[26] Lead in foods comes primarily from leaded-gasoline exhaust, which works its way through rainfall and soil into plants and animals used as food.[27]

A standard has been recommended for weekly acceptable intakes of lead, but no monitoring system keeps track of the amounts to which people are actually exposed.* Exposures are known to be higher in urban and industrial areas, near highways, and in slums, where children may accidentally ingest leaded paint by teething on old furniture, the railings of old buildings, or lead-tainted dirt. The reduction of the use of leaded gasoline for automobiles and the application of new technology and material to the canning process are helping to limit the amounts of lead in the environment.

Chelating agent a chemical that sequesters another chemical; in nutrition, an agent that binds minerals and makes them unavailable for absorption.

A popular new therapy to prevent or relieve poisoning by heavy metals is chelation therapy, in which a person ingests a **chelating agent**, expecting it to capture poisons and remove them from the body with the feces. The agent most often used is EDTA—ethylene diamine tetraacetic acid—a nonspecific chelating agent that grabs positively charged molecules based only on their electrical charges. The trouble is that many nutrients have such charges, and EDTA does not distinguish ions you might want to absorb, such as calcium, iron, magnesium, and copper, from those you do not want, such as lead or mercury. Long-term use has been known to remove so much calcium from the bones that the bones no longer can support the body's weight. EDTA has legitimate uses. It can save the life of a child afflicted with metal poisoning, but it is also sometimes advertised by quacks who claim to be able to leach plaques out of your arteries or do other such imaginary things.

It is generally accepted that the hazard from contamination of food by chemical agents is small; the chief risk to individuals is from accidental gross contamination. However, the example of chronic low-level lead poisoning warns us that more subtle effects may be occurring. It just happens that much of what we know about contaminants necessarily derives from episodes of acute contamination of limited populations. No one knows to what extent the total burden of contaminants accumulating in the environment may be reaching and posing a hazard to human beings. No one knows whether some individuals may be susceptible today to contamination levels in some areas.

Another unknown factor is the interaction among contaminants. A substance that poses no threat by itself is chlorine in drinking water. However, when chlorine combines with organic wastes in the water, the chemicals join to form potent carcinogens. Still another unknown is the time factor. Many

*The World Health Organization suggests not more than 3 mg/week for adults. Evaluation of mercury, lead, cadmium, and the food additives amaranth, diethylpyrocarbonate, and octyl gallate, in *WHO Food Additives Series No. 4,* (Geneva: WHO, 1972) as cited by D. G. Lindsay and J. C. Sherlock, Environmental contaminants, in *Adverse Effects of Foods,* E.F.P. Jelliffe and D.B. Jelliffe (Eds.) (New York: Plenum Press, 1982), pp. 85–110.

substances of concern have been around for only a short time. What are the effects of prolonged exposure to them? Contaminants are sometimes hard to identify. Sometimes it is not even known that they are present, so they are hard to regulate.

An in-depth understanding of nutrition is essential to understanding the risks from contaminants. Not 100 percent of the time, but more often than not, an adequate diet and optimal health help to protect against the toxicity of food contaminants and other environmental pollutants. If you want to be well protected against possible exposure to toxic environmental contaminants in the future, you should look to your own nutritional health today. If you want your children to be protected, you should make sure that they receive an adequate and varied diet. Variety in food choices and moderation in food intake ensures an adequate intake of essential nutrients, enhances the nutritional value of our diets, and minimizes exposure to environmental contaminants.

Safe Food Preparation

Commercially prepared, canned, or packaged food is usually, but not always, safe. Batch numbering makes it possible to recall contaminated foods through public announcements via newspapers, television, and radio. The chance that someone may tamper with grocery store food is remote. To protect against even this unlikely event, however, carefully inspect the seals and wrappers of packages. Jars should be firmly sealed (many have safety "buttons," areas of the lid designed to pop up once opened). Notice how the majority of the packages on the shelf appear. If the package you have chosen looks different or has holes or tears, do not buy it—turn the product in to the store manager. A broken seal or mangled package is not doing its job of protecting the product.

Most cases of food poisoning that arise from kitchen mistakes can be averted by doing three simple things: keep hot food hot; keep cold food cold; and keep your hands, the utensils, and the kitchen clean. Keeping hot food hot includes allowing sufficient cooking time for food to reach safe internal temperatures during cooking (these temperatures are listed on meat thermometers) and holding the food at a high enough temperature to prevent bacterial growth until served. Temperatures between 140 and 165 degrees Fahrenheit are usually safe for up to 2 hours. After that, all of the food should be chilled.

Keeping cold food cold starts when you leave the grocery store. If you are running errands, shop last so the groceries do not stay in the car too long. Pack foods into the refrigerator or freezer immediately upon arrival at home.

A clean kitchen prevents contamination of otherwise wholesome foods. Wash the countertops, your hands, and utensils in warm, soapy water before each step of food preparation. Microbes love to nestle down in the fibers of wood cutting boards, kitchen cloths, and sponges. A microwave oven is handy for sterilizing wet sponges and cloths—after using, cook them on "high" until they are steamy and hot. Laundering with bleach will do the same thing; sponging bleach solution over the cutting board is a way to sterilize two kitchen items at once. Wash wooden and plastic cutting boards in the dishwasher if possible.

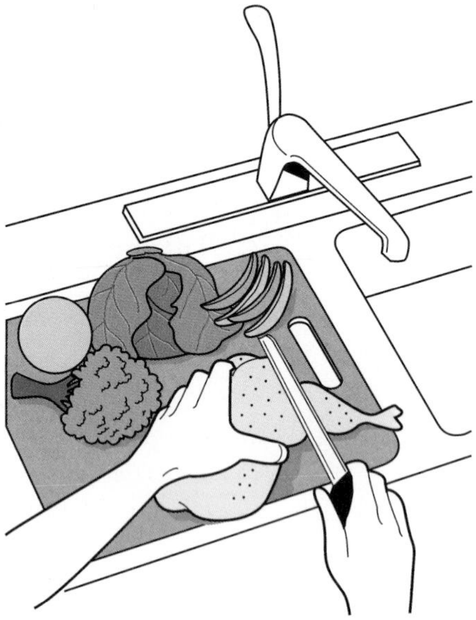

Never work with raw meat on the same surface that you use for other foods without thoroughly cleaning the surface after you've finished with the meat. Otherwise, bacteria on the meat can migrate to other foods and contaminate them.

Meat requires special handling. It may contain all sorts of bacteria, and it provides a moist, nutritious environment—just right for microbial growth. If raw meat has been marinated in a dish, don't put the meat back in the same dish after cooking it, and don't use the marinade unless it has been cooked thoroughly. Wash the dish in hot, soapy water before reusing it, or else the bacteria inevitably left in the dish from the raw meat can contaminate and grow in the cooked product or other food. This is a classic example of cross-contamination.

Especially susceptible to bacterial contamination is ground meat. It is handled more than other kinds of meat and has much more surface exposed to the air for bacteria to land on. It is best to cook hamburgers to at least medium well. For a meat loaf, use a thermometer to test the internal temperature.

Remember: fresh food smells fresh. It bears repeating that any food that has an off odor should not be used but should be returned to the grocery store or thrown out. That odor is probably the result of bacterial wastes and indicates that the number of bacteria in the food is dangerous. Not all types of food poisoning are detectable by odor, but if an abnormal odor exists, chances are excellent that the food is spoiled. Refer to Table 11–3; if you learn and follow the rules given there, you may save yourself the pain and inconvenience (and sometimes danger) of foodborne illness. (See the Kitchen Safety Scorecard at the end of this section to help you score your kitchen for safety.)

Picnics are fun and can be safe, too. Choose foods that last without refrigeration, such as fresh fruits and vegetables, breads and crackers, and canned spreads and cheeses that can be opened and used on the spot. Aged cheeses, such as cheddar and Swiss, do well for an hour or two, but they should be carried in an ice chest for longer periods. The advice not to add mayonnaise to picnic foods such as meat or pasta salad has been reversed by some, who cite a study that found that mayonnaise was resistant to spoilage because of its acid content. Still, whether or not mixed salads of chopped ingredients contain mayonnaise, they spoil easily because they have extensive surface area for bacteria to invade, and they have been in contact with cutting boards, hands, and kitchen utensils that easily transmit bacteria to food. Chill them well before, during, and after the picnic. It's best to keep mayonnaise itself cold, too.

Another danger concerns honey. Honey has been found to contain dormant bacterial spores, which can awaken in the human body to produce botulism, mentioned earlier. In adults this is not a hazard, but infants under one year of age should never be fed honey.[28] (Honey can also be contaminated with environmental pollutants picked up by the bees.) Honey has been implicated in several cases of sudden infant death.[29]

For adults and children alike, eating raw or lightly steamed seafood is a risky proposition. As the population density increases along the shores of seafood-harvesting waters, pollution of those waters inevitably invades the seafood living there. Watchdog agencies try to monitor the waters and keep harvesters out of the worst areas, but these efforts are often insufficient to ensure the wholesomeness of the food.[30]

The foodborne infections that lurk in normal-appearing seafood can be much worse than those of spoilage—hepatitis, worms and parasites, severe viral intestinal disorders, and other diseases. Hepatitis is a prolonged illness

Kitchen Safety Scorecard

Improper storage of food not only increases the risk of food poisoning but also almost always results in a loss of nutrients and good taste. The following quiz is designed to find out how your kitchen rates.

To take the quiz, answer whether each statement describes your kitchen, always, sometimes, or never. Then read the comments that follow for additional tips. Score each statement as follows:

Always: 2 points; Sometimes: 1 point; Never: 0 points

1. Highly perishable foods like milk are stored in the refrigerator, not in the refrigerator door.
2. Milk is kept in opaque, closed containers. Orange juice is kept tightly covered.
3. Eggs are stored in their original carton.
4. Fresh produce—especially leafy greens—are in plastic bags or in the vegetable bin.
5. Whole-wheat flour and wheat germ are stored in the refrigerator.
6. Refrigerated leftovers and frozen foods are marked to indicate their contents and the date they were stored.
7. Food is frozen in small containers.
8. Food is loosely packed in the freezer.
9. Dented cans are checked for seam damage or leaks.
10. Package and can labels are checked for storage directions before being stored.
11. Food is stored in cabinets, not under the sink.
12. Food is stored in cabinets away from the stove.
13. Refrigerator and freezer door seals are periodically cleaned and checked.

Read the following to find out how each of the previous statements relates to kitchen safety:

1. The refrigerator door does not stay as cold as the rest of the refrigerator, so highly perishable foods—especially milk—should not be stored there. Use the door for storing condiments like catsup and mayonnaise.
2. Milk is a good source of riboflavin, but much is lost if milk is exposed to light. Orange juice loses vitamin C upon exposure to air, so use closed containers, or prepare only as much juice as needed.
3. Eggs stay fresh longest when stored, large end up, in the carton in which they are sold. Use refrigerated eggs within a week for best flavor and cooking quality, although they're safe to eat for three to four weeks. Eggs that have cracked shells should be thrown out—they may be contaminated with *Salmonella* bacteria.
4. Most vegetables keep best when stored in the crisper drawer or in plastic bags on the lower shelf of the refrigerator. Either way helps keep in moisture which prevents wilting.
5. Most flours and grains can be kept at room temperature but should be tightly covered to prevent insect infestation. Whole grains, however, keep better in the refrigerator. Because of their higher fat content, they are more susceptible to rancidity and insect infestation. Wheat germ should always be refrigerated after opening.
6. Marking the contents of refrigerated and frozen foods eliminates the guessing game. Dating foods is also essential, so foods can be rotated—oldest foods can be used first.
7. The faster foods are cooled, the less time there is for bacteria to grow. Avoid putting hot foods into large containers. The center may be dangerously warm for too long.
8. Overpacking a freezer interferes with air circulation, making it work harder to keep low temperatures. If the temperature isn't low enough, food won't keep as long.
9. Buying dented cans is okay, but only if they are free of seam damage and leaks. Check again just before opening. A sticky ring left on the shelf under the can may be an indication of leakage.
10. Some dry packaged foods and canned foods require refrigeration once they are opened; some even before they are opened. Check labels for storage information.
11. Storing food under the sink is potentially dangerous for three reasons. First, cleaning products could leak and soak through cardboard boxes or bags. Second, leaking pipes can rust cans and damage boxes. Finally, openings in the walls for pipes give insects and rodents easy access.
12. Cabinets over the stove get hot. Most foods won't last long under such conditions.
13. Door gaskets should be periodically washed to ensure the cold is sealed in. As a test, close a dollar bill in the door. If the seal is tight, you shouldn't be able to pull it out.

Scoring:

24–26	Excellent food storage savvy.
20–23	Pretty good habits, but try to be more consistent.
15–19	Not so good. Better read the next section carefully.
0–14	Poor storage I.Q. Tape a copy of this quiz to the refrigerator as a reminder.

Source: Adapted from S. M. Smith, How to score a kitchen, *Environmental Nutrition* 11 (1988): 1–2. Used with permission.

of months' or years' duration and greatly increases the risk of liver cancer later. People who love raw seafood and have eaten it for years may try to brush these threats off because they have never experienced serious illness. Now, though, experts are suggesting that the risks are increasing to the point of being unacceptably high, and it may be time to warn people to cook all seafood thoroughly before eating it. Those who choose to indulge in sushi should do so only in reputable restaurants. At home, consumers should freeze the fish first for four to five days at −4° Fahrenheit to kill any mature parasitic worms (only cooking can kill all worm eggs and microorganisms).

Food Laws

How is a safe food supply achieved, especially given the potential for contamination in all phases of food production, processing, and preparation? How is a superior level of food safety maintained, what with new chemicals being introduced into the environment? Here in North America, stringent food laws currently regulate the food supply and enhance food safety, although things weren't always the way they are today.

During colonial times, Americans were primarily an agricultural society, with the seasons determining which foods were available. The standard colonial diet consisted of meat, salt pork, cornmeal, hominy, whole-wheat bread, and vegetables in season. The food supply was largely homegrown, because there were no satisfactory methods of refrigerating or storing large quantities of foods. Dehydrating or drying foods was the primary method of food preservation.

The few food laws in existence at that time were limited in scope. For example, a law passed by the Massachusetts Bay Colony in 1646 stipulated how much a loaf of bread must weigh to be sold for a penny and authorized official inspectors to enter small shops to check the weight of bread being sold. Most food laws applied to exported meat and imported tea. During colonial times, federal and state governments had little control over the food supply, with the result that many foods were **adulterated.** Milk was generally of extremely poor quality and often contained added chalk and water. Sand was sometimes added to cornmeal, chalk added as a whitener to flour, and lard added as an extender to butter. In some cases, animals dying of disease (for example, hog cholera) were sold as food.[31]

Adulterated food a lowering of the value or purity of a food product or any change that alters the food's composition or the meaning of the name under which it's sold.

Not until the efforts of Harvey W. Wiley in the late 1800s did a national movement emerge to protect food quality. Dr. Wiley, a physician, was appointed chief of the Bureau of Chemistry of the U.S. Department of Agriculture (USDA) in 1880. Described as the greatest name in food law history, he organized a "poison squad" (a title to which he objected strongly), whose mission was to test the health effects of commonly used food preservatives. Twelve young men working at USDA were selected to consume such preservatives as boric acid, benzoic acid, and formaldehyde. (Such experiments would not be allowed today because of stringent laws governing the health and safety of humans participating in research.) The experimental results showed that ingesting these preservatives was harmful to humans, whether the chemicals were consumed in small amounts for long periods of time or in large doses over short periods of time. The activities of the "poison squad" made national headlines and served to stimulate the public's interest in issues of food safety.

Another of Dr. Wiley's main goals was to accomplish the enactment of federal legislation regulating food composition. As a result of Dr. Wiley's efforts—which occurred in concert with farmers' complaints that their wholesome butter and milk products were being adulterated—Congress enacted the Food and Drugs Act in 1906. The Act established state departments of agriculture and prevented the manufacture, sale, or transportation of adulterated, **misbranded**, or poisonous foods, drugs, medicines, and liquors. It represented a major step forward in protecting the public health. Unfortunately, the law lacked clout in that it required the government to prove that alleged offenders had *intended* to deceive consumers. The government almost never won a case in court, because defendants merely claimed ignorance of the health effects of ingredients added to their food products. A lack of standards of purity related to ingredients and foods made enforcing the law almost impossible.

Misbranded food a food with a false or misleading label, one sold under the name of another food, or one sold in a container that isn't filled properly or is otherwise misleading.

Tolerances the limits on the amounts of substances allowed in foods.

These problems were overcome with the enactment in 1938 of the Food, Drug, and Cosmetic Act, the law that currently regulates the U.S. food supply. The Act differed from the 1906 law in that it placed the burden of proof of ingredient safety on the food processor or manufacturer. The new law prohibited the addition of poison to foods *except* where such an addition was required in food processing or could not be avoided by good manufacturing practices. It set **tolerances** for authorized poisons added during processing. It also required label declarations of artificial colorings, artificial flavorings, and chemical preservatives in foods and labeling of special dietary foods.

For the first time, standards were established to measure the quantity, quality, weight, or value of food products. A standard of identity, for example, defines a food product in specific terms, spelling out which ingredients are required and which are optional in the product. It also specifies how the label for the product should read. The standard of identity for canned peas, for example, indicates that the name of the food product is "peas" and that either shelled, succulent peas (*Pisum sativum*) of smooth skin varieties or those of sweet, wrinkled varieties can be used. Several optional ingredients can be added to canned peas and are outlined in the standard of identity: salt, monosodium glutamate, disodium inosinate, disodium guanylate, hydrolyzed vegetable protein, autolyzed yeast extract, sugar, spice, and flavoring (except artificial), to name a few. Because of standards of identity, consumers know that a food label showing a picture of peas and labeled "peas" has certain basic ingredients, whether it is sold by Company ABC or Company XYZ. Other standards also exist, namely standards for grade, standards of quality, and standards of fill of container. All are designed to assure the consumer that foods are safe to eat and that labels and containers are not deceptive or misleading.

Several important amendments to the Food, Drug, and Cosmetic Act of 1938 have been enacted. The first, in 1954, was the Pesticide Chemicals Amendment, which gave the Food and Drug Administration (FDA) responsibility for enforcing safety tolerances for registered **pesticides** in or on raw agricultural products. (The Environmental Protection Agency is responsible for setting the safety tolerances for pesticides used on foods.) The second was the Food Additives Amendment of 1958, which strengthened the regulation of **food additives** (described a little later). In 1960, the Color Additives Amendment was enacted which restricted the addition of **color additives** to cosmetics, drugs, and foods to those *listed* by FDA as safe. Finally, the Vitamin

Pesticides poisons used intentionally on food crops or in other situations where pests are a problem. Pests include all living organisms that destroy or spoil foods: bacteria, molds, and fungi, insects of all kinds, and rats and other rodents.

Food additives substances not normally consumed as foods by themselves, but added to food either intentionally or by accident.

Color additives natural and synthetic dyes and pigments that impart color to foods, drugs, and cosmetics.

Delaney Clause a clause in the Food Additive Amendment to the Food, Drug, and Cosmetic Act that states that no substance that is known to cause cancer in animals or humans at any dose level shall be added to foods.

and Mineral Amendment, passed in 1976, was designed to provide more FDA control over product formulation and labeling. Together, these laws specify which ingredients can be used in foods, which foods they can be used in, and the appropriate levels of use of added ingredients.

Special mention should be made here of the famous **Delaney clause** written into the Food Additives Amendment of 1958. As the food additives bill was being debated in Congress, James J. Delaney (U.S. Representative to New York) chaired the Delaney Committee, whose mandate was to study the use of chemicals in food in the early 1950s. Congressman Delaney sponsored a provision to the food additives bill that forbid the approval of any additive found to cause cancer in animals, no matter how small the dose. The rationale for the provision was based, in part, on the belief of many experts that it was possible to completely eliminate cancer-causing agents from the food supply. Following considerable debate in Congress about the implications of this provision, the clause made its way into the final bill that was passed and became law.

The significance of the Delaney clause for the regulatory agencies is that it is now believed that the elimination of all cancer-causing agents from the food supply is neither a realistic nor an achievable goal. Consider that many substances, even those found naturally in a number of foods, can cause cancer when given to animals in large enough amounts. In fact, the Delaney clause has been criticized for encouraging studies to be performed on animals, in which the animals are fed doses as large as 64,000,000 times the dose that humans would ingest. Experts ask how meaningful the results of such studies can be.

The challenge for the FDA and other regulatory agencies in light of the Delaney clause is how to realistically apply the anti-cancer principle to the regulation of the food supply. The agencies' approach must consider the degree to which humans are exposed to the cancer-causing agent and the level of intake at which the agent causes cancer and in which animals. Any potential risks to consumers of ingesting the carcinogen must be evaluated as well.

The FDA has moved toward a greater consideration of both the risks and the benefits of additives, with the realization that absolute safety of any component of food—whether naturally occurring or added during processing—cannot be guaranteed.

Regulatory Agencies

Several U.S. government agencies are responsible for safeguarding the food supply. The primary mission of the FDA, as mentioned previously, is enforcing the Food, Drug, and Cosmetic Act as a means of regulating the activities of producers of foods, drugs, cosmetics, and medical devices. The FDA has four major responsibilities where foods are concerned:

1. To ensure that foods are produced and stored under sanitary conditions.
2. To ensure that foods are free of toxic chemical contaminants and pesticides.
3. To ensure that foods are properly labeled.
4. To evaluate the safety of food additives.

The scope of the FDA's activities is enormous. Through its field staff, the FDA inspects imported foods and local food establishments; collects and analyzes food samples to determine whether they are contaminated with pesticides, industrial chemicals, toxic elements, and natural poisons; conducts research to assess the health concerns of additives currently being used in the marketplace; controls the spread of communicable diseases via interstate commerce by inspecting aircraft, buses, trains and vessels, and waste support systems; conducts surveys to help monitor and improve the nutritional quality of the food supply; regulates the labeling of food products; and searches out violators of the Food, Drug, and Cosmetic Act. The latter is accomplished by seizing or detaining adulterated or misbranded foods, recalling contaminated foods, and prosecuting violators.

A recently acquired function of the FDA is the regulation of domestic and imported seafood. Through a new Office of Seafood in its Center for Food Safety and Applied Nutrition, the FDA is responsible for monitoring the safety of seafood sold to retail establishments and consumers.

Virtually all foods come under the FDA's jurisdiction *except* red meat, poultry, and eggs, which are regulated by USDA. Through its Food Safety and Inspection Service (FSIS), USDA inspects both domestic and imported meat, poultry, and related products and monitors the meat and poultry industry for violations of inspection laws. FSIS inspects live animals for diseases, approves plans for slaughtering and processing meat and poultry, inspects slaughterhouses for safety and sanitation, and samples meat and poultry for bacteria and harmful residues. It also establishes ingredient standards for meat and poultry products and approves recipes and labels for processed products such as sausages, frozen dinners, canned meats, and soups made with meat and poultry.

The Environmental Protection Agency (EPA) sets the tolerance levels for pesticide residues that occur on or in foods and monitors these levels in foods and humans. It also specifies the conditions under which pesticides can be used. The EPA and FDA work together in regulating pesticide residues on foods.

Substances in Human Food

The Federal Food, Drug, and Cosmetic Act accounts for *all* substances that are or may become components of human food. Each substance is classified into one of six categories (discussed separately in the following sections) and is regulated depending on its classification.

Substances Generally Recognized as Safe (GRAS) Some background information will help you understand how this category came to be established. Before the enactment of the Food Additives Amendment of 1958, the food industry's approach to using additives was fairly simple—an added substance was either safe—and therefore permitted—or "poisonous and deleterious," and therefore banned. With the growing sophistication of the science of toxicology, however, the FDA realized that eventually it would be possible to show that virtually every substance has a toxic or harmful effect in some organism if the dose is large enough. It would therefore be possible to eliminate the addition of any ingredient to any food!

As Congress debated the bill that would later become the Food Additives Amendment, a question arose as to how to deal with additives already on the market and in use in 1958. One option was to exempt from regulation all additives already in use at the time. Some members of Congress were concerned, however, that not all additives in use then were, in fact, safe—for the simple reason that they had never been tested for safety. It was finally decided that a substance in use prior to January 1, 1958, and shown to be safe would be classified as a "Substance Generally Recognized as Safe" (a GRAS substance). Substances not in use before January 1, 1958, would automatically be classified as food additives and regulated under the new law.

GRAS (generally recognized as safe) list a list of ingredients, established by the FDA, that had long been in use and were believed safe. The list is subject to revision as new facts become known.

Thus, **GRAS substances** are those that had been in use—and in use *safely*—when the food additives amendment was passed in 1958. Hundreds of substances were placed on the GRAS list. Such ingredients as vegetable oils, salt, pepper, sugar, caffeine, vinegar, and baking powder, and such foods as meat, poultry, eggs, milk, seafoods, cereals, fruit, and vegetables were—and still are—classified as GRAS substances. In general, a food processor can claim that an ingredient is a GRAS substance; but if challenged by FDA, the food processor must provide proof of the ingredient's safety to the FDA.

In 1969, a problem developed with one of the GRAS substances—cyclamate, an artificial sweetener. A concern about its safety for use in human food resulted in its being removed from the GRAS list. After reviewing many studies in both humans and animals, the FDA decided to ban cyclamate from use in foods and beverages. As a result of this incident, President Richard Nixon ordered a reevaluation of the safety of all substances on the GRAS list to determine whether they should remain there. The FDA then reviewed the safety of all GRAS substances and removed about 300 substances from the GRAS list. Today, the more than 400 substances classified as GRAS are continually reviewed for safety in light of new research data.

Unavoidable Contaminants Unavoidable contaminants in foods are those that are either found naturally in foods or are added to foods and cannot be avoided by good manufacturing practices. Aflatoxins are an example of this type of substance in human food. Aflatoxins are a type of **mycotoxin** produced by certain molds, particularly *Aspergillus flavus* and *Aspergillus parasiticus*. They are powerful liver toxins in animals, are known to be carcinogenic in some species, and can be lethal if consumed in large doses. Aflatoxins have been found on peanuts, wheat, corn, meat pies, dry beans, and even refrigerated and frozen pastries. Growth of the molds that produce the aflatoxins typically occurs when commodities such as corn and peanuts become wet and are then stored in a warm place, such as a grain silo or railroad boxcar. Considerable effort is made to ensure that such foodstuffs do not become contaminated with molds during transport and storage. The control of aflatoxins and other mycotoxins in food is difficult but is taken seriously by the food industry and regulatory agencies.

Mycotoxin a poisonous compound produced by molds.

Pesticide Residues Pesticides are any substances used to prevent, destroy, or repel any pest *or* to regulate plant growth or defoliate plants. Pesticides are unique among manmade chemicals used in relation to food because they are intended specifically to poison living things. Pesticides do occur in nature—an example is the nicotine in tobacco, which serves to protect the tobacco plant from hungry insects—but they are far less lethal to other living things than are the manmade chemicals. The trouble with pesticides is, of course, that they can also be lethal to human beings. Table 11–6 lists a sampling of pesticides and shows how toxic they are.

When pesticides were first used, it was considered desirable to use persistent ones—chemicals that would keep on killing for as long as they remained in the soil. Unfortunately, this was based on a simplistic idea—that

Table 11–6

A Sampling of Pesticides and Their Biological Effects

Type of Use	Common Names (examples)	Biological Effects
Insecticides	Parathion, Malathion	Toxic to nerves; acute poisoning causes respiratory failure.
	Aldicarb, Zectran	Toxic to nerves.
	DDT, Dieldrin, Heptachlor, Chlordane, Mirex	Accumulate in fatty tissues, inhibit electrolyte transport, impair reproduction in birds.
	Ethylene dibromide (EDB)	Carcinogenic.
Herbicides	2,4,5-T	Toxic generally and to nerves.
	Paraquat	Toxic generally; causes edema in the lungs.
	Prophan	Allergenic.
	Simazine	Carcinogenic.
Fungicides	Captan	Causes birth defects.
	Pentachlorophenol (PCP)	Toxic generally.
Rodenticides	Warfarin	An anticoagulant.
	Red squill	Causes heart failure.
	Compounds 1080,1081	Inhibit cellular respiration.
	ANTU	Causes edema in the lungs.

Source: Adapted from M. G. Mustafa, Agricultural chemicals, in *Adverse Effects of Foods,* E. F. P. Jelliffe and D. B. Jelliffe (Eds.) (New York: Plenum Press, 1982), Table 1, pp. 112–113.

they *would* remain in the soil. They did not. They washed into waterways, contaminated wild animals, contaminated the food supply, and would not go away. DDT, now no longer in use, was such a persistent pesticide and after years of use began to show up in high concentrations in the body fat of animals. It threatened the survival of the American eagle by weakening eggshells to the point that they would collapse, killing the developing chicks. It showed up in big fish, carnivorous animals, human beings, and human breast milk. Finally, after years of widespread agricultural use, DDT was banned.

A lesson was learned in relation to substances like DDT: the extent to which a contaminant lingers in the body partly determines its potential harmfulness. If a contaminant enters the system and then is rapidly metabolized to some harmless compound, its ingestion may not give cause for concern. If the contaminant is rapidly and preferentially excreted, then, too, the body may be able to survive a brief exposure time. But if it enters the body, interacts with the body's systems, is not metabolized or excreted, and fools the cells' protein machinery into accepting it as part of their structure, it is dangerous. Additional doses will be piled on top of the first ones, and the substance will accumulate. All of these things were true of DDT, and that is why it was so deadly.

When a substance is resistant to breakdown either inside the body (by the body's enzymes) or outside (by microorganisms), and furthermore accumulates from one species to the next, it builds up in the food chain (refer to Figure 11–1 on page 326).

The ideal pesticide is one that destroys the pest and then quickly degenerates to other products that are nontoxic to people and other animals. The search for the perfect pesticide is not over. National and international agen-

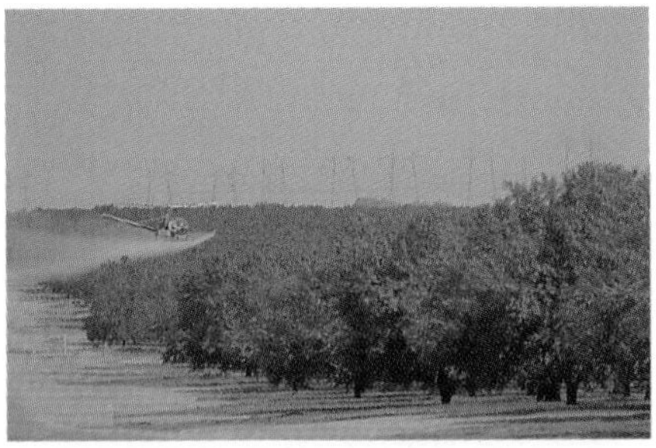

Pesticides require careful monitoring because they do not simply remain in the soil. They can easily find their way into waterways and thus contaminate the food supply.

cies such as the Food and Agriculture Organization (FAO), the World Health Organization (WHO), and, domestically, the EPA and the FDA have adopted standards and attempt to regulate pesticide use.

Pesticide use worldwide is increasing and is not well monitored. The hazards of many of the chemicals in use today may be considerable and are unknown. The EPA monitors pesticide levels in fish, birds, and mammals; in water, air, and food; and in human beings.[32] The monitoring does not guarantee consumer safety, though, because new pesticides keep appearing before the EPA can act to monitor them and because the maximum amounts allowed in food assume that a person will consume only moderate quantities of that food. In reality, people sometimes overeat certain specific foods. Also, other countries use pesticides that are illegal for use here—some, even exported from here to those countries—and imported foods may not be tested for the presence of those pesticides.

Diagnosing the toxic effects of pesticides is difficult. Many cause delayed reactions, especially those that poison the nerves. Toxins may collect in fatty tissues, sequestered away from the rest of the body. They are harmless until that fat becomes mobilized, such as may occur in animals when food is scarce or in people losing weight. The development of new pesticides and the monitoring of their use is an ongoing activity that will require continued vigilance on the part of government agencies and consumers. Consumers should read reliable literature, discuss it with others, advise their government representatives on how pesticides should be handled, and bring pressure to bear wherever it will help change procedures.

Meanwhile, how are consumers to avoid using foods containing unacceptably high levels of pesticides? Must they pay high prices for foods sold in special health food stores and labeled "organic"—meaning "pesticide-free"? If all grocery store foods were permeated with poisons and all organic foods were free of them, that might be the obvious choice, but such is not the case. Two important considerations bear on the presence of pesticide residues in foods.

The first is the quantity of the poison present. Anything, even water, can be toxic if you consume enough of it. Whether a food has been exposed to pesticides at some time in the past is not the right question to ask about that food's effect on your health. The question to ask is how much residue remains in the food at the time you eat it in relation to the threshold at which harm might occur. If a food has been sprayed and the poison has since evaporated, changed into a nontoxic compound, or been diluted below the point at which it can do any harm, the food may not be inferior to an unsprayed food. It may even be nutritionally superior because it has not been weakened by attacks of pests.

Second, even though so-called organic foods sold in special stores claim not to have been sprayed, testing shows that they sometimes contain pesticide residues in the same amounts as grocery store foods. Where these residues come from is not clear. Perhaps in some cases, farmers secretly spray their crops. Perhaps in other cases, pesticides drift onto farms that are not directly using them themselves. Perhaps in still other cases, organic farms may be situated on pesticide-contaminated soil. The question is not what is on the label, then; the question is what is really in the food. The terms "natural," "organic," or "health food" have never been legally defined. Thus they can appear on labels of foods that are actually quite unnatural or unhealthful. In other words, such foods may not be superior to ordinary grocery store foods in terms of pesticide residues—that is, the quantity of a pesticide that remains

Figure 11–2

Rank of Hazards from Eating Food

Public and expert perception of risks from eating food do not coincide. Whereas experts judge hazard based on known deaths or cases of illness, the public has different criteria.

Source: Adapted from K. Lee, Food neophobia: Major causes and treatments, *Food Technology* 43 (1989): 62–73.

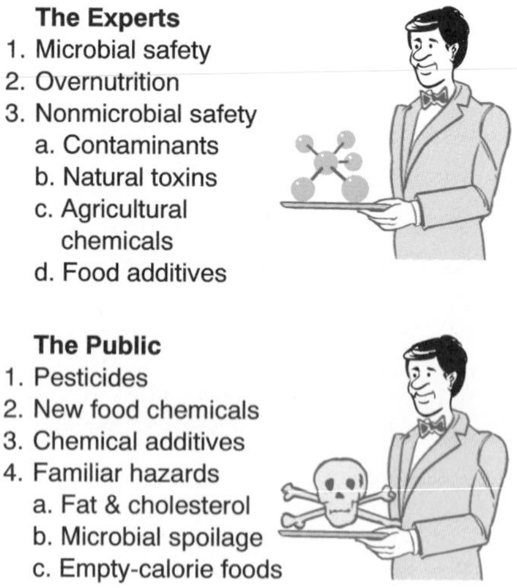

in a food after good manufacturing practices (such as rinse baths for vegetables) have been used to remove it. As indicated previously, the use of pesticides here in the United States is controlled by both the EPA, which is responsible for outlining how and in what manner a pesticide can be used and for establishing tolerances related to a pesticide's use, and the FDA, which enforces the tolerances set by the EPA.

Food Additives Food additives present the *least* hazard among the FDA's food-related concerns because they are closely regulated, although consumers tend to rank them high on their list of risks from eating food (see Figure 11–2). In addition, consumers tend to lump all kinds of substances, including pesticides, under the heading of "food additives." This is not appropriate. The term *food additives* has a very specific, legal meaning under the law: "any substance the intended use of which results or may reasonably be expected to result, directly or indirectly, in its becoming a component . . . of any food."[32]

Substances added to foods deliberately are called direct or **intentional additives**, while indirect or **incidental additives** are those that may get in by accident during processing. Intentional food additives are substances put into foods to give the foods some desirable characteristic: color, flavor, texture, stability, or resistance to spoilage. Some are nutrients added to foods to increase their nutritional value, such as vitamin C added to fruit drinks or potassium iodide added to salt. Many of the major categories of food additives are listed in Table 11–7. Incidental additives—packaging materials or processing chemicals, for example—are also regulated and food processors must

Intentional food additives additives intentionally added to food, such as nutrients or colors.

Incidental food additives substances that can get into food not through intentional introduction, but as a result of contact with the food during growing, processing, packaging, storing, or some other stage before the food is consumed. Other terms for the same thing are accidental additives or indirect additives.

Table 11–7 Common Food Additives[a]

Food Additive	Purpose	Some Foods in Which Used
Anticaking or free-flow agents: Calcium silicate	Prevent caking or lumping	Dessert mixes
Antimicrobial agents: Potassium benzoate, calcium propionate	Prevent the growth of microorganisms	Breads, rolls, fruit juices, jams, salad dressings
Antioxidants: Butylated hydroxyanisole (BHA), tocopherols (vitamin E), citric acid, ascorbic acid	Slow down the deterioration and discoloration of foods	Vegetable shortenings and oils, potato chips, pie and pudding fillings
Dough strengtheners: Benzoyl peroxide, calcium bromate	Produce a more stable dough	Breads, rolls
Flavor enhancers: Monosodium glutamate (MSG), disodium guanylate	Enhance or modify the taste or aroma of food	Salad dressing mixes, sauces, pudding and pie mixes
Formulation aids: Monoglycerides, lecithin	Promote a certain texture or physical state of food	Salad dressing mixes, cake mixes, chocolate
Fumigants	Control insects or pests	. . . .
Humectants: Glycerine, propylene glycol	Promote moisture retention	Salad dressing mixes, flaked coconut, dessert mixes
Leavening agents: Calcium phosphate	Stimulate carbon dioxide production in baked goods	Breads, rolls, baked goods
Nonnutritive sweeteners: Saccharin	Have less than 2% of the caloric value of sucrose	Soft drinks
pH control agents: Citric acid, lactic acid	Maintain the acid or base levels of a food	Gelatin desserts, baked goods
Stabilizers and thickeners: Carrageenan, cellulose gum, pectin, guar gum	Produce a viscous solution, give body, or improve the consistency of a food	Ice creams, cream cheese, jams and jellies, salad dressing mixes
Texturizers: Modified food starch	Enhance the appearance or feel of the food	Pudding mixes, pie fillings

[a]A complete list of categories of food additives appears in H. W. Schultz, *Food Law Handbook* (Westport, Conn.: Avi, 1981), pp. 573–574.

perform tests to discover whether they are present. Adverse effects are rare, with the exception of lead.

Safety the practical certainty that injury will not result from the use of a substance.

The FDA is charged with the responsibility of deciding which food additives shall be used. The FDA's authority over food additives hinges primarily on the additives' **safety**. A manufacturer has to go through a special procedure to get permission to use a new food additive in food products. The procedure puts the burden on the manufacturer to prove that the food additive is safe, and it may take several years to do so. First, the manufacturer must test the additive chemically to satisfy the FDA that the additive is effective (it does what it is supposed to do) and that it can be detected and measured in the final food product. Then the manufacturer has to feed the additive in large doses to certain animals under strictly controlled conditions and prove that the additive is safe (it causes no cancer, birth defects, or other injury). Finally, the manufacturer must submit all test results to the FDA.

The FDA responds to the manufacturer's petition by announcing a public hearing. Consumers are invited to participate at these hearings, where experts present testimony for and against the acceptance of the food additive for the proposed uses. The FDA's official publication, *FDA Consumer,* announces the hearings. Thus, the consumer's rights and responsibilities are written into the provisions for deeming additives safe.

Regulation a rule that has the force and the effect of a law; it must be observed and obeyed.

If the FDA approves the food additive's use, that does not mean the manufacturer can add it in any amount to any food. On the contrary: the FDA writes a **regulation** stating in what amounts and in what foods the additive may be used. No food additives are permanently approved; all are periodically reviewed.

A food additive's safety is determined based on a distinction between *toxicity* and *hazard* (refer to the previous discussion of the difference between these two terms). A food additive is not considered to be a hazard if some immense amount that people never consume is toxic. The food additive is a hazard only if it is toxic under the conditions of its actual use. Food additives are supposed to have wide margins of safety. (The safety evaluation described here applies equally to color additives, discussed below.)

Margin of safety when speaking of food additives, it is a zone between the concentration normally used and the zone at which a hazard exists. For common table salt, for example, the margin of safety is 1/5 (five times the concentration normally used would be hazardous).

Most additives that involve risk are allowed in foods only at levels 100 times below those at which the risk is still known to be zero; their **margin of safety** is 1/100. Experiments to determine the extent of risk involve feeding test animals the substance at different concentrations throughout the animals' lifetimes. The additive is then permitted in foods at 1/100 the level that can be fed under these conditions without any hazard whatever. In many foods, naturally occurring substances appear at levels that bring their margin of safety closer to 1/10. Even nutrients, as you have seen, present hazards at high dosage levels. For example, the margin of safety for vitamins A and D is 1/25 to 1/40; it may be less than 1/10 in infants. For some trace elements, it is about 1/5. People consume common table salt daily in amounts only three to five times less than those that present a serious hazard.

The margin of safety concept also applies to nutrients when they are used as food additives. Iodine has been added to salt to prevent iodine deficiency, but it has had to be added with care because it is a deadly poison in excess. Similarly, iron has been added to refined bread and other grains (enrichment) and has doubtless helped prevent many cases of iron-deficiency anemia in women and children who are prone to that disease. But the addition of too much iron could put men (who usually have enough dietary iron and who consume more calories than women do) at risk for iron overload. The upper limit has to be remembered.

All the food additives just named are in foods for a reason. They offer benefits in comparison with which the risks are deemed either small enough to ignore or worth taking. When the benefit to be gained from an additive is small, the risks may be deemed not worth taking. It is also the manufacturer's responsibility not to use more of a food additive than is necessary to get the needed effect. Additives should also not be used:

- To disguise faulty or inferior products.
- To deceive the consumer.
- Where they significantly destroy nutrients.
- Where their effects can be achieved by economical, sound manufacturing processes.

The regulations in force governing the management of intentional additives are well conceived and have been effective, on the whole. Cutbacks in funding in the mid-1980s limit the capabilities of watchdog agencies such as the FDA, however, and some mistakes and cases of false reporting are bound to slip by. All things considered, however, the Food Additives Amendment to the Food, Drug, and Cosmetic Act has worked successfully to safeguard the safety of the U.S. food supply.

Color Additives For hundreds, if not thousands, of years, people have been coloring foods to make them attractive. Today's food processor is no different: colors are added to foods to enhance their appeal and to meet consumers' expectations about the appearance of food. This is not a trivial consideration, since consumers often judge a food's quality by its color. Oranges are expected to be orange; cola drinks should be brown. In fact, if it were not for colors added during processing, some ripe oranges would be a mottled green and cola drinks would be clear. The color of food is often just as important as its flavor and quality.

Before the enactment of food laws to protect consumers, some unscrupulous food processors used colors to their advantage to sell foods that were spoiled or otherwise of poor quality. Pickles, for example, were "dyed" their traditional green with copper sulfate, a poison that killed some consumers outright. Used tea leaves were colored with black lead and other chemicals, then sold as a fresh, unused product. The special orange color of Gloucester cheese was due to the addition of a poison, red lead.[33]

The Color Additives Amendment of 1960 was enacted to prevent this kind of adulteration. Color additives are dyes and pigments that impart color to foods, drugs, and cosmetics. Some colorants are obtained from natural products—plants (particularly flowers and fruits), animals, minerals, and even insects. Examples of naturally occurring plant pigments are the anthocyanins that give grapes, strawberries, and blueberries their vibrant red and blue colors, and the yellow and orange carotenoids that give carrots, tomatoes, corn, and salmon their familiar colors.

Others are synthetic; they are called "certified food colors." Certified color additives are added to carbonated beverages, baked goods, dairy products, icings, cake and donut mixes, pet foods, and many other products. One of the better known certified food colors is FD&C Red No. 2 (commonly known as amaranth). A concern that this dye was carcinogenic prompted the FDA to ban it in 1976, with the result that many consumers were outraged that a popular chocolate candy (red M&M's®) would disappear from the U.S. market. As an example of how countries differ in their interpretation of research data, consider that Canada, Sweden, Denmark, West Germany, and Japan, among others, still allow FD&C Red No. 2 to be used. In the United States, replacements for "red dye no. 2"—namely, FD&C Red No. 40 and FD&C Red No. 3—have been approved by the FDA for use in foods.

As with the food additives and GRAS substances described previously, color additives must undergo a rigid safety evaluation and should be used at appropriate levels as dictated by good manufacturing practices. They can be used to ensure that foods are uniform in color, as with fruits harvested at different times during the season; to restore a food to its original color after heat processing (for example, canned vegetables); to enhance a natural color, as in fruit yogurts and soft drinks; and to help preserve the attractive appearance and identity of a food in keeping with consumers' expectations. A food processor who uses a color additive to conceal defective or spoiled food products is violating the Color Additives Amendment to the Food, Drug, and Cosmetic Act and is subject to fines and penalties.

Prohibited Substances With each of the previously mentioned categories of substances allowed in food, the risk of using a particular substance was weighed against the benefits to consumers of allowing the substance to be added to foods. Although in some cases, a potential hazard was identified, it was believed that the risk to human health could be minimized by using good manufacturing practices to keep the level of the hazardous substance in foods low. It didn't matter whether the substance was manmade, as in the case of synthetic pesticides, or naturally occurring in foods, as in the case of solanine in potatoes.

Prohibited substances compounds not allowed in foods.

In a few cases, however, the bulk of the research data indicates a potential risk to human health. These substances are called **prohibited substances** and are not safe for use in food. Specific examples of such substances include the cyclamates, dulcin, coumarin, safrole, and chlorofluorocarbon propellants. It is unlawful to add these compounds to foods and beverages.

Food Safety Risks

Whether consumers realize it or not, they make decisions every day on the basis of their judgment of the benefits compared with the risks inherent in an act being considered. In some cases consumers are able to grasp the benefits and risks fairly easily. For example, many consumers are aware of the increased risk of lung cancer associated with cigarette smoking and decide to continue smoking; for these individuals the perceived benefits of smoking seem to outweigh the risks. In other situations consumers are not able to evaluate the risks and benefits readily. What is the risk of death resulting from consuming mycotoxin residues in foods, when no deaths have actually been linked to mycotoxin consumption?

Just 30 years ago, cancer-causing agents were believed to be mostly manmade and found largely in industrial processes. The goal at that time was fairly straightforward; the chemicals that cause cancer in laboratory animals should be eliminated. However, as the technology of detecting minute levels of cancer-causing chemicals improved, it became apparent that cancer-causing agents were found widely in nature, both in foods and in the environment, and that trace amounts of these chemicals did not necessarily translate to an increased risk of cancer.

Consider the case of Alar, a chemical used widely in the processing of apples and reported to cause cancer in laboratory mice when fed in high doses. On hearing of this cancer connection, many consumers stopped giving their children apple juice to drink and threw out vast quantities of applesauce, apple butter, and other apple products. Was this a realistic response? No, if you consider that to consume the same level of Alar as the laboratory mice tested, you'd have to eat 500 pounds of apples at one sitting. In the emotionally-charged atmosphere surrounding the Alar controversy, several key points were overlooked: 1) The extremely high levels of Alar fed to mice cannot be duplicated in standard human diets; 2) Current levels of Alar in apples (when it can be detected at all) fall well below the limit established by the federal government; and 3) Alar has been used without ill effects since 1967.[34] The irony is that parents who would withhold apple juice from their children because of an Alar-related cancer risk are sometimes willing to accept much greater risks in other areas—allowing their children to ride a bicycle without a helmet or not wearing a seatbelt in the car.

The challenge for experts and consumers alike is to place the risks into perspective with the benefits, to balance real risks with perceived (and possibly "nonreal") risks. Being able to define food-related risks and benefits will ultimately enhance the safety and wholesomeness of our food supply.

Food and Nutrition in the Twenty-first Century

Consider for a moment the enormous changes in the "business of food" that have occurred over the past 100 years. Gone is the corner grocery store in many communities; it's been replaced by the mega-giant supermarket boasting shelf space for as many as 25,000 items. Where once consumers were familiar mainly with local or regional brands of food products, today food marketing and retailing is a multimillion-dollar industry, and brand names have national—if not international—recognition. Food packaging in the 1990s is a mere shadow of its former self. Where cans and bottles once dominated the packaging market, we now have aseptic and retort packaging, along with new plastic and flexible packaging materials such as blow-molded bottles and films.

What does the food industry say about future foods? Experts in marketing predict that the aging profile of the U.S. and Canadian populations will have an enormous effect on the kinds of foods in the marketplace. Because there will be more older people and more people living alone, we can expect to see more healthful foods, fresher foods, more microwaveable foods, and more single-serving packages. The "mature market" will also demand more ethnic foods and yet still look to traditional foods as the central focus of its diet. Low-fat foods are expected to lead the way into the twenty-first century as consumers become increasingly more health conscious. What's more, the ever-growing concern about the environment is likely to affect the way foods of the future are packaged and marketed (see the Nutrition Action feature).

The challenge for regulatory agencies and the food industry as the year 2001 approaches will be to maintain—and strive to surpass—the current food safety record. Because our food supply is complex and diverse, this effort will require increased monitoring of imported foods, new and existing ingredients, and domestic fresh and processed foods. The controversy surrounding the anti-cancer (Delaney) clause will probably heat up in the coming decade as technology tests the limits of detection of cancer-causing substances in food. More research will be required to improve the safety of our food supply and to ensure the nutritional value of the foods available in the marketplace. For consumers in North America, the dawn of the twenty-first century promises to bring new foods and flavors for their eating enjoyment and new challenges to eating a healthful, varied diet.

The Green Revolution at the Supermarket

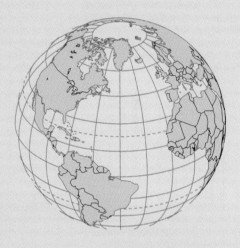

Before her death in 1978, famed anthropologist Margaret Mead wrote: "We are living beyond our means. As a people we have developed a lifestyle that is draining the earth of its priceless and irreplaceable resources without regard for the future of our children and people all around the world."[35] Hers was a vision ahead of its time. At the same time Ms. Mead offered her forecast, in fact, one social critic dubbed the era the "Throwaway Age." His description is fitting, given that the United States ranks as the world's top generator of garbage—pitching some 1,400 pounds of waste per person each year, an amount that has been rising since 1960.[36]

Fortunately, news of overflowing landfills, polluted waterways, and environmental disasters such as oil spills has begun to stir a growing environmental consciousness throughout mainstream America. In a 1990 survey conducted for the Food Marketing Institute (a trade group) and *Better Homes and Gardens Magazine,* consumers rated the problem of garbage disposal as more severe than problems with food safety, nuclear safety, and national defense.[37] What's more, nearly 80 percent of the respondents to a 1989 survey said they would pay more for products packaged in recyclable or biodegradable materials.[38] No wonder hundreds of products touted with claims including "degradable," "environmentally friendly," "recycled," and "safe for the environment" have been introduced into supermarkets since the beginning of this decade, creating a "green revolution" in the grocery store.

On the surface, such efforts on the part of manufacturers are definitely a move in the right direction. Nevertheless, questions have been raised about the legitimacy of placing environmental claims on grocery store items. Because the terms manufacturers use to sell "green" products have not been defined legally, they can sometimes mislead conservation-minded consumers. One manufacturer of garbage bags, for example, was sued by a group of attorneys general for selling an expensive version of bags boasted as being "biodegradable." That's because while the term suggested that the bags would break down fairly rapidly in garbage heaps, they turned out to be photodegradable. In other words, they degraded when exposed to sunlight but not in the middle of a landfill, making them no better from an environmental standpoint than regular trash bags.[39] The case illustrates why some experts contend that the widely used claims "biodegradable," "photodegradable," and "degradable" are relatively meaningless in practical terms.

Although virtually everything breaks down eventually upon exposure to air and water, about 80 percent of our trash ends up buried amid a heap of rubbish in a landfill, where air and moisture can barely penetrate, thereby preserving even substances that would otherwise degrade rapidly.[40] Consider that archeologists digging in landfills for the University of Arizona's Garbage Project have discovered perfectly legible newspapers, which tend to be highly degradable, dated as far back as 1949.[41] Similarly, the claim that a product is made with recycled paper or other materials can be confusing in some instances. Unless the package spells out what percentage of the item is truly recycled, manufacturers may use as little or as much of the recycled material as they like. A box made with recycled cardboard, for example, can be made of anywhere from 1 percent to 50 percent to 100 percent recycled material.

Another point of discrepancy is the oft-used claim that a product is "recyclable." Granted, recycling ranks as an excellent means of helping to preserve our resources. The problem is that many areas of the country lack facilities to recycle certain products, particularly those made of plastic. Hence, experts question whether it's fair to tout them as "recyclable" in the first place.

In addition, products advertised as "safe for the environment" or "environmentally friendly," without any explanation as to why they are superior, may be nothing more than hype. Those terms, like the others, have not been defined legally.

Chlorofluorocarbons substances once used to make aerosol sprays and styrofoam and that seem to contribute to the destruction of the earth's ozone layer.

Finally, items labeled "ozone friendly" or "no CFCs" are not necessarily good for the planet. It's true that substances called **chlorofluorocarbons** (CFCs), which appear to play a role in destroying the protective layer of ozone that surrounds the earth and helps filter out cancer-causing rays from the sun, were once used in most aerosol sprays and are still found in some styrofoam products. Still, since 1978, CFCs have been virtually eliminated from aerosol sprays sold in the United States. Furthermore, most styrofoam products no longer contain the substances. But while CFCs are no longer a significant issue, aerosol sprays and styrofoams may be made with other harmful substances. What it all boils down to is that "ozone friendly" products are not necessarily innocuous.[42]

Source reduction (also called precycling) reducing waste by using fewer materials to begin with.

Beyond the issue of environmental claims is the issue of whether recycling, as many consumers believe, is the solution to the garbage problem. While it can certainly help, the best option, say most experts, is **source reduction**—that is, reducing waste by using fewer materials to begin with, thereby eliminating the use of virgin materials, the need for disposal, and the energy and pollution generated by recycling. Given that about a third of the trash discarded by Americans comes from packaging (much of it for food), practicing source reduction at the supermarket, along with recycling whenever possible, can make a significant impact on the environment. The Earthworks Group, a California-based environmental organization, estimates that if 10 percent of Americans purchased products packaged with less plastic just 10 percent of the time, 144 million pounds of plastic would be eliminated from our landfills.[43]

Packaging accounts for one out of every $11 Americans spend on food.

Use the following tips to help practice source reduction and recycling at the supermarket or in the kitchen.

- Buy foods in bulk or in economy-size packages. The more food that fits into a single container, the better.
- Look for products sold in refillable bottles that can be washed and used again, or at least those that can be recycled. It takes much less energy to wash out an old bottle than to recycle it or make a new one from scratch. A 12-ounce refillable glass bottle, for example, requires 75 percent less

energy per use than a recycled aluminum can or glass bottle and as much as 90 percent less energy than a can or bottle used once and then tossed into the trash.[44]

- Find another use for glass jars or plastic containers. Use empty margarine tubs to store leftovers, for example.
- Purchase items made from recycled materials when possible. Check the labels or examine the box. Most cereal boxes that are gray inside are made from 100 percent recycled cardboard.
- Carry your groceries home in a reusable bag, not paper or plastic.
- Store food in reusable containers instead of wrapping it in aluminum foil or plastic wrap.
- Wipe spills with rags that can be washed and reused instead of using paper towels all the time. Then wash and use the rags again.
- Pack your sandwich in a plastic container that can be washed and reused rather than in a plastic bag that will wind up in the garbage.
- Call your local recycling center to find out where you can recycle. Look for it in the Yellow Pages, or call 1-800-CALLEDF, the Environmental Defense Fund, and ask them to help you find your nearest center.
- Remember your power as a consumer. Every purchase you make makes a statement to the manufacturer about your preferences. If no one buys heavily packaged products, companies will stop making them.

The recycling symbol.

Along with conserving material resources, ecology-minded consumers can save energy (and money) by using certain cooking techniques.[45]

- Use the smallest oven possible when you cook. The larger the oven, the more energy needed to heat it.
- Choose the smallest pan needed to cook a food. Smaller pans use less energy.
- Match pan size to the burner size on electric stove tops. Placing a 6-inch pan on an 8-inch burner will waste more than 40 percent of the heat generated by the burner.
- Keep the grease-catching metal pan underneath burners clean and shiny. Blackened burner pans absorb heat rather than reflect it, thereby reducing a burner's ability to heat efficiently.
- Cover pans with lids whenever possible. Consider that it takes about three times as much energy to cook a pot of spaghetti that's uncovered than one that's covered.
- Turn off electric burners just before heating is completed. The burner will keep putting out heat for a short time after it's shut off.
- Call your gas company if your gas stove's flames are not blue. A yellow flame means the gas might not be burning efficiently.
- Don't preheat your oven. Research indicates that there is little difference in the quality of products cooked in preheated versus non-preheated ovens, making preheating an unnecessary waste of energy.[46]
- Try not to peek in the oven. Each time you open the door, heat escapes and considerable energy is wasted. Check on foods by looking in the oven window instead.

- Cook foods in glass or ceramic pans in ovens. That will allow you to turn down the oven temperature about 25 degrees Fahrenheit without prolonging cooking time.
- Keep the inside surface of microwave ovens clean to keep the appliance working efficiently.

Consumer Tips

Microwaving the Safe Way

Some 75 percent of American kitchens have microwave ovens for use in thawing, cooking, and reheating foods quickly. Nevertheless, many consumers are not aware of certain safety measures that should be taken when using them to lower the risk of foodborne illness or other health problems. Using the following tips will help ensure that you microwave safely.[47]

- Prevent "cold spots" by arranging portions of meat or poultry evenly in a wide, shallow dish. After cooking, check the items' temperature in several places using a probe or meat thermometer. Meat should be at least 160 degrees Fahrenheit; poultry should reach 180 degrees Fahrenheit.
- Cut large pieces of meat or poultry into smaller portions when possible to ensure that all segments are heated thoroughly.
- Cook food that has been thawed in the microwave; don't refreeze it. Unlike defrosting meat or poultry in the refrigerator, thawing in the microwave subjects food to low cooking temperatures in which bacteria can multiply. Refreezing will prevent additional growth, but it won't kill the bacteria that are already present.
- Remember to remove casseroles and other items put in the microwave to thaw. According to the U.S. Department of Agriculture, consumers often forget to do this. If you accidentally do leave a product in the oven for more than two hours, throw it away.
- Don't partially cook a food ahead of time to speed microwave heating later. Partially cooking food may not generate enough heat to kill any bacteria present; the same goes for microwaving the product later.
- Don't put brown paper bags or recycled paper towels in the microwave. While some recipes suggest microwaving turkeys or ham in those materials to promote tenderness, the paper could start a fire or release dangerous chemicals into the food.
- Cook in dishes that are designed specifically for use in microwave ovens. Margarine tubs or plastic containers made for storing food may melt upon coming into contact with hot foods. In addition, they may leach dangerous chemicals into food during cooking.
- Allow foods to stand for the recommended period of time after cooking to ensure heating through and through. Foods keep cooking even after the microwave is turned off.
- Heat baby bottles on a stove rather than in the microwave. Liquids held in bottles heated in the microwave can be 20 degrees higher than the outside of the bottle. Thus, while the bottle may feel warm to the touch, the formula inside may be hot enough to scald an infant's mouth.[48]

Spotlight Domestic and World Hunger

This book has discussed the problems of *overnutrition*—obesity, heart disease, cancer, and others—diseases of economically developed nations. People in developing nations as well as people in the less privileged parts of developed nations suffer from problems of *undernutrition,* which is characterized by chronic debilitating hunger and malnutrition. These conditions are most visible in times of famine, but they are widespread and persistent even when famine does not occur. They have been with us throughout history, and despite numerous development programs, they are not disappearing; the number of hungry and malnourished people continues to grow.

Everyone has known the discomfort of hunger that signals time to eat and passes with the eating of the next meal. But many people know hunger as a constant companion because a meal does not follow to quiet the hunger signal. For these people, hunger is ceaseless. People who live with chronic hunger either have too little food to eat or do not receive an adequate intake of the essential nutrients from the foods available to them. Either way, malnutrition ensues.

• How are hunger and poverty related?

Hunger was once viewed as a problem of overpopulation and inadequate food production. Today many people recognize it as a problem of poverty. Poverty exists for many reasons, including overpopulation; greed; unemployment; and the lack of productive resources such as land, tools, and credit. If it is at all possible to provide adequate nutrition for all the earth's hungry people, it can be achieved only when the economic, political, and social structures that create a gap between rich and poor—and thereby limit food production, distribution, and consumption—become the targets of change.

Millions of children die each year from the diseases of poverty: parasitic and infectious diseases such as dysentery, whooping cough, measles, tuberculosis, cholera, and malaria. These diseases interact with poor nutrition to form a vicious cycle in which the outcome for many is death.

• Who are at highest risk for undernutrition?

When nutrient needs are high (as in times of rapid growth), the risk of undernutrition increases. If family food is limited, pregnant and lactating women, infants, and children are the first to show the signs of undernutrition. Effects of hunger can be devastating to this group of the population.

During pregnancy, healthy women in developed countries gain an average of about 27 pounds, while low-income women show a weight gain of only 11 to 15 pounds.[49] As a result, babies of these women tend to have low birthweights (less than 5½ pounds). A low-birthweight baby has a statistically greater-than-normal chance of having physical and mental birth defects, of contracting diseases, and of dying early in life. Low birthweight contributes to more than half of the deaths worldwide of children under five years of age.

Breastfeeding permits infants in many developing countries to achieve weight and height gains equal to those of children in developed countries until about six months of age, but then the majority of these children fall behind in their growth and development because of the inadequate addition of supplementary foods to their diets.

Replacing breast milk with infant formula in environments and economic circumstances that make it impossible to feed formula safely may lead to infant undernutrition. Breast milk, the recommended food for infants, is sterile and contains antibodies that enhance an infant's resistance to disease. In the absence of sterilization and refrigeration, formula in bottles is an ideal breeding ground for bacteria. Feeding infants formula made with contaminated water often causes infections leading to diarrhea, dehydration, and inability to absorb nutrients.

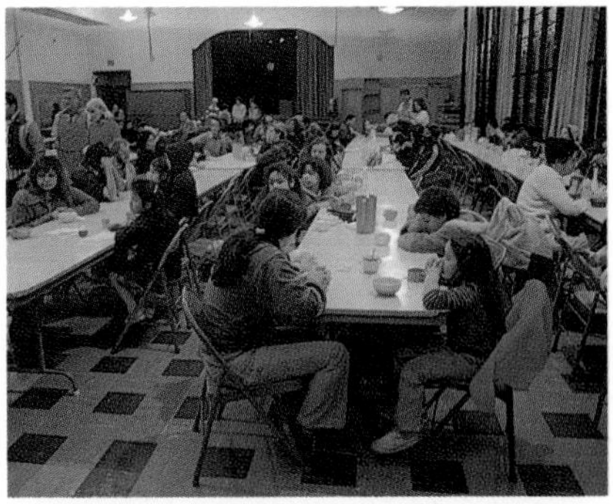

Feeding the hungry—in the United States.

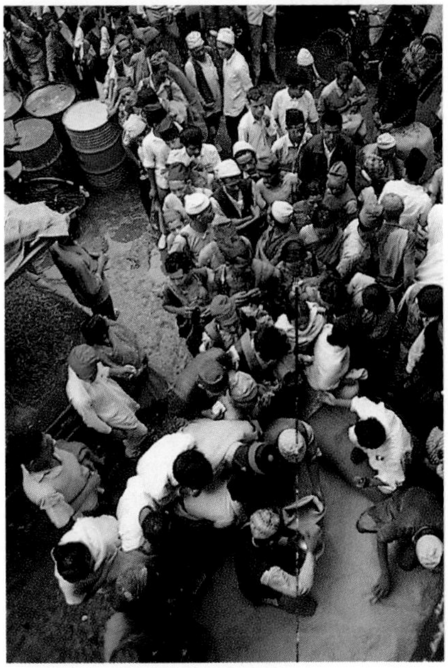

Feeding the hungry—in Nepal.

Even if infants are protected by breastfeeding at first, they must eventually be weaned. The weaning period is one of the most dangerous periods for children in developing countries for a number of reasons. Newly weaned infants often receive nutrient-poor diluted cereals or starchy root crops, and the infants' foods are often prepared with contaminated water, making infection almost inevitable.

Women are more susceptible than men to hunger and undernutrition because of increased needs during childbearing years, their families' lack of access to food, and unequal distribution of the food supply within their own families.

• What is the status of hunger in the United States?

Since the early 1980s, numerous studies on hunger have been conducted throughout the United States. Almost without exception, these studies find hunger to be a serious and rapidly growing problem. Approximately 20 million people in the United States—12 million children and 8 million adults—are suffering from chronic hunger, with the problems getting worse in all regions of the country. America has become a soup kitchen society to an extent unmatched since the bread lines of the Great Depression. Malnutrition and other health problems associated with chronic hunger—stunted growth, failure to thrive, low-birthweight babies, infant mortality, and anemia—are reported to be either escalating for the first time in many years or slowing in their long-term rates of improvement. In some of these conditions, the United States compares poorly with other industrialized countries.

• Who are the hungry in the United States?

Through the late 1960s and 1970s, hunger was evident among the chronic poor: migrant workers, Native Americans, southern blacks, unemployed minorities, and some of the elderly as well as the newly unemployed blue-collar workers during the 1970s. Now, hunger is reaching into other segments of the population, without regard for age, marital status, previous employment or successes, family ties, or efforts to change the situation. The U.S. farm economy has been burdened by chronic price-depressing surpluses, and available resources are failing to reach many groups. One in 12 goes hungry at least two days a month. The millions who experience hunger today in the United States include the young, the new poor, the elderly, the homeless, low-income women, and ethnic minorities. The most compelling single reason for this hunger is poverty.

• What are some of the causes of hunger in the United States?

Poverty and hunger share an interdependent relationship. Nutrition surveys investigating people's nutritional health in the United States have demonstrated consistently that the lower a family's income, the less adequate the family's nutrition status. Nationally, most studies conducted since 1980 attribute the increases in hunger throughout the country to worsening economic conditions among the poor. Major reductions in federal spending for antipoverty programs occurred throughout the 1980s. Severe reductions came in programs directly affecting those deepest in poverty, including Aid to Families with Dependent Children (AFDC), food stamps, low-income housing assistance, and child nutrition. Funding for the school lunch program was cut by one-third.[50] Cuts in college financial aid effectively blocked a pathway out of poverty taken by many in the past.

While poverty is the major cause of hunger in the United States, other causes also contribute, including alcoholism and chronic substance abuse; mental illness, loneliness, isolation, depression, and despair; the reluctance of people to accept what they perceive as "welfare" or "charity"; delays in receiving public assistance benefits; an increase in the number of single mothers without the means to care for their children; poor management of limited family financial resources; health problems of old age; lack of nutritional adequacy and balance in the food available to hungry people; lack of access to assistance programs; insufficient community food resources for the hungry; and insufficient community transportation systems, which are needed to deliver food to hungry people who have no transportation.[51]

As a result of the evidence accumulated during the 1960s and 1970s showing that hunger was a problem in the United States, the problems of poverty and hunger became national priorities. Old programs were revised and new programs were developed in an attempt to prevent malnutrition in those people found to be at greatest risk. The Food Stamp Program was expanded to serve more people. School lunch and breakfast programs were enlarged to support children nutritionally while they learned. Feeding programs to reach senior citizens were started. A supplemental food and nutrition program (WIC Program) was established for pregnant and breastfeeding women, infants, and children who were of low income and were nutritionally at risk, in order to provide food and nutrition education during the years when nutrition has the most crucial impact on growth, development, and future health. The result of these efforts was that hunger diminished as a serious problem for this country. Now, however, hunger is on the rise due to rising poverty and cuts in government aid.

• What are people doing to help reduce problems of hunger?

Concerned citizens are working through community programs and churches to provide meals to the hungry. The dramatic increases in the number of food banks, food pantries, soup kitchens, and other emergency food assistance programs across the nation, however, cannot keep pace with the growth in the number of hungry people seeking food assistance. Each day's worth of meals lasts only for that day, leaving the problem of poverty unsolved, as before. Moreover, one out of every five needy people is not even receiving meals. These people are left to scavenge garbage, steal food or money to buy food, or continue to starve.

● How are farm families affected by hunger?

The number of hungry farm families is not known, but agencies that provide aid to the rural poor say the demand for food assistance is increasing. Ironically, farm families do not generally grow fruits, vegetables, and other crops and animals to feed themselves. With modern practices aimed at efficiency, most farmers raise two or three crops—for example, feed corn, sorghum, and wheat—and buy most of the food they eat themselves from the grocery store. As a result, when crop prices drop, farmers struggle to survive under the sagging prices and realize no significant profits. Eventually, the farmers go out of business entirely from lack of profits, just as would happen in any other type of business in the United States.

● How does world hunger differ from hunger in the United States?

World hunger is more extreme than domestic hunger. In fact, most people would find it hard to imagine the severity of poverty in the developing world:

> Many hundreds of millions of people in the poorest countries are preoccupied solely with survival and elementary needs. For them, work is frequently not available, or pay is low, and conditions barely tolerable. Homes are constructed of impermanent materials and have neither piped water nor sanitation. Electricity is a luxury. Health services are thinly spread, and in rural areas only rarely within walking distance. Permanent insecurity is the condition of the poor. . . . In the wealthy countries, ordinary men and women face genuine economic problems. . . . But they rarely face anything resembling the total deprivation found in the poor countries.[52]

World hunger is a problem of supply and demand, of inappropriate technology, of environmental abuse, of demographic distribution, of unequal access to resources, of extremes in dietary patterns, and of unjust economic systems.

● How are international trade and debt connected to hunger?

Over the years, developing countries have seen the prices of imported fuels and manufactured items rise much faster than the prices they receive for their export goods on the international market. Their export commodities include items such as bananas, coffee, and various raw materials. The combination of high import costs with low export profits often pushes a developing country into accelerating international debt that sometimes leads to bankruptcy.

Debt and trade are closely related to the progress a country can make toward achieving adequate diets for its people. As import prices increase relative to export prices, more of a country's total money base moves abroad. As more and more of a country's money moves abroad, the country is forced to borrow money, usually at high interest rates, to continue functioning at home. Many of its financial resources must then go to pay the interest on the borrowed money, thus draining its economy further. Creditor nations may not demand much, or any, capital back, but they do require that interest be paid each year, and the interest can be equal to most of a country's gross national product. Large and growing debts can slow or halt a nation's attempt to deal effectively with its problems of local hunger. As more and more of its financial resources (money paid for imports and cash crops exported) are being used to pay off interest on the country's trade debts, less and less money is available to deal with hunger at home.[53] Each year, the debt crisis worsens and leads to further problems with hunger.

● What about the role of multinational corporations in this issue?

The competition for farmland on which to grow cash crops or food crops provides a classic example of the plight of the poor. Typically, large landowners and multinational corporations hire indigenous people for below-subsistence wages to work in the fertile farmlands growing crops to be exported for profit, leaving little fertile

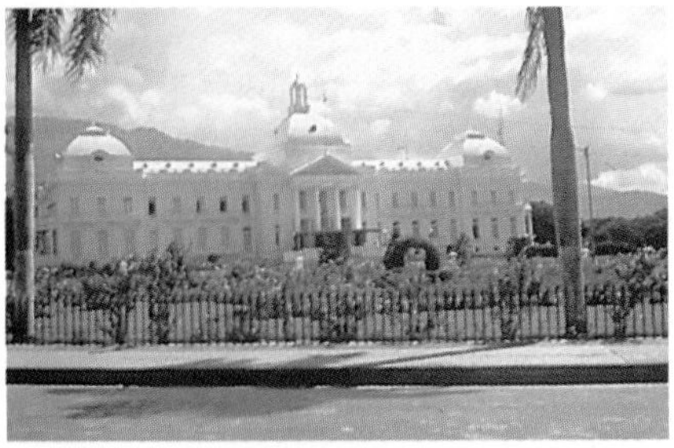
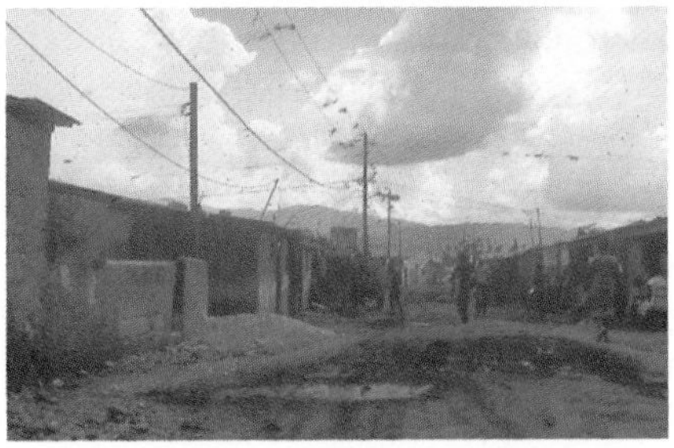
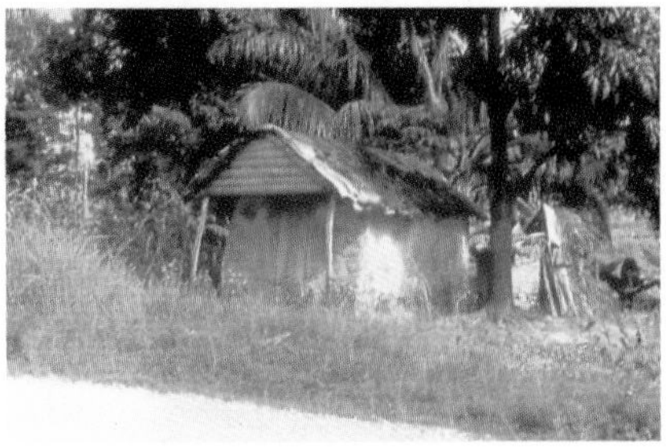

The stark contrasts between rich and poor within a single developing country are depicted here in the homes of the people. The ruler maintains a palace, while the majority of the population live in city tenements or rural huts.

land for the local farmers to use to grow food. The local people work hard cultivating cash crops for others, not food crops for themselves. The money they earn is not even enough to buy the products they help produce. The people do not adequately share in the profits realized from the marketing of products grown with their labor. The results: imported foods—bananas, beef, cocoa, coconuts, coffee, pineapples, sugar, tea, winter tomatoes, and others—fill the grocery stores of developed countries, while the poor who labored to grow these foods have less food and fewer resources than when they farmed the land for their own use. Additional cropland is diverted for nonfood cash crops—tobacco, rubber, cotton, and other agricultural products. These practices have also had an adverse effect on the financial status of many U.S. farmers. The foreign cash crops often undersell the same U.S.-grown produce. The U.S. farmer cannot compete against these lower-priced imported foods and may be forced out of business.

Besides diverting acreage away from the traditional staples of the local diet, some multinational corporations may also contribute to hunger as a result of their marketing techniques. Their advertisements lead many consumers with limited incomes to associate products like cola beverages, cigarettes, infant formulas, and snack foods with good health and prosperity. These promotions are tragically inappropriate for these people. A poor family's nutrition status suffers when its tight budget is pinched further by the purchase of such goods.

• How does overpopulation fit into the picture?

The current world population is approximately 5 billion, and for the year 2000, the projected United Nations figure is 6 billion. The earth may not be able to adequately support this many people. The world's present population is certainly of concern, as is the projected increase in that population. As important as the population question is, it is only one cause of the world food problem. Poverty seems to be at the root of both problems—hunger and overpopulation.

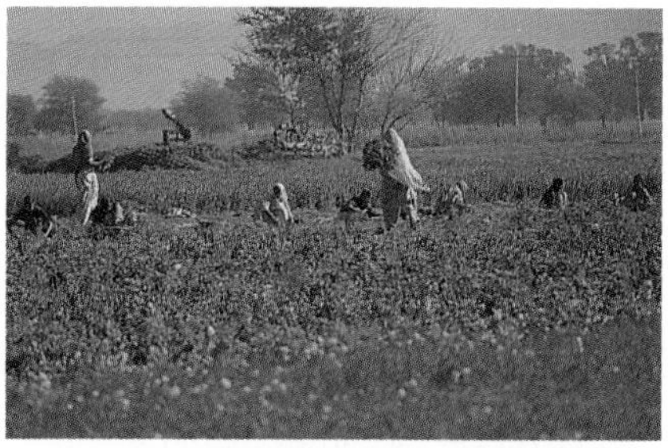

Families in developing countries depend on their children to help cultivate the land, to secure food and water, and to make the adults secure in their old age.

Three major factors affect population growth: birthrates, death rates, and standards of living. Low-income countries have high birthrates, high death rates, and low standards of living.

As the world's population continues to grow, it threatens the world's capacity to produce adequate food in the future. The activity of billions of human beings on the earth's limited surface is seriously and adversely affecting our planet: wiping out many of the varieties of plant life, heating up our climate, using up our freshwater supplies, and destroying the protective ozone layer that shields life from the sun's damaging rays—in short, overstraining the earth's ability to support life. Population control is one of the most pressing needs of this time in history.

• Is there a better way to distribute world resources?

Land reform—giving people a meaningful opportunity to produce food for local consumption, for example—can combine with population control to increase everyone's assets. Poor nations must be allowed to increase their agricultural productivity. Much is involved, but to put it simply, poor nations must gain greater access to five things simultaneously: land, capital, water, technology, and knowledge.[54] Equally important, each nation must adopt the political priority of improving the conditions of all its people. International food aid may be required temporarily during the development period, but eventually this aid will be less and less necessary.

• What about the role of agricultural technology in reducing world hunger?

Governments can learn from recent history the importance of developing local agricultural technology. A major effort made in the 1960s—the green revolution—demonstrated the potential for increased grain production worldwide. It was an effort to bring the agricultural technology of the industrial world to the developing countries; but the high-yielding strains of wheat and rice that were selected required irrigation, chemical fertilizers, and pesticides—all costly and beyond the economic means of too many of the farmers in the developing world.

Instead of transplanting industrial technology into the developing countries, small, efficient farms and local structures for marketing, credit, transportation, food storage, and agricultural education should be developed. International research centers need to examine the conditions of tropical countries and orient their research toward appropriate technology—labor-intensive rather than energy-intensive agricultural methods.

For example, labor-intensive technology, such as the use of manual grinders for grains, is appropriate in some places because it makes the best use of human, financial, and natural resources. A manual grinder can process 20 pounds of grain per hour, replacing the mortar and pestle, which in the same time can pound a maximum of only 3 pounds.[55] The specific technology that is appropriate for use varies from situation to situation.

Environmental concerns must be taken more seriously as well. As important as the amount of land available for crop production is the condition of the soil and the availability of water. Soil erosion is now accelerating on every continent at a rate that threatens the world's ability to continue feeding itself. Erosion of soil has always occurred; it is a natural process. But in the past it has been compensated for by processes that build the soil up—such as the growth of trees. Where forest has already been converted to farmland and there are no trees, farmers should alternate soil-devouring crops with soil-building crops, a practice known as crop rotation. When farmers must choose whether to make three times as much money planting corn year after year or to rotate crops and go bankrupt, many choose the short-term profits. Ruin may not follow immediately, but it will follow.[56]

• Is there hope for a world without hunger for women and children?

Women make up 50 percent of the world's population. Any solution to the problems of poverty and hunger is incomplete and even hopeless if it fails to address the role of women in developing countries, since women and their children represent the majority of those living in poverty.

In many countries, over 90 percent of the population live in rural areas. The life of a woman living in rural poverty is oppressive. In many countries, women in the rural areas not only are the primary food producers but also are responsible for child care and food preparation. Often they have to work as harvesters on other people's lands. Husbands are frequently required to be absent from their homes to seek employment.

Women play a vital role in the nutrition of their nation's people. Their nutrition during pregnancy and lactation determines the future health of their children. If women are weakened by malnutrition themselves or are ignorant about how to feed their families, the consequences ripple outward to affect many other individuals. The importance of the role women play in these countries is increasingly appreciated, and many countries now offer development programs with women in mind.

Seven basic strategies are at the heart of women's programs:

1. Removing barriers to financial credit.
2. Providing access to time-saving technologies.
3. Providing appropriate training to promote self-reliance.
4. Teaching management and marketing skills.
5. Making health and day-care services available.
6. Forming women's support groups.[57]
7. Providing of information and technology to promote planned pregnancies.

The recognition of women's needs by some development organizations is an encouraging trend in the efforts to contend with the world hunger crisis.

There is hopeful news for children in developing countries and in neglected parts of the United States. A plan set forth by UNICEF [GOBI, an acronym for growth charts, oral rehydration therapy (ORT), breast milk, and immunization] can cut the number of hunger-related child deaths from 40,000 to 20,000 a day.

A mother can learn to weigh her child every month and chart the child's growth on a specially designed paper growth chart. She can learn to detect for herself the early stages of hidden malnutrition that can leave a child irreparably retarded in mind and body. Then at least she can know she needs to take steps to remedy the malnutrition—if she can.

Most children who die of malnutrition don't starve to death—they die because their health has been compromised by dehydration from infections causing diarrhea. Until recently, there was no easy way of stopping the infection-diarrhea cycle and saving their lives. ORT is the administration of a simple solution using locally available ingredients, which increases a body's ability to absorb fluids 25-fold.[58] International development groups also provide mothers with packets of premeasured salt and sugar to be mixed with water in rural and urban areas. A safe and sanitary supply of drinking water is a prerequisite for the success of the ORT program.

The promotion of breastfeeding among mothers in developing countries has many benefits. Breast milk is hygienic, readily available, and nutritionally sound and provides infants with immunologic protection specific for their environment. In the developing world, its advantages over formula feeding can mean the difference between life and death.

Immunizations could prevent most of the 5 million deaths each year from measles, diphtheria, tetanus, whooping cough, poliomyelitis, and tuberculosis. However, adequate protein nutrition is necessary for vaccinations to be useful so that the vaccine itself is not used by the body as a source of protein.

• What can I do to help alleviate hunger problems?

The problems of hunger may appear so great that they seem approachable only by way of worldwide political decisions. But many individuals are working to improve the chances of the future well-being of the world and its people through a number of national and international organizations.*

Solutions to the hunger problem depend on the willingness of people to take action and to work together. Regardless of the type and level of involvement a person chooses, each person can make a difference. Individual people can do the following:

- Assist in government programs as volunteers.
- Help develop means of informing low-income people of food-related

*For information, contact Bread for the World, 802 Rhode Island Avenue N.E., Washington, D.C. 20018; or Oxfam America, 115 Broadway, Boston, MA 02116.

services and programs for which they are eligible.

- Help increase the accessibility of existing programs and services to those who need them.
- Document the needs that exist in their own communities.
- Join with others in the community who have similar interests (support groups that speak for the poor).
- Lobby to draw political attention to the need for more job opportunities and a higher minimum wage.

Individuals can also help change the world through the personal choices they make each day.[59] Our choices have an impact on the way the rest of the world's people live and die. Our nation, with 6 percent of the world's population, consumes about 40 percent of the world's food and energy resources. People in affluent nations have the freedom and means to choose their lifestyles. We can find ways to reduce our consumption of the world's nonrenewable resources; we can use only what is absolutely required.

Choosing a diet at the level of necessity rather than excess would reduce the resource demands made by our industrial agriculture. It would also produce humanitarian and economic benefits. In fact, those who study the future are convinced that the hope of the world lies in everyone's adopting a simple lifestyle. As one such person put it, "the widespread simplification of life is vital to the well-being of the entire human family."[60] Personal lifestyles do matter, for a society is nothing more than the sum of its individuals. As we go, so goes our world.

APPENDIX A
Nutrition Resources

People interested in nutrition often want to know where they can find reliable nutrition information in their own town or county. No matter where you live, there are several sources you can turn to:

- The Department of Health may have a nutrition expert such as a registered dietitian.
- The local extension agent is often a resource who can provide answers to questions regarding food and nutrition.
- The registered dietitians at your local hospital can serve as sources of reliable nutrition information.
- A nearby college or university may be staffed with knowledgeable professors of nutrition or biochemistry.

The syndicated column on nutrition by Jean Mayer and Jeanne Goldberg of Tufts University, which appears in many newspapers, presents well-researched, reliable information on current nutrition issues.

Books

- *Present Knowledge in Nutrition*, 6th ed. Washington, D.C.: International Life Sciences Institute—Nutrition Foundation, 1990.

This 532-page paperback has a chapter on each of 59 topics, including energy, obesity, vitamins and minerals, several diseases, malnutrition, growth and its assessment, immunity, alcohol, fiber, drugs, and toxins. Watch for an update; these come out every several years.

Another book that readers may wish to add to their libraries is the latest edition of *Recommended Dietary Allowances*, available from the National Academy of Sciences (see "Addresses" section that follows). The Canadian equivalent is *Recommended Nutrient Intakes for Canadians* available by mail from the Canadian Government Publishing Centre, Supply and Services Canada, Ottawa, Ontario K1A OS9 Canada.

Two excellent cookbooks for families wishing to prepare truly healthful meals are:

- White, A., and the Society for Nutrition Education. *The Family Health Cookbook*. New York: McKay, 1980.
- *American Heart Association Cookbook*, 5th ed. New York: Times Books, Random House, 1991.

Journals

Nutrition Today, the publication of the Nutrition Today Society, is an excellent magazine that makes a point of raising controversial issues and providing a forum for conflicting opinions. Six issues per year, from Williams & Wilkins. (See "Addresses" section that follows.)

The *Journal of the American Dietetic Association*, the official publication of the ADA, contains articles of interest to dietitians and nutritionists, news of legislative action on food and nutrition, and a very useful section of abstracts of articles from many other journals of nutrition and related areas. Twelve issues per year, from the American Dietetic Association. (See "Addresses" section that follows.)

Nutrition Reviews, a publication of the Nutrition Foundation, does much of the work for the library researcher, compiling recent evidence on current topics and presenting extensive bibliographies. Twelve issues per year, from the Nutrition Foundation. (See "Addresses" section that follows.)

The *Tufts University Diet & Nutrition Letter* is a monthly newsletter that provides up-to-date, easy-to-read, and practical information on nutrition for consumers. (See "Addresses" section that follows.)

Other publications that deserve mention here are *Nutrition and the MD*, the *Journal of Nutrition*, *Food Technology*, the *American Journal of Clinical Nutrition*, and the *Journal of Nutrition Education*. *FDA Consumer*, a government publication with many articles of interest to the consumer, is available from the Food and Drug Administration. (See "Addresses" section that follows.) Many other journals of value are referred to throughout this book.

Addresses

U.S. Government

The U.S. Department of Agriculture (USDA) has several divisions. The USDA's Food Safety and Inspection Service (FSIS) inspects and analyzes domestic and imported meat, poultry, and meat and poultry food products; establishes standards and approves recipes and labels of processed meat and poultry products; and monitors the meat and poultry industries for violations of inspection laws. To obtain publications or ask questions, write or call:

- FSIS, USDA
  Public Awareness
  Fourteenth and Independence Avenue
  1165 South
  Washington, D.C. 20250
  (202) 690-0351
  USDA also maintains a Meat and Poultry Hotline:
  1-800-535-4555.

The USDA's Agricultural Research Service (ARS) conducts research to fulfill the diverse needs of agricultural users—from farmers to consumers—in the areas of crop and animal production, protection, processing, and distribution; food safety and quality; and natural resources conservation. Write or call the information staff:

- ARS, USDA
  Information Staff
  Room 307, Building 005
  BARC - West
  Beltsville, MD 20705
  (301) 504-6264

The USDA's Human Nutrition Information Service (HNIS) maintains the USDA's Nutrient Data Bank, conducts the Nationwide Food Consumption Survey, monitors the nutrient content of the U.S. food supply, provides nutrition guidelines for education and action programs, collects and disseminates food and nutrition materials, and conducts nutrition education research. Write or call:

- HNIS, USDA
  5505 Belcrest Road
  Hyattsville, MD 20782
  (301) 436-8498

The USDA's Food and Nutrition Service (FNS) administers the food stamp program; the national school lunch and school breakfast programs; the special supplemental food program for women, infants, and children (WIC); and the food distribution, child care food, summer food service, and special milk programs. Write or call:

- FNS, USDA
  3101 Park Center Drive
  Alexandria, VA 22302
  (703) 756-3284

The USDA's Agricultural Marketing Service (AMS) operates a variety of marketing programs and services—several of interest to consumers—that include developing grades and standards for the trading of food and other farm products and carrying out grading services on request from packers and processors; inspecting egg products for wholesomeness; administering marketing orders that aid in the marketing of milk, fruits, vegetables, and related specialty crops like nuts; and administering truth-in-seed labeling and other regulatory programs. Write or call:

- AMS, USDA
  P.O. Box 96456
  Washington, DC 20090-6456
  (202) 447-8998

The USDA's *Food News for Consumers*, a quarterly newsletter, is available from the Government Printing Office. Other government addresses and telephone numbers follow:

- Food and Drug Administration
  5600 Fishers Lane
  Rockville, MD 20852
  (301) 443-1544

- The Food and Nutrition Information Center
  National Agriculture Library
  10301 Baltimore Boulevard, Room 304
  Beltsville, MD 20705-2351
  (301) 344-3719

- National Academy of Sciences/National Research Council (NAS/NRC)
  2101 Constitution Avenue, NW
  Washington, DC 20418
  (202) 334-2000
- National Center for Health Statistics
  U.S. Department of Health and Human Services
  Public Health Service
  6525 Belcrest Road
  Hyattsville, MD 20782
  (301) 436-8500
- U.S. Government Printing Office
  The Superintendent of Documents
  Washington, DC 20402
  (202) 783-3238

Canadian Government

- Bureau of Nutritional Sciences
  Food Directorate
  Health Protection Branch
  Department of National Health and Welfare
  Banting Building
  Tunney's Pasture
  Ottawa, Ontario K1A OL2 Canada
  (613) 957-0911
- Nutrition Programs Unit
  Health Promotion Directorate
  Department of National Health and Welfare
  Room 456, Jeanne Mance Building
  Tunney's Pasture
  Ottawa, Ontario K1A 1B4 Canada
  (613) 957-8328
- Nutrition Consultant
  Community Health, Indian and Northern Health Services
  Department of National Health and Welfare
  Room 1116, Jeanne Mance Building
  Tunney's Pasture
  Ottawa, Ontario K1A OL3 Canada
  (613) 954-7757
- Nutrition Coordinator
  Special Services
  Department of Health and Social Services
  16 Fitzroy St.
  P.O. Box 2000
  Charlottetown, Prince Edward Island C1A 7J9 Canada
  (902) 368-5004
- Home Economics Section
  2nd floor of Portage Avenue
  Winnipeg, Manitoba R3G OP1 Canada
  (204) 945-8564

Consumer and Advocacy Groups

- Center for Science in the Public Interest
  1875 Connecticut Avenue, NW
  Suite 300
  Washington, DC 20009-5728
  (202) 332-9110
- Children's Foundation
  725 Fifteenth Street, NW
  Suite 505
  Washington, DC 20005
  (202) 347-3300
- Community Nutrition Institute
  2001 S Street, NW
  Suite 530
  Washington, DC 20009
  (202) 462-4700
- The Consumer Information Center
  Pueblo, CO 81009
  (719) 948-3334
- Food Research and Action Center
  1875 Connecticut Avenue, NW
  Suite 540
  Washington, DC 20009
  (202) 986-2200
- National Council Against Health Fraud, Inc.
  P.O. Box 1276
  Loma Linda, CA 92354
  (714) 824-4690

Professional and Service Organizations

- Al-Anon Family Group Headquarters
  862 Midtown Station
  New York, NY 10018
  (212) 302-7240
- Alcoholics Anonymous World Services
  P.O. Box 459
  Grand Central Station
  New York, NY 10017
  (212) 686-1100

- American Academy of Pediatrics
  P.O. Box 927, 141 Northwest Point Boulevard
  Elk Grove Village, IL 60009-0927
  (708) 228-5005
- American Anorexia/Bulimia Association, Inc.
  418 East 76 Street
  New York, NY 10021
  (212) 734-1114
- American Council on Science and Health
  1995 Broadway
  New York, NY 10023
  (212) 362-7044
- American Dental Association
  211 East Chicago Avenue
  Chicago, IL 60611
  (312) 440-2500
- American Diabetes Association
  1660 Duke Street
  Alexandria, VA 22314
  (703) 549-1500
- American Dietetic Association
  216 West Jackson Boulevard, Suite 800
  Chicago, IL 60606-6995
  (312) 899-0040

  The American Dietetic Association's National Center on Nutrition and Dietetics operates a toll-free nutrition hot line for consumers. Call 1-800-366-1655.
- American Heart Association
  7320 Greenville Avenue
  Dallas, TX 75231
  (214) 373-6300
- American Institute for Cancer Research
  1759 R Street, NW
  Washington, DC 20009
  (202) 328-7744
- American Institute of Nutrition
  9650 Rockville Pike
  Bethesda, MD 20014
  (301) 530-7050
- American Medical Association
  515 North State Street
  Chicago, IL 60610
  (312) 464-5000
- American Red Cross
  National Headquarters
  431 Eighteenth Street, NW
  Washington, DC 20006
  (202) 737-8300
- American Public Health Association
  1015 Fifteenth Street, NW
  Washington, DC 20005
  (202) 789-5600
- American Society for Clinical Nutrition
  9650 Rockville Pike
  Bethesda, MD 20814
  (301) 530-7110
- Anorexia Nervosa and Related Eating Disorders, Inc.
  P.O. Box 5102
  Eugene, Oregon 97405
  (503) 344-1144
- Canadian Diabetes Association
  78 Bond Street
  Toronto, Ontario M5B 2J8 Canada
  (416) 362-4440
- Canadian Dietetic Association
  480 University Avenue
  Suite 601
  Toronto, Ontario M5G 1V2 Canada
  (416) 596-0857
- Institute of Food Technologists
  221 North LaSalle Street
  Chicago, IL 60601
  (312) 782-8424
- La Leche League International, Inc.
  9616 Minneapolis Avenue
  Franklin Park, IL 60131
  (708) 455-7730
- March of Dimes Birth Defects Foundation
  (National Headquarters)
  1275 Mamaroneck Avenue
  White Plains, NY 10605
  (914) 428-7100
- National Council on Alcoholism
  12 West Twenty-first Street
  New York, NY 10010
  (212) 206-6770
- Nutrition Foundation, Inc.
  1126 Sixteenth Street, NW, Suite 111
  Washington, DC 20036
  (202) 659-0074

- Office on Smoking and Health
  National Center for Chronic Disease
  Prevention and Health Promotion
  Mail Stop K-50
  Centers for Disease Control
  1600 Clifton Road, NE
  Atlanta, GA 30333
  (404) 488-5705
- Overeaters Anonymous (OA)
  P.O. Box 92870
  Los Angeles, CA 90009
  (213) 618-8835
- PM, Inc. (Publisher of *Nutrition and the MD*)
  P.O. Box 10172
  Van Nuys, CA 91410
  (818) 997-8011
- Society for Nutrition Education
  2001 Killebrew Drive
  Suite 340
  Minneapolis, MN 55425-1882
  (612) 854-0035
- *Tufts University Diet & Nutrition Letter*
  203 Harrison Avenue
  Boston, MA 02111
  (800) 274-7581
- Williams & Wilkins
  (Publisher of *Nutrition Today*)
  428 East Preston Street
  Baltimore, MD 21202
  (410) 528-4000

Trade Organizations

- American Egg Board
  1460 Renaissance Drive
  Park Ridge, IL 60068
  (708) 296-7043
- American Meat Institute
  1700 North Moore Street, Suite 1600
  Arlington, VA 22209
  (703) 841-2400
- Best Foods
  Consumer Service Department
  Division of CPC International
  International Plaza
  P.O. Box 8000
  Englewood Cliffs, NJ 07632
  (201) 894-4000
- Borden Farm Products
  Borden Company, Consumer Affairs
  180 East Broad Street
  Columbus, OH 43215
  (614) 225-4000
- Campbell Soup Company
  Campbell Place
  Camden, NJ 08103-1799
  (609) 342-4800
- General Mills
  P.O. Box 1113
  Minneapolis, MN 55440
  (612) 540-2311
- Gerber Products Company
  445 State Street
  Fremont, MI 49413
  (616) 928-2000
- H.J. Heinz
  Consumer Relations
  P.O. Box 57
  Pittsburgh, PA 15230
  (412) 456-5700
- Hunt-Wesson Foods
  1645 West Valencia Drive
  Fullerton, CA 92633
  (714) 680-1000
- Kellogg Company
  Battle Creek, MI 49016
  (616) 961-2000
- Kraft General Foods Consumer Center
  250 North Street
  White Plains, NY 10625
  (914) 335-2500
- Mead Johnson Nutritionals
  2400 West Lloyd Expressway
  Evansville, IN 47721
  (812) 429-5000
- National Dairy Council
  6300 North River Road
  Rosemont, IL 60018
  (708) 696-1860
- Nestle Company
  100 Manhattanville Road
  Purchase, NY 10577
  (914) 251-3000

- Oscar Mayer Company
  P.O. Box 7188
  Madison, WI 53707
  (608) 241-3311
- Pillsbury Company
  200 South Sixth Street
  Minneapolis, MN 55402-1464
  (612) 330-4966
- The Potato Board
  1385 South Colorado Boulevard, Suite 512
  Denver, Co 80222
  (303) 758-7783
- Rice Council
  P.O. Box 740123
  Houston, TX 77274
  (713) 270-6699
- Ross Laboratories
  625 Cleveland Avenue
  Columbus, OH 43215
  (614) 624-7900
- Sister Kenny Institute
  800 East Twenty-eighth Street
  Minneapolis, MN 55407
  (612) 863-4457
- Soy Protein Council
  1255 Twenty-third Street, NW
  Washington, DC 20037
  (202) 467-6610
- Sunkist Growers
  Consumer Service, Division BB
  Box 7888
  Valley Annex
  Van Nuys, CA 91409
  (818) 986-4800
- United Fresh Fruit and Vegetable Association
  727 N. Washington Street
  Alexandria, VA 22314
  (703) 836-3410

Organizations Concerned with World Hunger

- Bread for the World
  802 Rhode Island Avenue, NE
  Washington, DC 20018
  (202) 269-0200
- The Hunger Project
  1388 Sutter Street—4th Floor
  San Francisco, CA 94109
  (415) 928-8700
- Institute for Food and Development Policy
  145 Ninth Street
  San Francisco, CA 94103
  (415) 864-8555
- Oxfam America
  115 Broadway
  Boston, MA 02116
  (617) 482-1211
- Seeds
  P.O. Box 6170
  Waco, TX 76706
  (817) 755-7745
- Worldwatch Institute
  1776 Massachusetts Avenue, NW
  Washington, DC 20036
  (202) 452-1999

United Nations

- Food and Agriculture Organization (FAO)
  North American Regional Office
  1001 Twenty-second Street, NW
  Washington, DC 20437
  (202) 653-2402
- World Health Organization
  1211 Geneva 27
  Switzerland

APPENDIX B

An Introduction to the Human Body

The brief anatomy lesson that follows is a lesson in "anatomy for nutrition's sake" to review the body systems and terminology referred to in this book. To make the body's design understandable, the first few paragraphs are devoted to the life needs of the cells and the evolutionary mechanisms that ensure that they are met.

The Cells

The body is composed of millions of cells, and not one of them knows anything about food. While you get hungry for meat, milk, or bread, each cell of your body sits in its place waiting until the nutrients it needs pass by. Each of the body's **cells** is a self-contained, living entity (Figure B–1), although each depends on the rest of the body to supply its needs. Each cell keeps itself alive just as its single-celled ancestors did, living alone in the ocean 3 billion

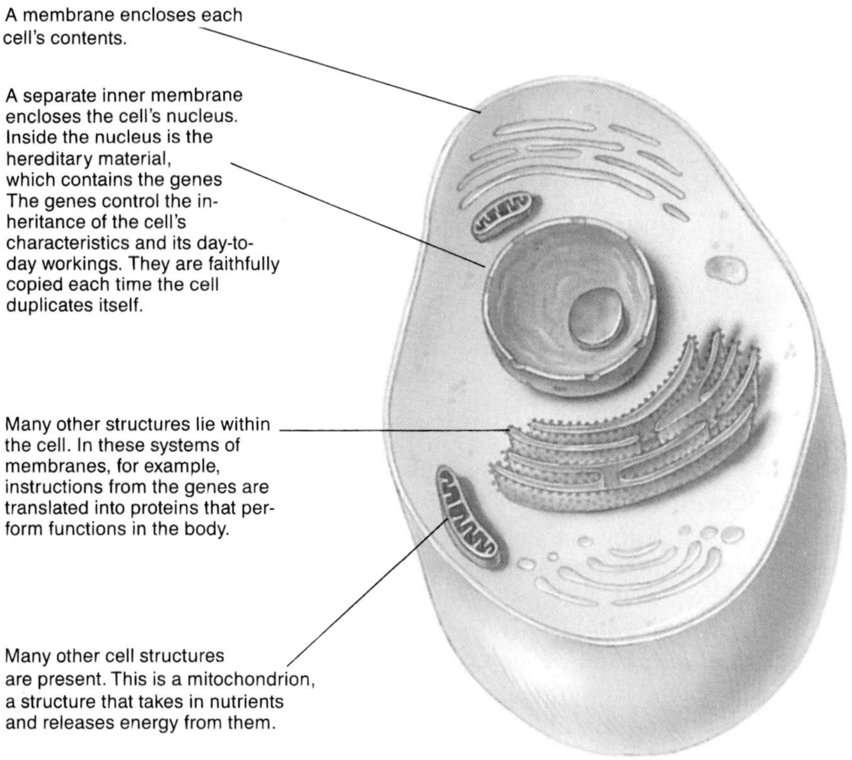

A membrane encloses each cell's contents.
A separate inner membrane encloses the cell's nucleus. Inside the nucleus is the hereditary material, which contains the genes The genes control the inheritance of the cell's characteristics and its day-to-day workings. They are faithfully copied each time the cell duplicates itself.
Many other structures lie within the cell. In these systems of membranes, for example, instructions from the genes are translated into proteins that perform functions in the body.
Many other cell structures are present. This is a mitochondrion, a structure that takes in nutrients and releases energy from them.

Figure B–1

A Typical Cell (Simplified Diagram)

years ago, by taking up the substances it needs from the surrounding fluid and releasing the wastes it produces into that fluid.

The body cells' most basic need, always, is for energy fuel and the oxygen with which to burn it. Next, they need water, the environment in which they live. Then they need building blocks to maintain themselves—especially the materials they can't make for themselves. These building blocks—the **essential nutrients**—must be supplied preformed from food. These are among the limitations of our heredity from which there is no appeal, and they underlie the first principle of diet planning. Whatever foods we choose, they must provide energy, water, and the essential nutrients. In a sense, the body is only a system organized to provide for these needs of its cells.

In the human body every cell works in cooperation with every other to support the whole. The cell's **genes** determine the nature of that work. Each gene is a blueprint that directs the making of a piece of protein machinery—most often an **enzyme**—that helps to do the cell's work. Each cell contains a complete set of genes, but different ones are active in different types of cells. For example, in some intestinal cells, the genes for making digestive enzymes are active; in some of the body's fat cells, the genes for making enzymes that make and break down fat are active.

Cells are organized into tissues that perform specialized tasks governed by the genes that are active in them. For example, some cells are joined together to form muscle tissue, which can contract. Tissues also are organized in sets to form whole organs. In the heart organ, for example, muscle tissues, nerve tissues, connective tissues, and other types all work together to pump blood. Some jobs around the body require that several related organs cooperate to perform them. The organs that join together to work on a function are parts of a body system. For example, the heart, lungs, and blood vessels all work to deliver oxygen and nutrients to the body tissues as parts of the cardiovascular system. The next few sections present some body systems with special significance to nutrition.

The Body Fluids

Every cell of the body needs a continuous supply of water, oxygen, energy, and building materials. The body fluids supply these necessities, bathing the outside of all the cells (see Figure B–2). Every cell continuously uses up oxygen (producing carbon dioxide) and nutrients (producing waste products). The body fluids are the transport canals for these materials, carrying oxygen and nutrients to the cells and carbon dioxide and waste away from them. These fluids must circulate to pick up fresh supplies and deliver the wastes to points of disposal.

The fluids that bathe the cells and circulate around the body are the extracellular fluids, the **blood** and **lymph** (Figure B–3). Blood travels within the **arteries**, **veins**, and **capillaries**, as well as within the heart's chambers (Figure B–4). Lymph is derived from the blood in the capillaries; it squeezes out across their walls and circulates around the cells, permitting exchange of materials. Some of the lymph returns to the blood farther along the capillaries, and the rest travels around the body by way of its own vessels, eventually returning to the bloodstream elsewhere.

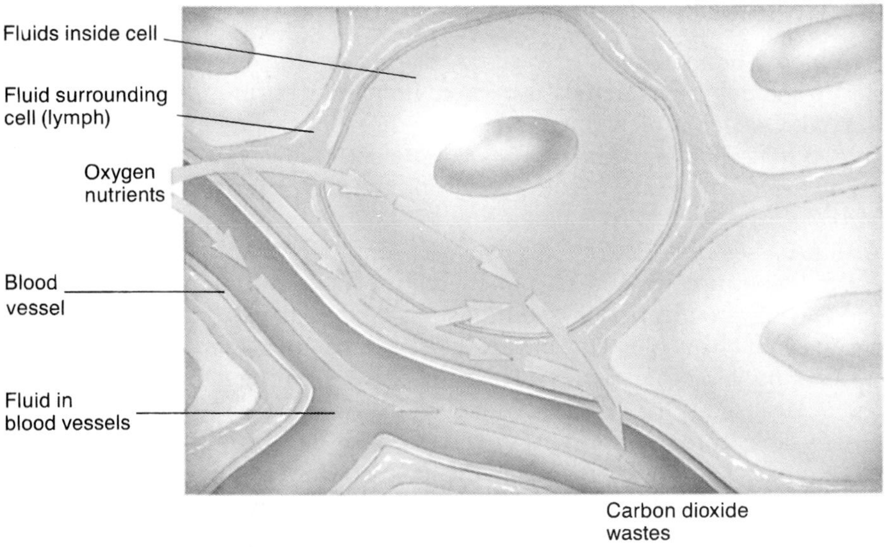

● *Figure B–2*

One Cell and the Associated Fluids

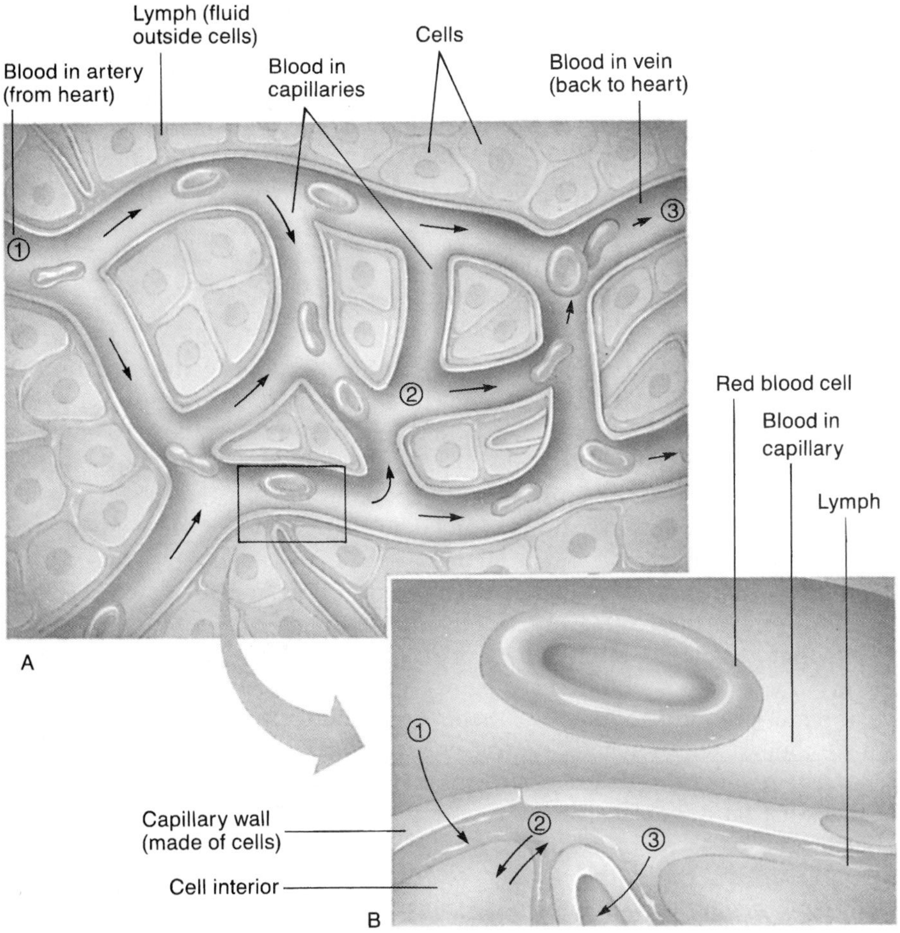

● *Figure B–3*

How the Body Fluids Circulate Around Cells

A. Portion of body tissue.
   1. Blood enters tissues by way of an artery.
   2. Blood circulates among cells by way of capillaries.
   3. Blood collects into veins for return to heart.

B. Detail of A.
   1. Lymph filters out of capillary.
   2. Exchange of materials takes place between cell fluid and lymph.
   3. Lymph circulates away, later reentering bloodstream in a vein.

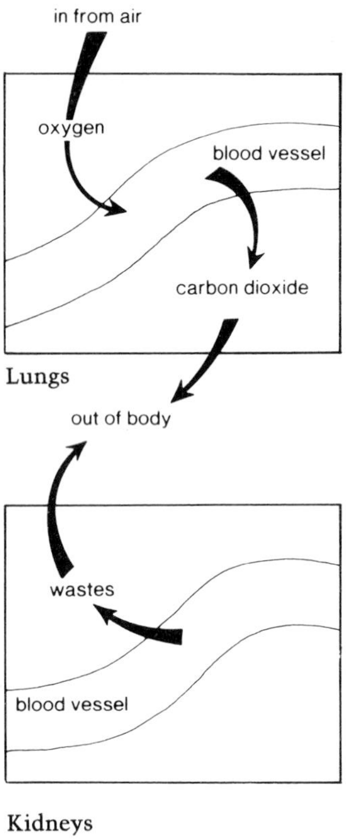

The Circulatory System

As the blood, pumped by the heart, travels through the circulatory system, it picks up and delivers materials as needed. Its routing ensures that all cells will be served. Oxygen is picked up and carbon dioxide released in the **lungs**, and all blood that circulates to the lungs is returned to the heart. From there, it must go to the other body tissues. Thus all tissues receive freshly oxygenated blood.

As it passes the digestive system, the blood delivers oxygen to the cells there and picks up nutrients from the **intestine** for distribution elsewhere. All blood leaving the digestive system must go next to the **liver**, which has the special task of chemically altering the absorbed materials to make them better suited for use by other tissues. Then, in passing through the **kidneys**, the blood is cleansed of its wastes.

As it flows through the skin, the blood is cooled by radiating heat to the surroundings, helping to maintain the temperature of the body's internal organs. Fluid leaving the blood as lymph may ultimately evaporate from the lungs and skin or be used to make body secretions, such as digestive juices, which will be used within the body for various purposes. On its return to the heart, the blood has delivered most of its oxygen and picked up carbon dioxide from the body cells. Its next stop is the lungs once again, to release its carbon dioxide and replenish its oxygen.

In summary, the routing of the blood is as shown in Figure B–4:

- Heart to body to heart to lungs to heart (repeat).

The portion of the blood that flows by the digestive tract travels from:

- Heart to digestive tract to liver to heart.

The Immune System

Many of the body's cells cooperate to maintain its defenses against infection. The skin presents a physical barrier, and the body's cavities (lungs, digestive tract, and others) are lined with membranes that resist penetration by invading **microbes** or unwanted substances. The body's linings are easily damaged by nutrient deficiencies, and clinicians inspect both the skin and the inside of the mouth to detect signs of malnutrition. (The chapters on protein, vitamins, and minerals present details of the signs of deficiencies.)

When a wound or infection penetrates these first lines of defense (the skin and linings), the lymph and blood present internal defenses: cells and proteins that can inactivate, remove, or destroy microbes and foreign substances. Special cells are able to recognize the chemical structures of some foreign materials and to remember them for a time so that they can quickly mobilize their defenses when they see them again. This ability confers **immunity** against many diseases that you have previously fought and conquered. Some immune cells produce proteins that act as ammunition (**antibodies**) designed to destroy specific targets (**antigens**), and still other cells can gobble up and digest the invaders.

Immune system components reside in tissues all over the body—in the linings of the bones, in the digestive tract, in the blood vessels, in the lymph glands, and in glands of their own. They are in constant flux, being made and

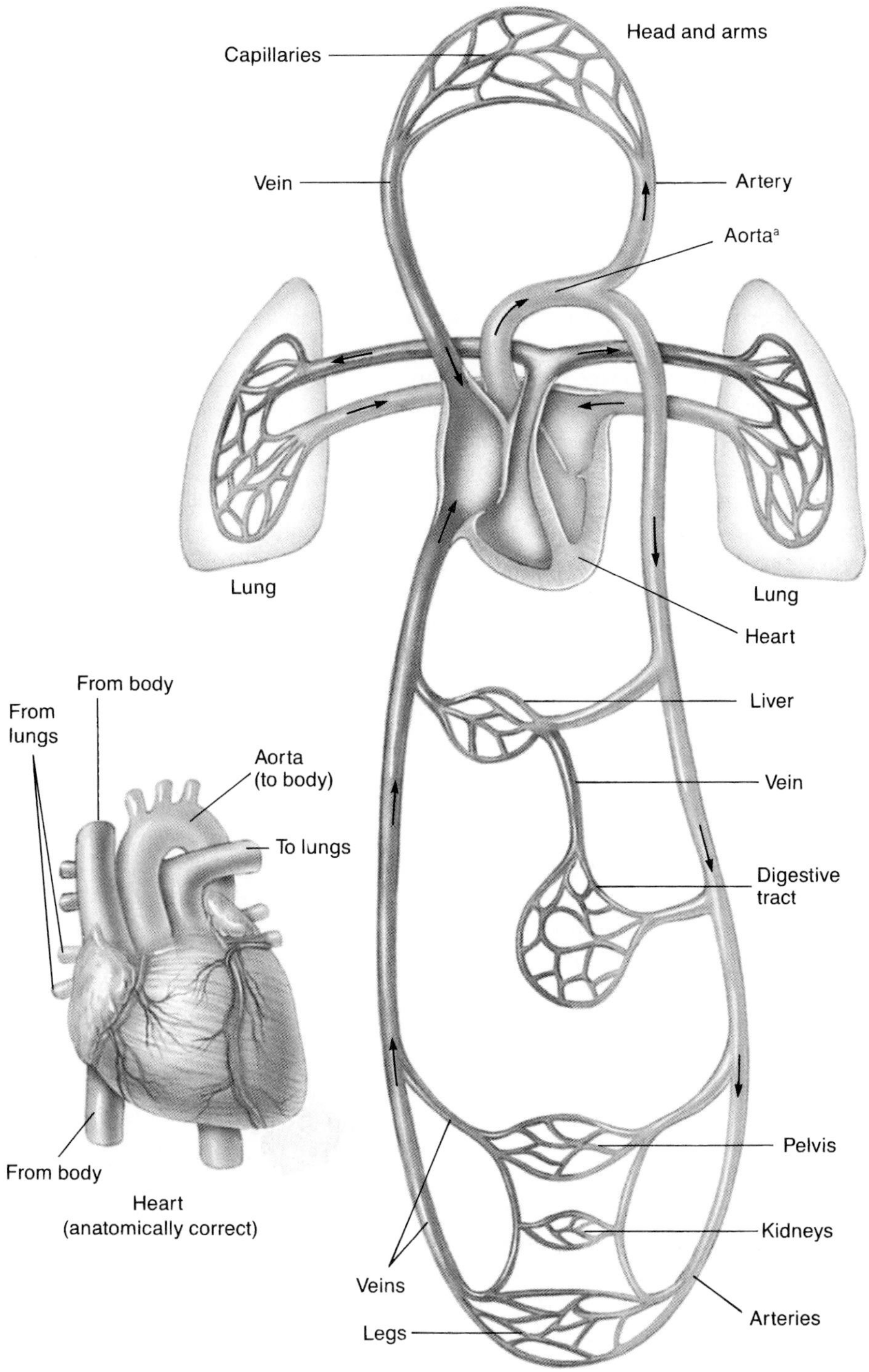

● *Figure B–4*

The Cardiovascular System

Blood leaves right side of heart, picks up oxygen in lungs, and returns to left side of heart. Blood leaves left side of heart, goes to head or digestive tract and then to liver or lower body, and then returns to right side of heart.

[a]The aorta is the main artery that launches blood on its course through the body. The picture is not anatomically correct but is drawn this way for clarity. The aorta actually arises behind the left side of the heart and arcs upwards, then divides. See detail of heart.

dismantled rapidly, and their maintenance requires a continuous supply of nutrients. A deficiency or an overdose of any nutrient is likely to affect the immune system adversely, and a deficiency of nutrients early in an infant's development can weaken that individual's immune defenses against infection for years.

The Hormonal and Nervous Systems

More about the blood glucose level—Chapter 3.

The blood also carries messages, chemical signals from one system of cells to another, that communicate the changing needs of the living system. These chemical messages, or **hormones**, are secreted and released into the blood by the **endocrine** glands. For example, when the **pancreas** (a gland) experiences a too-high concentration of glucose in the blood, it releases **insulin** (a hormone). Insulin stimulates the liver, muscles, and fat cells to remove glucose from the blood and put it away. When the blood glucose level falls too low, the pancreas secretes another hormone, glucagon. The liver responds by releasing glucose into the blood once again.

Glands and hormones abound in the body, each gland a detector system to monitor a condition in the body that needs regulation and each hormone a messenger to stimulate certain tissues to take appropriate action. Examples of the working of these hormones appear throughout this book.

The body's other major communication system is, of course, the nervous system. With the brain and spinal cord as central controllers, the system receives and integrates messages from sensory receptors all over the body—sight, hearing, touch, smell, taste, and others—which all communicate to the brain the state of both the outer and inner worlds, including the availability of food and the need to eat. The system then returns instructions to the muscles and glands, telling them what to do.

The nervous system's part in hunger regulation is coordinated by the brain. The sensations of hunger and appetite are experienced in the **cortex** of the brain, the thinking, outer layer. However, much of the brain's regulatory work goes on without the person's (or the cortex's) awareness in the deep brain centers. An organ there, the **hypothalamus** (Figure B–5), monitors many body conditions, including the availability of nutrients and water.

Figure B–5

The Brain's Hypothalamus and Cortex

The hypothalamus monitors the body's conditions and sends signals to the brain's thinking portion, the cortex, which decides on actions.

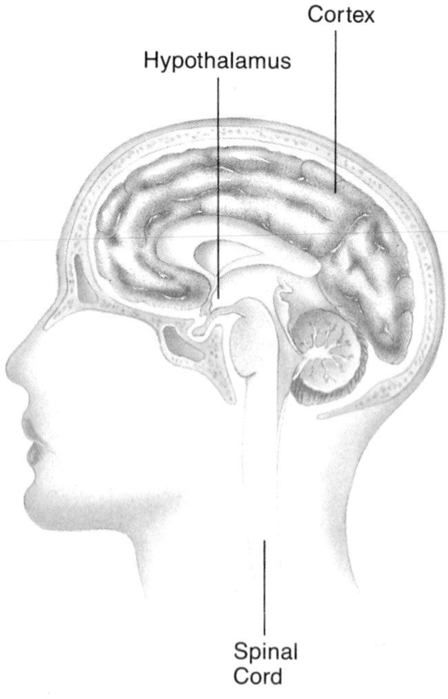

The Excretory System

To dispose of waste, the **kidneys** straddle the circulatory system and filter each pass of the blood (see Figure B–6). Waste materials removed with water are collected as urine in tubes that deliver them to the urinary bladder, which is periodically emptied. Thus the blood is purified continuously throughout the day, and dissolved minerals are excreted as necessary (including sodium, to keep blood pressure from rising too high). As you might expect, the kidneys' work is regulated by hormones secreted by glands responsive to conditions in the blood (such as the sodium concentration).

Temperature Regulation

All the body's cells obtain energy by breaking down the nutrients—carbohydrate, fat, and to some extent protein—and one of the ways this

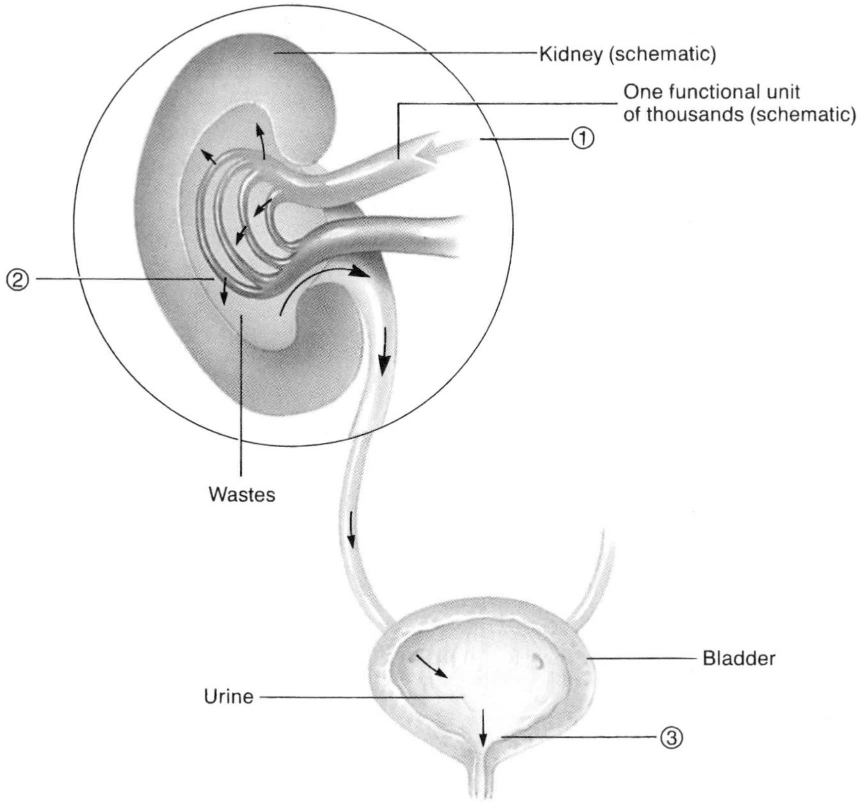

Figure B–6

The Excretory System

1. Blood enters kidney by way of arteries, and disperses into capillaries.
2. Kidney filters waste from blood and sends it as urine to the bladder.
3. Bladder periodically eliminates urine.

energy is released is as heat. The heat is lost to the air through the skin surface. Temperature regulation involves speeding up or slowing down cellular heat production (**metabolism**) and increasing or decreasing heat loss through the skin. Specialized nerve cells in an area of the brain called the hypothalamus serve as a thermostat, measuring the temperature of the blood. These cells signal other cells, near the body surface, to respond appropriately. When the body is too hot, blood vessels immediately under the skin dilate, allowing warm blood to flow near the surface, where its heat can radiate away. The sweat glands also are activated to secrete warm fluid onto the skin surface, where its heat can be lost by evaporation. When the body is cold, these mechanisms shut down and shivering is triggered, generating heat.

By means of these systems of transportation, communication, waste disposal, and heat regulation, the cells of the multicellular human animal cooperate to provide one another with a circulating bath of warm, clean, nutritive fluid whose composition is finely regulated to meet their needs.

The Digestive System

You may eat meals only two or three times a day, but your body's cells need their nutrients twenty-four hours a day. Providing the needed nutrients requires the cooperation of millions of specialized cells. When the body's cells are deprived of fuel, certain nerve cells in the brain (the hypothalamus) detect

Figure B–7

The Digestive System

FIBER	STARCH
	The salivary glands secrete a watery fluid into the mouth to moisten the food. An enzyme begins digestion by splitting starch into smaller polysaccharides and maltose. This digestion continues after the food is swallowed until stomach acid and enzymes start to digest the salivary enzymes.
The mechanical action of the mouth crushes and tears fiber in food and mixes it with saliva to moisten it for swallowing.	The pancreas produces carbohydrate-digesting enzymes and releases them through the common bile duct into the small intestine. These enzymes split polysaccharides into disaccharides. Then enzymes on the surface of the small intestinal cells break these into simple sugars (monosaccharides). The cells absorb the monosaccharides as they are freed.
Most fiber passes intact through the digestive tract to the large intestine. Here, some types of fiber are digested to glucose by bacterial enzymes, and the free glucose molecules are absorbed into the body. Fiber in the large intestine holds water and regulates bowel activity. Some fiber binds cholesterol and certain minerals and carries them out in the feces.	

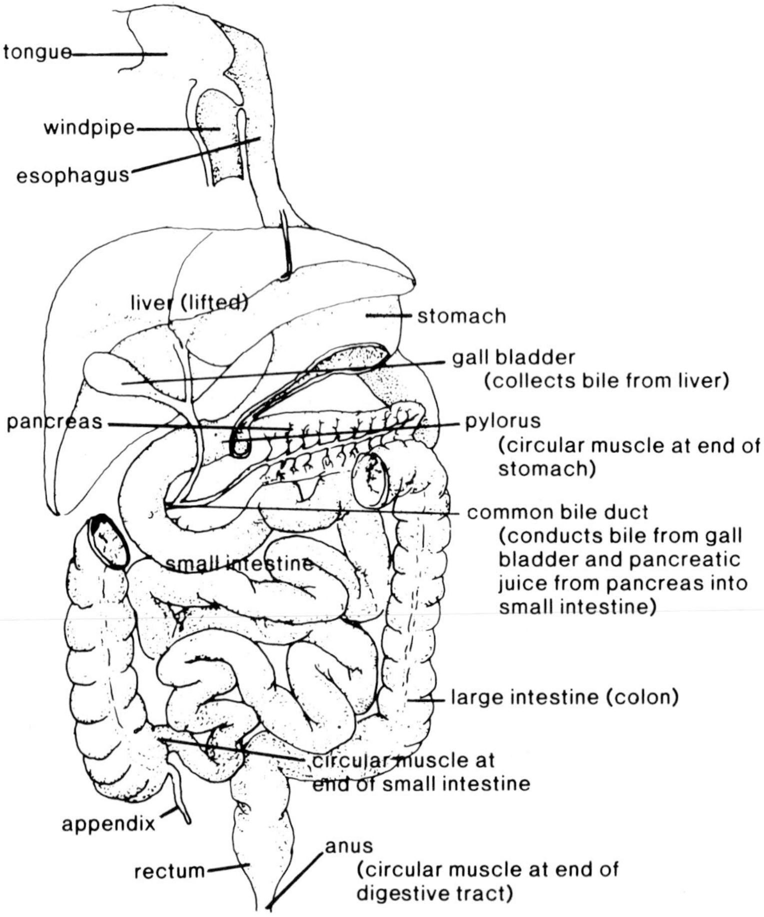

PROTEIN	FAT	VITAMINS	MINERALS AND WATER
			All digestive reactions take place in water secreted into the digestive tract by various organs. The salivary glands of the mouth are the first to contribute water.
In the mouth, chewing crushes and softens protein-rich foods and mixes them with saliva to be swallowed.			The stomach secretes enough watery fluid to turn a moist, chewed mass of swallowed food into a liquid.
Stomach acid works to uncoil protein strands and activate stomach enzymes. Then the enzymes break the strands into smaller fragments.	Fat floats up from the other foods in the watery stomach acid. The stomach digests a small percentage of fat. The liver secretes bile; the gallbladder stores it and releases it through the common bile duct into the small intestine when fat arrives there. The bile emulsifies the fat, making it ready for enzyme action.	Water-soluble vitamins need little action by the digestive organs except absorption in the small intestine. However, vitamin B_{12} requires "intrinsic factor" produced by the stomach in order to be absorbed.	Stomach acid acts on iron to make it more absorbable. Vitamin C and a factor in meat also increase iron absorption. Binders in vegetables and grains "tie up" zinc and calcium, making them unavailable for absorption. If a person's body has plenty of a certain mineral like iron, zinc, or calcium, then the small intestine absorbs a smaller percentage of that mineral from food than it would if the person was deficient.
	The pancreas produces fat-digesting enzymes and releases them through the common bile duct into the small intestine. These enzymes split triglycerides into monoglycerides, free fatty acids, and glycerol, which are absorbed. Some fatty materials escape absorption and are carried out of the body via the large intestine.	Bile from the liver, stored in the gallbladder, is released through the common bile duct into the small intestine when fat is present there. The bile emulsifies fat-soluble vitamins and aids in their absorption with other fats. The bacteria in the large intestine release vitamin K, which is absorbed there.	The small intestine, along with the pancreas and liver, secretes its own fluids for a total of about 2 gallons of water secreted into the digestive tract per day. This water is not lost, but is conserved by reabsorption in the large intestine.
In the small intestine, the fragments of protein are split into free amino acids, dipeptides, and tripeptides with the help of enzymes from the pancreas and small intestine. Enzymes on the surface of the small intestinal cells break these peptides into amino acids, and they are absorbed through the cells into the blood. The large intestine carries any undigested protein residue out of the body. Normally, practically all the protein is digested and absorbed.			Absorption of calcium depends on adequate vitamin D status. Other minerals, like sodium and potassium, are absorbed in the small and large intestines whether or not the person has sufficient amounts of the minerals in the body.

Digestive tract secretions:
- **Salivary glands:**
  - Saliva.
  - Salivary amylase (enzyme that breaks down starch).
- **Stomach (gastric) glands:**
  - Gastric juice.
  - Hydrochloric acid (uncoils protein).
  - Gastric protease (enzyme that breaks down protein).
  - Mucus (thick coating that protects the stomach wall from these secretions).
- **Intestinal cells:**
  - Enzymes (break down carbohydrate and protein).
  - Mucus (thin coating that protects the intestinal wall).
- **Liver and gallbladder:**
  - Bile (emulsifier that separates fat into small particles enzymes can attack).
- **Pancreas:**
  - Bicarbonate (neutralizes acid fluid from stomach so intestinal and pancreatic enzymes can work on its contents).
  - Enzymes (break down carbohydrate, fat, and protein).

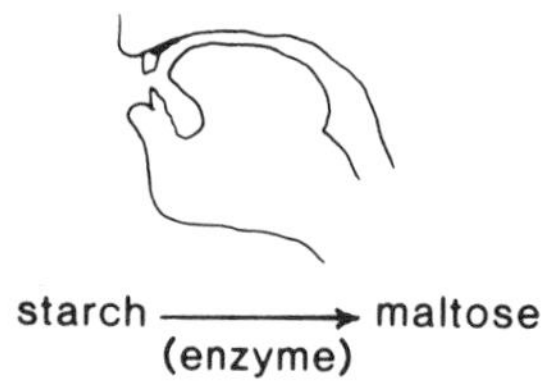

Digestion in the mouth.

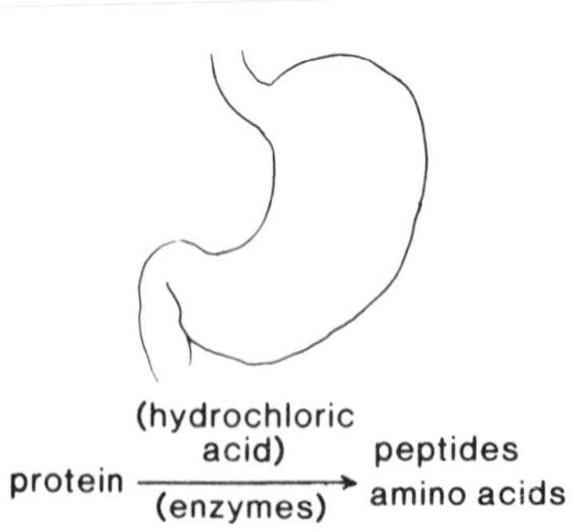

Digestion in the stomach.

this condition and generate nerve impulses that signal hunger to the conscious part of the brain, the cortex. They also stimulate the stomach to intensify its contractions, creating hunger pangs. Becoming conscious of hunger, then, you eat, delivering a complex mixture of chewed and swallowed food to the intestinal tract.

Many of the cells lining the intestinal tract secrete powerful juices and **enzymes** to disintegrate nutrients (especially carbohydrate and protein) into their component parts. Two organs outside the digestive tract—the liver with its associated gallbladder and the pancreas—also contribute digestive juices through a common duct into the small intestine. The presence of these digestive juices and enzymes requires that still other cells specialize in protecting the digestive system. They secrete a thick, viscous substance known as **mucus**, or the **mucous membrane**, which coats the intestinal tract lining and ensures that it will not itself be digested.

The process of digestion is diagrammed in Figure B–7. The first part, the mouth, is designed for physically breaking down foods. The teeth cut off a bite-size portion and then, aided by the tongue, grind it finely enough to be mixed with saliva and swallowed. The esophagus carries the mixture to the stomach. The stomach is supplied with several sets of muscles to mix and grind it further and secretes acid and enzymes that will begin to break it apart chemically.

During the preparatory stage, as the complex carbohydrate known as starch is released from a food (such as bread), an enzyme present in the saliva starts to break it down chemically to smaller units. But this action is stopped when the carbohydrate units reach the stomach, because glands in the stomach wall exude hydrochloric acid. The salivary enzyme that breaks up starch is digested in the stomach, together with other proteins. Further dismantling of carbohydrate occurs after it leaves the stomach.

Fats and oils, taken as part of such complex foods as meats or nuts or in relatively pure form as butter or oil, are not much affected until after leaving the stomach.

Proteins are eaten as part of such foods as meat, milk, and legumes. Although no chemical action on them takes place in the mouth, chewing and mixing protein with saliva is an important part of preparing it for the chemical action that begins in the stomach. There, enzymes and hydrochloric acid break apart the large, complex protein molecules into smaller pieces known as peptides and finally into dipeptides, tripeptides, and amino acids.

The complicated chemical dismantling that takes place beyond the stomach requires that only small amounts be processed at one time. To accomplish this, the **pylorus**, a circular muscle surrounding the lower end of the stomach, controls the exit of the contents, allowing only a little at a time to be squirted forcefully into the small intestine. Gradually the stomach empties itself by means of these powerful squirts.

The small intestine is "the" organ of digestion and absorption; it finishes the job the mouth and stomach have started. It is actually about 20 feet long, but it is called small because its diameter is small compared with that of the large intestine. Its contents must touch its walls in order to make contact with the secretions and in order to be absorbed at the proper places. At the end of the small intestine, a circular muscle (similar in function to the pylorus at the end of the stomach) controls the flow of the contents going into the large intestine (colon).

The small intestine works with the precision of a laboratory chemist. As the thoroughly liquefied and partially digested nutrient mixture arrives there, hormonal messages tell the gallbladder to send its **emulsifier, bile,** in amounts matched to the amount of fat present. Other hormones notify the **pancreas** to release **bicarbonate** in amounts precisely adjusted to neutralize the stomach acid as well as enzymes of the appropriate kinds and quantities to continue dismantling whatever large molecules remain. Such messages also keep the strong muscles imbedded in the walls of the intestine contracting, in a squeezing activity called **peristalsis,** so that the contents will be pressed along to the next region. Peristalsis is stimulated by the presence of roughage or fiber and is quieted by the presence of fat, which requires a longer time for digestion.

Meanwhile, as the pancreatic and intestinal enzymes act on the bonds that hold the large nutrients together, smaller and smaller units make their appearance in the intestinal fluids. Finally, units that cells can use—glucose, glycerol, fatty acids, and amino acids, among others—are released.

Once the digestive system has broken food down to its nutrient components, it must deliver them to the rest of the body. The cells of the intestinal lining absorb nutrients from the mixture within the intestine and deposit them in the blood and lymph. Every molecule of nutrient must traverse one of these cells if it is to enter the body fluids. The cells are selective: they can recognize the nutrients needed by the body. The cells are also extraordinarily efficient: they absorb enough nutrients to nourish all the body's other cells.

The intestinal tract lining is composed of a single sheet of cells, and the sheet pokes out into millions of finger-shaped projections (**villi**). Each villus has its own capillary network and a lymph vessel so that as nutrients move across the cells, they can immediately mingle into the body fluids. On every villus every cell has a brushlike covering of tiny hairs (**microvilli**) that can trap the nutrient particles. Figure B–8 and Figure B–9 provide a close look at these details.

The small intestine's lining, villi and all, is wrinkled into thousands of folds, so that its absorbing surface is enormous. If the folds, and the villi that cover them, were spread out flat, the total area would equal a third of a football field in size. The billions of cells of that surface, although they weigh only 4 to 5 pounds, absorb enough nutrients in a few hours a day to nourish the other 150 or so pounds of body tissues.

Nutrients released early in the digestive process, such as simple sugars, and those requiring no special handling, such as the water-soluble vitamins, are absorbed high in the small intestine; nutrients that are released more slowly are absorbed further down. The lymphatic and circulatory systems then take over the job of transporting them to the cell consumers. The lymph at first carries most of the products of fat digestion and the fat-soluble vitamins, later delivering them to the blood. The blood carries the products of carbohydrate and protein digestion, the water-soluble vitamins, and the minerals. By the time the remaining mixture reaches the end of the small intestine, little is left but water, indigestible residue (mostly fiber), and dissolved minerals. The cells lining the colon are specialized for absorbing these minerals and retrieving the water for recycling. The final waste product, the feces,

Figure B–8

Microvilli of the Small Intestine

The two dark objects are individual cells of two neighboring villi; the fingerlike projections that border them are microvilli. This photograph was taken through an electron microscope at a magnification of 51,000 times.

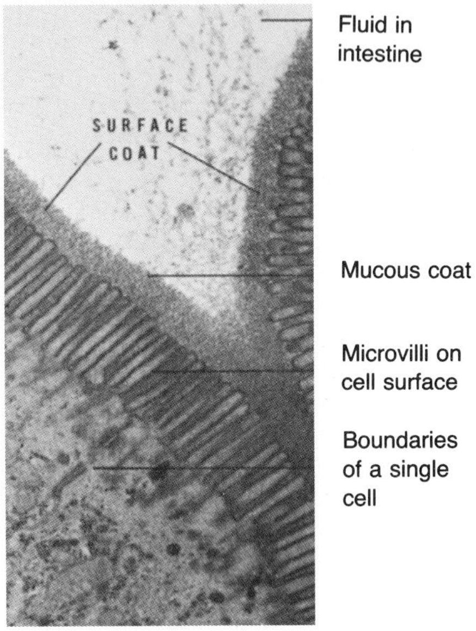

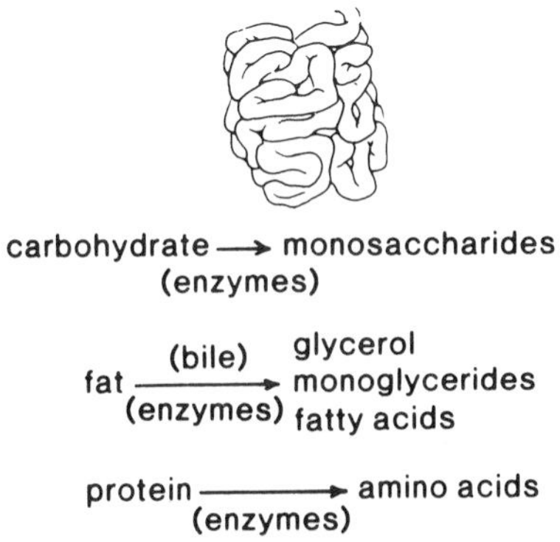

Digestion in the small intestine.

● *Figure B–9*

Details of the Lining of the Small Intestine

The wall of the small intestine is wrinkled into thousands of folds and is carpeted with villi (part A). Each villus, in turn (part B), is covered with even smaller projections, the microvilli (part C).

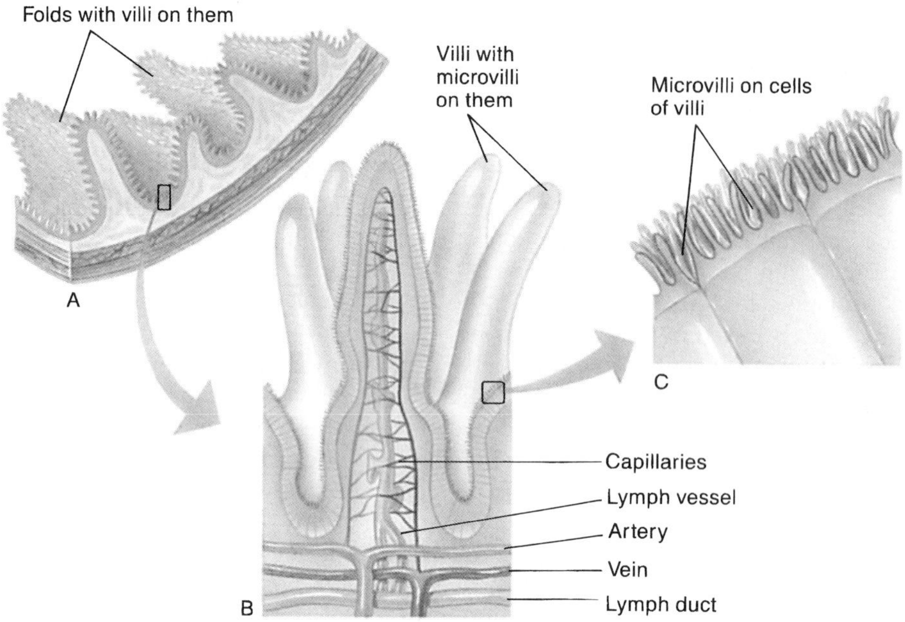

a smooth paste of a consistency suitable for excretion, is stored in the colon until excretion. Such a system can adjust to whatever mixture of foods is presented.

Although a meal may be eaten in half an hour, the nutrients it provides reach the body fluids over a span of about four hours. However, as already mentioned, the cells of the body need their nutrients around the clock. Providing a constant supply requires that there be systems of storage and release to meet the cells' needs between meals.

Storage Systems

Nutrients leave the digestive system by way of both circulatory systems—the blood and the lymph. The blood carries products of carbohydrate and protein digestion and some of the smaller fats; the lymph carries the larger fats in packages called chylomicrons (see Chapter 4).

All nutrients leaving the digestive system by way of the blood are collected in thousands of capillaries in the membrane that supports the intestine. These converge into veins and then into a single large vein. This vein conveys its contents to the liver and there breaks up once again into a vast network of capillaries that weave among the liver cells, allowing them access to the newly arriving nutrients. The liver cells process these nutrients. They convert the sugars from carbohydrate mostly into the body's sugar, glucose; and if there is a surplus, they store some as glycogen and convert the remainder to fat. They reassemble fatty acids and glycerol from fat into larger fats and package them with protein for transport to other parts of the body. As for the amino acids from protein, the liver cells alter these as needed, making glucose from some if necessary and fat from others if there is an excess, or converting one amino acid into another to use in making proteins.

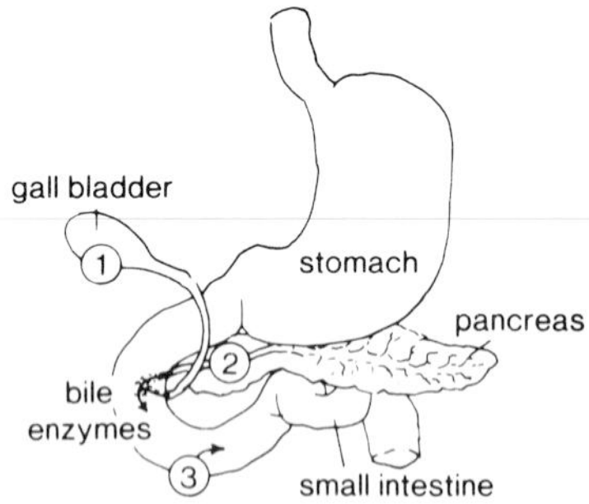

Small intestine—details.

1. The gallbladder sends bile into the small intestine by way of a duct.
2. The pancreas sends enzymes (and bicarbonate).
3. The small intestine also secretes enzymes.

The nutrients leaving the digestive tract by way of the lymph as chylomicrons circulate throughout the body, giving all cells the opportunity to withdraw fats from them. Some also find their way into the blood and circulate through the liver, which removes them, alters their components, and releases new products, including other lipoproteins.

The new products of liver metabolism—glucose, fat packaged with protein (lipoproteins), and amino acids—are released into the bloodstream again and circulated to all other cells of the body. Surplus fat is then removed by cells specialized for its storage; these fat cells are located in deposits all over the body.

The liver's glycogen provides a reserve supply of the body's sugar, glucose, and thus can sustain cell activities if the intervals between meals become so long that glucose absorbed from ingested food is used up. When the body is depending solely on liver glycogen, however, the supply is used up within three to six hours. Similarly, the fat cells store reserves of fat, the body's other principal energy nutrient. Unlike the liver, however, the fat cells have virtually infinite storage capacity and can continue to supply fat for days, weeks, or even months when no food is eaten.

More about liver glycogen—Chapter 3.

More about lipoproteins—Chapter 4.

More about fasting—Chapter 8.

More about protein deficiency—Chapter 5.

These storage systems for glucose and fat ensure that the cells will not go without energy nutrients even if the body is hungry for food, except under extreme conditions. Body stores also exist for many other nutrients, each with a characteristic capacity. For example, the third energy nutrient, protein, is held in an available pool (the amino acids in the liver and blood) that is rather rapidly depleted during protein deficiency. The liver and fat cells store many vitamins, and the bones provide reserves of calcium, sodium, and other minerals that can be drawn on to keep the blood levels constant and to meet cellular demands.

Other Systems

In addition to the systems described above, the body has many more: the bones, the muscles, the nerves, the lungs, the reproductive organs, and others. All of these cooperate so that each cell can carry on its own life. Each assures, through hormonal or nerve-mediated messages, that its needs will be met by the others, and each contributes to the welfare of the whole by doing the work it is specialized for.

Of the millions of cells in the body, only a small percentage comprise the cortex of the brain, in which the conscious mind resides. These receive messages from other cells when they require you to "become conscious" of a need for decision and action. In modern life the need may be as complex as, for example, to notice that you feel anxious and to decide to consult an advisor, or it may be such a "simple" need as "I'm tired, I think I'll go to bed," or "I'm hungry, I guess I'd better eat."

Most of the body's work is done automatically and is finely regulated to achieve a state of well-being. But when your cortex does become involved, you would do well to "listen" to your body and to cultivate an understanding and appreciation of its needs. Then when you make decisions you will act to promote your health.

Glossary

antibodies proteins made by the immune system, expressly designed to combine with and to inactivate specific antigens.

antigens microbes or substances that are foreign to the body.

arteries blood vessels that carry blood containing fresh oxygen supplies from the heart to the tissues.

bicarbonate a chemical that neutralizes acid; a secretion of the pancreas.

bile a compound made from cholesterol by the liver, stored in the gallbladder, and secreted into the small intestine. It emulsifies lipids to ready them for enzymatic digestion.

blood the fluid of the circulatory system—water, red and white blood cells and other formed particles, proteins, nutrients, oxygen, and other constituents.

capillaries minute, weblike blood vessels that connect arteries to veins and permit transfer of materials between blood and tissues.

cells the smallest units in which independent life can exist. All living things are single cells or organisms made of cells.

cortex an outer covering; in the brain, that part in which conscious thought takes place.

emulsifier (ee-MULL-sih-fire) a compound with both water-soluble and fat-soluble portions that can attract lipids into water solution.

endocrine (EN-doh-crin) a term to describe a gland secreting or a hormone being secreted into the blood (*endo* means "into").

enzyme a protein catalyst. A catalyst is a compound that facilitates (speeds up the rate of) a chemical reaction without itself being altered in the process.

essential nutrients compounds that can't be synthesized by the body in amounts sufficient to meet physiological needs.

gene a unit of a cell's inheritance, made of a chemical, DNA, that is copied faithfully so that every time the cell divides, both its offspring get identical copies. Genes direct the cells' machinery to make the proteins that form each cell's structures and do its work.

hormone a chemical messenger, secreted by one organ (a gland) in response to a condition in the body, that acts on another organ or organs to change that condition.

hypothalamus (high-poh-THALL-uh-mus) a part of the brain that senses a variety of conditions in the blood, such as temperature, salt content, glucose content, and others, and signals other parts of the brain or body to change those conditions when necessary.

immunity the ability to successfully resist a disease, conferred on the body by way of the immune system's memory of previous exposure to that disease and its ability to mount a specific defense promptly and swiftly.

insulin a hormone from the pancreas that helps glucose get into cells.

intestine a long, tubular organ of digestion and the site of nutrient absorption.

kidneys the organs that filter the blood to remove waste material and forward it to the bladder for excretion.

liver the large, many-lobed organ that lies under the ribs and filters the blood, removing, processing, and readying for redistribution many of its materials.

lungs the organs of gas exchange. Blood circulating through the lungs releases its carbon dioxide and picks up fresh oxygen to carry to the tissues.

Glossary—Continued

lymph (LIMF) the fluid outside the circulatory system that bathes the cells, derived from the blood by being pressed through the capillary walls; similar to the blood in composition but without red blood cells.

metabolism (meh-TAB-o-lism) total of all chemical reactions that go on in living cells.

microbes bacteria, viruses, or other organisms invisible to the naked eye; some cause disease.

microvilli (MY-croh-VILL-ee, MY-croh-VILL-eye) tiny hairlike projections on each cell of the intestinal tract lining that can trap nutrient particles and translocate them into the cells (singular: **microvillus**).

mucus (MYOO-cus) a thick, slippery coating of the intestinal tract lining (and other body linings) that protects the cells from exposure to digestive juices. The adjective form is *mucous*, and the coating is often called the **mucous membrane**.

mutation event that alters a gene so that it codes for a different protein; a very rare event but one that makes possible variation among organisms (*muta* means "change").

pancreas a gland that secretes the endocrine hormone insulin and also produces the exocrine secretions that aid digestion in the small intestine. (An *exocrine* secretion is one that is expelled through a duct into a body cavity or onto the surface of the skin; *exo* means "out." See also *endocrine*.)

peristalsis (perri-STALL-sis) the wavelike squeezing motions of the stomach and intestines that push their contents along.

pylorus (pye-LORE-us) muscle that regulates the opening at the bottom of the stomach.

veins blood vessels that carry used blood from the tissues back to the heart.

villi (VILL-ee, VILL-eye) poked-out parts of the sheet of cells that line the GI tract; the villi make the surface area much greater than it would otherwise be (singular: **villus**).

APPENDIX **C**

Nutrition Guidelines for Canadians

● *Table C–1*

Average Energy Requirements for Canadians

Age	Sex	Average Height (cm)	Average Weight (kg)	Requirements[a]					
				(kcal/kg)[b]	(MJ/kg)[b]	(kcal/day)	(MJ/day)	(kcal/cm)	(MJ/cm)
Months									
0–2	Both	55	4.5	120–100	0.50–0.42	500	2.0	9	0.04
3–5	Both	63	7.0	100–95	0.42–0.40	700	2.8	11	0.05
6–8	Both	69	8.5	95–97	0.40–0.41	800	3.4	11.5	0.05
9–11	Both	73	9.5	97–99	0.41	950	3.8	12.5	0.05
Years									
1	Both	82	11	101	0.42	1,100	4.8	13.5	0.06
2–3	Both	95	14	94	0.39	1,300	5.6	13.5	0.06
4–6	Both	107	18	100	0.42	1,800	7.6	17	0.07
7–9	M	126	25	88	0.37	2,200	9.2	17.5	0.07
	F	125	25	76	0.32	1,900	8.0	15	0.06
10–12	M	141	34	73	0.30	2,500	10.4	17.5	0.07
	F	143	36	61	0.25	2,200	9.2	15.5	0.06
13–15	M	159	50	57	0.24	2,800	12.0	17.5	0.07
	F	157	48	46	0.19	2,200	9.2	14	0.06
16–18	M	172	62	51	0.21	3,200	13.2	18.5	0.08
	F	160	53	40	0.17	2,100	8.8	13	0.05
19–24	M	175	71	42	0.18	3,000	12.6		
	F	160	58	36	0.15	2,100	8.8		
25–49	M	172	74	36	0.15	2,700	11.3		
	F	160	59	32	0.13	1,900	8.0		
50–74	M	170	73	31	0.13	2,300	9.7		
	F	158	63	29	0.12	1,800	7.6		
75+	M	168	69	29	0.12	2,000	8.4		
	F	155	64	23	0.10	1,500	6.3		

[a]Requirements can be expected to vary within a range of ± 30%.
[b]First and last figures are averages at the beginning and at the end of the 3-month period.

Source: Health and Welfare Canada, *Nutrition Recommendations: The Report of the Scientific Review Committee* (Ottawa: Canadian Government Publishing Centre, 1990), Tables 5 and 6, pp. 25, 27.

Table C–2

Recommended Nutrient Intakes for Canadians, 1990

Age	Sex	Weight (kg)	Protein (g/day)[a]	Fat-Soluble Vitamins: Vitamin A (RE/day)[b]	Vitamin D (μg/day)[c]	Vitamin E (mg/day)[d]
Months						
0–4	Both	6.0	12[f]	400	10	3
5–12	Both	9.0	12	400	10	3
Years						
1	Both	11	13	400	10	3
2–3	Both	14	16	400	5	4
4–6	Both	18	19	500	5	5
7–9	M	25	26	700	2.5	7
	F	25	26	700	2.5	6
10–12	M	34	34	800	2.5	8
	F	36	36	800	2.5	7
13–15	M	50	49	900	2.5	9
	F	48	46	800	2.5	7
16–18	M	62	58	1,000	2.5	10
	F	53	47	800	2.5	7
19–24	M	71	61	1,000	2.5	10
	F	58	50	800	2.5	7
25–49	M	74	64	1,000	2.5	9
	F	59	51	800	2.5	6
50–74	M	73	63	1,000	5	7
	F	63	54	800	5	6
75+	M	69	59	1,000	5	6
	F	64	55	800	5	5
Pregnancy (additional amount needed)						
1st trimester			5	0	2.5	2
2nd trimester			15	0	2.5	2
3rd trimester			24	0	2.5	2
Lactation (additional amount needed)			20	400	2.5	3

Recommended intakes of energy and of certain nutrients are not listed in this table because of the nature of the variables upon which they are based. The figures for energy are estimates of average requirements for expected patterns of activity (see Table C–1). For nutrients not shown, the following amounts are recommended: thiamin, 0.4 mg/1000 cal (0.48/5000 kJ); riboflavin, 0.5 mg/1000 cal (0.6 mg/5000 kJ); niacin, 7.2 NE/1000 cal (8.6 NE/5000 kJ); vitamin B_6, 15 μg, as pyridoxine, per gram of protein. Recommended intakes during periods of growth are taken as appropriate for individuals representative of the midpoint in each age group. All recommended intakes are designed to cover individual variations in essentially all of a healthy population subsisting upon a variety of common foods available in Canada.

Source: Health and Welfare Canada, *Nutrition Recommendations: The Report of the Scientific Review Committee* (Ottawa: Canadian Government Publishing Centre, 1990), Table 20, p. 204.

Table C–2 (continued)

Water-Soluble Vitamins			Minerals					
Vitamin C (mg/day)[e]	Folate (μg/day)	Vitamin B_{12} (μg/day)	Calcium (mg/day)	Phosphorus (mg/day)	Magnesium (mg/day)	Iron (mg/day)	Iodine (μg/day)	Zinc (mg/day)
20	25	0.3	250	150	20	0.3[g]	30	2[h]
20	40	0.4	400	200	32	7	40	3
20	40	0.5	500	300	40	6	55	4
20	50	0.6	550	350	50	6	65	4
25	70	0.8	600	400	65	8	85	5
25	90	1.0	700	500	100	8	110	7
25	90	1.0	700	500	100	8	95	7
25	120	1.0	900	700	130	8	125	9
25	130	1.0	1,100	800	135	8	110	9
30	175	1.0	1,100	900	185	10	160	12
30	170	1.0	1,000	850	180	13	160	9
40	220	1.0	900	1,000	230	10	160	12
30	190	1.0	700	850	200	12	160	9
40	220	1.0	800	1,000	240	9	160	12
30	180	1.0	700	850	200	13	160	9
40	230	1.0	800	1,000	250	9	160	12
30	185	1.0	700	850	200	13[i]	160	9
40	230	1.0	800	1,000	250	9	160	12
30	195	1.0	800	850	210	8	160	9
40	215	1.0	800	1,000	230	9	160	12
30	200	1.0	800	850	210	8	160	9
0	200	0.2	500	200	15	0	25	6
10	200	0.2	500	200	45	5	25	6
10	200	0.2	500	200	45	10	25	6
25	100	0.2	500	200	65	0	50	6

[a]The primary units are expressed per kilogram of body weight. The figures shown here are examples.
[b]One retinol equivalent (RE) corresponds to the biological activity of 1 μg of retinol, 6 μg of beta-carotene, or 12 μg of other carotenes.
[c]Expressed as cholecalciferol or ergocalciferol.
[d]Expressed as δ-α-tocopherol equivalents, relative to which β- and γ-tocopherol and α-tocotrienol have activities of 0.5, 0.1, and 0.3, respectively.
[e]Cigarette smokers should increase intake by 50 percent.
[f]The assumption is made that the protein is from breast milk or is of the same biological value as that of breast milk, and that between 3 and 9 months, adjustment for the quality of the protein is made.
[g]Based on the assumption that breast milk is the source of iron.
[h]Based on the assumption that breast milk is the source of zinc.
[i]After menopause, the recommended intake is 8 mg/day.

Table C–3

Canada's Food Guide

Milk and milk products—2 servings[a]
Meat, fish, poultry, and alternates—2 servings
Fruits and vegetables—4 to 5 servings[b]
Breads and cereals—3 to 5 servings

[a]A serving is 250 ml, or about 1 c. Milk group servings differ for children up to age 11—2 to 3 servings; adolescents—3 to 4 servings; pregnant and nursing women—3 to 4 servings.
[b]Include at least two vegetables.

Source: *Canada's Food Guide Handbook,* revised (Health and Welfare Canada, 1985).

Table C–4

Nutrition Recommendations for Canadians

THE CANADIAN DIET SHOULD:
1. Provide energy consistent with the maintenance of body weight within the recommended range.
2. Include essential nutrients in amounts recommended in the RNI.
3. Include no more than 30 percent of energy as fat and no more than 10 percent as saturated fat.
4. Provide 55 percent of energy as carbohydrate from a variety of sources.
5. Reduce sodium contents.
6. Include no more than 5 percent of total energy as alcohol, or two drinks daily, whichever is less.
7. Contain no more caffeine than the equivalent of four regular cups of coffee per day.
8. Provide 1 milligram fluoride per litre of water.

Source: Adapted from Scientific Review Committee and the Communications/Implementation Committee, *Nutrition Recommendations . . . A Call for Action* (Ottawa: Canadian Government Publishing Centre, 1989).

APPENDIX **D**

Aids to Calculation

Many mathematical problems have been worked out for you as examples at appropriate places in the text. This appendix aims to help with the use of the metric system and with those problems not fully explained elsewhere.

Conversion Factors*

Conversion factors are useful mathematical tools in everyday calculations, like the ones encountered in the study of nutrition. Skill in the use of conversion factors is especially desirable as the United States and Canada "go metric."

A conversion factor is a fraction in which the numerator (top) and the denominator (bottom) express the same quantity in different units. For example, 2.2 pounds and 1 kilogram are equivalent; they express the same weight. The conversion factor used to change pounds to kilograms or vice versa is:

$$\frac{2.2 \text{ lb}}{1 \text{ kg}} \text{ or } \frac{1 \text{ kg}}{2.2 \text{ lb}}$$

Because either of these factors equals 1, a measurement can be multiplied by the factor without changing the value of the measurement. Thus its units can be changed.

The correct factor to use in a problem is the one with the unit you are seeking in the numerator (top) of the fraction.

Following are three examples of problems commonly encountered in nutrition study; they illustrate the usefulness of conversion factors.

Example 1

Convert ¼ cup to an approximate number of milliliters for use in a recipe.

1. The conversion factor is:

$$\frac{1 \text{ c}}{250 \text{ ml}} \text{ or } \frac{250 \text{ ml}}{1 \text{ c}}$$

2. Multiply ¼ cup by the factor:

$$\frac{1}{4}\,\not{c} \times \frac{250 \text{ ml}}{1\,\not{c}} = 62.5 \text{ ml, or about 60 ml.}$$

*For information on conversion factors, see inside back cover.

Example 2

Convert the weight of 130 pounds to kilograms.

1. Choose the conversion factor in which the unit you are seeking is on top:

$$\frac{1 \text{ kg}}{2.2 \text{ lb}}$$

2. Multiply 130 pounds by the factor:

$$130 \text{ lb} \times \frac{1 \text{ kg}}{2.2 \text{ lb}} = \frac{130 \text{ kg}}{2.2} = 59 \text{ kg (rounded off to nearest whole number).}$$

Example 3

How many grams of saturated fat are contained in a 4-ounce hamburger? A 3-ounce hamburger contains 8 grams of saturated fat.

1. You are seeking grams of saturated fat; therefore, the conversion factor is:

$$\frac{8 \text{ g saturated fat}}{3 \text{ oz hamburger}}$$

2. Multiply 4 ounces of hamburger by the conversion factor:

$$4 \text{ oz hamburger} \times \frac{8 \text{ g saturated fat}}{3 \text{ oz hamburger}} = \frac{4 \times 8 \text{ g}}{3}$$

$$= 11 \text{ g saturated fat (rounded off to nearest whole number).}$$

Percentages

A percentage is a comparison between a number of items (perhaps your intake of calories) and a standard number (perhaps the number of calories recommended for your age and sex—your energy RDA). The standard number is the number you divide by. The answer you get after the division must be multiplied by 100 to be stated as a percentage (*percent* means "per 100").

Example 4

What percentage of the RDA for calories is your calorie intake?

1. Find your energy RDA (inside front cover). We'll use 2,100 calories to demonstrate.
2. Total your calorie intake for a day—for example, 1,200 calories.
3. Divide your calorie intake by the RDA calories:

$$1{,}200 \text{ cal (your intake)} \div 2{,}100 \text{ cal (RDA)} = 0.571.$$

4. Multiply your answer by 100 to state it as a percentage:

$$0.571 \times 100 = 57.1 = 57\% \text{ (rounded off to the nearest whole number).}$$

In some problems in nutrition, the percentage may be more than 100. For example, suppose your daily intake of vitamin A is 3,200 RE and your RDA (male) is 1,000 RE. Your intake as a percentage of the RDA is more than 100 percent (that is, you consume more than 100 percent of your vitamin A RDA). The following calculations show your vitamin A intake as a percentage of the RDA:

$$3{,}200 \div 1{,}000 = 3.2.$$
$$3.2 \times 100 = 320\% \text{ of RDA.}$$

Sometimes the comparison is between a part of a whole (for example, your calories from protein) and the total amount (your total calories). In this case, the total number is the one you divide by.

Example 5

What percentages of your total calories for the day come from protein, fat, and carbohydrate?

1. Using Appendix F and your diet record, find the total grams of protein, fat, and carbohydrate you consumed—for example, 60 grams protein, 80 grams fat, and 285 grams carbohydrate.
2. Multiply the number of grams by the number of calories from 1 gram of each energy nutrient (conversion factors):

$$60 \text{ g protein} \times \frac{4 \text{ cal}}{1 \text{ g protein}} = 240 \text{ cal.}$$

$$80 \text{ g fat} \times \frac{9 \text{ cal}}{1 \text{ g fat}} = 720 \text{ cal.}$$

$$285 \text{ g carbohydrate} \times \frac{4 \text{ cal}}{1 \text{ g carbohydrate}} = 1{,}140 \text{ cal.}$$

$$240 + 720 + 1{,}140 = 2{,}100 \text{ cal.}$$

3. Find the percentage of total calories from each energy nutrient (see Example 4):

$$\text{Protein: } 240 \div 2{,}100 = 0.114.$$
$$0.114 \times 100 = 11.4 = 11\% \text{ of calories.}$$

$$\text{Fat: } 720 \div 2{,}100 = 0.343.$$
$$0.343 \times 100 = 34.3 = 34\% \text{ of calories.}$$

$$\text{Carbohydrate: } 1{,}140 \div 2{,}100 = 0.543.$$
$$0.543 \times 100 = 54.3 = 54\% \text{ of calories.}$$

$$11\% + 34\% + 54\% = 99\% \text{ of calories (total).}$$

The percentages total 99 percent rather than 100 percent because a little was lost from each number in rounding off. Either 99 or 101 is a reasonable total in problems like this.

Ratios

A ratio is a comparison of two or three values in which one of the values is reduced to 1. A ratio compares identical units and so is expressed without units. For example, the P:S ratio is a comparison of the grams of polyunsaturated fat to grams of saturated fat in the diet.

Example 6

Find the P:S ratio of your diet.

1. Using Appendix F and your diet record, find the grams of linoleic acid (polyunsaturated fat) and grams of saturated fat that you consume. Say they are 32 grams linoleic acid and 25 grams saturated fat.
2. Divide the larger of the amounts above by the smaller—divide linoleic acid grams by saturated fat grams:

$$\text{Linoleic acid (g)} \div \text{saturated fat (g)}.$$
$$32\text{ g} \div 25\text{ g} = 1.28$$

3. The P:S ratio is usually expressed as correct to one decimal place: 1.28 = 1.3. The P:S ratio of your diet is 1.3:1 (read as "one point three to one" or simply "one point three"), meaning that you consumed 1.3 grams of polyunsaturated fat for each gram of saturated fat.

Research is beginning to find that diets low in saturated fats and high in monounsaturated fatty acids may protect against heart disease. Consequently, the polyunsaturated to monounsaturated to saturated (P:M:S) ratio may be more meaningful than the P:S ratio.

Nutrient Units

To convert IU (International Units) found on supplement labels to the units used in the RDA tables:

Vitamin A

From animal sources:

.3 μg = 1 IU
1 RE[a] = 3.33 IU

From vegetables and fruits:

.6 μg = 1 IU
1 RE = 10 IU

Vitamin D_3

1 μg = 40 IU

Vitamin E

1 mg = 1 IU
1 α TE[b] = 1 IU

Sodium

To convert milligrams of sodium to grams of salt:

mg sodium ÷ 400 = g of salt

The reverse is also true:

g salt × 400 = mg sodium

[a]Retinol equivalents
[b]Alpha-tocopherol equivalents

APPENDIX E
Chapter References

Chapter 1 Notes

1. H. A. Guthrie, *Introductory Nutrition* (St. Louis: The C. V. Mosby Company, 1983), pp. 2–4.
2. Position of the American Dietetic Association: Identifying food and nutrition misinformation, *Journal of the American Dietetic Association* 88 (1988): 1589–1591.
3. Top 10 health frauds, *FDA Consumer* (October 1989): 29–31.
4. M. Simonton, An overview—Advances in research and treatment of obesity, *Food and Nutrition News,* March/April 1982.
5. Health food store sales, *Nutrition Forum* (May/June 1991): 22.
6. Personal communication with Lynn Dornblaser, publisher, *Gorman's New Product News,* Chicago.
7. U.S. Department of Health and Human Services, Public Health Service, *The Surgeon General's Report on Nutrition and Health: Summary and Recommendations* (Washington, D.C.: U.S. Government Printing Office, 1988), pp. 2–4.
8. N. B. Belloc and L. Breslow, Relationship of physical health status and health practices, *Preventive Medicine* 1 (1972): 409–421.
9. Committee on Diet and Health, National Research Council, *Diet and Health: Implications for Reducing Chronic Disease Risk-Executive Summary* (Washington, D.C.: National Academy Press, 1989), pp. 10–15.
10. U.S. Department of Health and Human Services, Public Health Service, *The Surgeon General's Report on Nutrition and Health: Summary and Recommendations* (Washington, D.C.: U.S. Government Printing Office, 1988), p. 6.
11. U.S. Department of Health and Human Services, Public Health Service, *Healthy People 2000: National Health Promotion and Disease Prevention Objectives* (Washington, D.C.: U.S. Government Printing Office, 1990), pp. 93–94.
12. C. Roberts, Fast-food fare: Consumer guidelines, *New England Journal of Medicine* 321 (1989): 752–756.
13. S. L. Anderson, A look at the Japanese dietary guidelines, *Journal of the American Dietetic Association* 90 (1990): 1527.
14. U.S. Department of Agriculture, Human Nutrition Information Service, *Shopping for Food and Making Meals in Minutes Using the Dietary Guidelines* (Home and Garden Bulletin No. 232-10), p. 25.
15. Remarks of R. Wyden in *Deception and Fraud in the Diet Industry—Part 1: Hearing before the House of Representatives, Subcommittee on Regulation, Business Opportunities, and Energy, Committee on Small Business* (Washington, D.C.: U.S. Government Printing Office, March 26, 1990), p. 1.
16. Personal communication with staff of *The Lempert Report,* Belleville, New Jersey.
17. Oat bran's last gasp? . . ., *The Lempert Report,* January 24, 1990, p. 1.
18. A. Miller, D. Tsiantar, K. Springen, M. Hager, and K. Robins, Oat-bran heartburn, *Newsweek,* January 29, 1990, p. 50.
19. J. Seligmann, Is it still the right thing to do?, *Newsweek,* January 29, 1990, p. 52; C. Sugarman, The rise and fallacies of oat bran, *Washington Post,* January 31, 1990, p. E1.
20. J. F. Swain, I. L. Rouse, C. B. Curley, and F. M. Sacks, Comparison of the effects of oat bran and low-fiber wheat on serum lipoprotein levels and blood pressure, *New England Journal of Medicine* 322 (1990): 147–152.
21. Statement from Dr. James Anderson, University of Kentucky, in response to *New England Journal of Medicine's* article entitled "Comparison of the Effects of Oat Bran . . .," issued January 17, 1990.
22. *FDA Consumer,* October 1989.

Chapter 2 Notes

1. Improved nutrition, *Public Health Reports Supplement,* September/October 1983, p. 132.
2. U.S. Department of Health and Human Services, Public Health Service, *Promoting Health, Preventing Disease: Objectives for the Nation* (Washington, D.C.: U.S. Government Printing Office, 1980), p. 73.
3. U.S. Senate Select Committee on Nutrition and Human Needs, *Dietary Goals for the United States,* 2d ed. (Washington, D.C.: U.S. Government Printing Office, 1977), p. 4.
4. D. R. Davis, Clayton Foundation Biochemical Institute, University of Texas, Austin, Texas, unpublished data, 1983.
5. J. D. Gussow and K. L. Clancy, Dietary guidelines for sustainability, *Journal of Nutrition Education* 18 (1986): 1–5.
6. 1990 snack sales figures from the Snack Food Association, Alexandria, Virginia.
7. American Medical Association and American Dietetic Association, *Targets for Adolescent Health: Nutrition and Physical Fitness* (Chicago: American Medical Association, 1991), p. 2.
8. U.S. Department of Agriculture, *Making Bag Lunches, Snacks, & Desserts Using the Dietary Guidelines,* USDA HNIS Home and Garden Bulletin No. 232-9 (Washington, D.C.: U.S. Government Printing Office), pp. 2–25.
9. American Heart Association, *Nutritious Nibbles* (Dallas: American Heart Association, 1984), p. 5.
10. J. C. King and coauthors, Evaluation and modification of the basic four food guide, *Journalz of Nutrition Education* 10 (1978): 27–29.

Chapter 3 Notes

1. R. Levine, Monosaccharides in health and dzisease, *Annual Reviews of Nutrition* 6 (1986): z211–224.
2. D. A. T. Southgate, The relation between composition and properties of dietary fiber and physiological effects, in *Dietary Fiber: Basic and Clinical Aspects,* eds. G. V. Vahouny and D. Kritchevsky (New York: Plenum Press, 1986), pp. 35–48.
3. Personal communication with Packaged Facts Research Company, New York, N.Y.
4. Position of the American Dietetic Association: Appropriate use of nutritive and nonnutritive sweeteners, *Journal of the American Dietetic Association* 87 (1987): 1689–1694.
5. Council on Scientific Affairs, Saccharin: Review of safety issues, *Journal of the American Medical Association* 254 (1985): 2622–2624.
6. C. Lecos, Approval of acesulfame K (Food and Drug Administration press release, July 27, 1988).
7. S. S. Schiffman, C. E. Buckley, H. A. Sampson, E. W. Massey, J. N. Baraniuk, J. V. Follett, and Z. S. Warwick, Aspartame and susceptibility to headache, *New England Journal of Medicine* 317 (1987): 1181–1185.

8. Council on Scientific Affairs, Aspartame: Review of safety issues, *Journal of the American Medical Association* 254 (1985): 400–402.
9. B. J. Rolls, Effects of intense sweeteners on hunger, food intake, and body weight: a review, *American Journal of Clinical Nutrition* 53 (1991): 872–878.
10. American Diabetes Association, Use of noncaloric sweeteners, *Diabetes Care* 10 (1987): 526.
11. P. A. Crapo and M. A. Powers, Alias sugar, *Diabetes Forecast* (March 1990): 58–65.
12. E. Danforth, Diet and obesity, *American Journal of Clinical Nutrition,* 41 (1985): 1132–1145.
13. W. J. L. Chen and W. J. Anderson, Hypocholesterolemic effects of soluble fiber, in *Dietary Fiber: Basic and Clinical Aspects,* eds. G. V. Vahouny and D. Kritchevsky (New York: Plenum Press, 1986), pp. 275–286.
14. J. W. Anderson, Dietary fiber in nutrition management of diabetes, in *Dietary Fiber: Basic and Clinical Aspects,* eds. G. V. Vahouny and D. Kritchevsky (New York: Plenum Press, 1986), pp. 343–360.
15. D. J. A. Jenkins and coauthors, Simple and complex carbohydrates, *Nutrition Reviews* 44 (1986): 44–49.
16. Hypoglycemia: Evolving concepts, *Nutrition and the MD,* November 1986.
17. L. Warschoff, *What Betty Crocker doesn't tell you about sugar!* (Baltimore: American Friends Service Committee, 1976), p. 1.
18. K. K. Carroll, Experimental evidence of dietary factors and hormone-dependent cancers, *Cancer Research* 35, no. 2 (1975): 3374–3383; B. Modan, Role of diet in cancer etiology, *Cancer* 40 (1977): 1887–1891.
19. V. T. DeVita and S. M. Hubbard, Prevention of cancer, *NCI Monographs* 2 (1986): 15–24.
20. B. S. Drasar and D. Irving, Environmental factors and cancer of the colon and breast, *British Journal of Cancer* 27 (1973): 167–172.
21. W. C. Willett and coauthors, Relation of meat, fat, and fiber intake to the risk of colon cancer in a prospective study among women, *New England Journal of Medicine* 323 (1990): 1664–1672.
22. B. S. Reddy and coauthors, Nutrition and its relationship to cancer, *Advances in Cancer Research* 32 (1980): 238–345.
23. R. L. Prentice and coauthors, Dietary fat and breast cancer: A quantitative assessment of the epidemiological literature and a discussion of methodological issues, *Cancer Research* 49 (1989): 3147–3156.
24. W. C. Willett and coauthors, Dietary fat and the risk of breast cancer, *New England Journal of Medicine* 316 (1987): 22–28.
25. K. Katsouyanni and coauthors, Diet and breast cancer: A case-control study in Greece, *International Journal of Cancer* 38 (1986): 815–820.
26. F. Lubin and coauthors, Role of fat, animal protein, and dietary fiber in breast cancer etiology: A case-control study, *Journal of the National Cancer Institute* 77 (1986): 605–612.
27. D. P. Rose, Micronutrients in carcinogenesis, in *Environmental Aspects of Cancer: The Role of Macro and Micro Components of Foods* (Westport: Food & Nutrition Press, Inc., 1983), pp. 127–156.
28. P. Knekt and coauthors, Vitamin E and cancer prevention, *American Journal of Clinical Nutrition* 53 (1991, Suppl): 283S–286S.
29. E. L. Wynder, Dietary habits and cancer epidemiology, *Cancer* 43 (1979): 1955–1961, as cited by S. H. Brammer and R. L. DeFelice, Dietary advice in regard to risk for colon and breast cancer, *Preventive Medicine* 9 (1980): 544–549.
30. Reddy and coauthors, 1980.
31. J. L. Werther, Food and cancer, *New York State Journal of Medicine,* August 1980, pp. 1401–1408.
32. Werther, 1980.
33. L. W. Wattenberg and coauthors, Dietary constituents altering the responses to chemical carcinogens, *Federation Proceedings* 35 (1976): 1327–1331; L. W. Wattenberg and W. D. Loub, Inhibition of polycyclic aromatic hydrocarbon-induced neoplasia by naturally occurring indoles, *Cancer Research* 38 (1978): 1410–1413.
34. R. R. Butrum and coauthors, NCI dietary guidelines: Rationale, *American Journal of Clinical Nutrition* 48 (1988): 888–895.
35. J. M. Coon, Natural food toxicants: A perspective, in *Nutrition Reviews' Present Knowledge in Nutrition,* 4th ed. (Washington, D.C.: Nutrition Foundation, 1976), pp. 528–546.

Chapter 4 Notes

1. The following discussion is adapted from E. M. N. Hamilton, E. N. Whitney, and F. S. Sizer, *Nutrition: Concepts and Controversies,* 4th ed. (St. Paul, Minn.: West, 1988), pp. 111–113, and P. A. Anderson and H. W. Sprecher, Omega-3 fatty acids in nutrition and health, *Dietetic Currents* 14 (1987).
2. Lipid Research Clinics Program, The Lipid Research Clinics coronary primary prevention trial results: II. The relationship of reduction in incidence of coronary heart disease to cholesterol lowering, *Journal of the American Medical Association,* 251 (1984): 365–374.
3. D. Kromhout, E. B. Bosschieter, and C. D. Coulander, The inverse relation between fish consumption and 20-year mortality from coronary heart disease, *New England Journal of Medicine* 312 (1985): 1205–1209.
4. A. M. Fehily and coauthors, The effect of fatty fish on plasma lipid and lipoprotein concentrations, *American Journal of Clinical Nutrition* 38 (1983): 349–351; W. S. Harris and coauthors, in *Nutrition and Heart Disease* (London: Churchill Livingstone, 1983), as cited in Fish oils, serum lipids and platelet aggregation, *Nutrition and the MD,* January 1985.
5. E. M. Berry and J. Hirsch, Does dietary linolenic acid influence blood pressure? *American Journal of Clinical Nutrition* 44 (1986): 336–340.
6. Fehily and coauthors, 1983.
7. Personal communication with Lynn Dornblaser, publisher, *Gorman's New Product News,* Chicago.
8. Personal communication with Consumer Affairs, Entenmann's, Bay Shore, N.Y.
9. Personal communication with Media Relations, McDonald's Corporation, Oak Brook, IL.
10. Personal communication with Consumer Affairs, Kraft, Glenview, IL.
11. G. E. Ruoff, Reducing fat intake with fat substitutes, *American Family Physician* 43 (April 1991): 1235–1242.
12. *Simplesse All Natural Fat Substitute: A Scientific Overview* (Deerfield, IL: The Simplesse Company, 1991), pp. 3–10.
13. C. A. Bernhardt, Olestra—a non-caloric fat replacement, *Food Technology International—Europe* (1988).
14. J. L. Wood and R. G. Allison, Effects of consumption of choline and lecithin on neurological and cardiovascular systems, *Federation Proceedings* 41 (1982): 3015–3021; Choline and lecithin in the treatment of neurologic disorders, *Nutrition and the MD,* April 1980.
15. O. H. Ford, S. F. Knutsen, and E. Arnesen, The Tromso heart study: Coffee consumption and serum lipid concentrations in men with hypercholesterolaemia: A randomised intervention study, *British Medical Journal* 290 (1985): 893–895.
16. Data from S. M. Grundy, Cholesterol and coronary heart disease, *Journal of the American Medical Association* 256 (1986): 2849–2858.
17. Consensus conference: Lowering blood cholesterol to prevent heart disease, *Journal*

of the American Medical Association 253 (1985): 2080–2086.
18. Dozens of research articles now support this finding. A typical one: J. G. Brook and coauthors, High-density lipoprotein subfractions in normolipemic patients with coronary atherosclerosis, *Circulation* 66 (1982): 923–926.
19. R. Goor and coauthors, Nutrient intakes among selected North American populations in the Lipid Research Clinics Prevalence Study: Composition of fat intake, *American Journal of Clinical Nutrition* 41 (1985): 299–311.
20. Is it the olive oil? Cardiovascular benefits of the 'Mediterranean diet,' *Nutrition and the MD,* September, 1987, p. 4.
21. F. H. Mattson, A changing role for dietary monounsaturated fatty acids, *Journal of the American Dietetic Association,* 89 (1989): 387–391.
22. Lipid Research Clinics Program, The Lipid Research Clinics Coronary Primary Prevention Trial results: I. Reduction in incidence of coronary heart disease, *Journal of the American Medical Association,* 251 (1984): 351–364.
23. National Cholesterol Education Program, *Report of the Expert Panel on Population Strategies for Blood Cholesterol Reduction* (Bethesda: National Institutes of Health, 1990), pp. 1–13.
24. A. M. Stephen and N. J. Wald, Trends in individual consumption of dietary fat in the United States, 1920–1984, *American Journal of Clinical Nutrition* 52 (1990): 457–469.
25. P. A. Judd and A. S. Truswell, The effect of rolled oats on blood lipids and fecal steroid excretion in man, *American Journal of Clinical Nutrition* 34 (1981): 2061–2067; R. W. Kirby and coauthors, Oat-bran intake selectively lowers serum low-density lipoprotein cholesterol concentrations of hypercholesterolemic men, *American Journal of Clinical Nutrition* 34 (1981): 824–829; J. W. Anderson and coauthors, Cholesterol-lowering effects of psyllium hydrophilic mucilloid for hypercholesterolemic men, *Archives of Internal Medicine* 148 (1988): 292–296.
26. T. O. Von Lossonczy and coauthors, The effect of a fish diet on lipids in healthy human subjects, *American Journal of Clinical Nutrition* 31 (1978): 1340–1346.
27. J. W. Anderson and W. L. Chen, Plant fiber: Carbohydrate and lipid metabolism, *American Journal of Clinical Nutrition* 32 (1979): 346–363; Dietary fiber, exercise and selected blood lipid constituents, *Nutrition Reviews* 38 (1980): 207–209.
28. J. L. Marx, The HDL: The good cholesterol carriers? (Research News), *Science* 205 (1979): 677–679.
29. P. D. Wood and coauthors, The distribution of plasma lipoproteins in middle-aged male runners, *Metabolism* 25 (1976): 1249–1257; R. H. Dressendorfer and coauthors, High-density lipoprotein-cholesterol in marathon runners during a 20-day road race, *Journal of the American Medical Association* 247 (1982): 1715–1717.
30. T. R. Thomas, Effects of interval and continuous running on HDL-cholesterol, apoproteins A-1 and B, and LCAT, *Canadian Journal of Applied Sports Sciences* 10 (1985): 52–59; A. Weltman, S. Matter, and B. A. Stamford, Caloric restriction and/or mild exercise: Effects on serum lipids and body composition, *American Journal of Clinical Nutrition* 33 (1980): 1002–1009; J. A. Cauley, R. E. LaPorte, L. H. Kuller, and R. Black-Sandler, The epidemiology of high density lipoprotein cholesterol levels in post-menopausal women, *Journal of Gerontology* 37 (1982): 10–15.
31. Recommendations based on data in Tables H4B-3 and H4B-4 in E. N. Whitney, E. M. N. Hamilton, and M. A. Boyle, *Understanding Nutrition,* 4th ed. (St. Paul, Minn.: West, 1987), pp. 129–130.
32. Try a little TLC, *Science 80,* January/February 1980, p. 15.
33. National Institutes of Health, National Heart, Lung, and Blood Institute Press Release, *New Recommendations on Cholesterol and Children Released,* April 8, 1991, pp. 1–5.

Chapter 5 Notes

1. S. A. Laidlaw, Indispensable amino acids, *Nutrition and the M.D.,* August 1986, pp. 1–3; K. C. Hayes, Taurine requirements in primates, *Nutrition Reviews* 43 (1985): 65–70.
2. W. J. Visek, Arginine needs, physiological state and usual diets: A reevaluation, *Journal of Nutrition* 116 (1986): 36–46.
3. A. A. Albanese and L. A. Orto, The proteins and amino acids, in *Modern Nutrition in Health and Disease,* 5th ed., R. S. Goodhart and M. E. Shils, eds. (Philadelphia: Lea and Febiger, 1973), p. 59.
4. World Health Organization Technical Report No. 724, as cited in Energy and protein requirements, *Cereal Foods World* 31 (1986): 694–695.
5. Albanese and Orto, 1973, pp. 28–88; L. E. Holt, Jr., Protein economy in the growing child, *Postgraduate Medicine* 27 (1960): 783–798; Infections and undernutrition, *Nutrition Reviews* 40 (1982): 119–128.
6. J. Klug, Overeating possible cause of renal disease, *Internal Medicine News,* December 1–14, 1982, pp. 1, 30–31.
7. A. R. Sherman, L. Helyar, and I. Wolinsky, Effects of dietary protein concentration on trace minerals in rat tissues at different ages, *Journal of Nutrition* 115 (1985): 607–614.
8. H. H. Sandstead, Zinc: Essentiality for brain development and function, *Nutrition Today,* November/December 1984, pp. 26–30; B. Worthington-Roberts, Nutrition and maternal health, *Nutrition Today,* November-/December 1984, pp. 6–19; D. Rush, Z. Stein, and M. Susser in *Diet in Pregnancy: A Randomized Controlled Trial of Prenatal Nutritional Supplementation* (New York: Alan Liss, 1979).
9. E. Pollitt and N. Lewis, Nutritional and educational achievement, *Food and Nutrition Bulletin* 2 (1980): 33–37.
10. Dietary protein and body fat distribution, *Nutrition Reviews* 40 (1982): 89–90.
11. Urinary calcium increases with high protein intakes, perhaps because the protein makes the urine more acid than usual. A. A. Licata, Acute effects of increased meat protein on urinary electrolytes and cyclic adenosine monophosphate and serum parathyroid hormone, *American Journal of Clinical Nutrition* 34 (1981): 1779–1784; High protein diets and bone homeostasis, *Nutrition Reviews* 39 (1981): 11–13.
12. Personal communication with Gerald Gleich, M.D., Department of Immunology, Mayo Clinic, Rochester, MN.
13. W. J. Darby, The ban on tryptophan supplements, *Nutrition Today,* May/June 1990, p. 5.
14. E. A. Belongia and coauthors, An investigation of the cause of the eosinophilia-myalgia syndrome associated with tryptophan use, *New England Journal of Medicine* 323 (1990): 357–365.
15. C. Ballentine, The essential guide to amino acids, *FDA Consumer,* September 1985, pp. 23–25.
16. C. Ballentine, 1985.
17. P. J. Rasch, J. W. Hamby, and H. J. Burns, Protein dietary supplementation and physical performance, *Medicine and Science in Sports* 1 (1969): 195–199.
18. N. J. Smith and B. Worthington-Roberts, *Food for Sport* (Palo Alto, CA: Bull Publishing Company, 1989), p. 21.
19. R. M. Marston and B. B. Peterkin, Nutrient content of the national food supply, *National Food Review,* Winter 1980, pp. 21–25.
20. Position of the American Dietetic Association: Vegetarian Diets, *Journal of the Amer-*

ican Dietetic Association, 88 (1988): 351–355. 1988.

Chapter 6 Notes

1. J. Jaramillo-Arango, The conquest of nutritional diseases (vitamins), in *The British Contribution to Medicine* (Edinburgh: E. & S. Livingstone, Ltd., 1953), pp. 140–162.
2. R. Hill and coauthors, The discovery of vitamins, in *The Chemistry of Life* (Cambridge: Cambridge University Press, 1970), pp. 156–170.
3. K. Y. Guggenheim, Pellagra, in *Nutrition and Nutritional Diseases—The Evolution of Concepts* (Lexington: Collamore Press, 1981), pp. 245–264.
4. D. Lonsdale and R. J. Shamberger, Red cell transketolase as an indicator of nutritional deficiency, *American Journal of Clinical Nutrition* 33 (1980): 205–211.
5. L. C. Pauling, *Vitamin C and the Common Cold* (San Francisco: W. H. Freeman, 1970.)
6. H. Schaumberg and coauthors, Sensory neuropathy from pyridoxine abuse, *New England Journal of Medicine* 309 (1983): 445–448.
7. M. K. Berman and coauthors, Vitamin B-6 in premenstrual syndrome, *Journal of the American Dietetic Association* 90 (1990): 859–860.
8. More B_6 toxicity reported, *Nutrition Forum,* November 1985, p. 84.
9. C. J. Schorah, G. M. Sobala, M. Sanderson, N. Collis, and J. N. Primrose, Gastric juice ascorbic acid: Effects of disease and implications for gastric carcinogenesis, *American Journal of Clinical Nutrition* 53 (Suppl) (1991): 287S–293S. J. H. Weisburger, Nutritional approach to cancer prevention with emphasis on vitamins, antioxidants, and carotenoids, *American Journal of Clinical Nutrition* 53 (Suppl) (1991): 226S–237S.
10. B. S. N. Rao and C. Gopalan, *Present Knowledge in Nutrition* (Washington D.C.: The Nutrition Foundation, 1984), pp. 318–331.
11. S. H. Zeisel, K-A Da Costa, P. D. Franklin, E. A. Alexander, J. T. Lamont, N. F. Shread and A. Beiser, Choline, an essential nutrient for humans, *FASEB Journal* 5 (1991): 2093–2098.
12. J. L. Greger, Food, supplements, and fortified foods: Scientific evaluations in regard to toxicology and nutrient bioavailability, *Journal of the American Dietetic Association* 87 (1987): 1369–1373.
13. D. Walker and R. E. Beauchene, The relationship of loneliness, social isolation, and physical health to dietary adequacy of independently living elderly, *Journal of the American Dietetic Association* 91 (1991): 300–304.
14. J. E. Morley and coauthors, Nutrition in the elderly, *Annals of Internal Medicine* 109 (1988): 890–904.
15. D. M. Hegsted, Recommended dietary intakes of elderly subjects, *American Journal of Clinical Nutrition* 50 (1989): 1190–1194.
16. S. C. DeSouza and R. R. Eitenmiller, Effects of processing and storage on the folate content of spinach and broccoli, *Journal of Food Science* 51 (1986): 626–628.

Chapter 7 Notes

1. C. M. McCay, Anorganic substances, in *Notes on the History of Nutrition Research,* ed. F. Verzar (Vienna: Hans Huber Publishers, 1973), pp. 156–184.
2. L. H. Allen, Calcium bioavailability and absorption: A review, *American Journal of Clinical Nutrition* 35 (1982): 783–808.
3. Parts of the following discussion are adapted from E. N. Whitney, E.M.N. Hamilton, and M. A. Boyle, *Understanding Nutrition,* 4th ed. (St. Paul: West, 1987), pp. 391–398.
4. N. W. Solomons, An update on lactose intolerance, *Nutrition News,* February 1986.
5. R. R. Recker, Calcium absorption and achlorhydria, *New England Journal of Medicine* 313 (1985): 70–73.
6. L. D. McBean, Food versus pills versus fortified foods, *Dairy Council Digest* 58, March–April 1987; J. Mayer and J. Goldberg, Sufficient calcium intake still a major problem, *Tallahassee Democrat,* 5 November 1987.
7. Dietary potassium and hypertension, *Lancet,* 8 June 1985, pp. 1308–1309.
8. A. W. Voors and coauthors, Relation between ingested potassium and sodium balance in young Blacks and whites, *American Journal of Clinical Nutrition* 37 (1983): 583–594.
9. O. Ophir and coauthors, Low blood pressure in vegetarians: The possible role of potassium, *American Journal of Clinical Nutrition* 37 (1983): 755–762.
10. P. G. Lindner, Caution: All potassium supplements are not the same! *Obesity and Bariatric Medicine* 10 (1981): 87, 89, 92.
11. American Heart Association, *Salt, Sodium and Blood Pressure* (Dallas: American Heart Association, 1988).
12. D. Riccardella and J. Dwyer, Salt substitutes and medicinal potassium sources: Risks and benefits, *Journal of the American Dietetic Association* 85 (1985): 471–474.
13. N. M. Kaplan, Non-drug treatment of hypertension, *Annals of Internal Medicine* 102 (1985): 361.
14. National Heart, Lung, and Blood Institute, National Institutes of Health, *Nonpharmacologic Approaches to the Control of High Blood Pressure* (Bethesda, Md.: National Institutes of Health, 1984), p. 3.
15. National Heart, Lung, and Blood Institute, National Institutes of Health, *Nonpharmacologic Approaches to the Control of High Blood Pressure* (Bethesda, Md.: National Institutes of Health, 1984), p. 10.
16. 1988 Joint National Committee, The 1988 Report of the Joint National Committee on Detection, Evaluation, and Treatment of High Blood Pressure, *Archives of Internal Medicine* 148 (1988): 1023–1038.
17. National Research Council, *Diet and Health: Implications for Reducing Chronic Disease Risk—Executive Summary* (Washington, D.C.: National Academy Press, 1989), pp. 14–15.
18. R. Stamler and coauthors, Primary prevention of hypertension by nutritional-hygienic means, *Journal of the American Medical Association* 262 (1989): 1801–1807.
19. N. M. Kaplan, Non-drug treatment of hypertension, *Annals of Internal Medicine* 102 (1985): 363.
20. K. Clark, Calcium and hypertension: Does a relationship exist?, *Nutrition Today* July/August 1989, pp. 21–26.
21. F. C. Luft, Dietary sodium, potassium and chloride intake and arterial hypertension, *Nutrition Today,* May/June 1989, pp. 11–12.
22. 1988 Joint National Committee, 1988.
23. M. Moser, *High Blood Pressure & What You Can Do About It* (Elmsford, N.Y.: The Benjamin Company, 1989), pp. 4–7.
24. N. S. Scrimshaw, Functional consequences of iron deficiency in human populations, *Journal of Nutrition Science and Vitaminology* 30 (1984): 47–63.
25. E. R. Monsen and coauthors, Estimation of available dietary iron, *American Journal of Clinical Nutrition* 31 (1978): 134–141.
26. K. M. Hambidge and coauthors, Low levels of zinc in hair, anorexia, poor growth, and hypogeusia in children, *Pediatric Reserach* 6 (1972): 868–74.
27. M. A. Brown and coauthors, Food poisoning involving zinc contamination, *Archives of Environmental Health* 8 (1964): 657–60; Questions doctors ask, *Nutrition and the MD,* October 1978.
28. F. Taylor, Iodine—Going from hypo to hyper, *FDA Consumer,* April 1981, pp. 15–18.
29. H. A. Guthrie, *Introductory Nutrition* (St. Louis: C. V. Mosby, 1983), p. 214.
30. National Research Council, *Recommended Dietary Allowances—10th Edition* (Washington, D.C.: National Academy Press, 1989), pp. 248–249.
31. U.S. Environmental Protection Agency, Office of Water, *Is Your Drinking Water Safe?* (U.S. Environmental Protection Agency, 1989).

32. U.S. Environmental Protection Agency, Office of Water, *Lead and Your Drinking Water* (Washington, D.C.: U.S. Environmental Protection Agency, 1987).
33. Position of the American Dietetic Association: The impact of fluoride on dental health, *The Journal of the American Dietetic Association* 89 (1989): 971–974.
34. U.S. Department of Health and Human Services, Public Health Service, *The Surgeon General's Report on Nutrition and Health: Summary and Recommendations* (Washington, D.C.: U.S. Government Printing Office, DHHS (PHS) Publication No. 88-50211, 1988), p. 51.
35. American Council on Science and Health, *Fluoridation* (New York: American Council on Science and Health, 1990), p. 8.
36. U.S. General Accounting Office, *Food Safety and Quality: Stronger FDA Standards and Oversight Needed for Bottled Water* (Washington, D.C.: U.S. General Accounting Office, 1991), pp. 2–3.
37. U.S. General Accounting Office, *Food Safety and Quality: Stronger FDA Standards and Oversight Needed for Bottled Water* (Washington, D.C.: U.S. General Accounting Office, 1991), p. 17.
38. J. Stannard and coauthors, Fluoride content of some bottled waters and recommendations for fluoride supplementation, *The Journal of Pedodontics* 14 (1990): 103–107.
39. The International Bottled Water Association, *20 Questions About the Bottled Water Industry,* 1990.

Chapter 8 Notes

1. Parts of the following discussion are adapted from E. N. Whitney, E.M.N. Hamilton, and M. A. Boyle, *Understanding Nutrition,* 4th ed. (St. Paul: West, 1987), chap. 8.
2. M. Simonton, An overview—Advances in research and treatment of obesity, *Food and Nutrition News,* March/April 1982.
3. Consensus panel addresses obesity question, *Journal of the American Medical Association* 254 (1985): 1878.
4. S. Escott-Stump, *Nutrition and Diagnosis-Related Care* (Philadelphia: Lea & Febiger, 1988), p. 19.
5. L. Lapidus and coauthors, Distribution of adipose tissue and risk of cardiovascular disease and death: A twelve year follow-up of participants in the population study of women in Gothenburg, Sweden, *British Medical Journal* 289 (1984): 1257–1261.
6. M. Ashwell, T. J. Cole, and A. K. Dixon, Obesity: New insight into the anthropometric classification of fat distribution showed by computed tomography, *British Medical Journal* 290 (1985): 1692–1694.
7. Consensus panel, 1985.
8. T. B. Van Itallie and R. G. Campbell, Multidisciplinary approach to the problem of obesity, *Journal of the American Dietetic Association* 61 (1972): 385–390.
9. A. J. Stunkard, T. T. Foch, and Z. Hrubec, A twin study of human obesity, *Journal of the American Medical Association,* 256 (1986): 51–54; A. J. Stunkard and coauthors, An adoption study of human obesity, *New England Journal of Medicine* 314 (1986): 193–198. A. J. Stunkard and coauthors, The body-mass index of twins who have been reared apart, *New England Jounal of Medicine,* 322 (1990): 1483–1487.
10. S. M. Garn, Effect of parental fitness levels on the fitness of biological and adoptive children, *Ecology of Food and Nutrition* 6 (1977). 91–93.
11. C. Bouchard and coauthors, The response to long-term overfeeding in identical twins, *New England Journal of Medicine,* 322 (1990): 1477–1482.
12. T. B. Van Itallie, Obesity, the American disease, *Food Technology,* December 1979, pp. 43–47.
13. H. Bruch, Role of the emotions in hunger and appetite, *Annals of the New York Academy of Sciences* 63, part 1 (1955): 68–75.
14. J. Slochower and S. P. Kaplan, Anxiety, perceived control, and eating in obese and normal weight persons, *Appetite* 1 (1980): 75–83.
15. W. H. Griffith, Food as a regulator of metabolism, *American Journal of Clinical Nutrition* 17 (1965): 391–398.
16. J. Yudkin, Prevention of obesity, *Royal Society of Health Journal* 81 (1952): 221–224.
17. A. Tremblay and coauthors, Impact of dietary fat content and fat oxidation on energy intake in humans, *American Journal of Clinical Nutrition* 49 (1989): 799–805.
18. I. Romieu, Energy intake and other determinants of relative weight, *American Journal of Clinical Nutrition* 47 (1988): 406–412.
19. T. B. Van Itallie and M. U. Yang, Current concepts in nutrition and diet and weight loss, *New England Journal of Medicine* 297 (1977): 1158–1161; Evaluation of 3 weight-reducing diets, *Nutrition and the MD,* March 1978. An experiment in which fasting caused increased weight loss but decreased fat loss compared with a low-calorie mixed diet was reported in M. F. Ball, J. J. Canary, and L. H. Kyle, Comparative effects of caloric restriction and total starvation on body composition in obesity, *Annals of Internal Medicine* 67 (1967): 60–67.
20. J. Beedoe and coauthors, A review of low-calorie and very-low-calorie diet plans and possible metabolic consequences, *Topics in Clinical Nutrition* 6(1) (1990): 68–83; R. L. Atkinson, Very low calorie diets: getting sick or remaining healthy on a handful of calories, *Journal of Nutrition* 116 (1986): 18–21.
21. J. Stevens and coauthors, Effect of psyllium gum and wheat bran on spontaneous energy intake, *American Journal of Clinical Nutrition* 46 (1987): 812–817.
22. J. M. Davies and L. Strunin, Anesthesia in 1984: How safe is it? *Canadian Medical Association Journal* 131 (1984): 437–441.
23. The American Dietetic Association's nutrition recommendations for women, *Journal of the American Dietetic Association* 86 (1986): 1663–1664.
24. T. A. Wadden and coauthors, Long-term effects of dieting on resting metabolic rate in obese outpatients, *Journal of the American Medical Association* 264 (1990): 707–711.
25. K. Brownell, Yo-yo dieting, in C. C. Cook-Fuller (ed.) with S. Barrett, *Nutrition 91/92* (Guilford, CT: The Dushkin Publishing Group, 1991), pp. 132–134.
26. J. Rodin and coauthors, Weight cycling and fat distribution, *International Journal of Obesity* 14 (1990): 303–310.
27. Personal conversation with Vivian Meehan, President of National Association of Anorexia Nervosa and Associated Disorders, June 9, 1991.
28. H. Bruch, Anorexia nervosa, *Nutrition Today,* September/October 1978, pp. 14–18.
29. D. Williamson, *Assessment of Eating Disorders: Obesity, Anorexia, and Bulimia Nervosa* (New York: Pergamon Press, 1990).

Chapter 9 Notes

1. R. DeLorme and F. Stransky, *Fitness and Fallacies* (Kendal/Hunt, 1990), p. 1.
2. Part of the following discussion is adapted from F. S. Sizer and E. N. Whitney, *Life Choices: Health Concepts and Strategies* (St. Paul: West, 1988), Chapter 7.
3. S. Rainville and P. Vaccaro, Lipoprotein cholesterol levels, coronary artery disease and regular exercise: A review. *American Corrective Therapy Journal* 37 (1983): 161–165; B. Stamford, Improving coronary circulation, *The Physician and Sportsmedicine* 11 (1983): 163.
4. R. S. Paffenbarger and coauthors, Physical activity, all-cause mortality and longevity of college alumni, *New England Journal of Medicine* 314 (1986): 605–613.
5. The idea of positive addiction and this list of prerequisites for it originate with the psy-

chologist W. Glasser, *Positive Addiction* (New York: Harper & Row, 1976), p. 93.

6. DeLorme and Stransky, 1990; F. Katch and W. McArdle, *Nutrition, Weight Control, and Exercise* (Philadelphia: Lea and Febriger, 1988), p. 203.

7. American College of Sports Medicine, Position Paper: The Recommended Quantity and Quality of Exercise for Developing and Maintaining Cardiorespiratory and Muscular Fitness in Healthy Adults, *Medicine and Science in Sports and Exercise, 22 (1990): 265.*

8. American College of Sports Medicine, *Guidelines for Exercise Testing and Prescription (4th edition)* (Philadelphia: Lea and Febiger, 1991), Chapter 3.

9. PAR-Q Validation Report, British Columbia Department of Health, June 1975 (modified version). From American College of Sports Medicine, *Guidelines for Exercise Testing and Prescription (4th edition)* (Philadelphia: Lea and Febiger, 1991), Chapter 3.

10. Katch and McArdle, 1988, p. 59.

11. Katch and McArdle, 1988, p. 45.

12. E. Jequier, Carbohydrate: Energetics and performance, *Nutrition Reviews* 44 (1986): 55–59.

13. R. C. Hickson, Carbohydrate metabolism in exercise, in *Report of the Ross Symposium on Nutrient Utilization During Exercise* (Columbus, Ohio: Ross Laboratories, 1983), pp. 1–8.

14. S. Blair, *Living with Exercise* (American Health, 1991), p. 85; DeLorme and Stransky, 1990.

15. D. C. Nieman, *Fitness and Sports Medicine: An Introduction* (Palo Alto, Calif.: Bull, 1990), pp. 246–248.

16. P.W.R. Lemon, The importance of protein for athletes, *Sports Med* 1 (1984): 474–488.

17. S. Short and W. R. Short, Four-year study of university athletes' dietary intake, *Journal of the American Dietetic Association* 82 (1983): 632–645.

18. Katch and McArdle, 1988, pp. 115–136.

19. American College of Sports Medicine, 1990.

20. L. Hermansen, Post exercise elevation of resting oxygen uptake: Possible mechanisms and physiological significance, in *Physiological Chemistry of Training* (Macronnet and Poortmans, Eds.) (Basel, Karger, 1984); B. A. Brehm and B. Gutin, Recovery energy expenditure for steady state exercise in runners and nonexercisers, *Medicine and Science in Sports and Exercise* 18 (1986): 205–210; Nieman, 1990: 317–354.

21. K. B. Wheeler and A. M. Cameron, Plasma Volume: The hidden key to performance, *American Fitness Quarterly* (April 1990), pp. 24–26.

22. Wheeler and Cameron, 1990.

23. *Fluid Replacement in Athletics: Fluid and Energy Requirements during and after Exercise* (Columbus, Ohio: Ross Laboratories, 1986), pp. 2–27.

24. Wheeler and Cameron, 1990.

25. Wheeler and Cameron, 1990; R. S. Seiple, V. M. Vivian, and coauthors, Gastric emptying characteristics of two glucose polymers-electrolyte solutions, in *Report of the Ross Symposium on Nutrient Utilization during Exercise* (Columbus, Ohio: Ross Laboratories, 1983), pp. 85–87; W. A. Norris, A. D. Kanonchoff, and coauthors, Metabolic response to an experimental hydration solution in long-term exercise, in *Report of the Ross Symposium on Nutrient Utilization during Exercise* (Columbus, Ohio: Ross Laboratories, 1983), pp. 87–91.

26. Nieman, 1990; Katch and McArdle, 1988.

27. S. M. Blum, A. R. Sherman, and R. A. Boileau, The effects of fitness-type exertion on iron status in adult women, *American Journal of Clinical Nutrition* 43 (1986): 456–463.

28. Nutrition and physical performance, in Nieman, 1990, pp. 221–268.

29. "Anaemia" in athletes, *Lancet,* 29 June 1985, pp. 1491–1492.

30. M. E. Nelson and coauthors, Diet and bone status in amenorrheic runners, *American Journal of Clinical Nutrition* 43 (1986): 910–916.

31. Nelson and coauthors, 1986.

32. Osteoporosis Consensus Conference, *Journal of the American Medical Association* 252 (1984): 799–802.

33. P. Astrand, Something old and something new—very new, *Nutrition Today* June 1968, pp. 9–11.

34. H. C. McGill and G. E. Mott, Diet and coronary heart disease, in *Nutrition Reviews' Present Knowledge in Nutrition, (4th edition)* (New York: The Nutrition Foundation, Inc., 1976), pp. 376–391.

35. J. D. Cantwell, Questions and answers: Carbohydrate loading, *Journal of the American Medical Association* 256 (1986): 3024.

36. G. R. Hagerman, Nutrition in part-time athletes, *Nutrition and the MD,* August 1981.

37. K. Keller and R. Schwarzkopf, Preexercise snacks may decrease exercise performance, *The Physician and Sportsmedicine* 11 (1984): 89–91.

38. S. C. Costill and D. L. Maxwell, Impact of carbohydrate source and osmolality on gastric emptying rates of liquid nutritionals, abstracted, *Journal of Enteral and Parenteral Nutrition* 3 (1979): 32; J. T. Snook, V. M. Vivian, and A. L. Hecker, Stool characteristics resulting from defined formula diets, abstracted, *Journal of Enteral and Parenteral Nutrition* 5 (1981): 570.

39. T. H. Murray, The ethics of drugs in sports, in *Drugs & Performance in Sports,* R. H. Strauss (Ed.) (Philadelphia: W. B. Saunders Company, 1987), p. 11.

40. Position of the American Dietetic Association: Nutrition for physical fitness and athletic performance for adults, *Journal of the American Dietetic Association* 87 (1987): 933–939.

41. G. Mirkin, Can bee pollen benefit health?, *Journal of the American Medical Association* 262 (1989): 1854.

42. T. Larkin, Bee pollen as a health food, *FDA Consumer* (April 1984): 21–22.

43. A. Z. Belko, Vitamins and exercise—An update, *Medicine and Science in Sports and Exercise* 19 (1987): S191–S196; E. J. Vander Beek, Vitamins and endurance training: Food for running or faddish claims? *Sports Med* 2 (1985): 175–197; Nutrition and physical performance, in Nieman, 1990, pp. 221–268.

44. D. C. Nieman, *Fitness and Sports Medicine: An Introduction* (Palo Alto, Calif.: Bull, 1990), pp. 243–256.

45. American College of Sports Medicine, 1990.

46. D. C. Nieman, 1990.

47. Food and Drug Administration, *Anabolic Steroids: Losing at Winning,* DHHS Publication No. (FDA) 88-3171.

48. W. H. Griffith, Food as a regulator of metabolism, *American Journal of Clinical Nutrition* 17 (1965): 391–398.

49. A. S. Levine and J. E. Morley, Stress-induced eating, in *Food in Contemporary Society,* symposium sponsored by Stokely-Van Camp at the University of Tennessee, Knoxville, May 27–29, 1981, pp. 126–135; J Slochower and S. P. Kaplan, Anxiety, perceived control, and eating in obese and normal weight persons, *Appetite* 1 (1980): 75–83.

Chapter 10 Notes

1. N. B. Belloc and L. Breslow, Relationship of physical health status and health practices, *Preventive Medicine* 1 (1972): 409–421.

2. E. Hackman and coauthors, Maternal birth weight and subsequent pregnancy outcome, *Journal of the American Medical Association* 250 (1983): 2016–2019.

3. N. M. Lien, K. K. Meyer, and M. Winick, Early malnutrition and "late" adoption: A study of the effects on the development of Korean orphans adopted into American families, *American Journal of Clinical Nutrition* 30 (1977): 1734–1739.

4. R. Kumar, W. R. Cohen, and F. H. Epstein, Vitamin D and calcium hormones in pregnancy, *New England Journal of Medicine* 302 (1980): 1143–1145.

5. F. B. Glenn, W. D. Glenn, and R. C. Duncan, Fluoride tablet supplementation during pregnancy for caries immunity—A study of the offspring produced, *American Journal of Obstetrics and Gynecology* 143 (1982): 560–564.

6. C. W. Suitor, Perspectives on *Nutrition During Pregnancy: Part I, Weight Gain; Part II, Nutrient Supplements, Journal of the American Dietetic Association* 91 (1991): 96–98; Institute of Medicine, National Academy of Sciences, *Nutrition During Pregnancy* (Washington, D.C.: National Academy Press, 1990), p. 20.

7. K. K. Sulik, M. C. Johnston, and M. A. Webb, Fetal alcohol syndrome: Embryogenesis in a mouse model, *Science* 214 (1981): 936–938.

8. Even moderate drinking may be hazardous to maturing fetus (medical news), *Journal of the American Medical Association* 237 (1977): 2535.

9. M. H. Kaufman, Ethanol-induced chromosomal abnormalities at conception, *Nature* 302 (1983): 258–260.

10. *Nutrition Today* letter, April 8, 1981.

11. H. L. Rosett, L. Weiner, and K. C. Edelin, Treatment experience with pregnant problem drinkers, *Journal of the American Medical Association* 249 (1983): 2029–2033.

12. B. J. Myers, Mother-infant bonding: Rejoinder to Kennell and Klaus, *Developmental Review* 4 (1984): 283–288.

13. K. M. Shahani, A. J. Kwan, and B. A. Friend, Role and significance of enzymes in human milk, *American Journal of Clinical Nutrition* 33 (1980): 1861–1868; Thyroid hormones in human milk, *Nutrition Reviews* 37 (1979): 140–141; Prostaglandins in human milk, *Nutrition Reviews* 39 (1981): 302–303; J. J. Kabara, Lipids as host-resistance factors of human milk, *Nutrition Reviews* 38 (1980): 65–73. E. Hazum and coauthors, Morphine in cow and human milk: Could dietary morphine constitute a ligand for specific morphine (mu) receptors? *Science* 213 (1981): 1010–1012.

14. American Academy of Pediatrics, Committee on Nutrition, The use of whole cow's milk in infancy, *Pediatrics* 72 (1983): 253–255.

15. L. L. Clark and V. A. Beal, Age at introduction of solid foods to infants in Manitoba, *Journal of the Canadian Dietetic Association* 42 (1981): 72–78.

16. E. M. Widdowson, Mental contentment and physical growth, *Lancet* 1 (1951): 1316–1318.

17. J. Cravioto, Nutrition, stimulation, mental development and learning, *Nutrition Today* (September/October 1981): 4–8, 10–15.

18. H. R. Armstrong and D. B. Root, Managing a lean NET program, *Community Nutritionist* 2 (1983): 8–10.

19. J. H. Shaw, Causes and control of dental caries, *New England Journal of Medicine* 317 (1987): 996–1004.

20. B. G. Bibby, S. A. Mundorff, D. T. Zero, and K. J. Almekinder, Oral food clearance and the pH of plaque and saliva, *Journal of the American Dental Association* 112 (1986): 333–337.

21. M. E. Jensen, Responses of interproximal plaque pH to snack foods and effect of chewing sorbitol-containing gum, *Journal of the American Dental Association* 113 (1986): 262–266.

22. Councils on Dental Health and Health Planning, Dental Research, and Dental Therapeutics, Statement on diet and dental caries, *Journal of the American Dental Association* 107 (1983): 78.

23. American Dental Association, *Diet & Dental Health* (Chicago: American Dental Association, 1986), pp. 1–8.

24. J. C. Greene, R. Louie, and S. J. Wycoff, Preventive dentistry, *Journal of the American Medical Association* 262 (1989): 3459–3463.

25. A. E. Harper, Nutrition, aging, and longevity, *American Journal of Clinical Nutrition* (supplement) 36 (October 1982): 737–749.

26. Harper, 1982.

27. The items shown in the margin were listed by K. A. Meister, Can diet cure arthritis? *ACSH News and Views* (September/October 1980): 10; and in Morsels and tidbits, *Nutrition and the MD,* January 1982.

28. B. Kowsari and coauthors, Assessment of the diet of patients with rheumatoid arthritis and osteoarthritis, *Journal of the American Dietetic Association* 82 (1983): 657–659; P. A. Simkin, Oral zinc sulphate in rheumatoid arthritis, *Lancet,* September 11, 1976, pp. 539–542.

29. Dr. Charles P. Lucas, internist at Wayne State University School of Medicine, has observed a low-fat diet, adequate in all essential nutrients and emphasizing fruits, vegetables, and whole grains, to relieve the symptoms of rheumatoid arthritis in a few clients (personal communication, February 1984).

30. S. R. Gambert and A. R. Guansing, Protein-calorie malnutrition in the elderly, *Journal of the American Geriatrics Society* 28 (1980): 272–275.

31. G. E. Gray, A. Paganini-Hill, and R. K. Ross, Dietary intake and nutrient supplement use in a Southern California retirement community, *American Journal of Clinical Nutrition* 38 (1983): 122–128.

32. A. A. Sorensen, D. I. Sorensen, and J. G. Zimmer, Appropriateness of vitamin and mineral prescription orders for residents of health related facilities, *Journal of the American Geriatrics Society* 27 (1979): 425–430.

33. E. Luros, A rational approach to geriatric nutrition, *Dietetic Currents, Ross Timesaver* 8 (November-December 1981).

34. E. Luros, 1981.

35. R. Tannahil, *Food in History* (New York: Crown Publishers, 1988), p. 275.

36. S. Eisenberg, Looking for the perfect brew, *Food Technology* 43 (1989): 44–45.

37. Quantum Sufficit, *American Family Physician* 43 (1991): 1499.

38. A.A.A. Bak and D. E. Grobbee, The effect on serum cholesterol levels of coffee brewed by filtering or boiling, *New England Journal of Medicine* 321 (1989): 1432–1437.

39. E. M. Puccio and others, Clustering of atherogenic behavior in coffee drinkers, *American Journal of Public Health* 80 (1990): 1310–1313.

40. S. G. Oei, R.P.L. Vosters, and N.L.J. van der Hagen, Fetal arrhythmia caused by excessive intake of caffeine by pregnant women, *British Medical Journal* 298 (1989): 568.

41. N. L. Benowitz, S. M. Hall, and G. Modin, Persistent increase in caffeine concentrations in people who stop smoking, *British Medical Journal* 298 (1989): 1075–1076.

42. Committee on Diet and Health, *Diet and Health* (Washington, D.C.: National Academy Press, 1989), pp. 16, 431–464.

43. R. A. Dietrich, Genetics of alcoholism: How do we find the answers and what do we do then? *Alcohol & Alcoholism* 25 (1990): 571–572.

44. P. Avogaro, Alcohol—A risk or protective factor in aging, *Sedentary Life and Nutrition,* F. Fabris, L. Pernigotti, and E. Farrario, eds. (New York: Raven Press, Ltd., 1990), pp. 163–172.

45. M. J. Stampfer and co-authors, A prospective study of moderate alcohol consumption and the risk of coronary disease and stroke in women, *New England Journal of Medicine* 319 (1988): 267–273.

46. M. Frezza and co-authors, High blood alcohol levels in women—The role of decreased gastric alcohol dehydrogenase activity and first-pass metabolism, *New England Journal of Medicine* 322 (1990): 95–99.

47. Luros, 1981.

48. A. B. Eisenstein, Nutritional and metabolic effects of alcohol, *Journal of the American Dietetic Association* 81 (1982), 247–251.

49. J.J.B. Anderson and B. R. Switzer, Effects of alcohol on nutritional status: Part I—Minerals, *Internal Medicine* 8 (1987): 69, 73–75, 81–82, 85.
50. F. Iber, In alcoholism, the liver sets the pace, *Nutrition Today* (January-February 1971): 2–9.

Chapter 11 Notes

1. M. Kroger and J. S. Smith, An overview of chemical aspects of food safety, *Food Technology* 38 (1984): 62–64.
2. J. D. Dziezak (ed.), International foods—A growing market in the U.S., *Food Technology* 41 (1987): 120, 120–123, 125–132, 134.
3. J. D. Dziezak (ed.), Fats, oils, and fat substitutes, *Food Technology* 43 (1989): 66–74.
4. J. J. Albrecht, Business and technology issues in U.S. food science and technology, *Food Technology* 40 (1986): 122–127.
5. Food Technologists' Expert Panel on Food Safety and Nutrition, A scientific status summary—Bacteria associated with foodborne disease, *Food Technology* 42 (1988): 181–200.
6. National Dairy Council, A perspective on food safety concerns, *Dairy Council Digest* 58 (1987): 1–6.
7. N. H. Mermelstein (ed.), New bacteria in the news—a special symposium, *Food Technology* 40 (1986): 16–26.
8. Food Technologists' Expert Panel on Food Safety and Nutrition, 1988.
9. R. J. I. Bain, Accidental digitalis poisoning due to drinking herbal tea (letter to the editor), *British Medical Journal* 290 (1985): 1624.
10. E. N. Whitney, E. M. N. Hamilton, and M. A. Boyle, *Understanding Nutrition,* 4th ed. (St. Paul: West, 1987), p. 451.
11. R. W. Miller, Honey: Making sure it's pure, *FDA Consumer,* September 1979, pp. 12–13; I. B. Vyhmeister, What about honey? *Life and Health,* August 1980, pp. 5–7.
12. A. A. Brynjolfsson, Food irradiation and nutrition, *Professional Nutritionist,* Fall 1979, pp. 7–10.
13. R. Dubos, The intellectual basis of nutrition science and practice. Paper presented at the NIH conference on the biomedical and behavioral basis of clinical nutrition, 19 June 1978, in Bethesda, Maryland, and reprinted in *Nutrition Today,* July–August 1979, pp. 31–34.
14. N. D. Vietmeyer, The preposterous puffer, *National Geographic* 166 (1984): 260–270.
15. W. A. Krehl, Mercury, the slippery metal, *Nutrition Today,* November/December 1972, pp. 4–15.
16. W. A. Krehl, 1972.
17. M. A. Wessel and A. Dominski, Our children's daily lead, *American Scientist* 65 (1977): 294–298.
18. 97% of Michigan population contaminated by 1973 spills, *Tallahassee Democrat,* 16 April 1982.
19. F. M. Strong, Toxicants occurring naturally in foods, in *Nutrition Reviews' Present Knowledge in Nutrition,* 4th ed. (Washington, D.C.: Nutrition Foundation, 1976), pp. 516–527.
20. K. R. Mahaffey, Nutrition factors in lead poisoning, *Nutrition Reviews* 39 (1981): 353–362.
21. M. B. Rabinowitz, J. D. Kopple, and G. W. Wetherill, Effect of food intake and fasting on gastrointestinal lead absorption in humans, *American Journal of Clinical Nutrition* 33 (1980): 1784–1788.
22. R. W. Miller, The metal in our mettle, *FDA Consumer,* December 1988–January 1989, pp. 24–27.
23. Getting the lead out, *Science News,* 24 October 1987, p. 269.
24. D. Faust and J. Brown, Moderately elevated blood lead levels: Effect on neuropsychological functioning in children, *Pediatrics* 80 (1987): 623–629.
25. Getting the lead out, 1987.
26. D. Blumenthal, The canning process: Old preservation technique goes modern, *FDA Consumer,* September 1990, p. 17.
27. Update: Childhood lead poisoning, *Journal of the American Dietetic Association* 80 (1982): 592, 594.
28. Corn syrup can also be contaminated with *C. botulinum* spores. D. A. Kautter and coauthors, *Clostridium botulinum* spores in infant foods—a survey, *Journal of Food Protection* 45 (1982): 1028–1029.
29. I. B. Vyhmeister, What about honey? *Life and Health,* August 1980, pp. 5–7; R. W. Miller, Honey: Making sure it's pure, *FDA Consumer* 13 (September 1979): 12–13.
30. D. L. Morse and coauthors, Widespread outbreaks of clam- and oyster-associated gastroenteritis: role of Norwalk virus, *New England Journal of Medicine* 314 (1986): 678–681; H. L. Dupont, Consumption of raw shellfish—is the risk now unacceptable? (editorial), *New England Journal of Medicine* 314 (1986): 707–708; Sushi lovers: beware of parasites, *Science News,* 2 March 1985, p. 141.
31. H. W. Schultz, *Food Law Handbook* (Westport, Conn.: Avi, 1981), pp. 573–574.
32. M. G. Mustafa, Agricultural chemicals, in *Adverse Effects of Foods* by E. F. P. Jelliffe and D. B. Jelliffe (New York: Plenum Press, 1982), pp. 111–128.
33. Food Technologists Expert Panel on Food Safety and Nutrition, A scientific status summary—food colors, *Food Technology* 40 (1986): 49–56.
34. F. J. Stare and coauthors, *Balanced Nutrition* (Holbrook: Bob Adams, Inc., 1989), pp. 81–99.
35. *The Macmillan Dictionary of Quotations* (New York: Macmillan, 1989), p. 175.
36. J. E. Young, Reducing Waste, Saving Materials in *State of the World 1991,* Worldwatch Institute (New York: W. W. Norton, 1991), pp. 42–49.
37. *The Green Shopping Revolution: How Solid Waste Issues Are Affecting Consumer Behavior* (Washington, D.C. and New York: The Food Marketing Institute and *Better Homes and Gardens Magazine,* 1990), p. 5.
38. Michael Peters Group Press Release, American Consumers Going "Green," As Environment Plays Large Role in Purchase Decisions (New York: July 20, 1989), p. 1.
39. Personal communication with Cheryl Sutton, Assistant Communications Director for Attorney General Hubert H. Humphrey III, St. Paul, Minnesota.
40. The Office of the Attorney General Hubert Humphrey III, *The "Environmentally Friendly" Consumer: A Shopper's Guide.*
41. Personal communication with Douglas Wilson, Research Associate with the Garbage Project, University of Arizona, Tucson.
42. The Office of the Attorney General Hubert Humphrey III, *The "Environmentally Friendly" Consumer: A Shopper's Guide.*
43. The Earthworks Group, *50 Simple Things You Can Do to Save the Earth* (Berkeley, Calif.: The Earthworks Press, 1989), p. 66–67.
44. J. E. Young, 1991.
45. A. Wilson, *Consumer Guide to Home Energy Savings* (Washington, D.C.: The American Council for an Energy-Efficient Economy, 1990), pp. 183–187.
46. D. Odland and C. Davis, Products cooked in preheated versus non-preheated ovens, *Journal of the American Dietetic Association* 81 (1982): 135–145.
47. U.S. Department of Agriculture News Division, News Feature, *Quick, Safe Microwave Technique,* April 17, 1989; U.S. Department of Agriculture—FSIS, *Food News for Consumers,* Hotline Calling, But the Recipe Says . . . , Winter 1989.
48. R. A. Hibbard and R. Blevins, Palatal Burn Due to Bottle Warming in a Microwave Oven, *Pediatrics* 82 (1988): 382–384.
49. M. Cameron and Y. Hofvander, *Manual on Feeding Infants and Young Children,* 2nd ed. (New York: Protein Advisory Board of the United Nations, 1976), p. 1.

50. Physician Task Force on Hunger in America, *Hunger in America: The Growing Epidemic* (Middletown, Conn.: Wesleyan University Press, 1985), p. 17.
51. Department of Health and Rehabilitative Services and the Florida Task Force on Hunger, *Hunger in Florida: A Report to the Legislature* (Tallahassee, Fla.: Department of Health and Rehabilitative Services, April 1986), pp. 32–33.
52. Independent Commission on International Issues, *North-South: A Program for Survival* (Cambridge, Mass.: MIT Press, 1980), pp. 49–50.
53. The Hunger Project, *Ending Hunger: An Idea Whose Time Has Come* (New York: Praeger, 1985), pp. 314–315.
54. T. Peterson, Hunger and the environment, *Seeds,* October 1987, pp. 6–13.
55. E. O'Kelly, Appropriate technology for women, *Development Forum,* June 1976, p. 2.
56. National Agricultural Lands Study, *Soil Degradation: Effects on Agricultural Productivity,* Interium Report No. 4 (Washington, D.C.: U.S. Department of Agriculture, November 1980), as cited by L. R. Brown, World population growth, soil erosion, and food security, *Science* 214 (1981): 995–1002.
57. Oxfam America, *Facts for Action: Women Creating a New World,* No. 3 (Boston: Oxfam America, 1986), p. 3.
58. Oral rehydration therapy, *World Health* (Geneva: World Health Organization), June, 1985.
59. The case for optimism, in E. Cornish and members and staff of the World Future Society, *The Study of the Future: An Introduction to the Art and Science of Understanding and Shaping Tomorrow's World* (Washington, D.C.: World Future Society, 1977), pp. 34–37.
60. D. Elgin, *Voluntary Simplicity: Toward a Way of Life That Is Outwardly Simple, Inwardly Rich* (New York: Morrow, 1981), p. 25.

APPENDIX F

Table of Food Composition

This table of food composition is not the standard table found in most nutrition textbooks. The list of foods chosen is an expanded version of that presented in the 1986 edition of the USDA *Home and Garden Bulletin Number 72, Nutritive Value of Foods*. The *Bulletin,* however, does not contain the values for dietary fiber, vitamin B_6, folate, magnesium, or zinc. Also, many additional foods have been added (such as frozen yogurt, canola oil, and imitation seafood items) to reflect current food patterns. The latest data for beef is also included. It is from the USDA data tapes and reflects the leaner cuts of beef now sold.

To achieve a complete and reliable listing of nutrients for all the foods, many sources of information had to be researched. Government sources of information is the primary base for all of the data: USDA *Handbooks 8–1* through *8–18*; *Handbook 8–21*; prepublication material on cereals, grains, and pasta; current supplemental data on vegetables and other foods; and provisional USDA information of nutrient values—both published and unpublished. Many conversations with professional staff members at the USDA Human Nutrition Information Service in Hyattsville, Maryland, also contributed professional assistance to the refinement and completion of the data.

Even with all the government sources available, there are still many missing nutrient values; and, as the various government data are updated, conflicting values are often reported from the USDA. To fill in the missing values and resolve discrepancies, other sources of reliable information were used: journal articles, food composition tables from Canada and England, information from other nutrient data banks and publications, unpublished scientific data, and manufacturers' data.

Estimates of nutrient amounts for foods include all possible adjustments. When multiple values are reported for a nutrient, the numbers are averaged and weighted with consideration of the original number of samples in the separate sources. Whenever water percentages are available, estimates of nutrient amounts are adjusted for water content. When no water is given, water percentage is assumed to be that shown in the table. Whenever a reported weight appears inconsistent (cooked eggplant and collards, for example), many kitchen tests are made, and the average weight of the typical product is given as tested.

When estimates of nutrient amounts in cooked foods are derived from reported amounts in raw foods, published retention factors are applied. Some reported data for combination foods are modified in this table to include newer data available for major ingredients. For example, since the "pies" were analyzed and reported, newer data on fruits has been published. Older reported data on certain bakery items are updated for the new enrichment levels for certain nutrients.

Considerable effort has been made to report the most accurate data available and to eliminate missing values. There will always be future changes and the authors welcome any suggestions or comments from readers.

It is important to know

that there can be many different values reported for the same nutrient. Many factors influence the amounts of nutrients in foods: the mineral content of the soil, the method of processing, genetics, the diet of the animal or the fertilizer of the plant, the season of the year, methods of analysis, the differences in moisture contents of the samples analyzed, the length and method of storage, and methods of cooking the food.

Even reliable sources report conflicting data. Although each nutrient from USDA government data is presented as a single number in some USDA publications, each number is actually an average of a range of data. In the more detailed reports (Handbook 8 series), the number of samples is identified, and the standard deviation is also noted. USDA data will report different values for foods as well because old information is being updated in the more recent publications. Therefore, nutrient data should be used only as a guide, a close approximation of nutrient content.

Dietary fiber deserves a special word. It is important to remember that changes will be made to the dietary fiber data, as research continues and analytical techniques are modified. Estimates of dietary fiber are included for all the foods in this table. The sources of this information are primarily extensive published and unpublished information from the USDA Human Nutrition Information Service in Hyattsville, Maryland; *Composition of Foods by Southgate* (England); and many journal articles.

Dietary fiber is composed of cellulose, hemicellulose, lignin, pectin, gums, and mucilages. Very little data is available for gum and mucilage, but there is considerable data on the other components.

Many different analytical techniques are used to measure various components of fiber, and these methods are undergoing their own review of accuracy in the scientific community. In this table, either an estimate of the total dietary fiber (a specific analytical technique) or a combination of measures for the insoluble components and pectin, when available, are used.

Vitamin A is reported in retinol equivalents. The amount of this vitamin can vary with the season of the year. Reported values in both dairy products and plants are higher in summer and early fall than in winter. The values reported here represent year-round averages. In the organ meats of all animal products (liver especially), there are large amounts of vitamin A, and these amounts vary widely with the background of the animal. The vitamin is present in very small amounts in regular meat and is often reported as a trace.

Newer reported vitamin A values for some plant foods have increased significantly due to additional information and sometimes to newer plant genetics. New vitamin A values for canned pumpkin, for example, are 3.5 times greater than the previously reported values. This information was used to modify the vitamin A value of pumpkin pie, which had not yet been updated.

The energy and nutrients in recipes and combination foods vary widely, depending on the ingredients. The various fatty acids and cholesterol are influenced by the type of fat used (the specific type of oil, vegetable shortening, butter, margarine, etc.).

Total fat, as well as the breakdown of total fat to saturated, monounsaturated, and polyunsaturated fat, is listed in the table. The fatty acids seldom add up exactly to the total. This is due to rounding and to the existence of small amounts of other fatty acid components that are not included in the three basic categories.

Niacin values are for preformed niacin and do not include additional niacin that may form in the body from the conversion of tryptophan.

The items in this table have been organized into several categories, which are listed at the head of each right-hand page. As the key shows, each group has a number and that number is indicated in the first column. For ease in paging through this table, the category listed on the page you are on is printed in bold type. Thus if 7-GRAIN has bold type and you are looking for dairy foods, turn back a few pages; if you are looking for sweets, turn forward.

Note: This table has been prepared for West Publishing Company and is copyrighted by ESHA Research in Salem, Oregon—the developer and publisher of "The Food Processor®" computerized nutrition systems. The major sources for the data from the U.S. Department of Agriculture are supplemented by over 450 additional sources of information. Because the list of references is so extensive, it is not provided here, but it is available from the publisher.

• *Table F–1* Food Composition

Grp	Computer Code No.	Food Description	Measure	Wt (g)	H_2O (%)	Ener (cal)	Prot (g)	Carb (g)	Dietary Fiber (g)	Fat (g)	Fat Breakdown (g)		
											Sat	Mono	Poly
BEVERAGES													
		Alcoholic:											
		Beer:											
1	1	Regular (12 fl oz)	1½ c	356	92	146	1	13	1	0	0	0	0
1	2	Light (12 fl oz)	1½ c	354	95	100[1]	1	5	1	0	0	0	0
		Gin, rum, vodka, whiskey:											
1	3	80 proof	1½ fl oz	42	67	97	0	<.1	0	0	0	0	0
1	4	86 proof	1½ fl oz	42	64	105	0	<.1	0	0	0	0	0
1	5	90 proof	1½ fl oz	42	62	110	0	<.1	0	0	0	0	0
		Liqueur:											
1	1359	Coffee Liqueur, 53 proof	1½ fl oz	52	31	174	0	24	0	<1	.1	t	.1
1	1360	Coffee & cream liqueur, 34 proof	1½ fl oz	47	47	154	1	10	0	7	4.5	2.1	.3
1	1361	Creme de menthe, 72 proof	1½ fl oz	50	28	186	0	21	0	<1	t	t	.1
		Wine:											
1	6	Dessert (4 fl oz)	½ c	118	72	181[2]	<1	14[2]	0	0	0	0	0
1	7	Red	3½ fl oz	103	88	74	<1	2	0	0	0	0	0
1	8	Rosé	3½ fl oz	103	89	73	<1	2	0	0	0	0	0
1	9	White medium	3½ fl oz	103	90	70	<1	1	0	0	0	0	0
		Carbonated[3]:											
1	10	Club soda (12 fl oz)	1½ c	355	100	0	0	0	0	0	0	0	0
1	11	Cola beverage (12 fl oz)	1½ c	370	89	151	0	39	0	0	0	0	0
1	12	Diet cola (12 fl oz)	1½ c	355	100	2	0	<1	0	0	0	0	0
1	13	Diet soda pop–average (12 fl oz)	1½ c	355	100	2	0	<1	0	0	0	0	0
1	14	Ginger ale (12 fl oz)	1½ c	366	91	124	0	32	0	0	0	0	0
1	15	Grape soda (12 fl oz)	1½ c	372	89	161	0	42	0	0	0	0	0
1	16	Lemon-lime (12 fl oz)	1½ c	368	90	149	0	38	0	0	0	0	0
1	17	Orange (12 fl oz)	1½ c	372	88	177	0	46	0	0	0	0	0
1	18	Pepper-type soda (12 fl oz)	1½ c	368	89	151	0	38	0	0	0	0	0
1	19	Root beer (12 fl oz)	1½ c	370	89	152	<1	39	0	0	0	0	0
		Coffee[3]:											
1	20	Brewed	1 c	240	99	2[4]	<1	1	<1	0	0	0	0
1	21	Prepared from instant	1 c	240	99	2[4]	<1	1	0	0	0	0	0
		Fruit drinks, noncarbonated[5]:											
1	22	Fruit punch drink, canned	1 c	253	88	118	<1	30	0	<1	t	t	t
1	1358	Gatorade	1 c	230	99	39	0	11	0	0	0	0	0
1	23	Grape drink, canned	1 c	250	88	112	0	35	<1	<1	t	t	t
1	1304	Koolade, sweetened with sugar	1 c	240	100	100	0	25	0	0	0	0	0
1	1356	Koolade, sweetened with nutrasweet	1 c	240	100	4	0	0	0	0	0	0	0
		Lemonade, frozen:											
1	26	Concentrate (6-oz can)	¾ c	219	52	397	1	103	1	<1	.1	t	.1
1	27	Lemonade prepared from frozen concentrate	1 c	248	89	100	<1	26	<1	<1	t	t	t
		Limeade, frozen:											
1	28	Concentrate (6-oz can)	¾ c	218	50	408	<1	108	1	<1	t	t	.1
1	29	Limeade prepared from frozen concentrate	1 c	247	89	102	<1	27	<1	<1	t	t	t
1	24	Pineapple grapefruit, canned	1 c	250	88	117	1	29	0	<1	t	t	.1
1	25	Pineapple orange, canned	1 c	250	87	125	3	29	0	<1	t	t	.1
		Fruit and vegetable juices: see Fruit and Vegetable sections											

(1)Calories can vary from 78 to 131 for 12 fl oz.
(2)Values are for sweet dessert wine. Dry dessert wines contain 149 cal and 5 g of carbohydrate.
(3)Mineral content varies depending on water source.
(4)Calorie values from USDA vary from 1 to 4 calories per cup.
(5)Usually less than 10% fruit juice.

GRP KEY: **1 = BEV** 2 = DAIRY 3 = EGGS 4 = FAT/OIL 5 = FRUIT 6 = BAKERY 7 = GRAIN 8 = FISH 9 = BEEF 10 = POULTRY 11 = SAUSAGE 12 = MIXED/FAST 13 = NUTS/SEEDS 14 = SWEETS 15 = VEG/LEG 16 = MISC 22 = SOUP/SAUCE

Chol (mg)	Calc (mg)	Iron (mg)	Magn (mg)	Phos (mg)	Pota (mg)	Sodi (mg)	Zinc (mg)	VT-A (RE)	Thia (mg)	Ribo (mg)	Niac (mg)	V-B6 (mg)	Fola (μg)	VT-C (mg)
0	18	.11	23	44	89	19	.07	0	.02	.09	1.61	.18	21	0
0	18	.14	18	43	64	10	.11	0	.03	.11	1.39	.12	15	0
0	0	.02	0	2	1	<1	.02	0	<.01	<.01	<.01	t	0	0
0	0	.02	0	2	1	<1	.02	0	<.01	<.01	<.01	0	0	0
0	0	.02	0	2	1	<1	.02	0	<.01	<.01	<.01	0	0	0
0	1	.03	1	3	15	4	.01	0	<.01	.01	.08	—	0	0
—	7	.06	1	23	15	43	.08	—	0	.03	.04	—	0	0
0	0	.04	0	0	0	3	—	0	0	0	<.01	0	0	—
0	9	.24	11	11	109	11	.08	0	.02	.02	.25	0	<1	0
0	8	.44	13	14	115	6	.10	0	<.01	.03	.08	.04	2	0
0	9	.39	10	15	102	5	.06	0	<.01	.02	.08	.03	1	0
0	9	.33	11	14	82	5	.07	0	<.01	<.01	.07	.01	<1	0
0	17	.15	4	0	6	75	.36	0	0	0	0	0	0	0
0	9	.13	3	46	4	15	.05	0	0	0	0	0	0	0
0	12	.11	4	30	0	21[6]	.28	0	.02	.08	0	0	0	0
0	14	.14	3	38	7	21[6]	.10	0	0	0	0	0	0	0
0	12	.66	3	1	5	25	.18	0	0	0	0	0	0	0
0	12	.31	4	0	3	57	.26	0	0	0	0	0	0	0
0	9	.25	2	1	4	41	.18	0	0	0	.06	0	0	0
0	19	.23	4	4	9	46	.38	0	0	0	0	0	0	0
0	12	.14	1	41	2	38	.15	0	0	0	0	0	0	0
0	19	.19	4	2	3	49	.26	0	0	0	0	0	0	0
0	4	.12	14	3	130	5	.08	0	0	.02	.53	0	<1	0
0	8	.12	9	8	87	8	.07	0	0	<.01	.69	0	0	0
0	19	.52	5	3	64	56	.31	4	.06	.06	.05	0	3	75
0	23	—	—	0	23	123	—	0	—	—	—	—	—	—
0	3	.41	5	3	13	16	.28	<1	.08	.02	.07	.02	1	85
0	0	0	0	0	0	0	0	0	0	0	0	0	0	6
0	0	0	0	0	0	0	0	0	0	0	0	0	0	6
0	15	1.58	11	19	148	8	.17	21	.06	.21	.16	.06	22	39[7]
0	4	.41	3	5	38	8	.05	5	.02	.95	.04	.02	6	10[7]
0	11	.22	60	13	129	<1	.11	<1	.02	.02	.22	.11	25	26
0	3	.06	15	3	33	<1	.03	<1	<.01	<.01	.05	.03	6	7
0	18	.77	15	14	154	34	.15	9	.08	.04	.67	.10	26	115
0	13	.67	14	10	116	9	.14	133	.08	.05	.52	.12	27	56

(6)Value for product sweetened with aspartame only; sodium is 32 mg if a blend of aspartame and sodium saccharin is used; 75 mg if just sodium saccharin is used.

(7)Vitamin C can range from 5 to 72 mg in a small can of frozen concentrate, and from 1 to 18 mg in 1 c of prepared lemonade.

• *Table F–1* Food Composition

Grp	Computer Code No.	Food Description	Measure	Wt (g)	H_2O (%)	Ener (cal)	Prot (g)	Carb (g)	Dietary Fiber (g)	Fat (g)	Fat Breakdown (g)		
											Sat	Mono	Poly
BEVERAGES—Con.													
1	1357	Perrier® bottled water, 6.5 fl oz bottle	1 ea	192	100	0	0	0	0	0	0	0	0
		Tea[8]:											
1	30	Brewed	1 c	240	100	2	<.01	1	0	0	0	0	0
1	31	From instant, unsweetened	1 c	237	100	2	0	<1	0	0	0	0	0
1	32	From instant, sweetened	1 c	262	91	86	0	22	0	0	0	0	0
DAIRY													
		Butter: see Fats and Oils, #158, 159, 160											
		Cheese, natural:											
2	33	Blue	1 oz	28	42	100	6	1	0	8	5.3	2.2	.2
2	34	Brick	1 oz	28	41	105	6	1	0	8	5.3	2.4	.2
2	35	Brie	1 oz	28	48	95	6	<1	0	8	5.0	2.3	.3
2	36	Camembert	1 oz	28	52	85	6	<1	0	7	4.3	2.0	.2
		Cheddar:											
2	37	Cut pieces	1 oz	28	37	114	7	<1	0	9	6.0	2.7	.3
2	38	1″ cube	1 ea	17	37	69	4	<1	0	6	3.6	1.6	.2
2	39	Shredded	1 c	113	37	455	28	1	0	37	24	11	1
		Cottage:											
2	40	Creamed, large curd	1 c	225	79	235	28	6	0	10	6.4	3.0	.3
2	41	Creamed, small curd	1 c	210	79	215	26	6	0	9	6.0	2.7	.3
2	42	With fruit	1 c	226	72	279	22	30	0	8	4.9	2.2	.3
2	43	Low fat 2%	1 c	226	79	205	31	8	0	4	2.8	1.2	.1
2	44	Low fat 1%	1 c	226	82	164	28	6	0	2	1.5	.7	.1
2	45	Dry curd	1 c	145	80	123	25	3	0	1	.4	.2	<.1
2	46	Cream	1 oz	28	54	99	2	1	0	10	6.2	2.8	.4
2	47	Edam	1 oz	28	42	101	7	<1	0	8	5.0	2.3	.2
2	48	Feta	1 oz	28	55	75	5	1	0	6	4.2	1.3	.2
2	49	Gouda	1 oz	28	42	101	7	1	0	8	5.0	2.2	.2
2	50	Gruyère	1 oz	28	33	117	8	<1	0	9	5.4	2.9	.5
2	51	Gorgonzola	1 oz	28	39	111	7	0	0	9	5.5	2.4	.5
2	52	Liederkranz	1 oz	28	53	87	5	0	0	8	5.3	2.2	.2
2	53	Monterey jack	1 oz	28	41	106	7	<1	0	9	5.4	2.4	.2
		Mozzarella, made with:											
2	54	Whole milk	1 oz	28	54	80	5	1	0	6	3.7	1.9	.2
2	55	Part skim milk, low moisture	1 oz	28	49	80	8	1	0	5	3.1	1.4	.1
2	56	Muenster	1 oz	28	42	104	6	<1	0	8	5.4	2.5	.2
		Parmesan, grated:											
2	57	Cup, not pressed down	1 c	100	18	455	42	4	0	30	19	8.7	.7
2	58	Tablespoon	1 tbsp	5	18	23	2	<1	0	2	1	.4	<.1
2	59	Ounce	1 oz	28	18	129	12	1	0	9	5.4	2.5	.2
2	60	Provolone	1 oz	28	41	100	7	1	0	8	4.8	2.1	.2
		Ricotta, made with:											
2	61	Whole milk	1 c	246	72	428	28	7	0	32	20	8.9	1
2	62	Part skim milk	1 c	246	74	340	28	13	0	19	12	5.7	.6
2	63	Romano	1 oz	28	31	110	9	1	0	8	4.9	2.2	.2
2	64	Swiss	1 oz	28	37	107	8	1	0	8	5.0	2.1	.3
		Pasteurized processed cheese products:											
2	65	American	1 oz	28	39	106	6	<1	0	9	5.6	2.5	.3
2	66	Swiss	1 oz	28	42	95	7	1	0	7	4.6	2.0	.2
2	67	American cheese food	1 oz	28	44	93	6	2	0	7	4.4	2.0	.2
2	68	American cheese spread	1 oz	28	48	82	5	2	0	6	3.8	1.8	.2

(8)Mineral content varies depending on water source.

(Computer code number is for West Diet Analysis program)

GRP KEY: **1 = BEV** 2 = DAIRY 3 = EGGS 4 = FAT/OIL 5 = FRUIT 6 = BAKERY 7 = GRAIN 8 = FISH 9 = BEEF 10 = POULTRY 11 = SAUSAGE 12 = MIXED/FAST 13 = NUTS/SEEDS 14 = SWEETS 15 = VEG/LEG 16 = MISC 22 = SOUP/SAUCE

Chol (mg)	Calc (mg)	Iron (mg)	Magn (mg)	Phos (mg)	Pota (mg)	Sodi (mg)	Zinc (mg)	VT-A (RE)	Thia (mg)	Ribo (mg)	Niac (mg)	V-B6 (mg)	Fola (μg)	VT-C (mg)
0	26	0	1	0	0	3	0	0	0	0	0	0	0	0
0	0	.05	7	1	89	7	.05	0	0	.03	.1	0	12	0
0	5	.05	5	3	47	8	.07	0	0	<.01	<.01	<.09	1	0
0	1	.04	3	3	49	1	.06	0	0	.04	.09	0	5	0
21	150	.09	7	110	73	396	.75	65	.01	.11	.29	.05	10	0
27	191	.13	7	128	38	159	.73	86	<.01	.1	.03	.02	6	0
28	52	.14	6	53	43	178	.7	57	.02	.15	.11	.07	18	0
20	110	.09	6	98	53	236	.68	71	.01	.14	.18	.06	18	0
30	204	.20	8	146	28	176	.92	86	.01	.11	.02	.02	5	0
18	124	.12	5	88	17	107	.54	52	<.01	.07	.01	.01	3	0
119	815	.77	31	579	111	701	3.51	342	.03	.42	.09	.08	21	0
34	135	.26	11	297	190	911	.8	108	.05	.37	.30	.14	27	<1
31	126	.30	11	277	177	850	.8	101	.04	.34	.27	.14	26	<1
25	108	.25	9	236	151	915	.66	81	.04	.29	.23	.12	22	<1
19	155	.36	14	340	217	918	.95	45	.05	.42	.33	.17	30	0
10	138	.32	12	302	193	918	.86	25	.05	.37	.29	.15	28	t
10	46	.33	6	151	47	19	.68	12	.04	.21	.23	.12	21	0
31	23	.34	2	30	34	84	.33	124	<.01	.06	.03	.01	4	0
25	207	.13	8	152	53	274	1.06	72	.01	.11	.02	.02	5	0
25	140	.18	5	96	18	316	.81	36	.04	.23	.29	.02	3	0
32	198	.07	8	155	34	232	1.1	49	<.01	.10	.02	.02	6	0
31	287	.06	4	172	23	95	1	98	.02	.08	.03	.02	3	0
25	149	.12	8	121	26	513	.57	103	.01	.09	.2	.04	9	0
21	110	.12	7	100	68	390	.7	91	.01	.18	.1	.04	34	0
26	212	.2	8	126	23	152	.85	81	<.01	.11	.02	.02	3	0
22	147	.05	5	105	19	106	.7	68	<.01	.07	.02	.02	2	0
15	207	.08	8	149	27	150	.83	54	<.01	.1	.03	.02	3	0
27	203	.13	8	133	38	178	.84	90	<.01	.09	.03	.02	3	0
79	1376	.95	51	807	107	1862	3.19	173	.04	.39	.32	.11	8	0
4	69	.05	3	40	5	93	.16	9	<.01	.02	.02	<.01	<1	0
22	390	.27	14	229	30	528	1	49	.01	.11	.09	.03	2	0
20	214	.15	8	141	39	248	.89	75	<.01	.09	.04	.02	3	0
124	509	.94	28	389	257	207	2.85	330	.03	.48	.26	.11	14	0
76	669	1.09	4	449	307	307	3.29	278	.05	.46	.19	.05	14	0
29	302	.23	12	215	26	340	1	40	.01	.11	.02	.03	2	0
26	272	.05	10	171	31	74	1.1	72	<.01	.1	.03	.02	2	0
27	174	.11	6	211	46	406	.93	82	.01	.1	.02	.02	2	0
24	219	.17	8	216	61	388	1.02	65	<.01	.08	.01	.01	2	0
18	163	.24	9	130	79	337	.85	62	.01	.13	.04	.02	2	0
16	159	.09	8	201	69	381	.78	54	.01	.12	.04	.03	2	0

(For purposes of calculations, use "0" for t, <1, <.1, <.01, etc.)

Table F–1 Food Composition

Grp	Computer Code No.	Food Description	Measure	Wt (g)	H_2O (%)	Ener (cal)	Prot (g)	Carb (g)	Dietary Fiber (g)	Fat (g)	Fat Breakdown (g) Sat	Mono	Poly
		DAIRY—Con.											
		Cream, sweet:											
		Half and half (cream and milk):											
2	69	Cup	1 c	242	81	315	7	10	0	28	17	8	1
2	70	Tablespoon	1 tbsp	15	81	20	<1	1	0	2	1.1	.5	.1
		Light, coffee or table:											
2	71	Cup	1 c	240	74	469	6	9	0	46	29	13	1.7
2	72	Tablespoon	1 tbsp	15	74	30	<1	1	0	3	1.8	.8	.1
		Light whipping cream, liquid:											
2	73	Cup	1 c	239	64	699	5	7	0	74	46	22	2.1
2	74	Tablespoon	1 tbsp	15	64	44	<1	<1	0	5	2.9	1.4	.1
		Heavy whipping cream, liquid[9]:											
2	75	Cup	1 c	238	58	821	5	7	0	88	55	25	3.3
2	76	Tablespoon	1 tbsp	15	58	51	<1	<1	0	6	3.5	1.6	.2
		Whipped cream, pressurized[9]:											
2	77	Cup	1 c	60	61	154	2	7	0	13	8.3	3.9	.5
2	78	Tablespoon	1 tbsp	4	61	10	<1	<1	0	1	.5	.2	<.1
		Cream, sour, cultured:											
2	79	Cup	1 c	230	71	493	7	10	0	48	30	14	1.8
2	80	Tablespoon	1 tbsp	14	71	30	<1	1	0	3	1.8	.9	.1
		Cream products—imitation and part dairy:											
		Coffee whitener:											
2	81	Frozen or liquid	1 tbsp	15	77	20	<1	2	0	2	1.4	t	t
2	82	Powdered	1 tsp	2	2	11	<1	1	0	1	.6	t	t
		Dessert topping, frozen:											
2	83	Cup	1 c	75	50	239	1	17	0	19	16	1.2	.4
2	84	Tablespoon	1 tbsp	5	50	15	<1	1	0	1	1.0	.1	t
		Dessert topping from mix:											
2	85	Cup	1 c	80	67	151	3	13	0	10	8.6	.7	.2
2	86	Tablespoon	1 tbsp	5	67	9	<1	1	0	1	.5	<.1	t
		Dessert topping, pressurized:											
2	87	Cup	1 c	70	60	185	1	11	0	16	13	1.4	.2
2	88	Tablespoon	1 tbsp	4	60	11	<1	1	0	1	.8	.1	t
		Sour cream imitation:											
2	91	Cup	1 c	230	71	479	6	15	0	45	41	1.4	.1
2	92	Tablespoon	1 tbsp	14	71	29	<1	1	0	3	2.5	.1	t
		Sour dressing, part dairy:											
2	89	Cup	1 c	235	75	416	8	11	0	39	31	4.6	1.1
2	90	Tablespoon	1 tbsp	15	75	25	<1	1	0	2	2.0	.3	.1
		Milk, fluid:											
2	93	Whole milk	1 c	244	88	150	8	11	0	8	5.1	2.4	.3
2	94	2% low-fat milk	1 c	244	89	121	8	12	0	5	2.9	1.4	.2
2	95	2% milk solids added[10]	1 c	245	89	125	9	12	0	5	2.9	1.4	.2
2	96	1% low-fat milk	1 c	244	90	102	8	12	0	3	1.6	.8	.1
2	97	1% milk solids added[10]	1 c	245	90	105	9	12	0	2	1.5	.7	.1
2	98	Skim milk	1 c	245	91	86	8	12	0	<1	.3	.1	t
2	99	Skim milk solids added[10]	1 c	245	90	91	9	12	0	1	.4	.2	t
2	100	Buttermilk	1 c	245	90	99	8	12	0	2	1.3	.6	.1

(9) For whipped cream, (non-pressurized), double the liquid cream volume of codes 75,76 or 73,74. One tablespoon liquid cream becomes 2 Tablespoons when "whipped".

(10) Milk solids added, label claims less than 10 g protein per cup.

(Computer code number is for West Diet Analysis program)

GRP KEY: 1=BEV **2=DAIRY** 3=EGGS 4=FAT/OIL 5=FRUIT 6=BAKERY 7=GRAIN 8=FISH 9=BEEF 10=POULTRY 11=SAUSAGE 12=MIXED/FAST 13=NUTS/SEEDS 14=SWEETS 15=VEG/LEG 16=MISC 22=SOUP/SAUCE

Chol (mg)	Calc (mg)	Iron (mg)	Magn (mg)	Phos (mg)	Pota (mg)	Sodi (mg)	Zinc (mg)	VT-A (RE)	Thia (mg)	Ribo (mg)	Niac (mg)	V-B6 (mg)	Fola (µg)	VT-C (mg)
89	254	.17	25	230	314	98	1.23	259	.09	.36	.19	.09	6	2
6	16	.01	2	14	20	6	.08	16	.01	.02	.01	<.01	<1	<1
159	231	.1	21	192	292	95	.65	437	.08	.36	.14	.08	6	2
10	14	.01	1	12	18	6	.04	27	<.01	.02	.01	<.01	<1	<1
265	166	.07	17	146	231	82	.60	705	.06	.30	.1	.07	9	1
17	10	<.01	1	9	15	5	.04	44	<.01	.02	.01	<.01	1	<1
326	154	.07	17	149	179	89	.55	1002	.05	.26	.09	.06	10	1
20	10	<.01	1	9	11	6	.03	63	<.01	.02	.01	<.01	1	<1
46	61	.03	6	54	88	78	.22	124	.02	.04	.04	.03	1	0
3	4	<.01	<1	3	5	5	.01	8	<.01	<.01	<.01	<.01	<1	0
102	268	.14	26	195	331	123	.69	448	.08	.34	.15	.04	25	2
6	16	.01	2	12	20	7	.04	27	<.01	.02	.01	<.01	2	<1
0	1	<.01	<1	10	29	12	<.01	1[10]	0	0	0	0	0	0
0	<1	.02	<1	8	16	4	.01	<1[10]	0	<.01	0	0	0	0
0	5	.09	1	6	14	19	.03	65[11]	0	0	0	0	0	0
0	<1	.01	<1	<1	1	1	<.01	4[11]	0	0	0	0	0	0
8	72	.03	8	69	121	53	.22	39[11]	.02	.09	.05	.02	3	1
<1	5	<.01	<1	4	8	3	.14	3[11]	<.01	<.01	<.01	<.01	<1	<1
0	4	.01	1	13	13	43	.01	33[11]	0	0	0	0	0	0
0	<1	<.01	<1	1	1	3	<.01	2[11]	0	0	0	0	0	0
0	6	.01	—	102	369	235	0	0	0	0	0	0	0	0
0	<1	<.01	—	6	23	14	0	0	0	0	0	0	0	0
213	266	.07	23	205	381	113	.87	5[11]	.09	.38	.17	.04	28	2
1	17	<.01	2	13	24	7	.05	<1[11]	.01	.02	.01	<.01	2	<1
33	291	.12	33	228	370	120	.94	76	.09	.4	.2	.1	12	2
22	297	.12	33	232	377	122	.96	140	.1	.4	.21	.1	12	2
18	314	.12	35	245	397	128	.98	140	.1	.42	.22	.11	12	2
10	300	.12	34	235	381	123	.96	145	.1	.41	.21	.11	12	2
10	314	.12	35	245	397	128	.98	145	.1	.42	.22	.11	12	2
4	302	.1	28	247	406	126	.92	149	.09	.34	.22	.1	14	2
5	316	.12	37	255	419	130	1	149	.1	.43	.22	.11	12	2
9	285	.12	26	219	371	257	1.03	20	.08	.38	.14	.08	12	2

(11) Vitamin A value is from beta-carotene used for coloring.

(For purposes of calculations, use "0" for t, <1, <.1, <.01, etc.)

Table F–1 Food Composition

Grp	Computer Code No.	Food Description	Measure	Wt (g)	H_2O (%)	Ener (cal)	Prot (g)	Carb (g)	Dietary Fiber (g)	Fat (g)	Fat Breakdown (g) Sat	Mono	Poly
DAIRY—Con.													
		Milk, canned:											
2	101	Sweetened condensed	1 c	306	27	982	24	166	0	27	17	7.4	1
2	102	Evaporated, whole	1 c	252	74	340	17	25	0	20	12	5.9	.6
2	103	Evaporated, skim	1 c	255	79	200	19	29	0	1	.3	.2	t
		Milk, dried:											
2	104	Buttermilk	1 c	120	3	464	41	59	0	7	4.3	2.0	.3
		Instant, nonfat:											
2	105	Envelope[12]	1 ea	91	4	326	32	48	0	1	.4	.2	t
2	106	Cup	1 c	68	4	244	24	36	0	1	.3	.1	t
2	107	Goat milk	1 c	244	87	168	9	11	0	10	6.5	2.7	.4
2	108	Kefir[13]	1 c	233	82	122	9	9	0	5	2.9	1.2	.1
		Milk beverages and powdered mixes:											
		Chocolate:											
2	109	Whole	1 c	250	82	210	8	26	4	8	5.3	2.5	.3
2	110	2% fat	1 c	250	84	180	8	26	4	5	3.1	1.5	.2
2	111	1% fat	1 c	250	84	160	8	26	4	3	1.5	.8	.1
		Chocolate-flavored beverages:											
2	112	Powder containing nonfat dry milk:	1 oz	28	1	100	4	23	<1	1	.7	.4	t
2	113	Drink prepared with water	¾ c	206	86	100	4	23	<1	1	.7	.4	t
2	114	Powder without nonfat dry milk:	¾ oz	22	<1	75	1	20	<1	1	.4	.2	t
2	115	Drink prepared with whole milk	1 c	266	81	226	9	31	<1	9	5.5	2.6	.3
2	116	Eggnog, commercial	1 c	254	74	342	10	34	0	19	11	5.7	.9
		Instant Breakfast:											
2	1027	Envelope, dry powder only	1 ea	37	3	130	7	23	0	0	0	0	0
2	1028	Prepared with whole milk	1 c	281	87	280	15	34	0	8	5.1	2.4	.3
2	1029	Prepared with 2% milk	1 c	281	88	251	15	35	0	5	2.9	1.4	.2
2	1283	Prepared with 1% milk	1 c	281	89	232	15	35	0	3	1.5	.7	.1
2	1284	Prepared with skim milk	1 c	282	89	216	15	35	0	<1	.3	.1	t
		Malted milk, chocolate flavor:											
2	117	Powder[14], 3 heaping tsp:	¾ oz	21	1	79	1	18	<1	1	.5	.2	.1
2	118	Drink prepared with whole milk	1 c	265	81	229	9	30	<1	9	5.2	2.6	.4
		Malted milk, natural flavor:											
2	119	Powder[14], 3 heaping tsp:	¾ oz	21	2	87	2	16	<1	2	.9	.4	.3
2	120	Drink prepared with whole milk	1 c	265	81	237	10	27	<1	10	6.0	2.8	.6
		Milk shakes:											
2	121	Chocolate (10 fl oz)	1¼ c	283	72	360	10	58	<1	11	6.6	3.0	.4
2	122	Vanilla (10 fl oz)	1¼ c	283	75	314	10	51	<1	8	5.3	2.4	.3
		Milk desserts:											
2	134	Custard, baked	1 c	265	77	305	14	29	0	15	6.8	5.4	.7
		Ice cream, regular vanilla (about 11% fat):											
		Hardened:											
2	123	½ gallon	½ gal	1064	61	2153	38	254	0	115	71	33	4
2	124	Cup	1 c	133	61	269	5	32	0	14	8.3	4.1	.5
2	125	Fluid ounces	3 oz	50	61	101	2	12	0	5	3.3	1.6	.2
2	126	Soft serve	1 c	173	60	377	7	38	0	22	14	6.7	1.0
		Ice cream, rich vanilla (about 16% fat):											
		Hardened:											
2	127	½ gallon	½ gal	1188	59	2805	33	256	0	190	118	55	7
2	128	Cup	1 c	148	59	349	4	32	0	24	15	6.8	.9

(12)Yields 1 qt fluid milk when reconstituted according to package directions.
(13)Most values provided by product labeling.
(14)The latest USDA data from *Handbook 8–14* on beverages updates previous USDA data.

(Computer code number is for West Diet Analysis program)

GRP KEY: 1=BEV **2=DAIRY** 3=EGGS 4=FAT/OIL 5=FRUIT 6=BAKERY 7=GRAIN 8=FISH 9=BEEF 10=POULTRY 11=SAUSAGE 12=MIXED/FAST 13=NUTS/SEEDS 14=SWEETS 15=VEG/LEG 16=MISC 22=SOUP/SAUCE

Chol (mg)	Calc (mg)	Iron (mg)	Magn (mg)	Phos (mg)	Pota (mg)	Sodi (mg)	Zinc (mg)	VT-A (RE)	Thia (mg)	Ribo (mg)	Niac (mg)	V-B6 (mg)	Fola (µg)	VT-C (mg)
104	868	.58	78	775	1136	389	2.88	248	.28	1.27	.64	.16	34	8
74	657	.48	60	510	764	267	1.94	136	.12	.8	.49	.13	18	5
10	738	.7	68	497	845	293	2.18	300	.11	.8	.4	.14	22	3
83	1421	.36	131	1119	1910	621	4.82	65	.47	1.9	1.05	.41	57	7
16	1120	.28	107	896	1552	500	4.01	646[15]	.38	1.59	.81	.31	45	5
12	837	.21	80	670	1160	373	3.06	483[15]	.28	1.19	.61	.24	34	4
28	326	.12	34	270	499	122	.73	137	.12	.34	.68	.11	2	3
10	350	.5	28	319	205	50	.9	155	.45	.44	.3	.09	20	6
31	280	.6	33	251	417	149	1.02	73	.09	.41	.31	.1	12	2
17	284	.6	33	254	422	151	.91	143	.09	.41	.32	.1	12	2
7	287	.6	33	256	425	152	1.02	148	.1	.42	.32	.1	12	2
1	89	.29	23	88	223	139	1.26	1	.03	.17	.18	.04	3	1
1	89	.29	23	88	223	139	1.26	1	.03	.17	.18	.04	3	1
0	8	.68	21	28	128	45	.33	1	.01	.03	.11	<.01	4	<1
33	300	.8	54	256	498	165	1.26	76	.1	.43	.32	.1	12	3
149	330	.51	47	278	420	138	1.17	203	.09	.48	.27	.13	2	4
0	10	7.9	80	15	0	166	3.00	175	.30	.07	5.00	.40	100	27
33	301	8.0	113	243	370	286	3.95	251	.39	.46	5.20	.50	112	29
18	307	8.0	113	247	377	289	3.96	315	.40	.47	5.21	.51	112	29
10	310	8.0	124	250	381	289	3.96	315	.40	.48	5.21	.51	112	29
4	312	8.0	108	262	406	292	3.96	327	.39	.41	5.22	.50	113	29
1	13	.48	15	37	130	53	.17	4	.04	.04	.42	.03	4	<1
34	304	.6	47	265	499	172	1.09	80	13	.44	.63	.14	16	3
4	63	.16	20	75	159	103	.21	19	.11	.19	1.1	.09	10	1
37	354	.27	52	303	529	223	1.14	94	.2	.59	1.31	.19	22	3
37	319	.88	47	288	567	273	1.15	64	.16	.69	.46	.14	10	1
32	344	.26	35	289	492	232	1.01	90	.13	.52	.52	.15	9	2
213	297	1.1	37	310	387	209	1.53	146	.11	.5	.3	.13	24	1
478	1405	.96	149	1075	2053	926	11.3	1064	.42	2.63	1.08	.49	22	6
59	176	.12	18	134	257	116	1.41	133	.05	.33	.13	.06	3	1
23	66	.05	7	50	97	44	.53	50	.02	.12	.05	.02	1	<1
153	236	.43	25	199	338	153	1.99	199	.08	.45	.18	.1	9	1
701	1212	.83	131	927	1770	867	9.74	1758	.36	2.27	.93	.43	23	5
88	151	.1	16	115	221	108	1.21	219	.04	.28	.12	.05	2	1

(15)With added vitamin A.

• *Table F–1* Food Composition

Grp	Computer Code No.	Food Description	Measure	Wt (g)	H_2O (%)	Ener (cal)	Prot (g)	Carb (g)	Dietary Fiber (g)	Fat (g)	Fat Breakdown (g) Sat	Mono	Poly
DAIRY—Con.													
		Milk Desserts—Con.											
		Ice milk, vanilla (about 4% fat):											
		Hardened:											
2	129	½ gallon	½ gal	1048	69	1467	41	232	0	45	28	13	1.7
2	130	Cup	1 c	131	69	184	5	29	0	6	3.5	1.6	.2
2	131	Soft serve (about 3% fat)	1 c	175	70	223	8	38	0	5	2.9	1.3	.2
		Pudding, canned, 5 oz can = .55 cup:											
2	135	Chocolate	1 ea	142	68	205	3	30	<1	11	9.5	.5	.1
2	136	Tapioca	1 ea	142	74	160	3	28	0	5	4.8	t	t
2	137	Vanilla	1 ea	142	69	220	2	33	0	10	9.5	.3	.1
		Puddings, prepared from dry mix with whole milk:											
2	138	Chocolate, instant	1 c	260	71	310	8	54	<1	8	4.6	2.2	.4
2	139	Chocolate, regular, cooked	½ c	130	73	150	4	25	<1	4	2.4	1.1	.1
2	140	Rice, cooked	½ c	132	73	155	4	27	<1	4	2.3	1.1	.1
2	141	Tapioca, cooked	½ c	130	75	145	4	25	0	4	2.3	1.1	.1
2	142	Vanilla, instant	½ c	130	73	150	4	27	0	4	2.2	1.1	.2
2	143	Vanilla, regular, cooked	½ c	130	74	145	4	25	0	4	2.3	1	.1
		Sherbet (2% fat):											
2	132	½ gallon	½ gal	1542	66	2158	17	469	0	31	19	8.8	1.1
2	133	Cup	1 c	193	66	270	2	59	0	4	2.4	1.1	.1
2	144	Soy milk	1 c	240	93	79	7	4	0	5	.5	.8	2.0
2	1584	Yogurt, frozen, low fat[16]	½ c	87	70	110	4	17	0	2	1.1	.5	<1
		Yogurt, low fat:											
2	145	Fruit added[17]	1 c	227	74	231	10	43	<1	2	1.6	.7	.1
2	146	Plain	1 c	227	85	144	12	16	0	3	2.3	1.0	.1
2	147	Vanilla or coffee flavor	1 c	227	79	193	11	31	0	3	1.8	.8	.1
2	148	Yogurt, made with nonfat milk	1 c	227	85	127	13	17	0	<1	.3	.1	t
2	149	Yogurt, made with whole milk	1 c	227	88	138	8	11	0	7	4.8	2.0	.2
EGGS[18]													
		Raw, large:											
3	150	Whole, without shell	1 ea	50	75	75	6	1	0	5	1.6	1.6	.7
3	151	White	1 ea	33.4	88	17	4	<1	0	0	0	0	0
3	152	Yolk	1 ea	16.6	49	59	3	<1	0	5	1.6	1.9	.7
		Cooked:											
3	153	Fried in margarine	1 ea	46	69	91	6	1	0	7	1.9	2.7	1.3
3	154	Hard-cooked, shell removed	1 ea	50	75	79	6	1	0	5	1.6	2.0	.7
3	155	Hard-cooked, chopped	1 c	136	75	211	17	2	0	14	4.5	5.5	2.0
3	156	Poached, no added salt	1 ea	50	75	75	6	1	0	5	1.5	1.9	.7
3	157	Scrambled with milk and margarine	1 ea	61	73	100	7	1	0	7	2.2	2.9	1.3
FATS and OILS													
		Butter:											
4	158	Stick	½ c	113	16	813	1	<1	0	92	57	27	3.4
4	159	Tablespoon	1 tbsp	14	16	100	<1	<1	0	12	7.2	3.3	.4
4	160	Pat (about 1 tsp)[19]	1 ea	5	16	34	<1	<1	0	4	2.5	1.2	.2

(16) Data is a composite of USDA information and several manufacturers.

(17) Carbohydrate and calories vary widely—consult label if more precise values are needed.

(18) This data is newest revised information from the USDA with 24% less cholesterol.

(19) Pat is 1″ square, ⅓″ thick; about 1 tsp; 90 per lb.

GRP KEY: 1=BEV **2=DAIRY** 3=EGGS 4=FAT/OIL 5=FRUIT 6=BAKERY 7=GRAIN 8=FISH 9=BEEF 10=POULTRY 11=SAUSAGE 12=MIXED/FAST 13=NUTS/SEEDS 14=SWEETS 15=VEG/LEG 16=MISC 22=SOUP/SAUCE

Chol (mg)	Calc (mg)	Iron (mg)	Magn (mg)	Phos (mg)	Pota (mg)	Sodi (mg)	Zinc (mg)	VT-A (RE)	Thia (mg)	Ribo (mg)	Niac (mg)	V-B6 (mg)	Fola (µg)	VT-C (mg)
146	1404	1.47	147	1035	2117	838	4.40	419	.61	2.78	.94	.68	21	6
18	176	.18	19	129	265	105	.55	52	.08	.35	.12	.09	3	1
13	274	.28	29	202	412	163	.86	44	.12	.54	.18	.13	5	1
1	74	1.2	24	117	254	285	.70	31	.04	.17	.6	.03	3	<1
1	119	.3	24	113	212	252	.70	<1	.03	.14	.4	.03	3	<1
1	79	.2	24	94	155	305	.70	<1	.03	.12	.6	.03	3	<1
28	260	.6	48	658	352	880	1.18	66	.08	.36	.22	.13	10	2
15	146	.2	24	120	190	167	.59	34	.05	.2	.13	.06	4	1
15	133	.5	16	110	165	140	.60	33	.10	.18	.6	.05	6	1
15	131	.1	16	103	167	152	.50	34	.04	.18	.1	.05	6	1
15	129	.1	16	273	164	375	.50	33	.04	.17	.1	.05	6	1
15	132	.1	16	102	166	178	.50	34	.04	.18	.1	.05	6	1
113	827	2.47	124	594	1588	709	10.6	308	.26	.71	1.05	.2	108	31
14	103	.31	15	74	198	88	1.33	39	.03	.09	.13	.03	14	4
0	10	1.38	45	117	338	30	.54	8	.39	.17	.35	.10	4	0
7	120	.05	5	980	148	45	.56	17	.03	.14	.07	.03	7	<1
10	345	.16	31	325	442	125	1.68	25	.08	.4	.22	.09	21	2
14	415	.18	40	326	531	159	2.02	36	.10	.49	.26	.11	25	2
11	388	.16	36	306	497	150	1.88	30	.10	.46	.24	.10	23	2
4	452	.2	43	354	579	173	2.20	5	.11	.53	.28	.12	28	2
30	275	.11	27	216	352	104	1.34	68	.07	.32	.17	.07	16	1
213	25	.72	5	89	60	61	.55	97	.03	.25	.04	.07	25	0
0	2	.01	4	4	48	55	<.1	0	<.01	.15	.03	<.01	1	0
213	23	.7	1	81	16	7	.54	97	.03	.11	.01	.07	24	0
211	25	.72	5	89	61	162	.55	114	.03	.24	.04	.07	18	0
215	25	.72	5	86	63	62	.55	84	.03	.26	.03	.06	22	0
574	68	1.95	14	233	171	169	1.5	227	.09	.70	.09	.16	61	0
212	25	.72	5	89	60	61	.55	95	.03	.22	.03	.06	18	0
215	44	.72	7	104	84	171	.6	119	.03	.26	.05	.07	18	0
247	27	.18	2	26	29	933[20]	.06	852[21]	.01	.04	.05	<.01	3	0
31	3	.02	<1	3	4	116[20]	.01	106[21]	<.01	<.01	.01	t	<1	0
11	1	.01	<1	1	1	41[20]	<.01	38[21]	t	<.01	<.01	t	<1	0

(20)For salted butter; unsalted butter contains 12 mg sodium per stick or ½ c, 1.5 mg/tbsp, or .5 mg/pat.

(21)Values for vitamin A are a year-round average.

(For purposes of calculations, use "0" for t, <1, <.1, <.01, etc.)

Table F–1 Food Composition

Grp	Computer Code No.	Food Description	Measure	Wt (g)	H_2O (%)	Ener (cal)	Prot (g)	Carb (g)	Dietary Fiber (g)	Fat (g)	Fat Breakdown (g) Sat	Mono	Poly
FATS and OILS—Con.													
		Fats, cooking:											
4	1363	Bacon fat	1 tbsp	14	<1	126	0	0	0	14	5.0	6.7	1.7
4	1362	Beef fat/tallow	1 c	205	0	1837	0	0	0	205	102	85.6	8.2
4	1364	Chicken fat	1 c	205	<1	1846	0	0	0	205	61.2	92.0	43.0
		Vegetable shortening:											
4	161	Cup	1 c	205	0	1812	0	0	0	205	51	91	54
4	162	Tablespoon	1 tbsp	13	0	15	0	0	0	13	3.3	5.8	3.4
		Lard:											
4	163	Cup	1 c	205	0	1849	0	0	0	205	80	93	23
4	164	Tablespoon	1 tbsp	13	0	115	0	0	0	13	5.1	5.9	1.5
		Margarine:											
		Imitation (about 40% fat), soft:											
4	165	8-oz container	8 oz	227	58	785	1	1	0	88	18	36	31
4	166	Tablespoon	1 tbsp	14	58	50	<.1	<.1	0	6	1.1	2.2	2.0
		Regular, hard (about 80% fat):											
4	167	Cup	½ c	113	16	812	1	1	0	91	18	41	29
4	168	Tablespoon	1 tbsp	14	16	100	<1	<1	0	11	2.3	5.1	3.6
4	169	Pat[19]	1 ea	5	16	36	<.1	<.1	0	4	.8	1.8	1.3
		Regular, soft (about 80% fat):											
4	170	8-oz container	8 oz	227	16	1626	2	1	0	183	31	65	79
4	171	Tablespoon	1 tbsp	14	16	100	1	<.1	0	11	2.0	4.0	4.9
		Spread (about 60% fat), hard:											
4	172	Cup	½ c	113	37	610	1	0	0	69	16	29	20
4	173	Tablespoon	1 tbsp	14	37	75	<.1	0	0	9	2.0	3.6	2.5
4	174	Pat[19]	1 ea	5	37	25	<.1	0	0	3	.7	1.3	.9
		Spread (about 60% fat), soft:											
4	175	8 oz container	8 oz	227	37	1225	1	0	0	138	29	72	31
4	176	Tablespoon	1 tbsp	14	37	75	<.1	0	0	9	1.8	4.4	1.9
		Oils:											
		Canola:											
4	1585	Cup	1 c	218	0	1927	0	0	0	218	13.1	128	65
4	1586	Tablespoon	1 tbsp	14	0	125	0	0	0	14	.8	8.2	4.1
		Corn:											
4	177	Cup	1 c	218	0	1927	0	0	0	218	28	53	128
4	178	Tablespoon	1 tbsp	14	0	125	0	0	0	14	1.8	3.4	8.2
		Olive:											
4	179	Cup	1 c	216	0	1909	0	0	0	216	29	159	18
4	180	Tablespoon	1 tbsp	14	0	125	0	0	0	14	1.9	10	1.2
		Peanut:											
4	181	Cup	1 c	216	0	1909	0	0	0	216	36	100	69
4	182	Tablespoon	1 tbsp	14	0	125	0	0	0	14	2.4	6.5	4.5
		Safflower:											
4	183	Cup	1 c	218	0	1927	0	0	0	218	20	26	162
4	184	Tablespoon	1 tbsp	14	0	125	0	0	0	14	1.3	1.7	10
		Soybean:											
4	185	Cup	1 c	218	0	1927	0	0	0	218	33	94	82
4	186	Tablespoon	1 tbsp	14	0	125	0	0	0	14	2	6	5
		Soybean/cottonseed:											
4	187	Cup	1 c	218	0	1927	0	0	0	218	39	64	105
4	188	Tablespoon	1 tbsp	14	0	125	0	0	0	14	2.5	4	7

(19) Pat is 1″ square, ⅓″ thick; about 1 tsp; 90 per lb.

GRP KEY: 1 = BEV 2 = DAIRY 3 = EGGS **4 = FAT/OIL** 5 = FRUIT 6 = BAKERY 7 = GRAIN 8 = FISH 9 = BEEF 10 = POULTRY 11 = SAUSAGE 12 = MIXED/FAST 13 = NUTS/SEEDS 14 = SWEETS 15 = VEG/LEG 16 = MISC 22 = SOUP/SAUCE

Chol (mg)	Calc (mg)	Iron (mg)	Magn (mg)	Phos (mg)	Pota (mg)	Sodi (mg)	Zinc (mg)	VT-A (RE)	Thia (mg)	Ribo (mg)	Niac (mg)	V-B6 (mg)	Fola (μg)	VT-C (mg)
84	—	—	—	—	—	140	—	<1	—	—	—	0	—	—
223	2	.41	—	27	0	0	—	<1	<.01	<.01	<.01	<.01	<1	0
174	—	—	—	—	—	—	—	350	—	—	—	0	0	0
0	0	0	0	0	0	0	.10	0	0	0	0	0	0	0
0	0	0	0	0	0	0	0	0	0	0	0	0	0	0
195	<1	0	<1	6	<1	<1	.23	0	0	0	0	0	0	0
12	<1	0	<1	<1	<1	<1	.01	0	0	0	0	0	0	0
0	40	0	3	31	57	2178[22]	.23	2254[23]	.01	.05	.03	.01	2	<1
0	3	0	<1	2	4	136[22]	.03	141[23]	<.01	<.01	<.01	<.01	<1	<1
0	34	.07	3	26	48	1066[22]	.23	1122[23]	.01	.04	.03	.01	1	<1
0	4	.01	<1	3	6	133[22]	.03	139[23]	<.01	<.01	<.01	<.01	<1	<1
0	2	.01	<1	1	2	47[22]	.01	50[23]	t	<.01	<.01	t	<1	<1
0	60	0	5	46	86	2448[22]	.46	2254[23]	.02	.07	.05	.02	2	<1
0	4	0	<1	3	5	153[22]	.03	140[23]	<.01	<.01	<.01	<.01	<1	<1
0	24	0	2	18	34	1123[22]	.17	1122[23]	<.01	.03	.02	.01	1	<1
0	3	0	<1	2	4	139[22]	.02	139[23]	<.01	<.01	<.01	<.01	<1	<1
0	1	0	<1	1	2	50[22]	.01	50[23]	t	<.01	<.01	t	<1	<1
0	47	0	4	37	68	2256[22]	.35	2254[23]	.16	.06	.04	.01	2	<1
0	3	0	<1	2	4	139[22]	.02	139[23]	.01	<.01	<.01	<.01	<1	<1
0	0	0	0	0	0	0	—	0	0	0	0	0	0	0
0	0	0	0	0	0	0	—	0	0	0	0	0	0	0
0	0	.01	0	2	0	0	.02	0	0	0	0	0	<1	0
0	0	0	0	0	0	0	.03	0	0	0	0	0	0	0
0	<1	.83	<1	3	0	0	.13	0	0	0	0	0	<1	0
0	<1	.05	<1	<1	0	0	.01	0	0	0	0	0	0	0
0	t	.06	<1	0	0	0	.02	t	0	0	0	0	<1	0
0	t	<.01	<1	0	0	0	<.01	t	0	0	0	0	0	0
0	0	0	—	0	0	0	.41	0	0	0	0	0	0	0
0	0	0	—	0	0	0	.03	0	0	0	0	0	0	0
0	<1	.05	<1	1	0	0	.4	0	0	0	0	0	<1	0
0	t	0	<1	t	0	0	.03	0	0	0	0	0	t	0
0	0	0	—	0	0	0	.4	0	0	0	0	0	<1	0
0	0	0	—	0	0	0	.03	0	0	0	0	0	0	0

(22)For salted margarine.
(23)Based on average vitamin A content of fortified margarine. Federal specifications require a minimum of 15,000 IU/lb.

(For purposes of calculations, use "0" for t, <1, <.1, <.01, etc.)

Table F–1 Food Composition

Grp	Computer Code No.	Food Description	Measure	Wt (g)	H_2O (%)	Ener (cal)	Prot (g)	Carb (g)	Dietary Fiber (g)	Fat (g)	Fat Breakdown (g) Sat	Mono	Poly
		FATS and OILS—Con.											
		Oils—Con.											
		Sunflower:											
4	189	Cup	1 c	218	0	1927	0	0	0	218	23	43	143
4	190	Tablespoon	1 tbsp	14	0	125	0	0	0	14	1.4	2.7	9.2
		Salad dressings/ sandwich spreads:											
4	191	Blue cheese salad dressing	1 tbsp	15	32	75	1	1	<1	8	1.5	1.9	4.3
		French salad dressing:											
4	192	Regular	1 tbsp	16	35	85	<.1	1	<1	9	1.4	4	3.5
4	193	Low calorie	1 tbsp	16	75	24	<.1	2	<1	2	.2	.3	1
		Italian salad dressing:											
4	194	Regular	1 tbsp	14	34	80	<1	1	<1	9	1.3	3.7	3.2
4	195	Low calorie	1 tbsp	15	86	5	<.1	1	<1	1.5	.2	.3	.9
		Mayonnaise:											
4	196	Regular	1 tbsp	14	15	100	<1	<1	0	11	1.7	3.2	5.8
4	197	Imitation, low calorie	1 tbsp	15	63	35	0	2	0	3	.5	.7	1.6
4	198	Ranch style salad dressing	½ c	119	35	435	4	6	0	45	6.7	19	17
		Mayo type salad dressing:											
4	199	Regular	1 tbsp	15	40	58	<1	4	0	5	.7	1.4	2.7
4	1030	Low calorie	1 tbsp	15	63	35	<1	2	0	3	.5	.8	1.4
4	200	Tartar sauce	1 tbsp	14	34	74	<1	1	<1	8	1.2	2.6	3.9
		Thousand Island salad dressing:											
4	201	Regular	1 tbsp	16	46	60	<1	2	<1	6	1.0	1.3	3.2
4	202	Low calorie	1 tbsp	15	69	25	<1	2	<1	2	.2	.4	.9
		Salad dressings, prepared from home recipe:											
4	203	Cooked type[24]	1 tbsp	16	69	25	1	2	0	2	.5	.6	.3
4	204	Vinegar and oil	1 tbsp	16	47	70	0	0	0	8	1.5	2.4	3.9
		FRUITS and FRUIT JUICES											
		Apples:											
		Fresh, raw, with peel:											
5	205	2¾″ diam (about 3 per lb with cores)	1 ea	138	84	80	<1	21	3	<1	.1	t	.1
5	206	3¼″ diam (about 2 per lb with cores)	1 ea	212	84	125	<1	32	5	1	.1	t	.2
5	207	Raw, peeled slices	1 c	110	84	65	<1	16	3	<1	.1	t	.1
5	208	Dried, sulfured	10 ea	64	32	155	1	42	8	<1	t	t	.1
5	209	Apple juice, bottled or canned	1 c	248	88	116	<1	29	<1	<1	.1	t	.1
		Applesauce:											
5	210	Sweetened	1 c	255	80	195	<1	51	4	<1	<.1	t	.1
5	211	Unsweetened	1 c	244	88	106	<1	28	4	<1	<.1	t	<.1
		Apricots:											
5	212	Raw, without pits (about 12 per lb with pits)	3 ea	106	86	51	1	12	2	<1	t	.2	.1
		Canned (fruit and liquid):											
5	213	Heavy syrup	1 c	258	78	214	1	55	4	<1	t	.1	t
5	214	Halves	3 ea	85	78	70	<1	18	1	<.1	t	t	t
5	215	Juice pack	1 c	248	87	119	2	31	4	<.1	t	t	t
5	216	Halves	3 ea	84	87	40	1	10	1	<.1	t	t	t
		Dried:											
5	217	Dried halves	10 ea	35	31	83	1	22	3	<1	t	.1	t
5	218	Cooked, unsweetened, with liquid	1 c	250	75	210	3	55	7	<1	t	.2	.1
5	219	Apricot nectar, canned	1 c	251	85	141	1	36	2	<1	t	.1	t

(24) Fatty acid values apply to product made with regular margarine.

GRP KEY: 1=BEV 2=DAIRY 3=EGGS **4=FAT/OIL** 5=FRUIT 6=BAKERY 7=GRAIN 8=FISH 9=BEEF 10=POULTRY 11=SAUSAGE 12=MIXED/FAST 13=NUTS/SEEDS 14=SWEETS 15=VEG/LEG 16=MISC 22=SOUP/SAUCE

Chol (mg)	Calc (mg)	Iron (mg)	Magn (mg)	Phos (mg)	Pota (mg)	Sodi (mg)	Zinc (mg)	VT-A (RE)	Thia (mg)	Ribo (mg)	Niac (mg)	V-B6 (mg)	Fola (µg)	VT-C (mg)
0	0	0	0	0	0	0	—	0	0	0	0	0	0	0
0	0	0	0	0	0	0	—	0	0	0	0	0	0	0
3	12	.03	11	11	6	164	.04	10	<.01	.02	.01	<.01	4	t
0	2	.06	<1	1	2	188	.01	t	t	t	t	<.01	0	t
0	6	.07	—	5	3	306	.03	t	t	t	t	0	t	t
0	1	.03	<1	1	5	162	.02	3	t	t	t	.03	0	t
0	1	.03	<1	1	4	136	0	t	t	t	t	0	t	t
8	2	.07	<1	4	5	80	.02	12	<.01	<.01	<.01	<.01	<1	0
4	0	0	—	0	2	75	—	0	0	0	0	0	t	0
47	119	.31	12	100	158	522	.43	86	.04	.17	.08	.05	6	1
4	2	.03	<1	4	1	105	0	13	<.01	<.01	t	<.01	t	0
4	3	.03	—	4	1	75	.02	10	.03	t	t	—	t	—
4	3	.1	<1	4	11	182	.02	9	<.01	<.01	<.01	<.01	<1	t
4	2	.09	<1	3	18	110	.03	15	<.01	<.01	.03	<.01	6	t
2	2	.09	<1	3	17	153	0	14	<.01	<.01	.03	<.01	<1	t
9	13	.08	—	14	19	117	0	20	.01	.02	.04	0	<1	t
0	0	0	—	0	1	0	—	0	0	0	0	0	—	0
0	10	.25	6	10	159	1	.05	7	.02	.02	.11	.07	4	8
0	15	.38	9	23	244	1	.08	11	.04	.03	.16	.1	6	12
0	4	.1	3	8	124	1	.04	5	.02	.01	.1	.05	<1	4
0	9	.9	10	24	288	56[25]	.13	0	0	.1	.59	.08	1	3
0	17	.92	8	17	295	7	.07	<1	.05	.04	.25	.07	1	2[26]
0	10	1	7	18	156	8	.1	3	.03	.07	.50	.07	2	4[26]
0	7	.29	7	18	183	5	.06	7	.03	.06	.46	.06	2	3[26]
0	15	.58	8	21	313	1	.28	166	.03	.04	.64	.06	9	11
0	23	.77	18	33	361	10	.27	317	.05	.06	.97	.14	4	8
0	7	.26	6	10	119	3	.09	105	.02	.02	.32	.05	1	3
0	30	.74	24	50	409	9	.27	419	.05	.05	.85	.18	5	12
0	10	.25	8	17	139	3	.1	142	.02	.02	.29	.06	2	4
0	16	1.65	16	41	482	4	.26	253	<.01	.05	1.05	.06	4	1
0	40	4.2	42	103	1222	8	.66	591	.02	.08	2.36	.28	0	4
0	18	.96	13	23	286	8	.23	330	.02	.04	.65	.16	3	2[27]

(25)Sodium bisulfite used to preserve color; unsulfured product would contain lower levels of sodium.

(26)Value based on products without added vitamin C. Bottled apple juice with added vitamin C usually contains 41.6 mg/100 g, or 103 mg per cup. Check label for specific vitamin C values.

(27)Without added vitamin C. Products with added vitamin C contain 136 mg per cup. Check label.

(For purposes of calculations, use "0" for t, <1, <.1, <.01, etc.)

Table F–1 Food Composition

Grp	Computer Code No.	Food Description	Measure	Wt (g)	H_2O (%)	Ener (cal)	Prot (g)	Carb (g)	Dietary Fiber (g)	Fat (g)	Fat Breakdown (g) Sat	Mono	Poly
		FRUITS and FRUIT JUICES—Con.											
		Avocados, raw, edible part only:											
5	220	California (½ lb with refuse)	1 ea	173	73	305	4	12	17	30	4.5	19	3.5
5	221	Florida (1 lb with refuse)	1 ea	304	80	340	5	27	29	27	5	15	5
5	222	Mashed, fresh, average	1 c	230	74	370	5	17	22	35	6	22	5
		Bananas, raw, without peel:											
5	223	Whole, 8¾″ long (weighs 175 g w/peel)	1 ea	114	74	105	1	27	2	1	.2	<.1	.1
5	224	Slices	1 c	150	74	138	2	35	3	1	.3	.1	.1
5	1285	Bananas, dehydrated slices	1 c	100	3	346	4	88	8	2	.7	.2	.3
5	225	Blackberries, raw	1 c	144	86	74	1	18	10	1	.3	.1	.1
		Blueberries:											
5	226	Fresh	1 c	145	85	82	1	21	4	1	<.1	.2	.3
		Frozen, sweetened:											
5	227	10-oz container	10 oz	284	77	230	1	62	7	<1	.1	.1	.2
5	228	Cup	1 c	230	77	185	1	51	5	<1	.1	.1	.2
		Cherries:											
5	229	Sour, red pitted, canned water pack	1 c	244	90	90	2	22	3	<1	.1	.1	.1
5	230	Sweet, raw, without pits	10 ea	68	81	49	1	11	1	1	.1	.2	.2
5	231	Cranberry juice cocktail[28]	1 c	253	85	145	<1[29]	36	1	<1	t	t	.1
5	232	Cranberry-apple juice	1 c	253	86	169	<1	43	1	1[30]	.2	.1	.4
5	233	Cranberry sauce, canned, strained	1 c	277	61	419	1	108	6	<1	<.1	.1	.2
		Dates:											
5	234	Whole, without pits	10 ea	83	22	228	2	61	7	<1	.2	.1	t
5	235	Chopped	1 c	178	22	489	4	131	15	1	.3	.2	.1
5	236	Figs, dried	10 ea	187	28	477	6	122	21	2	.4	.5	1.1
		Fruit cocktail, canned, fruit and liquid:											
5	237	Heavy syrup pack	1 c	255	80	185	1	48	3	<1	<.1	<.1	.1
5	238	Juice pack	1 c	248	87	115	1	29	3	<1	t	t	t
		Grapefruit:											
		Raw 3¾″ diam-weight with rind is 241 g for one-half											
5	239	Pink/red, half fruit, edible part	1 half	123	91	37	1	9	2	<1	t	t	<.1
5	240	White, half fruit, edible part	1 half	118	90	39	1	10	2	<1	t	t	<.1
5	241	Canned sections with liquid	1 c	254	84	152	1	39	3	<1	<.1	<.1	.1
		Grapefruit juice:											
5	242	Fresh, raw	1 c	247	90	96	1	23	1	<1	<.1	<.1	.1
		Canned:											
5	243	Unsweetened	1 c	247	90	93	1	22	1	<1	<.1	<.1	.1
5	244	Sweetened	1 c	250	87	115	1	28	1	<1	<.1	<.1	.1
		Frozen concentrate, unsweetened:											
5	245	Undiluted, 6-fl-oz can	¾ c	207	62	300	4	72	3	1	.2	.2	.3
5	246	Diluted with 3 cans water	1 c	247	89	102	1	24	1	<1	<.1	<.1	.1
		Grapes, raw, European type (adherent skin):											
5	247	Thompson seedless	10 ea	50	81	35	<1	9	1	<1	.1	t	.1
5	248	Tokay/Emperor, seeded types	10 ea	57	81	40	<1	10	1	<1	.1	t	.1
		Grape juice:											
5	249	Bottled or canned	1 c	253	84	155	1	38	1	<1	.1	t	.1
		Frozen concentrate, sweetened:											
5	250	Undiluted, 6-fl-oz can	¾ c	216	54	385	1	96	4	1	.2	<.1	.2
5	251	Diluted with 3 cans water	1 c	250	87	128	<1	32	1	<1	.1	t	.1

(28) Data here are from the newest USDA *Handbook 8–14* on beverages. These data are somewhat different from that presented in *Handbook 8–9* on fruits and fruit juices.

(29) The newest USDA *Handbook 8–14* data on beverages indicates "0" for protein.

(30) The newest USDA *Handbook 8–14* data on beverages indicates "0" for fat.

GRP KEY: 1=BEV 2=DAIRY 3=EGGS 4=FAT/OIL **5=FRUIT** 6=BAKERY 7=GRAIN 8=FISH 9=BEEF 10=POULTRY 11=SAUSAGE 12=MIXED/FAST 13=NUTS/SEEDS 14=SWEETS 15=VEG/LEG 16=MISC 22=SOUP/SAUCE

Chol (mg)	Calc (mg)	Iron (mg)	Magn (mg)	Phos (mg)	Pota (mg)	Sodi (mg)	Zinc (mg)	VT-A (RE)	Thia (mg)	Ribo (mg)	Niac (mg)	V-B6 (mg)	Fola (µg)	VT-C (mg)
0	19	2.04	70	73	1097	21	.73	106	.19	.21	3.32	.48	113	14
0	33	1.6	104	119	1484	14	1.28	186	.33	.37	5.84	.85	162	24
0	25	2.3	90	95	1378	24	.97	141	.25	.28	4.42	.64	142	18
0	7	.35	32	22	451	1	.19	9	.05	.11	.62	.66	24	10
0	9	.46	43	29	593	1	.25	12	.07	.15	.81	.87	31	14
0	22	1.15	108	74	1491	3	.61	31	.18	.24	2.80	.54	40	7
0	46	.8	29	30	282	0	.39	24	.04	.06	.58	.08	49	30
0	9	.24	7	15	129	9	.16	15	.07	.07	.7	.05	9	20
0	16	1.11	7	20	169	4	.14	12	.06	.15	.72	.17	19	3
0	13	.9	6	16	138	3	.14	10	.05	.12	.58	.14	16	2
0	27	3.34	15	25	240	17	.17	184	.04	.1	.43	.11	20	5
0	10	.3	8	13	152	0	.04	15	.03	.04	.3	.02	3	5
0	8	.38	5	5	45	5	.18	1	.02	.02	.09	.05	<1	90[31]
0	18	.15	5	7	68	5	.1	<1	.01	.05	.15	.06	<1	81[31]
0	11	.61	8	17	72	80	.09	6	.04	.06	.28	.05	3	6
0	27	1	29	33	541	2	.24	4	.08	.08	1.83	.16	14	0
0	58	2.14	63	70	1161	5	.52	9	.16	.18	3.92	.34	29	0
0	269	4.18	111	128	1331	21	.94	25	.13	.17	1.3	.42	16	1
0	16	.73	14	28	224	15	.21	52	.05	.05	.95	.11	1	5
0	20	.53	17	34	235	10	.21	76	.03	.04	0	.13	2	7
0	13	.15	10	11	158	0	.09	32[32]	.04	.03	.24	.05	15	47
0	14	.07	11	9	175	0	.08	1	.04	.02	.32	.05	12	39
0	36	1.02	25	25	328	4	.21	0	.1	.05	.62	.05	22	54
0	22	.49	30	37	400	2	.13	2[33]	.1	.05	.49	.11	52	94
0	17	.49	24	27	378	2	.22	2	.1	.05	.57	.05	26	72
0	20	.9	24	28	405	5	.15	2	.1	.06	.8	.05	26	67
0	56	1.02	78	101	1002	6	.38	6	.3	.16	1.6	.32	26	248
0	20	.34	26	34	337	2	.12	2	.1	.05	.54	.11	52	83
0	5	.13	3	7	92	1	.03	4	.05	.03	.15	.06	4	5
0	6	.15	4	8	105	1	.03	4	.05	.03	.17	.06	4	6
0	22	.61	24	27	334	8	.13	2	.07	.09	.66	.16	7	<1
0	28	.78	32	32	160	15	.28	6	.11	.2	.93	.32	9	179[34]
0	10	.26	11	11	53	5	.10	2	.04	.07	.31	.11	4	60[34]

(31) Nutrient added.
(32) Vitamin A in Texas red grapefruit would be 74 RE.
(33) This is Vitamin A for white grapefruit juice; pink or red grapefruit juice = 109 RE per cup.
(34) With added Vitamin C (ascorbic acid).

Table F–1 Food Composition

Grp	Computer Code No.	Food Description	Measure	Wt (g)	H_2O (%)	Ener (cal)	Prot (g)	Carb (g)	Dietary Fiber (g)	Fat (g)	Fat Breakdown (g) Sat	Mono	Poly
		FRUITS and FRUIT JUICES—Con.											
5	252	Kiwi fruit, raw, peeled (88g with peel)	1 ea	76	83	46	1	11	3	<1	t	.2	.2
5	253	Lemons, raw, without peel and seeds (about 4 per lb whole)	1 ea	58	89	17	1	5	1	<1	t	t	.1
		Lemon juice:											
		Fresh:											
5	254	Cup	1 c	244	91	60	1	21	1	t	t	t	t
5	255	Tablespoon	1 tbsp	15	91	4	<.1	1	<1	t	t	t	t
		Canned or bottled, unsweetened:											
5	256	Cup	1 c	244	92	52	1	16	1	<1	.1	<.1	.2
5	257	Tablespoon	1 tbsp	15	92	3	<1	1	<1	<.1	t	t	t
		Frozen, single strength, unsweetened:											
5	258	Cup	1 c	244	92	54	1	16	1	<1	.1	<.1	.2
5	259	Tablespoon	1 tbsp	15	92	3	<1	1	<1	<.1	t	t	t
		Lime juice:											
		Fresh:											
5	260	Cup	1 c	246	90	65	1	22	1	<1	<.1	<.1	.1
5	261	Tablespoon	1 tbsp	15	90	4	<1	1	<1	<.1	t	t	t
5	262	Canned or bottled, unsweetened	1 c	246	92	50	1	16	1	1	.1	.1	.2
5	263	Mangos, raw, edible part (weighs 300 g with skin and seeds)	1 ea	207	82	135	1	35	7	1	.1	.2	.1
		Melons, raw, without rind and cavity contents:											
5	264	Cantaloupe, 5″ diam (2⅓ lb whole with refuse), orange flesh	½ ea	267	90	94	2	22	3	1	.1	.1	.2
5	265	Honeydew, 6½″ diam (5¼ lb whole with refuse), slice = 1⁄10 melon	1 slice	129	90	45	1	12	1	<1	t	t	<.1
5	266	Nectarines, raw, without pits, 2½″ diam	1 ea	136	86	67	1	16	3	1	.1	.2	.3
		Oranges, raw:											
5	267	Whole without peel and seeds, 2⅝″ dm. (weighs 180 g with peel and seeds)	1 ea	131	87	60	1	15	3	<1	t	<.1	<.1
5	268	Sections, without membranes	1 c	180	87	85	2	21	4	<1	<.1	<.1	<.1
		Orange juice:											
5	269	Fresh, all varieties	1 c	248	88	111	2	26	1	<1	.1	.1	.1
5	270	Canned, unsweetened	1 c	249	89	105	1	25	<1	<1	<.1	.1	.1
5	271	Chilled	1 c	249	88	110	2	25	<1	1	.1	.1	.2
		Frozen concentrate:											
5	272	Undiluted (6-oz can)	¾ c	213	58	339	5	81	2	<1	.1	.1	.1
5	273	Diluted with 3 parts water by volume	1 c	249	88	110	2	27	<1	<1	t	<.1	<.1
5	1345	Orange juice, from dry crystals	1 c	248	89	114	2	27	0	<1	.1	.1	.1
5	274	Orange and grapefruit juice, canned	1 c	247	89	105	1	25	<1	<1	<.1	<.1	.1
		Papayas, raw:											
5	275	½″ slices	1 c	140	89	60	1	14	2	<1	.1	.1	<.1
5	276	Whole fruit, 3½″ diam by 5⅛″, without seeds and skin (1 lb with refuse)	1 ea	304	89	117	2	30	5	<1	.1	.1	.1
5	1031	Papaya nectar, canned	1 c	250	85	142	<1	36	2	<1	.1	.1	.1
		Peaches:											
5	277	Raw, whole, 2½″ diam, peeled, pitted (about 4 per lb whole)	1 ea	87	88	37	1	10	2	<1	t	<.1	<.1

(Computer code number is for West Diet Analysis program)

GRP KEY: 1=BEV 2=DAIRY 3=EGGS 4=FAT/OIL **5=FRUIT** 6=BAKERY 7=GRAIN 8=FISH 9=BEEF 10=POULTRY 11=SAUSAGE 12=MIXED/FAST 13=NUTS/SEEDS 14=SWEETS 15=VEG/LEG 16=MISC 22=SOUP/SAUCE

Chol (mg)	Calc (mg)	Iron (mg)	Magn (mg)	Phos (mg)	Pota (mg)	Sodi (mg)	Zinc (mg)	VT-A (RE)	Thia (mg)	Ribo (mg)	Niac (mg)	V-B6 (mg)	Fola (µg)	VT-C (mg)
0	20	.3	23	30	252	4	.08[35]	13	.02	.04	.4	.05[35]	17[35]	75
0	15	.35	2	9	80	1	.06	2	.02	.01	.06	.05	7	31
0	18	.08	16	14	303	2	.12	5	.07	.02	.24	.12	32	112
0	1	<.01	1	1	19	<1	.01	<1	<.01	<.01	.02	.01	2	7
0	26	.31	22	21	248	50[36]	.15	4	.10	.02	.48	.11	25	61
0	2	.02	1	1	15	3[36]	.01	<1	.01	<.01	.03	.01	2	4
0	19	.30	20	20	218	4	.12	4	.14	.03	.33	.15	23	77
0	1	.02	1	1	14	<1	.01	<1	.01	<.01	.02	.01	1	5
0	22	.08	14	18	268	2	.15	3	.05	.03	.25	.11	21	72
0	1	<.01	1	1	17	<1	.01	<1	<.01	<.01	.02	.08	1	5
0	30	.6	16	25	185	39[36]	.15	4	.08	.01	.4	.07	20	16
0	21	2.6	18	22	323	4	.07	806	.12	.12	1.21	.28	39	57
0	29	.56	19	45	825	24	.43	861	.1	.06	1.53	.31	80	113
0	8	.09	9	13	350	13	.11	5	.1	.02	.77	.08	39	32
0	6	.21	11	22	288	0	.12	100	.02	.06	1.35	.03	5	7
0	52	.14	13	18	237	<1	.09	27	.11	.05	.37	.08	40	70
0	72	.19	18	25	326	<1	.4	37	.16	.07	.51	.11	83	96
0	27	.50	27	42	496	2	.12	50	.22	.07	.99	.1	109	124
0	20	1.1	27	35	436	5	.17	44	.15	.04	.4	.1	15	86
0	25	.42	28	27	473	2	.11	19[37]	.28	.05	.7	.13	45[37]	82[37]
0	68	.75	73	121	1436	6	.38	59	.6	.14	1.53	.33	331	294
0	22	.27	24	40	474	2	.13	19	.2	.04	.5	.11	109	97
0	40	.02	5	31	50	1	—	.50	.20	.07	1.00	0	0	80
0	20	1.1	24	35	390	7	.18	29	.14	.07	.83	.06	20	72
0	33	.3	14	12	247	9	.10	282	.04	.05	.47	.03	26	92
0	72	.3	31	16	780	8	.22	612	.08	.10	1.03	.06	48	188
0	24	.86	8	1	78	14	.38	28	.02	.01	.38	.02	5	8
0	4	.1	6	10	171	0	.12	47	.02	.04	.86	.02	3	6

(35)Data are estimated from other fruit data.

(36)Sodium benzoate and sodium bisulfite added as preservatives.

(37)Values for juice from California oranges indicate the following values for 1 c: 36 RE of vitamin A, 72µg of folacin, and 106 mg of vitamin C.

Table F–1 Food Composition

Grp	Computer Code No.	Food Description	Measure	Wt (g)	H_2O (%)	Ener (cal)	Prot (g)	Carb (g)	Dietary Fiber (g)	Fat (g)	Fat Breakdown (g) Sat	Mono	Poly
		FRUITS and FRUIT JUICES—Con.											
		Peaches—Con.											
5	278	Raw, sliced	1 c	170	88	73	1	19	3	<1	t	.1	.1
		Canned, fruit and liquid:											
		Heavy syrup pack:											
5	279	Cup	1 c	256	79	190	1	51	3	<1	<.1	.1	.1
5	280	Half	1 ea	81	79	60	<1	16	1	<1	t	<.1	<.1
		Juice pack:											
5	281	Cup	1 c	248	88	109	2	29	3	<1	t	<.1	<.1
5	282	Half	1 ea	77	88	34	<1	9	1	<1	t	t	t
		Dried:											
5	283	Uncooked	10 ea	130	32	311	5	80	11	1	.1	.4	.5
5	284	Cooked, fruit and liquid	1 c	258	78	200	3	51	4	1	.1	.2	.3
		Frozen, sliced, sweetened:											
5	285	10-oz package	1 ea	284	75	267	2	68	6	<1	<.1	.1	.2
5	286	Cup, thawed measure	1 c	250	75	235	2	60	4	<1	<.1	.1	.2
5	1032	Peach nectar, canned	1 c	249	86	134	1	35	1	<1	t	<.1	<.1
		Pears:											
		Fresh, with skin, cored:											
5	287	Bartlett, 2½″ diam (about 2½ per lb)	1 ea	166	84	98	1	25	5[38]	1	<.1	.1	.2
5	288	Bosc, 2½″ diam (about 3 per lb)	1 ea	141	84	85	1	21	4[38]	1	<.1	.1	.1
5	289	D'Anjou, 3″ diam (about 2 per lb)	1 ea	200	84	120	1	30	6[38]	1	<.1	.2	.2
		Canned, fruit and liquid:											
		Heavy syrup pack:											
5	290	Cup	1 c	255	80	188	1	49	4[38]	<1	t	.1	.1
5	291	Half	1 ea	79	80	59	<1	15	1[38]	<1	t	t	t
		Juice pack:											
5	292	Cup	1 c	248	86	123	1	32	4[38]	<1	t	<.1	<.1
5	293	Half	1 ea	77	86	38	<1	10	1[38]	<1	t	t	t
5	294	Dried halves	10 ea	175	27	459	3	122	19	1	.1	.2	.3
5	1033	Pear nectar, canned	1 c	250	84	149	<1	39	2	<1	t	t	t
		Pineapple:											
5	295	Fresh chunks, diced	1 c	155	86	76	1	19	2	1	<.1	<.1	.2
		Canned, fruit and liquid:											
		Heavy syrup pack:											
5	296	Crushed, chunks, tidbits	1 c	255	79	199	1	52	2	<1	t	<.1	.1
5	297	Slices	1 ea	58	79	45	<1	12	1	<.1	t	t	<.1
		Juice Pack:											
5	298	Crushed, chunks, tidbits	1 c	250	84	150	1	39	2	<1	t	<.1	.1
5	299	Slices	1 ea	58	84	35	<1	9	1	<.1	t	t	t
5	300	Pineapple juice, canned, unsweetened	1 c	250	86	140	1	34	1	<1	t	t	.1
		Plantains, without peel:											
5	301	Raw slices (one whole plantain weighs 179 g without peel)	1 c	148	65	181	2	47	7[39]	1	.2	.1	.1
5	302	Cooked, boiled, sliced	1 c	154	67	179	1	48	7	<1	.1	<.1	.1
		Plums, canned:											
		Fresh:											
5	303	Medium 2⅛″ diam	1 ea	66	85	36	1	9	1	<1	<.1	.3	.1
5	304	Small, 1½″ diam	1 ea	28	85	15	<1	4	1	<1	t	.1	<.1

(38) Dietary fiber data vary 2.4 to 3.4 g/100 g for fresh pears; 1.6 to 2.6 g/100 g for canned pears.

(39) Dietary fiber value partially derived from data for bananas.

GRP KEY: 1=BEV 2=DAIRY 3=EGGS 4=FAT/OIL **5=FRUIT** 6=BAKERY 7=GRAIN 8=FISH 9=BEEF 10=POULTRY 11=SAUSAGE 12=MIXED/FAST 13=NUTS/SEEDS 14=SWEETS 15=VEG/LEG 16=MISC 22=SOUP/SAUCE

Chol (mg)	Calc (mg)	Iron (mg)	Magn (mg)	Phos (mg)	Pota (mg)	Sodi (mg)	Zinc (mg)	VT-A (RE)	Thia (mg)	Ribo (mg)	Niac (mg)	V-B6 (mg)	Fola (µg)	VT-C (mg)
0	9	.19	11	20	335	1	.18	91	.03	.07	1.68	.03	6	11
0	8	.69	13	29	235	16	.22	85	.03	.06	1.57	.05	8	7
0	3	.22	4	9	75	5	.07	27	.01	.02	.5	.01	3	2
0	15	.72	18	43	317	11	.26	94	.02	.04	1.44	.05	8	9
0	5	.21	6	13	98	3	.09	29	.01	.01	.45	.02	3	3
0	37	5.28	54	155	1295	9	.74	281	<.01	.28	5.69	.09	6	6
0	23	3.37	35	99	825	6	.46	51	.01	.05	3.92	.1	<1	10
0	9	1.05	14	31	369	17	.14	81	.04	.10	1.9	.05	9	268[40]
0	8	.93	12	28	325	16	.13	71	.03	.09	1.63	.04	8	236[40]
0	13	.47	11	16	101	10	.20	64	.01	.04	.72	.03	2	13
0	19	.42	9	18	208	1	.20	3	.03	.07	.17	.03	12	7
0	16	.40	8	16	176	<1	.17	3	.03	.06	.1	.03	10	6
0	22	.50	11	22	250	<1	.24	4	.04	.08	.2	.04	14	8
0	13	.56	11	18	166	13	.21	1	.03	.06	.62	.04	3	3
0	4	.17	3	5	51	4	.06	<1	.01	.02	.19	.01	1	1
0	22	.71	17	29	238	10	.22	1	.03	.03	.5	.04	5	4
0	7	.22	5	9	74	3	.07	<1	.01	.01	.15	.01	2	1
0	59	3.68	58	103	932	10	.68	1	.01	.25	2.4	.01	21	12
0	11	.65	6	7	33	8	.16	<1	<.01	.03	.32	.03	2	3
0	11	.57	21	11	175	2	.12	4	.14	.06	.65	.14	16	24
0	36	.97	40	18	265	3	.31	4	.23	.06	.73	.19	12	19
0	8	.22	9	4	60	1	.70	1	.05	.02	.17	.04	3	4
0	35	.70	35	15	305	3	.25	10	.24	.05	.71	.19	12	24
0	8	.16	8	4	71	1	.06	2	.06	.02	.17	.04	3	6
0	43	.65	34	20	335	3	.28	1	.14	.06	.64	.24	58	27[41]
0	4	.89	55	50	739	6	.27	167[42]	.08	.08	1.02	.44	33	27
0	3	.89	49	43	716	8	.21	140	.07	.08	1.16	.37	40	17
0	3	.07	4	7	114	<1	.07	21	.03	.06	.33	.05	3	6
0	1	.03	2	3	48	<1	.03	9	.01	.03	.14	.02	1	3

(40)With added vitamin C (ascorbic acid).
(41)If vitamin C is added, it contains 96 mg per cup.
(42)Vitamin A values range from 1.5 RE for white-fleshed varieties to 178 RE for yellow-fleshed varieties.

Table F–1 Food Composition

Grp	Computer Code No.	Food Description	Measure	Wt (g)	H_2O (%)	Ener (cal)	Prot (g)	Carb (g)	Dietary Fiber (g)	Fat (g)	Fat Breakdown (g) Sat	Mono	Poly
		FRUITS—Con.											
		Plums—Con.											
		Canned, purple, with liquid:											
		Heavy Syrup pack:											
5	305	Cup	1 c	258	76	230	1	60	4	<1	t	.2	.1
5	306	Plums	3 ea	110	76	98	<1	25	2	<1	t	.1	t
		Juice pack:											
5	307	Cup	1 c	252	84	146	1	38	4	<.1	t	<.1	t
5	308	Plums	3 ea	95	84	55	<1	14	2	<.1	t	t	t
		Prunes, dried, pitted:											
5	309	Uncooked (10 prunes weigh 97 g with pits, 84 g without pits.)	10 ea	84	32	201	2	53	8[43]	<1	<.1	.3	.1
5	310	Cooked, unsweetened, fruit and liquid (250 g with pits)	1 c	212	70	227	2	60	9	<1	<.1	.3	.1
5	311	Prune juice, bottled or canned	1 c	256	81	181	2	45	3	<.1	t	<.1	t
		Raisins, seedless:											
5	312	Cup, not pressed down	1 c	145	15	435	5	115	9	1	.2	<.1	.2
5	313	One packet, ½ oz	½ oz	14	15	41	<1	11	1	<.1	t	t	t
		Raspberries:											
5	314	Fresh	1 c	123	87	60	1	14	8	1	t	.1	.4
		Frozen, sweetened:											
5	315	10-oz container	10 oz	284	73	293	2	74	15	<1	t	<.1	.3
5	316	Cup, thawed measure	1 c	250	73	255	2	65	12	<1	t	<.1	.2
5	317	Rhubarb, cooked, added sugar	1 c	240	68	279	1	75	5	<1	t	t	.1
		Strawberries:											
5	318	Fresh, whole, capped	1 c	149	92	45	1	11	4	1	<.1	.1	.3
		Frozen, sliced, sweetened:											
5	319	10-oz container	10 oz	284	73	273	2	74	6	<1	t	.1	.2
5	320	Cup, thawed measure	1 c	255	73	245	1	66	8	<1	t	.1	.2
		Tangerines, without peel and seeds:											
5	321	Fresh (2⅜" whole) 116g with refuse	1 ea	84	88	37	1	9	2	<1	t	<.1	<.1
5	322	Canned, light syrup, fruit and liquid	1 c	252	83	154	1	41	4	<1	<.1	<.1	.1
5	323	Tangerine juice, canned, sweetened	1 c	249	87	125	1	30	1	<1	<.1	<.1	.1
		Watermelon, raw, without rind and seeds:											
5	324	Piece, 1" thick by 10" diam (weighs 2 lb with refuse or 926g)	1 pce	482	92	152	3	35	2	2	.3	.2	1
5	325	Diced	1 c	160	92	50	1	12	1	1	.1	.1	.4
		BAKED GOODS:											
		BREADS, CAKES, COOKIES, CRACKERS, PIES, PANCAKES, TORTILLAS											
6	326	Bagels, plain, enriched, 3½" diam	1 ea	68	32	180	7	35	1	1	.2	.3	.4
		Biscuits:											
6	327	From home recipe	1 ea	28	28	100	2	13	1	5	1.2	2	1.3
6	328	From mix	1 ea	28	29	94	2	14	1	3	.8	1.4	.9
6	329	From refrigerated dough	1 ea	20	30	65	1	10	<1	2	.6	.9	.6
6	330	Bread crumbs, dry grated (see 364, 365 for soft crumbs)	1 c	100	7	390	13	73	4	5	1.5	1.6	1
		Breads:											
6	331	Boston brown bread, canned, 3¼" slice	1 pce	45	45	95	2	21	2	1	.26	.13	.14
		Cracked wheat bread (¼ cracked-wheat flour, ¾ enr wheat flour):											
6	332	1-lb loaf	1 ea	454	35	1190	42	227	23	16	3.1	4.3	5.7
6	333	Slice (18 per loaf)	1 pce	25	35	65	2	13	1	1	.2	.2	.3
6	334	Slice, toasted	1 pce	21	26	65	2	13	1	1	.2	.2	.3

(43) Dietary fiber data can vary between 8 and 13 g for 10 prunes.

GRP KEY: 1 = BEV 2 = DAIRY 3 = EGGS 4 = FAT/OIL **5 = FRUIT** 6 = BAKERY 7 = GRAIN 8 = FISH 9 = BEEF 10 = POULTRY 11 = SAUSAGE 12 = MIXED/FAST 13 = NUTS/SEEDS 14 = SWEETS 15 = VEG/LEG 16 = MISC 22 = SOUP/SAUCE

Chol (mg)	Calc (mg)	Iron (mg)	Magn (mg)	Phos (mg)	Pota (mg)	Sodi (mg)	Zinc (mg)	VT-A (RE)	Thia (mg)	Ribo (mg)	Niac (mg)	V-B6 (mg)	Fola (µg)	VT-C (mg)
0	23	2.17	13	34	235	49	.18	67	.04	.1	.75	.07	7	1
0	10	.92	6	14	100	21	.08	29	.02	.04	.32	.03	3	<1
0	25	.86	20	38	388	3	.28	254	.06	.15	1.19	.1	8	7
0	10	.32	8	15	147	1	.11	96	.02	.06	.45	.04	3	3
0	43	2.08	38	66	626	3	.45	167	.07	.14	1.65	.22	3	3
0	49	2.35	43	74	708	4	.51	65	.05	.21	1.53	.46	<1	6
0	31	3.02	36	64	707	10	.54	1	.04	.18	2.01	.56	1	11
0	71	3.02	48	140	1089	17	.46	1	.23	.13	1.19	.36	5	5
0	7	.29	5	14	105	2	.05	<1	.02	.01	.12	.04	1	<1
0	27	.7	22	15	187	0	.57	16	.04	.11	1.11	.07	32	31
0	43	1.85	37	48	324	3	.51	17	.05	.13	.65	.1	74	47
0	38	1.62	32	43	285	3	.45	15	.05	.11	1.5	.09	65	41
0	348	.5	30	19	230	2	.19	17	.04	.06	.48	.05	13	8
0	21	.57	16	28	247	2	.19	4	.03	.1	.34	.09	28	85
0	31	1.7	20	37	278	9	.17	7	.05	.14	1.1	.09	47	118
0	28	1.5	18	33	250	8	.15	6	.04	.13	1.02	.08	42	106
0	12	.08	10	8	132	1	.38	77	.09	.02	.13	.06	17	26
0	18	.93	19	25	197	15	.60	212	.13	.11	1.1	.11	34	50
0	45	.5	20	35	443	2	.08	105	.15	.05	.25	.08	8	55
0	38	.82	52	41	560	10	.34	176	.39	.1	.96	.69	10	47
0	13	.27	17	14	186	3	.11	59	.13	.03	.32	.23	3	15
0	20	2.1	15	61	65	300	.61	0	.26	.20	2.4	.03	16	0
t	48	.7	6	36	32	195	.15	3	.08	.08	.8	.01	2	t
t	59	.58	7	129	57	265	.18	4	.12	.11	.85	.01	2	t
1	4	.47	4	78	18	249	.09	0	.08	.05	.67	.01	1	0
5	122	4.1	31	141	152	736	.50	0	.35	.35	4.8	.02	28	0
3	41	.90	40	72	131	113	.35	0	.06	.04	.7	.06	8	0
0	295	12.1	218	581	608	1966	6.36	0	1.73	1.73	15.3	.42	218	t
0	16	.67	12	32	34	106	.35	0	.1	.1	.84	.02	12	t
0	16	.67	12	32	34	106	.35	0	.07	.1	.84	.02	9	t

(For purposes of calculations, use "0" for t, <1, <.1, <.01, etc.)

Table F–1 Food Composition

Grp	Computer Code No.	Food Description	Measure	Wt (g)	H_2O (%)	Ener (cal)	Prot (g)	Carb (g)	Dietary Fiber (g)	Fat (g)	Fat Breakdown (g) Sat	Mono	Poly
		BAKED GOODS—Con.											
		Breads—Con.											
		French/Vienna bread, enriched:											
6	335	1-lb loaf	1 ea	454	34	1270	43	230	8	18	4	6	6
6	336	French, slice, 5 × 2½ × 1″	1 pce	35	34	100	3	18	1	1	.3	.4	.5
6	337	Vienna, slice 4¾ × 4 × ½″	1 pce	25	34	70	2	13	1	1	.2	.3	.3
		French toast: see Mixed Dishes, and Fast Foods, code # 691											
		Italian bread, enriched:											
6	338	1-lb loaf	1 ea	454	32	1255	41	256	5	4	.6	.3	1.6
6	339	Slice, 4½ × 3¼ × ¾″	1 pce	30	32	83	3	17	<1	<1	<.1	t	.1
		Mixed grain bread, enriched:											
6	340	1-lb loaf	1 ea	454	37	1165	45	212	18	17	3	4	7
6	341	Slice (18 per loaf)	1 pce	25	37	65	2	12	2	1	.2	.2	.4
6	342	Slice, toasted	1 pce	23	27	65	2	12	2	1	.2	.2	.4
		Oatmeal bread, enriched:											
6	343	1-lb loaf	1 ea	454	37	1145	38	212	16	20	4	7	8
6	344	Slice (18 per loaf)	1 pce	25	37	65	2	12	1	1	.2	.4	.5
6	345	Slice, toasted	1 pce	23	30	65	2	12	1	1	.2	.4	.5
6	346	Pita pocket bread, enr, 6½″ round	1 ea	60	31	165	6	33	1	1	.1	.1	.4
		Pumpernickel bread (⅔ rye flour, ⅓ enr. wheat flour):											
6	347	1-lb loaf	1 ea	454	37	1160	42	218	19	16	3	4	6
6	348	Slice, 5 × 4 × ⅜″	1 pce	32	37	80	3	15	2	1	.2	.3	.5
6	349	Slice, toasted	1 pce	29	28	80	3	15	1	1	.2	.3	.5
		Raisin bread, enriched:											
6	350	1-lb loaf	1 ea	454	33	1260	37	239	12	18	4	7	7
6	351	Slice (18 per loaf)	1 pce	25	33	68	2	13	1	1	.2	.4	.4
6	352	Slice, toasted	1 pce	21	24	68	2	13	1	1	.2	.4	.4
		Rye bread, light (⅓ rye flour, ⅔ enr. wheat flour):											
6	353	1-lb loaf	1 ea	454	37	1190	38	218	30	17	3.3	5.2	5.5
6	354	Slice, 4¾ × 3¾ × 7/16″	1 pce	25	37	65	2	12	2	1	.2	.3	.3
6	355	Slice, toasted	1 pce	22	28	65	2	12	2	1	.2	.3	.3
		Wheat bread (blend of enr. wheat flour and whole-wheat flour):[44]											
6	356	1-lb loaf	1 ea	454	37	1160	43	213	25	19	3.9	7.3	4.5
6	357	Slice (18 per loaf)	1 pce	25	37	65	2	12	1	1	.2	.4	.3
6	358	Slice, toasted	1 pce	23	28	65	2	12	1	1	.2	.4	.3
		White bread, enriched:											
6	359	1-lb loaf	1 ea	454	37	1210	38	222	12	18	5.6	6.5	4.2
6	360	Slice (18 per loaf)	1 pce	25	37	65	2	12	<1	1	.3	.4	.2
6	361	Slice, toasted	1 pce	22	28	65	2	12	<1	1	.3	.4	.2
6	362	Slice (22 per loaf)	1 pce	20	37	55	2	10	<1	1	.2	.3	.2
6	363	Slice, toasted	1 pce	17	28	55	2	10	<1	1	.2	.3	.2
		White bread cubes, crumbs:											
6	364	Cubes, soft	1 c	30	37	80	2	15	1	1	.4	.4	.3
6	365	Crumbs, soft	1 c	45	37	120	4	22	1	2	.6	.6	.4
		Whole-wheat bread:											
6	366	1-lb loaf	1 ea	454	38	1110	44	206	51	20	6	7	5
6	367	Slice (16 per loaf)	1 pce	28	38	70	3	13	2	1	.4	.4	.3
6	368	Slice, toasted	1 pce	25	29	70	3	13	2	1	.4	.4	.3

(44)A blend of white and whole-wheat flour—no official ratio specified.

GRP KEY: 1=BEV 2=DAIRY 3=EGGS 4=FAT/OIL 5=FRUIT **6=BAKERY** 7=GRAIN 8=FISH 9=BEEF 10=POULTRY 11=SAUSAGE 12=MIXED/FAST 13=NUTS/SEEDS 14=SWEETS 15=VEG/LEG 16=MISC 22=SOUP/SAUCE

Chol (mg)	Calc (mg)	Iron (mg)	Magn (mg)	Phos (mg)	Pota (mg)	Sodi (mg)	Zinc (mg)	VT-A (RE)	Thia (mg)	Ribo (mg)	Niac (mg)	V-B6 (mg)	Fola (µg)	VT-C (mg)
0	499	14	91	386	409	2633	2.9	0	2.09	1.59	18.2	.24	168	t
0	39	1.08	7	30	32	203	.22	0	.16	.12	1.4	.02	13	t
0	28	.77	5	21	23	145	.16	0	.12	.09	1	.01	9	t
0	77	12.7	106	350	336	2656	3.1	0	1.86	1.06	15.1	.24	160	0
0	5	.8	7	23	22	176	.21	0	.12	.07	1	.02	11	0
0	472	14.8	222	962	990	1870	5.45	t	1.77	1.73	18.9	.47	295	0
0	27	.8	12	55	56	106	.3	t	.1	.1	1.1	.03	16	t
0	27	.8	12	55	56	106	.3	t	.08	.1	1.1	.02	12	t
0	267	12	154	563	707	2231	4.45	0	2.09	1.2	15.4	.07	15	0
0	15	.7	9	31	39	124	.25	0	.12	.07	.85	<.01	1	0
0	15	.7	9	31	39	124	.25	0	.09	.07	.85	<.01	1	0
0	49	1.45	16	60	71	339	.50	0	.27	.13	2.32	.01	12	0
0	322	12.4	309	990	1966	2461	5.18	0	1.54	2.36	15	.72	222	0
0	23	.88	22	71	141	177	.4	0	.11	.17	1.06	.05	16	0
0	23	.88	22	71	141	177	.4	0	.09	.17	1.06	.05	12	0
0	463	14.1	114	395	1058	1657	2.81	1	1.5	2.81	18.6	.15	159	t
0	25	.78	6	22	59	92	.16	t	.08	.16	1.02	.01	9	t
0	25	.80	6	22	59	92	.16	t	.06	.16	1.02	.01	8	t
0	363	12.3	109	658	926	3164	5.77	0	1.86	1.45	15	.43	177	0
0	20	.68	8	36	51	175	.38	0	.1	.08	.83	.02	10	0
0	20	.68	6	36	51	175	.38	0	.08	.08	.83	.02	8	0
0	572	15.8	209	835	627	2447	4.77	t	2.09	1.45	20.5	.50	204	t
0	32	.87	12	47	35	135	.26	t	.12	.08	1.13	.03	11	t
0	32	.87	12	47	35	135	.26	t	.10	.08	1.20	.02	8	t
0	572	12.9	95	490	508	2334	2.81	t	2.13	1.41	17.0	.15	159	t
0	32	.71	5	27	28	129	.16	t	.12	.08	.94	.01	9	t
0	32	.71	5	27	28	129	.16	t	.09	.08	.94	.01	9	t
0	25	.57	4	22	22	103	.12	t	.09	.06	.75	.01	7	t
0	25	.6	4	21	22	103	.12	t	.07	.06	.75	.01	7	t
0	38	.85	6	32	34	154	.19	t	.14	.09	1.13	.01	11	t
0	57	1.28	9	49	50	231	.28	t	.21	.14	1.69	.02	16	t
0	327	15.5	422	1180	799	2887	7.63	t	1.59	.95	17.4	.85	250	t
0	20	.97	26	74	50	180	.50	t	.10	.06	1.09	.05	16	t
0	20	.97	26	74	50	180	.50	t	.08	.06	1.08	.05	12	t

(For purposes of calculations, use "0" for t, <1, <.1, <.01, etc.)

Table F–1 Food Composition

Grp	Computer Code No.	Food Description	Measure	Wt (g)	H_2O (%)	Ener (cal)	Prot (g)	Carb (g)	Dietary Fiber (g)	Fat (g)	Fat Breakdown (g) Sat	Mono	Poly
BAKED GOODS—Con.													
		Bread stuffing, prepared from mix:											
6	369	Dry type	1 c	140	33	500	9	50	4	31	6	13	10
6	370	Moist type, with egg	1 c	203	61	420	9	40	4	26	5	11	8
		Cakes, prepared from mixes:[45]											
		Angel food cake:											
6	371	Whole cake, 9 ¾″ diam tube	1 ea	635	38	1510	38	342	3	2	.4	.2	1
6	372	Piece, 1/12 of cake	1 pce	53	38	125	3	29	<1	<1	t	t	.1
6	373	Boston cream pie, ⅛ of cake	1 pce	120	35	260	3	44	1	8	2.8	3.1	1.5
		Coffee cake:											
6	374	Whole cake, 7¾ × 5⅛ × 1¼″	1 ea	430	30	1385	27	225	3	41	12	17	10
6	375	Piece, ⅙ of cake	1 pce	72	30	230	5	38	2	7	2.0	2.8	1.6
		Devil's food with chocolate frosting:											
6	376	Whole cake, 2 layer, 8 or 9″ diam	1 ea	1107	24	3755	49	645	5	136	56	51	20
6	377	Piece, 1/16 of cake	1 pce	69	24	235	3	40	1	8	3.5	3.2	1.2
6	378	Cupcake, 2½″ diam	1 ea	42	24	143	2	25	<1	5	2.1	2.0	.7
		Gingerbread:											
6	379	Whole cake, 8″ square	1 ea	570	37	1575	18	291	3	39	10	16	11
6	380	Piece, 1/9 of cake	1 pce	63	37	174	2	32	2	4	1.1	1.8	1.2
		Yellow, with chocolate frosting, 2 layer:											
6	381	Whole cake, 8 or 9″ diam	1 ea	1108	26	3735	45	638	5	125	48	49	22
6	382	Piece, 1/16 of cake	1 pce	69	26	235	3	40	<1	8	3	3.1	1.4
		Cakes from home recipes with enriched flour:											
		Carrot cake, cream cheese frosting:[46]											
6	383	Whole, 9 × 13″ cake	1 ea	1792	23	6496	63	832	20	328	69	135	114
6	384	Piece, 1/16 of 9 × 13″ cake 2¼ × 3¼″	1 pce	112	23	406	4	52	1	21	4.3	8.5	7.1
		Fruitcake, dark, 7½″ diam tube, 2¼″ high:[46]											
6	385	Whole cake	1 ea	1361	18	5185	74	783	38	228	48	113	52
6	386	Piece, 1/32 of cake, ⅔″ arc	1 pce	43	18	165	2	25	2	7	1.5	3.6	1.6
		Sheet cake, plain, no frosting:[47]											
6	387	Whole cake, 9″ square	1 ea	777	25	2830	35	434	3	108	30	45	26
6	388	Piece, 1/9 of cake	1 pce	86	25	315	4	48	<1	12	3.3	5	2.8
		Sheet cake, plain, uncooked white frosting:[48]											
6	389	Whole cake, 9″ square	1 ea	1096	21	4020	37	694	3	129	42	50	26
6	390	Piece, 1/9 of cake	1 pce	121	21	445	4	77	<1	14	5	6	3
		Pound cake:[48]											
6	391	Loaf, 8½ × 3½ × 3¼″	1 ea	514	22	2025	33	265	4	94	21	41	27
6	392	Piece, 1/17 of loaf, ½″ slice	1 pce	30	22	120	2	15	<1	5	1.2	2.4	1.6
		Cakes, commercial:											
		Pound cake:											
6	393	Loaf, 8½ × 3½ × 3″	1 ea	500	24	1935	26	257	4	94	52	30	4
6	394	Slice, 1/17 of loaf, ½″ slice	1 pce	29	24	110	2	15	<1	5	3.0	1.7	.2
		Snack cakes:											
6	395	Chocolate w/creme filling, 2 small cakes per package	1 ea	28	20	105	1	17	<1	4	1.7	1.5	.6
6	396	Sponge cake w/creme filling, 2 small cakes per package	1 ea	42	19	155	1	27	<1	5	2.3	2.1	.5

(45)Excepting angel food cake, cakes were made from mixes containing vegetable shortening, and frostings were made with margarine. All mixes use enriched flour.
(46)Made with vegetable oil.
(47)Cake made with vegetable shortening.
(48)Made with margarine.

GRP KEY: 1=BEV 2=DAIRY 3=EGGS 4=FAT/OIL 5=FRUIT **6=BAKERY** 7=GRAIN 8=FISH 9=BEEF 10=POULTRY 11=SAUSAGE 12=MIXED/FAST 13=NUTS/SEEDS 14=SWEETS 15=VEG/LEG 16=MISC 22=SOUP/SAUCE

Chol (mg)	Calc (mg)	Iron (mg)	Magn (mg)	Phos (mg)	Pota (mg)	Sodi (mg)	Zinc (mg)	VT-A (RE)	Thia (mg)	Ribo (mg)	Niac (mg)	V-B6 (mg)	Fola (μg)	VT-C (mg)
0	92	2.2	30	136	126	1254	.55	273	.17	.20	2.50	.02	14	0
67	81	2.03	45	134	118	1023	.78	256	.10	.18	1.62	.04	20	t
0	527	2.73	51	1086	845	3226	.82	0	.32	1.27	1.6	.08	51	0
0	44	.23	4	91	71	269	.07	0	.03	.11	.13	.01	4	0
20	26	.6	11	70	40	225	.23	70	.01	.18	.7	.05	7	0
279	262	7.30	27	748	469	1853	3.70	194	.82	.90	7.70	.12	30	1
47	44	1.22	5	125	78	310	.62	32	.14	.15	1.29	.02	5	t
598	653	22.1	200	1162	1439	2900	7.95	498	1.11	1.66	10	.32	82	1
37	41	1.40	12	72	90	181	.53	31	.07	.1	.6	.02	1	t
23	25	.85	7	44	55	110	.40	19	.04	.06	.37	.01	3	t
6	513	10.8	41	570	1562	1733	5.52	0	.86	1.03	7.4	.07	36	1
1	57	1.20	5	63	173	192	.61	0	.10	.11	.82	.01	4	t
576	1008	15.5	72	2017	1208	2515	3.31	465	1.22	1.66	11.1	.45	80	1
36	63	.97	5	126	75	157	.21	29	.08	.10	.69	.03	5	t
912	440	20	185	1040	1856	2336	7.2	10,600	1.92	1.97	15.0	1.12	192	23
57	27	1.2	12	65	116	146	.45	663	.11	.14	1.0	.06	12	1
640	1293	37.6	340	1592	6138	2123	6.8	422	2.41	2.55	17	1.72	54	504
20	41	1.2	11	50	194	67	.22	13	.08	.08	.5	.05	2	16
552	497	11.7	108	793	614	2331	2.75	373	1.24	1.40	10.1	.26	54	2
61	55	1.3	12	88	68	258	.31	41	.14	.15	1.1	.03	15	t
636	548	11	108	822	669	2488	2.90	647	1.21	1.42	9.9	.27	110	2
70	61	1.2	12	91	74	275	.32	71	.13	.16	1.1	.03	12	t
555	339	9.3	48	473	483	1645	2.69	1033	.93	1.08	7.8	.39	55	1
32	20	.5	3	28	28	98	.16	60	.05	.06	.5	.02	3	t
1100	146	9.3	48	517	443	1857	1.95	715	.96	1.12	8.1	.38	55	1
64	8	.5	3	30	26	108	.11	41	.06	.06	.5	.02	3	t
15	21	1.0	3	26	34	105	.17	4	.06	.09	.7	.01	3	0
7	14	.6	3	44	37	155	.21	9	.07	.06	.6	.02	4	0

(For purposes of calculations, use "0" for t, <1, <.1, <.01, etc.)

Table F–1 Food Composition

Grp	Computer Code No.	Food Description	Measure	Wt (g)	H_2O (%)	Ener (cal)	Prot (g)	Carb (g)	Dietary Fiber (g)	Fat (g)	Fat Breakdown (g) Sat	Mono	Poly
		BAKED GOODS—Con.											
		Cakes—Con.											
		White cake with white frosting, 2-layer:											
6	397	Whole cake, 8 or 9″ diam	1 ea	1140	24	4170	43	670	5	148	33	62	42
6	398	Piece, 1/16 of cake	1 pce	71	24	260	3	42	<1	9	2.1	3.8	2.6
		Yellow cake with chocolate frosting, 2-layer:											
6	399	Whole cake, 8 or 9″ diam	1 ea	1108	23	3895	40	620	5	175	92	59	10
6	400	Piece, 1/16 of cake	1 pce	69	23	245	3	39	<1	11	5.7	3.7	.6
		Cheesecake:											
6	401	Whole cake, 9″ diam	1 ea	1110	46	3350	60	317	5	213	120	66	15
6	402	Piece, 1/12 of cake	1 pce	92	46	278	5	26	1	18	9.9	5.4	1.2
6	1035	Cheese puffs/Cheetos®	1 oz	28.4	1	158	2	14	<1	10	4.8	3.4	.6
		Cookies made with enriched flour:											
		Brownies with nuts:											
6	403	Commercial with frosting, 1½ × 1¾ × ⅞	1 ea	25	13	100	1	16	<1	4	1.6	2	.8
6	404	Home recipe, 1¾ × 1¾ × ⅞″[49]	1 ea	20	10	95	1	11	<1	6	1.4	2.8	1.2
		Chocolate chip cookies:											
6	405	Commercial, 2¼″ diam	4 ea	42	4	180	2	28	<1	9	2.9	3.1	2.6
6	406	Home recipe, 2¼″ diam[50]	4 ea	40	3	185	2	26	1	11	3.9	4.3	2
6	407	From refrigerated dough, 2¼″ diam	4 ea	48	5	225	2	32	1	11	4	4.4	2
6	408	Fig bars	4 ea	56	12	210	2	42	3	4	1	1.5	1
6	409	Oatmeal raisin cookies, 2⅝″ diam	4 ea	52	4	245	3	36	1	10	2.5	4.5	2.8
6	410	Peanut butter cookies, home recipe, 2⅝″ diam[50]	4 ea	48	3	245	4	28	1	14	4	5.8	2.8
6	411	Sandwich-type cookies, all	4 ea	40	2	195	2	29	<1	8	2	3.6	2.2
		Shortbread cookies:											
6	412	Commercial, small	4 ea	32	6	155	2	20	1	8	2.9	3	1.1
6	413	From home recipe, large[51]	2 ea	28	3	145	2	17	1	8	1.3	2.7	3.4
6	414	Sugar cookies from refrigerated dough, 2½″ diam	4 ea	48	4	235	2	31	<1	12	2.3	5	3.6
6	415	Vanilla wafers	10 ea	40	4	185	2	29	<1	7	1.8	3	1.8
6	416	Corn chips	1 oz	28	1	155	2	16	1	9	1.8	3.4	3.7
		Crackers:[52]											
6	1034	Armenian cracker bread	4 pce	28.4	4	117	5	19	4	2	.4	.7	1.1
6	417	Cheese crackers	10 ea	10	4	50	1	5	<1	3	.9	1.2	.3
6	418	Cheese crackers with peanut butter	4 ea	30	3	150	4	19	<1	8	1.6	3.2	1.2
6	419	Graham crackers	2 ea	14	4	60	1	11	<1	1	.4	.6	.4
6	420	Melba toast, plain	1 pce	5	4	20	1	4	<1	<1	.1	.1	.1
6	421	Rye wafers, whole grain	2 ea	14	5	55	1	10	2	1	.3	.4	.3
6	422	Saltine® crackers[53]	4 ea	12	4	50	1	9	<1	1	.5	.4	.2
6	423	Snack-type crackers, round	3 ea	9	3	45	1	6	<1	3	.6	1.2	.3
6	424	Wheat crackers, thin	4 ea	8	3	35	1	5	1	1	.4	.5	.4
6	425	Whole wheat wafers	2 ea	8	4	35	1	5	1	2	.5	.6	.4
6	426	Croissants, 4½ × 4 × 1¾″	1 ea	57	22	235	5	27	1	12	3.5	6.7	1.4
		Danish pastry:											
6	427	Packaged ring, plain, 12 oz	1 ea	340	27	1305	21	152	3	71	22	29	16
6	428	Round piece, plain, 4¼″ diam 1″ high	1 ea	57	27	220	4	26	1	12	3.6	4.8	2.6

(49) Made with vegetable oil.
(50) Made with vegetable shortening.
(51) Made with margarine.
(52) Crackers made with enriched white (wheat) flour except for rye wafers and whole-wheat wafers.
(53) Made with lard.

GRP KEY: 1 = BEV 2 = DAIRY 3 = EGGS 4 = FAT/OIL 5 = FRUIT **6 = BAKERY** 7 = GRAIN 8 = FISH 9 = BEEF 10 = POULTRY 11 = SAUSAGE 12 = MIXED/FAST 13 = NUTS/SEEDS 14 = SWEETS 15 = VEG/LEG 16 = MISC 22 = SOUP/SAUCE

Chol (mg)	Calc (mg)	Iron (mg)	Magn (mg)	Phos (mg)	Pota (mg)	Sodi (mg)	Zinc (mg)	VT-A (RE)	Thia (mg)	Ribo (mg)	Niac (mg)	V-B6 (mg)	Fola (µg)	VT-C (mg)
46	536	15.5	60	1585	832	2827	1.77	194	3.19	2.05	27.6	.16	64	0
3	33	1	4	99	52	176	.11	12	.2	.13	1.7	.01	4	0
609	366	19.9	72	1884	1972	3080	3.3	488	.78	2.22	10	.45	80	0
38	23	1.24	5	117	123	192	.21	30	.05	.14	.62	.03	5	0
2053	622	5.33	111	977	1088	2464	4.66	833	.33	1.44	5.11	.71	200	56
170	52	.44	9	81	90	204	.39	69	.03	.12	.42	.06	17	5
5	18	.20	7	29	23	344	—	26	.01	.03	.20	—	—	0
14	13	.61	14	26	50	59	.36	18	.08	.07	.33	.04	5	t
18	9	.40	11	26	35	51	.31	6	.05	.05	.3	.04	4	t
5	16	.8	10	41	56	140	.3	15	.1	.23	.9	.02	4	t
18	13	1	14	34	82	82	.22	5	.06	.06	.58	.03	4	0
22	13	1.04	10	34	62	173	.24	8	.06	.10	.89	.01	4	0
27	40	1.36	15	34	162	180	.36	6	.08	.07	.73	.07	4	t
2	18	1.1	26	58	90	148	.53	12	.09	.08	1	.03	6	0
22	21	1.1	19	60	110	142	.36	5	.07	.07	1.9	.04	12	0
0	12	1.4	15	40	66	189	.21	0	.09	.07	.8	.01	1	0
27	13	.8	4	39	38	123	.15	8	.10	.09	.9	.01	3	0
0	6	.55	4	31	18	125	.13	89	.08	.06	.71	.01	2	t
29	50	.9	8	91	33	261	.24	11	.09	.06	1.1	.02	4	0
25	16	.8	6	36	50	150	.12	14	.07	.1	1	.01	4	0
0	35	.5	21	52	52	233	.44	11	.04	.05	.4	.04[54]	3[55]	1
0	21	.45	41	1	77	—	.90	1	.06	.04	1.05	.03	12	2
6	11	.35	3	17	17	112	.07	5	.05	.04	.4	.01	—	0
4	26	1.2	2	94	64	338	.06	3	.16	.12	2.4	.03	—	0
0	6	.37	6	20	36	86	.11	0	.02	.03	.6	.01	2	0
0	6	.1	1	10	11	44	—	0	.01	.01	.1	.01	.7	0
0	7	.5	16	44	65	115	1.60	0	.06	.03	.5	.03	10	0
4	3	.5	3	12	17	165	.09	0	.06	.05	.6	<.01	2	0
0	9	.3	2	18	12	90	.05	t	.03	.03	.3	<.01	1	0
.6	3	.25	6[56]	15	17	69	.24[56]	t	.04	.03	.4	.01	3[55]	0
0	3	.24	8[56]	22	31	59	.23	0	.02	.03	.4	.01	3[55]	0
13	20	2.1	9	64	68	452	.32	13	.17	.13	1.3	.03	18	0
292	360	6.5	68	347	316	1302	2.86	99	.95	1.02	8.5	.12	84	t
49	60	1.1	11	58	53	218	.48	17	.16	.17	1.4	.02	14	t

(54) B_6 values vary from 0 to .04 g between various brands—check label.

(55) Folacin values estimated and derived from values for cornmeal and corn tortillas.

(56) Values derived from whole-wheat recipes and retention values.

(For purposes of calculations, use "0" for t, <1, <.1, <.01, etc.)

Table F–1 Food Composition

Grp	Computer Code No.	Food Description	Measure	Wt (g)	H_2O (%)	Ener (cal)	Prot (g)	Carb (g)	Dietary Fiber (g)	Fat (g)	Fat Breakdown (g) Sat	Mono	Poly
		BAKED GOODS—Con.											
		Danish Pastry—Con.											
6	429	Ounce, plain	1 oz	28	28	110	2	13	<1	6	1.8	2.4	1.3
6	430	Round piece with fruit	1 pce	65	30	235	4	28	1	13	3.9	5.2	2.9
		Desserts, 3 × 3 inch piece:											
6	1348	Apple crisp	1 pce	78	58	146	1	25	1	5	1.0	2.3	1.7
6	1353	Apple cobbler	1 pce	104	56	201	2	35	2	6	1.4	2.7	1.9
6	1349	Cherry crisp	1 pce	138	73	157	2	27	2	5	1.0	2.3	1.7
6	1352	Cherry cobbler	1 pce	129	65	199	2	34	1	6	1.4	2.7	1.9
6	1350	Peach crisp	1 pce	139	72	166	2	30	2	5	1.0	2.3	1.7
6	1351	Peach cobbler	1 pce	130	64	130	2	37	2	6	1.4	2.7	1.9
		Doughnuts:											
6	431	Cake type, plain, 3¼″ diam	1 ea	50	21	210	2	25	1	12	3.4	5.8	2
6	432	Yeast-leavened, glazed, 3¾″ diam	1 ea	60	27	235	4	26	1	13	5.2	5.5	.9
		English muffins:											
6	433	Plain, enriched	1 ea	57	42	140	5	26	2	1	.3	.2	.3
6	434	Toasted	1 ea	50	29	140	5	26	2	1	.3	.2	.3
		Muffins, 2½″ diam, 1½″ high:											
		From home recipe:											
6	435	Blueberry[57]	1 ea	45	37	135	3	20	2	5	1.5	2.1	1.2
6	436	Bran, wheat[58]	1 ea	45	35	125	3	19	3	6	1.4	1.6	2.3
6	437	Cornmeal	1 ea	45	33	145	3	21	2	5	1.5	2.2	1.4
		From commercial mix:											
6	438	Blueberry	1 ea	45	33	140	3	22	2	5	1.4	2	1.2
6	439	Bran	1 ea	45	28	140	3	24	3	4	1.3	1.6	1
6	440	Cornmeal	1 ea	45	30	145	3	22	2	6	1.7	2.3	1.4
		Pancakes, 4″ diam:											
6	441	Buckwheat, from mix with egg and milk	1 ea	27	58	55	2	6	1	2	.9	.9	.5
6	442	Plain, from home recipe	1 ea	27	50	60	2	9	1	2	.5	.8	.5
6	443	Plain, from mix; egg, milk, oil added	1 ea	27	54	60	2	8	1	2	.5	.9	.5
		Piecrust, with enriched flour, vegetable shortening, baked:											
6	444	Home recipe, 9″ shell	1 ea	180	15	900	11	79	4	60	15	26	16
		From mix:											
6	445	Piecrust for 2-crust pie	1 ea	320	19	1485	21	141	6	93	23	41	25
6	446	1 pie shell	1 ea	180	19	835	12	79	4	52	13	23	14
		Pies, 9″ diam; pie crust made with vegetable shortening, enriched flour:											
		Apple pie:[59]											
6	447	Whole pie	1 ea	945	48	2420	22	360	19	105	25	46	29
6	448	Piece, ⅙ of pie	1 pce	158	48	405	4	60	3	18	4.1	7.6	4.9
		Banana cream pie:[60]											
6	449	Whole pie	1 ea	1190	66	1915	38	282	10	77	27	29	15
6	450	⅙ of pie	1 pce	198	66	319	6	47	2	13	4.5	4.9	2.5
		Blueberry pie:[59]											
6	451	Whole pie	1 ea	945	51	2285	23	330	22	102	24	45	28
6	452	Piece, ⅙ of pie	1 pce	158	51	380	4	55	4	17	4.0	7.5	4.7

(57)Made with vegetable shortening.
(58)Made with vegetable oil.
(59)Recipes updated for latest USDA values for fruits/nuts/fruit juice.
(60)Recipe based on pie crust, cooked vanilla pudding, 2 bananas.

GRP KEY: 1 = BEV 2 = DAIRY 3 = EGGS 4 = FAT/OIL 5 = FRUIT **6 = BAKERY** 7 = GRAIN 8 = FISH 9 = BEEF 10 = POULTRY 11 = SAUSAGE 12 = MIXED/FAST 13 = NUTS/SEEDS 14 = SWEETS 15 = VEG/LEG 16 = MISC 22 = SOUP/SAUCE

Chol (mg)	Calc (mg)	Iron (mg)	Magn (mg)	Phos (mg)	Pota (mg)	Sodi (mg)	Zinc (mg)	VT-A (RE)	Thia (mg)	Ribo (mg)	Niac (mg)	V-B6 (mg)	Fola (μg)	VT-C (mg)
24	30	.55	6	29	27	109	.24	9	.08	.09	.7	.01	7	t
56	17	1.3	13	80	57	233	.55	11	.16	.14	1.4	.02	16	t
0	20	.77	12	15	112	66	.09	65	.05	.04	.41	.03	3	4
1	32	.76	7	42	86	305	.17	76	.08	.07	.70	.04	3	<1
0	29	2.16	16	22	163	73	.14	144	.06	.08	.56	.05	10	3
1	39	1.78	10	46	113	311	.21	135	.09	.10	.81	.05	9	2
0	24	.997	18	30	197	71	.19	104	.05	.05	1.01	.03	5	5
1	35	.90	11	52	139	309	.24	105	.08	.08	1.15	.03	5	3
20	23	.8	12	111	58	192	.25	5	.12	.12	1.1	.02	4	t
21	17	1.4	13	55	64	222	.30	<1	.28	.12	1.8	.28	13	0
0	96	1.7	11	67	331	378	.41	0	.26	.18	2.14	.02	18	0
0	96	1.7	11	67	331	378	.41	0	.23	.18	2.14	.02	15	0
19	54	.9	11	46	47	198	.29	9	.10	.11	.9	<.01	12	1
24	60	1.4	34	125	99	189	.37	30	.11	.13	1.3	.01	9	3
23	66	.9	11	59	57	169	.31	15	.11	.11	.9	.04	5	t
45	15	.9	7	90	54	225	.21	11	.11	.13	1.17	<.01	14	<1
28	27	1.7	28	182	50	385	.95	14	.08	.12	1.9	.12	19	0
42	30	1.3	11	128	31	291	.34	16	.09	.09	.8	.04	5	t
20	59	.4	18	91	66	125	.5	17	.04	.05	.2	.06	6	t
16	27	.5	7	38	33	115	.23	10	.06	.07	.5	.02	4	t
16	36	.7	7	71	43	160	.23	7	.09	.12	.8	.01	3	t
0	25	4.5	31	90	90	1100	1.50	0	.54	.40	5.0	.17	32	0
0	131	9.3	44	272	179	2600	1.19	0	1.07	.79	9.89	.27	57	0
0	74	5.23	25	153	101	1462	.79	0	.60	.44	5.57	.15	32	0
0	170	10	69	300	600	2844	1.6	28	1.04	.76	9.5	.5	48	2
0	28	1.67	12	50	100	476	.27	5	.18	.13	1.6	.08	8	<1
90	880	6.54	186	809	2000	2532	4.17	222	.94	1.75	7.40	1.77	116	26
15	147	1.09	31	135	333	422	.69	37	.16	.29	1.23	.30	19	4
0	155	12.3	60	274	756	2533	1.68	85	1.04	.85	10.4	.43	84	36
0	26	2.1	10	46	126	423	.28	14	.17	.14	1.73	.07	14	6

(For purposes of calculations, use "0" for t, <1, <.1, <.01, etc.)

Table F–1 Food Composition

Grp	Computer Code No.	Food Description	Measure	Wt (g)	H_2O (%)	Ener (cal)	Prot (g)	Carb (g)	Dietary Fiber (g)	Fat (g)	Fat Breakdown (g) Sat	Mono	Poly
		BAKED GOODS—Con.											
		Pies—Con.											
		Cherry pie:[59]											
6	453	Whole pie	1 ea	945	47	2465	26	363	15	107	25	47	30
6	454	Piece, ⅙ of pie	1 pce	158	47	410	4	61	2	18	4.2	7.8	4.9
		Chocolate cream pie:[61]											
6	455	Whole pie	1 ea	1051	63	1863	45	255	4	76	27	30	15
6	456	Piece, ⅙ of pie	1 pce	175	63	311	7	42	1	13	4.5	5.0	2.5
		Custard pie:											
6	457	Whole pie	1 ea	910	58	1760	46	204	4	84	28	35	17
6	458	Piece, ⅙ of pie	1 pce	152	58	293	8	34	1	13	.9	5.8	2.8
		Lemon meringue pie:[59]											
6	459	Whole Pie	1 ea	840	47	2140	31	317	5	84	21	37	22
6	460	Piece, ⅙ of pie	1 pce	140	47	355	5	53	1	14	3.5	6.2	3.7
		Peach pie:[59]											
6	461	Whole pie	1 ea	945	48	2410	24	361	17	105	25	46	29
6	462	Piece, ⅙ of pie	1 pce	158	48	405	4	61	3	17	4.1	7.7	4.8
		Pecan pie:[59]											
6	463	Whole pie	1 ea	825	20	3500	38	551	10	142	24	75	34
6	464	Piece, ⅙ of pie	1 pce	138	20	583	6	92	5	24	3.9	13	5.7
		Pumpkin pie:[59]											
6	465	Whole Pie	1 ea	910	59	2200	54	308	15	94	34	37	17
6	466	Piece, ⅙ of pie	1 pce	152	59	367	9	51	5	16	5.7	6.1	2.8
		Pies, fried, commercial:											
6	467	Apple	1 ea	85	43	255	2	32	2	14	5.8	6.6	.6
6	468	Cherry	1 ea	85	43	250	2	32	1	14	5.8	6.7	.6
		Pretzels, made with enriched flour:											
6	469	Thin sticks, 2¼″ long	10 ea	3	2	10	<1	2	<1	<1	t	<.1	<.1
6	470	Dutch twists, 2¾ × 2⅝″	1 ea	16	2	65	2	13	<1	1	.1	.2	.2
6	471	Thin twists, 3¼ × 2¼ × ¼″	10 ea	60	3	240	6	48	2	2	.4	.8	.6
		Rolls and buns, enriched:											
		Commercial:											
6	472	Cloverleaf rolls, 2½″ diam, 2″ high	1 ea	28	32	85	2	14	1	2	.5	.8	.6
6	473	Hotdog buns	1 ea	40	34	115	3	20	1	2	.5	.8	.6
6	474	Hamburger buns	1 ea	45	34	129	4	23	1	2	.6	.9	.7
6	475	Hard rolls, white, 3¾″ diam, 2″ high	1 ea	50	25	155	5	30	1	2	.4	.5	.6
6	476	Submarine rolls or hoagies, 11½ × 3 × 2½	1 ea	135	31	400	11	72	2	8	1.8	3	2.2
		From home recipe:											
6	477	Dinner rolls 2½″ diam, 2″ high	1 ea	35	26	120	3	20	1	3	.8	1.2	.9
6	478	Toaster pastries, fortified	1 ea	54	13	210	2	38	1	6	1.7	3.6	.4
		Tortilla chips:											
6	1271	Plain	1 oz	28	4	139	2	17	1	8	1.1	3.1	3.1
6	1036	Nacho flavor	1 oz	28	1	139	2	18	1	7	1.4	2.5	2.8
6	1037	Taco flavor	1 oz	28	1	140	3	18	1	7	1.4	2.5	2.7
		Tortillas:											
6	479	Corn, enriched, 6″ diam	1 ea	30	45	65	2	13	2	1	.1	.3	.6
6	480	Flour, 8″ diam	1 ea	35	27	105	3	19	1	3	.4	1.2	1.0
6	1301	Flour tortilla, 10.5″ diam.	1 ea	57	27	168	4	31	2	4	.6	1.9	1.6
6	481	Taco shells	1 ea	14	4	59	1	9	1	2	.2	.6	1.2

(59) Recipes updated for latest USDA values for fruits/nuts/fruit juice.

(61) Based on value for pie crust, cooked chocolate pudding with meringue.

GRP KEY: 1=BEV 2=DAIRY 3=EGGS 4=FAT/OIL 5=FRUIT **6=BAKERY** 7=GRAIN 8=FISH 9=BEEF 10=POULTRY 11=SAUSAGE 12=MIXED/FAST 13=NUTS/SEEDS 14=SWEETS 15=VEG/LEG 16=MISC 22=SOUP/SAUCE

Chol (mg)	Calc (mg)	Iron (mg)	Magn (mg)	Phos (mg)	Pota (mg)	Sodi (mg)	Zinc (mg)	VT-A (RE)	Thia (mg)	Ribo (mg)	Niac (mg)	V-B6 (mg)	Fola (µg)	VT-C (mg)
0	220	19	91	350	920	2873	1.87	416	1.13	.85	9.50	.50	93	5
0	37	3.17	15	58	153	480	.31	70	.19	.14	1.58	.08	16	1
90	958	6.46	176	881	1332	2565	4.46	204	.91	1.80	6.38	.54	66	3
15	160	1.08	29	147	222	427	.74	34	.15	.30	1.06	.09	11	<1
705	742	8.64	110	880	1040	2000	4.75	573	.82	1.60	5.50	.51	91	1
118	124	1.44	18	147	173	333	.79	96	.14	.27	.92	.08	15	4
822	150	8.4	54	412	420	2369	3.06	395	.59	.84	.50	.30	78	25
137	25	1.4	9	69	70	395	.51	66	.10	.14	.83	.05	13	4
0	160	11.3	98	332	1408	2533	2.11	690	1.04	.93	13.9	.39	72	28
0	27	1.90	16	55	235	423	.35	115	.18	.16	2.30	.07	12	5
822	210	12.0	192	777	781	1823	8.8	248	1.63	.99	6.6	.51	110	0
137	35	1.85	32	130	130	304	1.47	41	.22	.17	1.1	.08	18	0
655	1273	15.8	240	1269	2400	2029	5.96	11170[62]	.82	1.76	7.3	.64	120	6
109	212	2.63	40	211	400	338	.99	1861[62]	.14	.29	1.22	.11	20	1
14	12	.94	6	34	42	326	.14	3	.09	.06	1.0	.03	4	1
13	11	.70	7	41	61	371	.15	19	.06	.06	.60	.04	8	1
0	1	.06	1	3	3	48	.03	0	.01	.01	.13	<.01	<1	0
0	4	.32	4	15	16	258	.17	0	.05	.04	.70	<.01	3	0
0	16	1.2	15	55	61	966	.42	0	.19	.15	2.6	.01	10	0
t	33	.81	6	44	36	155	.22	t	.14	.09	1.10	.01	11	<1
0	54	1.19	8	44	56	241	.36	t	.20	.13	1.58	.01	15	<1
0	61	1.34	9	50	63	271	.41	t	.22	.15	1.78	.02	17	<1
0	24	1.40	14	46	49	313	.44	0	.20	.12	1.70	.02	17	0
0	100	3.80	31	115	128	683	1.17	0	.54	.33	4.50	.09	49	0
12	16	1.10	10	36	41	98	.32	8	.12	.12	1.20	.01	12	0
0	104	2.16	10	104	91	248	.31	150[63]	.17	.18	2.27	.2	43	4
0	82	1.00	22	74	30	140	.42	1	.01	.02	.20	.08	<1	<1
0	17	.40	13	98	109	107	.42	13	.04	.03	.40	.10	—	0
0	45	.70	27	91	72	191	.42	15	.08	.09	.80	.10	—	0
0	42	.60	19	55	43	1	.36	8	.05	.03	.40	.09	6	0
0	21	.55	12	59	35	134	.27	0	.13	.08	1.20	.01	16	0
0	34	.88	19	94	56	215	.43	0	.21	.13	1.93	.02	25	0
0	26	.26	9	33	25	62	.22	1	<.01	.01	.25	.02	2	0

(62) Latest USDA values of Vitamin A for canned pumpkin are almost 3.5 times greater than previously published values. Canned pumpkin is usually a blend of pumpkin and winter squash.

(63) Vitamin A values from label declaration varies from 100 to 150 RE for major brands.

Table F–1 Food Composition

Grp	Computer Code No.	Food Description	Measure	Wt (g)	H_2O (%)	Ener (cal)	Prot (g)	Carb (g)	Dietary Fiber (g)	Fat (g)	Fat Breakdown (g) Sat	Mono	Poly
		BAKED GOODS—Con.											
		Waffles, 7″ diam:											
6	482	From home recipe	1 ea	75	37	245	7	26	1	13	4	4.9	2.6
6	483	From mix, egg/milk added	1 ea	75	42	205	7	27	1	8	2.7	2.9	1.5
		GRAIN PRODUCTS: CEREAL, FLOUR, GRAIN, PASTA and NOODLES, POPCORN											
		Barley, pearled:											
7	484	Dry, uncooked	1 c	200	11	700	16	158	31	2	.4	.3	1.1
7	485	Cooked	1 c	157	69	193	4	44	4	1	.1	.1	.3
		Breakfast cereals, hot, cooked:											
		Corn grits (hominy) enriched cooked:											
7	486	Regular and quick, prepared	1 c	242	85	146	4	31	5	<1	t	.1	.3
7	487	Instant, prepared from packet, white	1 pkt	137	85	80	2	18	3	<1	t	.1	.1
		Cream of Wheat®, cooked:											
7	488	Regular, quick, instant	1 c	244	86	140	4	29	3	1	.1	.1	.2
7	489	Mix and eat, plain, packet	1 ea	142	82	100	3	21	2	<1	<.1	<.1	.1
7	490	Malt-O-Meal® cereal, cooked	1 c	240	88	122	4	26	3	<1	<.1	<.1	.1
		Oatmeal or rolled oats, cooked:											
7	491	Regular, quick, instant, nonfortified	1 c	234	85	145	6	25	4	2	.4	.8	1
		Instant, fortified:											
7	492	Plain, from packet	¾ c	177	86	104	4	18	3	2	.3	.6	.7
7	493	Flavored, from packet	¾ c	164	76	160	5	31	3	2	.3	.7	.8
7	494	Whole wheat cereal, cooked	1 c	242	84	150	5	33	4	1	.1	.1	.3
		Breakfast cereals, ready to eat:											
7	495	All-Bran®	⅓ c	28	3	70	4	22	9	<1	.1	.1	.3
7	1306	Alpha Bits®	1 c	28	1	111	2	25	1	1	.1	.2	.3
7	1307	Apple Jacks®	1 c	28	2	110	2	26	<1	<1	<.1	<.1	<.1
7	1308	Bran Buds®	1 c	84	3	217	12	64	23	2	.4	.3	1.1
7	1305	Bran Chex®	1 c	49	2	156	5	39	9	1	.2	.2	.8
7	1309	Buc Wheats®	¾ c	28	3	110	2	24	2	1	.1	.1	.5
7	1310	C.W. Post® plain	1 c	97	2	432	9	69	2	15	11.3	1.7	1.4
7	1311	C.W. Post® with raisins	1 c	103	4	446	9	74	2	15	11.0	1.7	1.4
7	496	Cap'n Crunch®	1 c	37	2	156	2	30	1	3	2.2	.4	.5
7	1312	Cap'n Crunchberries®	1 c	35	3	146	2	29	<1	3	1.9	.4	.5
7	1313	Cap'n Crunch®, peanut butter	1 c	35	2	154	3	27	<1	5	1.9	1.4	1.0
7	497	Cheerios®	1 c	23	5	89	3	16	2	1	.3	.5	.6
7	1314	Cocoa Krispies®	1 c	36	3	139	2	32	<1	<1	.2	.2	.2
7	1316	Cocoa Pebbles®	⅔ c	21	2	87	1	18	<1	1	<.1	<.1	<.1
7	1315	Corn Bran®	1 c	36	3	124	3	30	7	1	.2	.3	.7
7	1317	Corn Chex®	1 c	28	2	111	2	25	<1	<1	.1	.3	.6
7	498	Corn Flakes, Kellogg's®	1¼ c	28	3	110	2	24	1	<1	t	t	.1
7	499	Corn Flakes, Post Toasties®	1¼ c	28	3	110	2	24	1	<1	t	t	.1
7	1318	Cracklin' Oat Bran®	1 c	60	4	229	6	41	9	9	2.1	2.3	3.5
7	1038	Crispy Wheat 'N Raisins®	1 c	43	7	150	3	35	2	1	.1	.1	.4
7	1319	Fortified oat flakes	1 c	48	3	177	9	35	1	1	.1	.3	.3
7	500	40% Bran Flakes, Kellogg's®	1 c	39	3	125	5	35	5	1	.14	.14	.4
7	501	40% Bran Flakes, Post®	1 c	47	3	152	5	37	6	1	.2	.2	.3
7	502	Froot Loops®	1 c	28	2	111	2	25	<1	1	.2	.1	.1

(Computer code number is for West Diet Analysis program)

GRP KEY: 1 = BEV 2 = DAIRY 3 = EGGS 4 = FAT/OIL 5 = FRUIT **6 = BAKERY** 7 = GRAIN 8 = FISH 9 = BEEF 10 = POULTRY 11 = SAUSAGE 12 = MIXED/FAST 13 = NUTS/SEEDS 14 = SWEETS 15 = VEG/LEG 16 = MISC 22 = SOUP/SAUCE

Chol (mg)	Calc (mg)	Iron (mg)	Magn (mg)	Phos (mg)	Pota (mg)	Sodi (mg)	Zinc (mg)	VT-A (RE)	Thia (mg)	Ribo (mg)	Niac (mg)	V-B6 (mg)	Fola (µg)	VT-C (mg)
102	154	1.50	17	135	129	445	.65	39	.18	.24	1.50	.03	13	t
59	179	1.20	14	257	146	515	.52	49	.14	.23	.90	.03	4	t
0	32	4.2	51	378	320	6	4.47	0	.24	.1	7.9	.45	40	0
0	17	2.1	35	85	146	5	1.29	0	.13	.1	3.2	.18	25	0
0	1	1.55[64]	11	29	54	0[65]	.18	15[66]	.24[64]	.15[64]	1.96[64]	.06	2	0
0	7	1[64]	5	16	29	343	.08	0	.18[64]	.08[64]	1.3[64]	.03	1	0
0	54[64]	10.9[64]	12	43[67]	46	5[67, 68]	.35	0	.24[64]	.07[64]	1.5[64]	.02	9	0
0	20[64]	8.10[64]	7	20[64]	38	241	.20	376[64]	.43[64]	.28[64]	5.0[64]	.01	5	0
0	5	9.6[64]	14	24[64]	31	2[68]	.17	0	.48[64]	.24[64]	5.8[64]	.02	5	0
0	19	1.59	56	178	131	2[68]	1.15	5	.26	.05	.3	.05	9	0
0	163[64]	6.32[64]	51	133	99	285[64]	1	453[64]	.53[64]	.29[64]	5.49[64]	.74	150	0
0	168[64]	6.7[64]	51	148	137	254[64]	1	460[64]	.53[64]	.38[64]	5.9[64]	.77	150	<1
0	17	1.5	53	168	171	3	1.16	0	.17	.12	2.13	.07	25	0
0	23	4.5[64]	106	264	320	260	3.7	375[64]	.37[64]	.43[64]	5.0[64]	.5	100	15[64]
0	8	1.80	17	51	100	219	1.50	375	.40	.40	5.0	.50	100	—
0	3	4.50	6	30	23	125	3.70	375	.40	.40	5.0	.50	100	15
0	56	13.4	267	729	930	516	11.1	1112	1.10	1.30	14.8	1.50	297	45
0	29	7.80	126	327	394	455	2.14	11	.60	.26	8.6	.90	173	26
0	60	8.10	24	60	—	235	.30	682	.68	.77	9.0	.90	—	27
0	47	15.4	67	224	198	167	1.64	1284	1.30	1.50	17.1	1.70	342	—
0	51	16.4	74	232	260	160	1.64	1364	1.30	1.50	18.1	1.90	364	—
0	6	9.83[64]	15	47	48	278	4.01	5[64]	.66[64]	.71[64]	8.64[64]	1	238	0
0	11	9.04	14	47	49	243	3.56	0	.59	.67	8.14	.93	128	—
0	7	9.10	19	49	57	268	3.79	0	.60	.70	8.97	1.04	244	—
0	38	3.6[64]	31	109	82	246	.63	304[64]	.32[64]	.32[64]	4.0[64]	.4	5	12[64]
0	6	2.30	12	47	53	275	1.90	477	.50	.50	6.3	.60	127	19
0	4	1.30	9	16	35	102	1.10	282	.30	.30	3.7	.40	75	—
0	41	12.2	18	52	70	310	4.00	—	.38	.70	10.9	.86	232	—
0	3	1.80	4	11	23	271	.10	14	.40	.07	5.0	.50	100	15
0	1	1.8[64]	3	18	26	351	.06	375[64]	.37[64]	.43[64]	5.0[64]	.51	100	15[64]
0	1	.7[64]	3	12	33	297	.06	375[64]	.37[64]	.43[64]	5.0[64]	.51	100	0
0	40	3.80	116	241	355	402	3.20	794	.80	.90	10.6	1.10	212	32
0	71	6.80	35	117	174	204	.51	569	.60	.60	7.6	.80	40	—
0	68	13.7	58	176	343	429	1.50	636	.60	.70	.39	.90	169	—
0	19	11.2[64]	71	192	248	363	5.15	522[64]	.51[64]	.59[64]	6.86[64]	.7	138	0
0	21	7.47[64]	102	296	251	431	2.5	629[64]	.62[64]	.72[64]	8.3[64]	.85	166	0
0	3	4.5[64]	9	28	30	125	3.7	225[64]	.4[64]	.4[64]	5.0[64]	.5	100	15[64]

(64)Nutrient added (values sometimes based on label declaration).

(65)Cooked without salt. If salt is added according to label recommendation, sodium content is 540 mg.

(66)Value for yellow corn grits; cooked white corn grits contain 0 RE of Vitamin A.

(67)Values for regular and instant cereal. For quick cereal, phosphorus is 102 mg, and sodium is 142 mg.

(68)Cooked without salt. If added according to label recommendations, sodium content is 390 mg for Cream of Wheat; 324 mg for Malt-O-Meal; 374 mg for oatmeal.

(For purposes of calculations, use "0" for t, <1, <.1, <.01, etc.)

Table F–1 Food Composition

Grp	Computer Code No.	Food Description	Measure	Wt (g)	H_2O (%)	Ener (cal)	Prot (g)	Carb (g)	Dietary Fiber (g)	Fat (g)	Fat Breakdown (g) Sat	Mono	Poly
		GRAIN PRODUCTS—Con.											
		Cereals—Con.											
7	1320	Frosted Mini-Wheats®	4 ea	31	5	111	3	26	2	<1	.1	<.1	.2
7	1321	Frosted Rice Krispies®	1 c	28	3	109	1	26	1	<1	<.1	<.1	<.1
7	1323	Fruit & Fiber® w/apples	½ c	28	2	90	3	22	4	1	.2	.2	.6
7	1324	Fruit & Fiber® w/dates	½ c	28	2	90	3	21	4	1	.2	.2	.6
7	1325	Fruitful Bran® cereal	¾ c	34	3	110	3	27	5	0	0	0	0
7	1322	Fruity Pebbles® cereal	⅞ c	28	3	113	1	24	<1	2	.3	.2	.4
7	503	Golden Grahams®	1 c	39	2	156	2	33	2	2	1.0	.1	.2
7	504	Granola, homemade	1 c	122	3	595	15	67	13	33	5.8	9.4	17
7	505	Grape Nuts®	½ c	57	3	210	6	46	5	<1	t	t	.2
7	1326	Grape Nuts® flakes	⅞ c	28	3	102	3	23	2	<1	<.1	<.1	.1
7	1327	Honey & Nut Corn flakes	¾ c	28	4	113	2	23	<1	2	.2	.5	.7
7	506	Honey Nut Cheerios®	1 c	33	3	127	4	27	1	1	.2	.4	.5
7	1328	Honey Bran	1 c	35	3	119	3	29	4	1	.1	.1	.4
7	1329	Honeycomb®	1 c	22	1	86	1	20	<1	<1	.1	.1	.2
7	1330	King Vitamin® cereal	1 c	21	2	85	1	18	<1	1	.7	.2	.2
7	1039	Kix®	1 c	19	3	73	2	16	<1	<1	.1	.1	.2
7	1331	Life®	1 c	44	5	162	8	32	1	1	.1	.2	.4
7	507	Lucky Charms®	1 c	32	3	125	3	26	1	1	.2	.4	.5
7	508	Nature Valley® Granola	1 c	113	4	503	12	76	12	20	13	2.8	2.8
7	1332	Nutri-Grain™—Barley	1 c	41	3	153	5	34	2	<1	<.1	<.1	.1
7	1333	Nutri-Grain™—Corn	1 c	42	3	160	3	36	3	1	.1	.3	.6
7	1334	Nutri-Grain™—Rye	1 c	40	3	144	4	34	3	<1	.1	.1	.1
7	1335	Nutri-Grain™—Wheat	1 c	44	3	158	4	37	3	<1	.1	.1	.3
7	1336	100% Bran	1 c	66	3	178	8	48	20	3	.6	.6	1.9
7	509	100% Natural® cereal, plain	¼ c	28	2	135	3	18	3	6	4.1	1.2	.5
7	1337	100% Natural® with apples	1 c	104	2	478	11	70	5	20	15.5	1.8	1.3
7	1338	100% Natural® with raisins & dates	1 c	100	4	496	11	72	4	20	13.7	3.7	1.7
7	510	Product 19®	1 c	33	3	126	3	27	<1	<1	t	t	.1
7	1339	Quisp®	1 c	30	2	124	2	25	<1	2	1.5	.3	.3
7	511	Raisin Bran, Kellogg's®	1 c	49	8	158	5	37	6	1	.2	.1	.4
7	512	Raisin Bran, Post®	1 c	56	9	170	5	42	6	1	.2	.2	.4
7	1040	Raisins, Rice & Rye™	1 c	46	9	155	3	39	<1	<1	<.1	<.1	<.1
7	1041	Rice Chex®	¾ c	19	3	75	1	17	1	1	.2	.2	.3
7	513	Rice Krispies, Kellogg's®	1 c	29	2	112	2	25	<1	<1	t	t	.1
7	514	Rice, puffed	1 c	14	3	55	1	13	<1	<1	t	t	<.1
7	515	Shredded Wheat®	¾ c	32	5	115	3	25	4	1	.1	.1	.3
7	516	Special K®	1½ c	32	2	125	6	24	<1	<1	t	t	t
7	1340	Sugar Corn Pops®	1 c	28	3	108	1	26	<1	<1	t	<.1	.1
7	518	Sugar Frosted Flakes®	1 c	35	3	133	2	32	1	<1	t	t	t
7	517	Super Sugar Crisp®	1 c	33	2	123	2	30	<1	<1	t	t	.1
7	519	Sugar Smacks®	¾ c	28	3	106	2	25	<1	<1	.1	.1	.2
7	1341	Tasteeos®	1 c	24	2	94	3	19	1	1	.2	.2	.3
7	1342	Team®	1 c	42	4	164	3	36	<1	1	.2	.2	.3
7	520	Total®, wheat, with added calcium	1 c	33	4	122	3	26	2	1	.1	.1	.4
7	521	Trix®	1 c	28	2	109	1	25	<1	1	.2	.1	.1
7	1042	Wheat & Raisin Chex®	1 c	54	7	185	5	43	4	<1	.1	.1	.2
7	1344	Wheat Chex®	1 c	46	3	169	5	38	3	1	.2	.2	.6
7	1043	Wheat, puffed	1 c	12	3	44	2	10	2	<1	t	t	.1
7	522	Wheaties®	1 c	29	5	101	3	23	3	1	.1	.1	.2

GRP KEY: 1=BEV 2=DAIRY 3=EGGS 4=FAT/OIL 5=FRUIT 6=BAKERY **7=GRAIN** 8=FISH 9=BEEF 10=POULTRY 11=SAUSAGE 12=MIXED/FAST 13=NUTS/SEEDS 14=SWEETS 15=VEG/LEG 16=MISC 22=SOUP/SAUCE

Chol (mg)	Calc (mg)	Iron (mg)	Magn (mg)	Phos (mg)	Pota (mg)	Sodi (mg)	Zinc (mg)	VT-A (RE)	Thia (mg)	Ribo (mg)	Niac (mg)	V-B6 (mg)	Fola (µg)	VT-C (mg)
0	10	2.00	26	81	106	9	1.60	410	.40	.50	5.5	.60	109	16
0	1	1.80	5	27	21	240	.31	375	.40	.40	5.0	.50	100	15
0	10	4.50	60	150	168	195	1.50	375	.38	.43	5.0	.50	100	0
0	10	4.50	60	100	168	170	1.50	378	.38	.43	5.0	.50	100	0
0	10	8.10	60	150	150	240	3.75	378	.38	.43	5.0	.50	100	0
0	4	1.80	6	16	22	157	2	375	.40	.40	5.0	.50	100	0
0	24	6.2[64]	16	56	82	476	.34	521[64]	.5[64]	.6[64]	6.9[64]	.7	136	21[64]
0	76	4.84	141	494	612	12	4.47	4	.73	.31	2.14	.43	99	1
0	20	16	52	153	183	341	2	753[64]	.7[64]	.9[64]	10.0[64]	1	200	0
0	11	4.50	31	84	99	218	.57	375	.40	.40	5.0	.50	100	—
0	3	1.80	6	13	36	225	.11	375	.40	.40	5.0	.50	100	15
0	23	5.2[64]	39	122	115	299	.87	437[64]	.4[64]	.5[64]	5.8[64]	.6	4	17[64]
0	16	5.60	46	132	151	202	.90	463	.50	.50	6.2	.60	23	19
0	4	1.40	8	22	70	166	1.20	291	.30	.30	3.9	.40	78	—
0	—	12.7	7	—	26	161	.16	717	.09	1.06	12.9	1.18	286	33
0	23	5.40	8	26	29	226	.17	250	.27	.27	3.33	.33	2	10
0	154	11.6	55	238	197	229	1.55	0	.95	1.00	11.6	.05	37	—
0	36	5.1[64]	27	88	66	227	.56	424[64]	.4[64]	.5[64]	5.6[64]	.6	—	17[64]
0	71	3.78	116	354	389	232	2.19	8	.39	.19	.83	.32	85	0
0	11	1.45	32	126	108	277	5.40	540	.50	.60	7.2	.70	145	22
0	1	.89	27	120	98	276	5.50	556	.50	.60	7.4	.75	148	22
0	8	1.13	31	104	72	272	5.30	530	.50	.60	7.0	.70	141	21
0	12	1.24	34	164	120	299	5.80	583	.60	.70	7.7	.80	155	23
0	46	8.12	312	801	824	457	5.74	0	1.60	1.80	20.9	2.10	200	63
0	49	.83	34	104	138	12	.63	2	.09	.15	.6	.64	8	0
0	157	2.89	71	350	513	52	2.00	8	.33	.58	1.88	.11	17	—
0	160	3.12	124	347	538	47	2.11	8	.30	.64	2.08	.17	45	—
0	4	21[64]	12	47	51	378	.5	1769[64]	1.7[64]	2[64]	23.3[64]	2.3	466	70[64]
0	9	6.31	12	25	45	241	.18	—	.54	.76	5.80	.91	8	—
0	25	24[64]	73	200	307	293	5.0	500[64]	.51[64]	.57[64]	6.67[64]	.67	133	0
0	27	9.01[64]	96	237	349	370	3.01	750[64]	.74[64]	.85[64]	10[64]	1.02	200	0
0	10	5.60	20	50	144	350	4.70	467	.50	.60	6.30	.60	125	0
0	3	1.20	5	19	22	158	.26	1	.27	.20	3.34	.33	67	10
0	4	1.8[64]	10	34	30	340	.48	388[64]	.4[64]	.4[64]	5.0[64]	.5	100	15[64]
0	1	.15[64]	4	14	16	<1	.14	0	.02[64]	.01[64]	.42[64]	.01	3	0
0	12	1.35	42	112	115	3	1.05	0	.08	.09	1.67	.08	16	0
0	9	5.06[64]	18	62	55	298	4.16	429[64]	.45[64]	.45[64]	5.63[64]	.56	112	17[64]
0	2	1.80	2	8	20	90	1.50	225	.40	.40	5.00	.50	100	15
0	1	2.2[64]	3	26	22	284	.05	463[64]	.5[64]	.5[64]	6.2[64]	.6	124	19[64]
0	7	2.1[64]	20	60	123	29	1.7	437[64]	.4[64]	.5[64]	5.8[64]	.6	116	0
0	3	1.8[64]	13	31	42	75	.28	375[64]	.37[64]	.43[64]	5[64]	.5	100	15[64]
0	11	3.80	26	96	71	183	.69	318	.30	.40	4.20	.40	9	13
0	6	2.57	19	65	71	259	.58	556	.55	.63	7.40	.80	—	22
0	200	21[64]	34	137	123	330	.15	1769[64]	1.7[64]	2[64]	23.3[64]	2.3	400	70[64]
0	6	4.5[64]	6	22	27	169	.13	379[64]	.4[64]	.4[64]	4.9[64]	.5	99	15[64]
0	—	7.70	53	163	174	306	1.19	<1	.50	.60	7.10	.70	143	2
0	18	7.30	58	182	174	308	1.23	0	.60	.17	8.10	.80	162	24
0	3	.57	17	43	42	0	.30	0	.02	.03	1.30	.02	4	0
0	44	4.6[64]	32	100	108	363	.65	388[64]	.4[64]	.4[64]	5.1[64]	.5	9	15[64]

[64] Nutrient added (values sometimes based on label declaration).

(For purposes of calculations, use "0" for t, <1, <.1, <.01, etc.)

Table F–1 Food Composition

Grp	Computer Code No.	Food Description	Measure	Wt (g)	H_2O (%)	Ener (cal)	Prot (g)	Carb (g)	Dietary Fiber (g)	Fat (g)	Fat Breakdown (g) Sat	Mono	Poly
		GRAIN PRODUCTS—Con.											
		Buckwheat:											
		Flour:											
7	523	Dark	1 c	98	12	338	12	71	8	3	.5	.8	.9
7	524	Light	1 c	98	12	340	6	78	6	1	.2	.4	.4
7	525	Whole grain, dry	1 c	175	11	586	23	128	16	4	.8	1.4	1.5
		Bulgar:											
7	526	Dry, uncooked	1 c	140	9	479	17	106	31	2	.3	.2	.8
7	527	Cooked	1 c	182	78	151	6	34	11	<1	.1	.1	.2
		Cornmeal:											
7	528	Whole-ground, unbolted, dry	1 c	122	10	442	10	94	13	4	.6	1.2	2
7	529	Bolted, nearly whole, dry	1 c	122	10	441	10	91	12	4	.6	1.2	2
7	530	Degermed, enriched, dry	1 c	138	12	505	12	107	10	2	.3	.6	1
7	531	Degermed, enriched, cooked	1 c	240	88	120	3	26	3	<1	.1	.1	.3
		Macaroni, cooked:											
7	532	Enriched	1 c	140	66	197	7	40	2	1	.1	.1	.4
7	533	Vegetable, enriched	1 c	134	68	172	6	36	2	.1	<.1	<.1	<.1
7	534	Whole wheat	1 c	140	67	174	8	37	2	1	.1	.1	.3
7	535	Millet, cooked	½ c	120	71	143	4	28	1	1	.2	.2	.6
		Noodles:											
7	536	Egg noodles, cooked	1 c	160	69	213	8	40	4	2	.5	.7	.6
7	537	Chow mein, dry	1 c	45	.73	237	4	26	2	14	2	4	8
7	538	Spinach noodles, dry	3½ oz	100	8	372	13	75	7	2	1.0	1.1	1.1
7	1343	Oat bran, dry	¼ c	25	6	61	4	17	4	2	.3	.6	.7
		Popcorn:											
7	539	Air popped, plain	1 c	8	4	30	1	6	1	<1	t	.1	.2
7	540	Popped in veg oil/salted	1 c	11	3	55	1	6	1	3	.5	1.4	1.2
7	541	Sugar-syrup coated	1 c	35	4	135	2	30	1	1	.1	.3	.6
		Rice:											
7	542	Brown rice, cooked	1 c	195	73	217	5	45	3	2	.3	.6	.6
		White, enriched, all types:											
7	543	Regular/long grain, dry	1 c	185	12	675	13	148	2	1	.3	.4	.3
7	544	Regular/long grain, cooked	1 c	205	69	264	6	57	1	<1	.2	.2	.2
7	545	Instant, prepared without salt	1 c	165	76	162	3	35	1	<1	.1	.1	.1
		Parboiled/converted rice:											
7	546	Raw, dry	1 c	185	10	686	13	151	4	1	.3	.3	.3
7	547	Cooked	1 c	175	73	200	4	43	1	<1	.1	.2	<.1
7	548	Wild rice, cooked	1 c	164	74	166	4	35	3	<1	.1	.1	<.1
7	549	Rye flour, medium	1 c	102	10	361	10	79	15	2	.2	.2	.8
7	1044	Soy flour, low fat	1 c	88	3	370	51	34	12	6	.9	1.3	3.3
		Spaghetti, cooked:											
7	550	without salt, enriched	1 c	140	66	197	7	40	2	1	.5	.1	.4
7	551	with salt, enriched	1 c	140	66	197	7	40	2	1	.5	.1	.4
7	552	Whole wheat spaghetti, cooked	1 c	140	94	174	7	37	5	1	.1	.1	.3
7	1302	Tapioca, dry	1 c	152	11	518	.3	135	2	<.1	<.1	<.1	<.1
7	553	Wheat bran	½ c	30	10	65	5	19	8	1	.2	.2	.7
		Wheat germ:											
7	554	Raw	1 c	100	11	360	23	52	12	10	1.7	1.4	6
7	555	Toasted	1 c	113	6	432	33	56	16	12	2.1	1.7	7.5
7	556	Rolled wheat, cooked	1 c	240	80	142	4	32	5	1	.1	.1	.3
7	557	Whole-grain wheat, cooked	⅓ c	50	86	28	1	7	1	<1	<.1	<.1	.1

(Computer code number is for West Diet Analysis program)

GRP KEY: 1=BEV 2=DAIRY 3=EGGS 4=FAT/OIL 5=FRUIT 6=BAKERY **7=GRAIN** 8=FISH 9=BEEF 10=POULTRY 11=SAUSAGE 12=MIXED/FAST 13=NUTS/SEEDS 14=SWEETS 15=VEG/LEG 16=MISC 22=SOUP/SAUCE

Chol (mg)	Calc (mg)	Iron (mg)	Magn (mg)	Phos (mg)	Pota (mg)	Sodi (mg)	Zinc (mg)	VT-A (RE)	Thia (mg)	Ribo (mg)	Niac (mg)	V-B6 (mg)	Fola (µg)	VT-C (mg)
0	32	2.5	135	298	490	1	2.65	0	.58	.16	2.75	.41	125	0
0	11	1	47	86	314	1	2.56	0	.09	.05	.47	.09	100	0
0	200	6.7	335	560	740	3	4.4	0	1.05	.26	7.7	.37	53	0
0	49	3.4	230	420	574	24	2.7	0	.33	.16	7.2	.48	38	0
0	18	1.8	58	73	124	9	1.04	0	.1	.05	1.8	.15	33	0
0	7	4.2	155	294	350	43	2.22	57	.47	.25	4.4	.37	31	0
0	21	4.2	154	272	303	43	2.22	57	.37	.1	2.3	.56	29	0
0	7	5.7	55	116	224	4	1	57	1	1	7	.35	66	0
0	2	1.48	17	34	38	1	.23	14	.14	.1	1.2	.06	6	0
0	10	2	25	76	43	1	.74	0	.29	.14	2.34	.05	10	0
0	15	1	26	67	42	8	.59	7	.15	.08	1.4	.03	4	0
0	21	1.5	42	125	62	4	1.1	0	.2	.1	1	.11	7	0
0	4	1	53	120	74	2	1.1	0	.1	.1	1.6	.13	23	0
50	19	2.5	30	110	45	11	1	10	.3	.13	2.4	.06	11	0
0	14	2.1	23	72	54	197	1	4	.3	.2	3	.05	10	0
0	58	2.1	174	322	376	36	2.8	46	.37	.2	4.6	.32	48	0
0	15	1.4	59	184	142	1	.78	0	.29	.05	.23	.04	13	—
0	1	.2	23	22	20	<1	.22	1	.03	.01	.2	.02	3	0
0	3	.27	25	31	19	86	.28	2	.01	.02	.1	.02	3	0
0	2	.5	29	47	90	<1	.29	3	.13	.02	.4	.03	3	0
0	20	1	84	162	84	10	1.23	0	.19	.05	3	.28	8	0
0	52	8	46	213	213	9	2.02	0	1	1	7.76	.3	15	0
0	23	2.3	27	96	80	4	.94	0	.33	.03	3.03	.19	6	0
0	13	1.04	8	23	6.6	5[69]	.4	0	.12	.08	1.45	.017	6.6	0
0	111	7	57	252	222	9.3	1.78	0	1.1	.13	6.7	.65	32	0
0	33	2	21	74	65	5	.54	0	.44	.03	2.5	.03	7	0
0	5	1	53	135	166	5	2.2	0	.1	.14	2.1	.221	43	0
0	25	2.16	77	211	347	3	2	0	.29	.11	1.76	.273	38	0
0	165	5.27	202	522	2262	16	1.04	4	.33	.25	1.90	.46	361	0
0	10	2.00	25	76	43	1	.74	0	.29	.14	2.34	.05	10	0
0	10	2	25	76	43	140	.74	0	.29	.14	2.34	.05	10	0
0	21	1.5	42	125	62	4	1.14	0	.15	.06	1	.11	7	0
0	30	2.4	1.5	10.6	17	2	.182	0	.01	.15	0	0	6	0
0	22	3.2	183	304	355	.6	2.18	0	.16	.17	4.07	.39	24	0
0	39	6.3	239	842	892	12	12	0	1.88	.5	6	1.3	281	0
0	51	10.3	362	1295	1070	5	18.9	0	1.89	.93	6.32	1.11	398	0
0	17	1.5	58	130	165	2	1.22	0	.17	.06	2.2	.08	27	0
0	3	.3	12	26	33	<1	.24	0	.04	.01	.5	.03	4	0

[69] If prepared with salt according to label recommendation, sodium would be 608 mg.

(For purposes of calculations, use "0" for t, <1, <.1, <.01, etc.)

Table F–1 Food Composition

Grp	Computer Code No.	Food Description	Measure	Wt (g)	H_2O (%)	Ener (cal)	Prot (g)	Carb (g)	Dietary Fiber (g)	Fat (g)	Fat Breakdown (g) Sat	Mono	Poly
		GRAIN PRODUCTS—Con.											
		Wheat flour (unbleached):											
		All-purpose white flour, enriched:											
7	558	Sifted	1 c	115	12	419	12	88	3	1	.2	.1	.5
7	559	Unsifted	1 c	125	12	455	13	95	3	1	.2	.1	.5
7	560	Cake or pastry flour, enriched, sifted	1 c	96	12	348	8	75	3	1	.1	.1	.4
7	561	Self-rising, enriched, unsifted	1 c	125	11	442	12	93	3	1	.2	.1	.5
7	562	Whole wheat, from hard wheats	1 c	120	10	407	16	87	15	2	.4	.3	1
		MEATS: FISH and SHELLFISH											
8	1045	Bass, baked or broiled	3.5 oz.	100	70	125	24	0	0	4	.9	1.6	1.2
		Bluefish:											
8	1046	Baked or broiled	3.5 oz.	100	68	159	26	0	0	5	1.1	2.1	1.3
8	1047	Fried in bread crumbs	3.5 oz.	100	61	205	23	5	0	10	2.1	4.3	2.5
		Clams:											
8	563	Raw meat only	3 oz	85	82	63	11	2	<1	1	.1	.1	.2
8	564	Canned, drained	3 oz	85	64	126	22	4	t	2	.2	.2	.5
8	1290	Steamed, meat only	20 ea	90	64	133	23	5	<1	2	.2	.2	.5
		Cod:											
8	565	Baked with butter	3½ oz	100	75	132	23	0	0	3	.4	.3	.5
8	566	Batter fried	3½ oz	100	61	199	20	8	0	10	3.9	5.5	.9
8	567	Poached, no added fat	3½ oz	100	76	102	22	0	0	1	.2	.1	.3
		Crab, meat only:											
8	1048	Blue crab, cooked	1 c	135	77	138	27	0	0	2	.3	.4	.9
8	1049	Dungeness Crab, cooked	.75 c	101	74	85	18	<1	0	2	.3	.6	1.1
8	568	Canned	1 c	135	76	133	28	0	0	2	.3	.3	.6
8	1587	Crab, imitation, from surimi	3 oz	85	74	87	10	9	0	1	—	—	—
8	569	Fish sticks, breaded pollock	2 ea	57	46	155	9	14	<1	7	1.8	2.9	1.8
		Flounder/sole, baked with lemon juice:											
8	570	With butter	3 oz	85	73	120	16	<1	0	6	3.2	1.5	.5
8	571	With margarine	3 oz	85	73	120	16	<1	0	6	1.2	2.3	1.9
8	572	Without added fat	3 oz	85	78	99	21	0	0	1	.3	.3	.4
		Haddock:											
8	573	Breaded, fried[70]	3 oz	85	61	175	17	7	<1	9	2.4	3.9	2.4
8	1050	Smoked	3.5 oz	100	72	116	25	0	0	1	.2	.2	.3
8	574	Broiled with butter and lemon juice	3 oz	85	72	140	23	0	0	6	3.3	1.6	.7
8	1051	Smoked	3.5 oz	100	49	224	21	0	0	15	2.5	4.8	6.9
8	1054	Raw	3.5 oz	100	78	110	21	0	0	2	.3	.7	.8
8	575	Herring, pickled	3 oz	85	55	223	12	8	0	15	2.0	10	1.4
8	1052	Lobster meat, cooked w/ moist heat	1 c	145	77	142	30	2	0	1	.2	.2	1
8	576	Ocean perch, breaded/fried	3 oz	85	59	185	16	7	<1	11	3	5	3
8	1056	Octopus, raw	3.5 oz.	100	80	82	15	2	0	1	.2	.2	.2
		Oysters:											
8	577	Raw, Eastern	1 c	248	85	170	18	10	0	6	1.6	.6	1.8
8	578	Raw, Pacific	1 c	248	82	200	23	12	0	6	1.3	.9	2.2
		Cooked:											
8	579	Eastern, breaded, fried, medium	6 ea	88	65	173	8	10	<1	11	2.8	4.1	2.9
8	580	Western, simmered	3½ oz	100	71	135	19	7	0	2	.5	.4	.9
		Pollock, cooked:											
8	581	Baked or broiled	3 oz	85	74	96	20	0	0	1	.2	.1	.6
8	1055	Moist heat, poached	3.5 oz	100	72	128	23	0	0	1	.2	.1	.6

(70) Dipped in egg, milk and bread crumbs; fried in vegetable shortening.

(Computer code number is for West Diet Analysis program)

GRP KEY: 1 = BEV 2 = DAIRY 3 = EGGS 4 = FAT/OIL 5 = FRUIT 6 = BAKERY **7 = GRAIN** 8 = FISH 9 = BEEF 10 = POULTRY 11 = SAUSAGE 12 = MIXED/FAST 13 = NUTS/SEEDS 14 = SWEETS 15 = VEG/LEG 16 = MISC 22 = SOUP/SAUCE

Chol (mg)	Calc (mg)	Iron (mg)	Magn (mg)	Phos (mg)	Pota (mg)	Sodi (mg)	Zinc (mg)	VT-A (RE)	Thia (mg)	Ribo (mg)	Niac (mg)	V-B6 (mg)	Fola (µg)	VT-C (mg)
0	17	5.34	25	124	123	2	.8	0	.90	.57	6.8	.05	30	0
0	19	5.8	28	135	134	3	.88	0	1.0	.62	7.4	.06	33	0
0	13	7	15	82	101	2	.6	0	.90	.41	6.5	.032	18	0
0	423	5.8	24	744	155	1587	.78	0	.80	.50	7.29	.06	53	0
0	41	4.7	166	415	486	6	3.52	0	.54	.26	7.6	.41	53	0
80	86	1.61	32	216	385	75	.70	35	.10	.03	2.40	.35	9	0
63	9	.62	42	290	477	77	1.04	127	.08	.11	7.78	.53	2	<1
60	8	.53	37	285	413	67	.90	120	.06	.08	5.50	.37	2	<1
29	39	11.9	8	144	267	47	1.16	77	.09	.18	1.5	.07	13	9
57	78	23.8	16	287	534	95	2.32	145	.01	.36	2.85	.07	4	3
60	83	25.2	17	304	565	100	2.46	154	.01	.38	3.02	.08	4	4
60	20	.49	42	140	245	224	.58	30	.09	.08	2.51	.28	10	<1
55	80	.5	36	200	370	100	.5	26	.04	.04	2.2	.24	9	<1
55	14	.49	42	138	244	78	.58	14	.09	.08	2.51	.28	11	<1
135	140	1.22	45	278	437	376	5.70	20	.14	.12	3.00	.33	20	2
64	46	.37	46	184	359	299	4.33	14	.04	.16	2.92	.33	20	2
120	137	1.13	52	351	505	450	5.42	14	.11	.11	1.85	.41	22	0
17	11	.33	—	—	77	715	—	—	—	.02	.15	—	—	—
64	11	.42	14	103	149	332	.38	18	.07	.1	1.21	.03	10	0
68	16	.28	50	187	272	145	.53	54	.07	.1	1.85	.20	10	1
55	16	.28	50	187	273	151	.53	69	.07	.1	1.85	.20	10	1
58	16	.28	50	246	292	89	.53	10	.07	.1	1.85	.20	10	1
55	34	1.15	26	183	270	123	.85	20	.06	.1	2.9	.13	14	0
77	49	1.40	54	251	415	763	.50	22	.05	.05	5.07	.40	3	<1
45	51	.91	91	242	490	100	.43	174	.06	.08	6.06	.34	6	<1
100	48	.84	83	222	450	480	.42	45	.05	.07	5.80	.33	5	<1
32	47	.84	83	222	450	54	.42	47	.06	.08	5.85	.34	12	<1
11	65	1.04	8	76	59	740	.45	219	.03	.12	2.8	.11	2	0
104	88	.57	51	268	510	551	4.23	38	<1	1	1.55	.112	16	t
46	92	1.2	26	191	241	138	.41	20	.10	.11	2	.22	6	0
48	53	5.30	—	186	—	—	1.68	<1	.03	.04	2.10	.36	—	<1
136	111	16.6	135	344	568	277	226[71]	223	.34	.41	3.3	.12	25	24
136	20	12.7	55	402	417	262	41.2[71]	223	.17	.58	5	.12	25	72
72	54	6.12	51	140	215	367	76.7[71]	86	.13	.18	1.45	.06	12	7
48	16	10.2	44	322	334	210	33[71]	81	.14	.46	3.82	.10	17	7
82	5	.24	31	250	329	98	.51	19	.06	.07	1.4	.06	4	t
70	60	.53	1	252	400	98	.54	9	.04	.18	3.14	.27	12	0

(71) Value varies widely.

(For purposes of calculations, use "0" for t, <1, <.1, <.01, etc.)

Table F–1 Food Composition

Grp	Computer Code No.	Food Description	Measure	Wt (g)	H_2O (%)	Ener (cal)	Prot (g)	Carb (g)	Dietary Fiber (g)	Fat (g)	Fat Breakdown (g) Sat	Mono	Poly
		MEATS: FISH and SHELLFISH—Con.											
		Salmon:											
8	582	Canned pink, solids and liquid	3 oz	85	69	118	17	0	0	5	1.3	1.5	1.7
8	583	Broiled or baked	3 oz	85	62	183	23	0	0	9	1.6	4.5	2.1
8	584	Smoked	3 oz	85	72	99	16	0	0	4	.8	1.7	.8
8	585	Atlantic sardines, canned, drained, 2=24 g	3 oz	85	60	177	21	0	0	11	1.4	3.6	4.7
8	586	Scallops, breaded, cooked from frozen	6 ea	93	59	200	17	9	<1	10	2.5	4.2	2.7
8	1588	Scallops, imitation, from surimi	3 oz	85	74	84	11	9	0	<1	—	—	—
		Shrimp:											
8	587	Cooked, boiled, 18 large shrimp	3½ oz	100	77	99	21	0	0	1	.3	.2	.4
8	588	Canned, drained	⅔ c	85	73	102	20	1	0	2	.3	.3	.6
8	589	Fried, 4 large = 30g[70]	12 ea	90	53	218	19	10	<1	11	1.9	3.4	4.6
8	1057	Raw, large, about 7 g each	14 ea	100	76	106	20	1	0	2	.3	.3	.7
8	1589	Shrimp, imitation, from surimi	3 oz	85	75	86	11	8	0	1	—	—	—
8	1053	Snapper, baked or broiled	3.5 oz	100	70	128	26	0	0	2	.4	.3	.6
8	1060	Squid, fried in flour[72]	3 oz	85	65	149	15	7	<1	6	1.6	2.3	1.8
8	1590	Surimi[73]	3 oz	85	76	84	13	6	0	1	—	—	—
		Swordfish:											
8	1058	Baked or broiled	3.5 oz	100	76	121	20	0	0	4	1.1	1.6	.9
8	1059	Raw	3.5 oz	100	69	155	25	0	0	5	1.4	2.0	1.2
8	590	Trout, baked or broiled	3 oz	85	63	129	22	<1	0	4	.7	1.1	1.3
		Tuna, light, canned, drained solids:											
8	591	Oil pack	3 oz	85	60	163	25	0	0	7	1.2	1.4	3.1
8	592	Water pack	3 oz	85	71	111	25	0	0	1	.2	.1	.3
8	1061	Tuna, raw, average	3.5 oz	100	68	144	23	0	0	5	1.3	1.4	1.7
		MEATS: BEEF, LAMB, PORK and others											
		BEEF, cooked:[74]											
		Braised, simmered, pot roasted:											
		Relatively fat, like choice chuck blade:											
9	593	Lean and fat, piece 2½ × 2½ × ¾″	3 oz	85	47	295	23	0	0	22	9	9	.8
9	594	Lean only	3 oz	85	55	223	26	0	0	12	5	5	.4
		Relatively lean, like choice round:											
9	595	Lean and fat, piece 4⅛ × 2¼ × ¾″	3 oz	85	52	233	24	0	0	14	5	6	.5
9	596	Lean only	3 oz	85	57	187	27	0	0	8	2.7	3.5	.3
		Ground beef, broiled, patty 3 × ⅝″:											
9	597	Extra lean, about 16% fat	3 oz	85	57	225	24	0	0	13	5.3	6.0	.5
9	598	Lean, 21% fat	3 oz	85	53	238	24	0	0	15	6	6.7	.6
		Roasts, oven cooked, no added liquid:											
		Relatively fat, prime rib:											
9	601	Lean and fat, piece 4⅛ × 2¼ × ½″	3 oz	85	46	319	19	0	0	27	11	11	1
9	602	Lean only	3 oz	85	58	204	23	0	0	12	5	5	.4
		Relatively lean, choice round:											
9	603	Lean and fat, piece 2½ × 2½ × ¾″	3 oz	85	59	204	23	0	0	12	5	5	.4
9	604	Lean only	3 oz	85	65	148	25	0	0	5	2	2	.15
		Steak, broiled, relatively lean, choice sirloin:											
9	605	Lean and fat, piece 2½ × 2½ × ¾″	3 oz	85	52	240	23	0	0	16	7	7	.6
9	606	Lean only	3 oz	85	62	171	26	0	0	7	3.0	3	.3

(70)Dipped in egg, bread crumbs, and flour; fried in vegetable shortening.
(72)Recipe is 94.6% squid, 4.9% flour, and 0.6% salt.
(73)Surimi is processed from Walleye (Alaska) pollock. Also see Imitation crab, shrimp, scallops.
(74)Outer layer of fat removed to about 1/2″ of the lean. Deposits of fat within the cut remain.

GRP KEY: 1=BEV 2=DAIRY 3=EGGS 4=FAT/OIL 5=FRUIT 6=BAKERY 7=GRAIN **8=FISH** 9=BEEF 10=POULTRY 11=SAUSAGE 12=MIXED/FAST 13=NUTS/SEEDS 14=SWEETS 15=VEG/LEG 16=MISC 22=SOUP/SAUCE

Chol (mg)	Calc (mg)	Iron (mg)	Magn (mg)	Phos (mg)	Pota (mg)	Sodi (mg)	Zinc (mg)	VT-A (RE)	Thia (mg)	Ribo (mg)	Niac (mg)	V-B6 (mg)	Fola (μg)	VT-C (mg)
37	181[75]	.72	29	279	277	471	.78	14	.02	.16	5.6	.10	13	0
74	6	.47	26	234	319	56	.43	53	.18	.14	5.67	.19	14	0
20	9	.72	15	139	149	666	.26	22	.02	.09	4.01	.24	2	0
121	325[75]	2.5	33	417	337	429	1.11	57	.07	.19	4.5	.14	10	0
57	39	.76	55	219	310	431	.99	21	.04	.10	1.4	.18	11	0
18	7	.26	—	—	88	676	—	—	.01	.01	.26	—	—	—
195	39	3.09	34	137	182	224	1.56	18	.03	.03	2.59	.13	4	<1
147	50	2.32	35	198	179	143	1.07	15	.02	.03	2.34	.09	2	0
159	60	1.13	36	196	213	310	1.24	50	.12	.12	2.76	.09	7	1.4
152	52	2.41	37	205	185	148	1.11	3	.03	.03	2.55	.10	3	2
31	16	.51	—	—	76	599	—	—	.02	.03	.15	—	—	—
47	40	.24	37	201	522	57	.44	12	.05	.08	3.46	.27	9	<1
221	33	.86	33	213	237	260	1.5	0	.05	.39	2.21	.05	—	4
25	7	.22	—	—	95	122	—	—	.02	.02	.19	—	—	—
39	4	.81	27	263	288	90	1.15	36	.04	.10	9.68	.33	14	1
50	6	1.04	34	337	369	115	1.47	41	.04	.12	11.8	.38	16	1
62	73	2.07	33	272	539	29	1.18	19	.07	.19	2.3	.42	6	3
27	11	1.2	26	265	176	301	.77	20	.03	.09	10.1	.32	5	0
28	10	2.7	26	158	267	303	.77	20	.03	.10	13.2	.32	5	0
38	16	1.02	38	191	252	39	.60	18	.24	.25	8.65	.46	25	0
84	9	2.6	16	183	206	50	5.7	0	.06	.20	2.66	.24	8	0
90	11	3.13	20	199	223	60	8.73	0	.07	.24	2.27	.25	5	0
82	5	2.65	19	208	239	43	4.18	0	.06	.21	3.17	.28	9	0
82	4	2.94	21	231	262	43	4.66	0	.06	.22	3.47	.31	9	0
84	8	2.36	21	162	314	70	5.47	0	.06	.27	5	.27	9	0
86	10	2.08	20	155	297	76	5.27	0	.05	.2	5	.27	9	0
72	9	2	16	146	251	54	4.5	0	.06	.15	2.9	.22	6	0
69	9	2.2	21	181	319	63	5.90	0	.07	.18	3.5	.26	7	0
61	5	1.6	20	175	305	50	3.7	0	.07	.14	2.95	.3	5	0
58	4	3	23	192	335	53	4	0	.08	.15	3.2	.31	6	0
77	9	2.6	24	185	305	53	5	0	1	.22	3.3	.34	8	0
76	9	3	27	208	343	56	6	0	.1	.25	3.6	.38	9	0

[75]If bones are discarded, calcium value is greatly reduced.

(For purposes of calculations, use "0" for t, <1, <.1, <.01, etc.)

Table F–1 Food Composition

Grp	Computer Code No.	Food Description	Measure	Wt (g)	H_2O (%)	Ener (cal)	Prot (g)	Carb (g)	Dietary Fiber (g)	Fat (g)	Fat Breakdown (g) Sat	Mono	Poly
		MEATS: BEEF, LAMB, PORK and others—Con.											
		BEEF, cooked—Con.											
		Steak, broiled, relatively fat, choice T-bone:											
9	1063	Lean and fat	3 oz	85	50	253	21	0	0	18	7	7.5	.7
9	1064	Lean only	3 oz	85	60	182	24	0	0	9	3.5	3.5	.3
		Variety meats:											
9	1086	Brains, pan fried	3 oz	85	71	167	11	0	0	13	3.2	3.4	2.0
9	599	Heart, simmered	3 oz	85	64	149	25	<1	0	5	1.4	1.1	1.2
9	600	Liver, fried	3 oz	85	56	185	23	7	0	7	2.3	1.4	1.5
9	1062	Tongue, cooked	3 oz	85	56	241	19	<1	0	18	7.6	8.1	.7
9	607	Beef, canned, corned	3 oz	85	58	213	23	0	0	13	5	5	.5
9	608	Beef, dried, cured	1 oz	28	57	47	8	<1	0	1	.4	.5	.1
		LAMB, domestic, cooked:											
		Chop, arm, braised (5.6 oz raw with bone):											
9	609	Lean and fat	2.5 oz	70	44	244	21	0	0	17	7	7	1
9	610	Lean part of #609	1.9 oz	55	49	152	19	0	0	8	2.8	3.4	.5
		Chop, loin, broiled (4.2 oz raw with bone):											
9	611	Lean and fat	2.3 oz	64	52	201	16	0	0	15	6	6	1
9	612	Lean part of #611	1.6 oz	46	61	100	14	0	0	5	1.6	2.0	.3
9	1067	Cutlet, avg of lean cuts, cooked	3 oz	85	62	175	24	0	0	8	2.9	3.6	.5
		Leg, roasted, 3 oz piece = 4⅛ × 2¼ × ½″:											
9	613	Lean and fat	3 oz	85	57	219	22	0	0	14	5.9	5.9	1.0
9	614	Lean only	3 oz	85	64	162	24	0	0	7	2.4	2.9	.4
		Rib, roasted, 3 oz piece = 2½ × 2½ × ¾″:											
9	615	Lean and fat	3 oz	85	48	305	18	0	0	25	11	11	1.9
9	616	Lean only	3 oz	85	60	197	22	0	0	11	4	5	1
		Shoulder, roasted:											
9	1065	Lean and fat	3 oz	85	56	235	19	0	0	17	7.4	7.1	1.4
9	1066	Lean only	3 oz	85	64	163	22	0	0	8	3.1	3.2	.7
		Variety meats:											
9	1069	Brains, pan-fried	3 oz	85	61	232	14	0	0	19	4.8	3.4	1.9
9	1068	Heart, braised	3 oz	85	64	158	22	2	0	7	2.7	1.9	.66
9	1070	Sweetbreads, cooked	3 oz	85	62	196	16	0	0	13	6.3	5.1	.7
9	1071	Tongue, cooked	3 oz	85	58	234	18	0	0	17	6.7	8.5	1.1
		PORK, CURED, cooked (see also #669–672):											
9	617	Bacon, medium slices	3 pce	19	13	109	6	<1	0	9	3.3	4.5	1.1
9	1087	Breakfast strips, cooked	3 pce	34	27	156	10	<1	0	13	4.3	5.6	1.9
9	618	Canadian-style bacon	2 pce	47	62	86	11	1	0	4	1.3	1.9	.4
		Ham, roasted:											
9	619	Lean and fat, 2 pieces 4⅛ × 2¼ × ¼″	3 oz	85	58	207	18	0	0	14	5.1	7	2
9	620	Lean only	3 oz	85	66	133	21	0	0	5	1.6	2.2	.5
9	621	Ham, canned, roasted	3 oz	85	66	140	18	<1	0	7	2.4	3.5	.8
		PORK, fresh, cooked:											
		Chops, loin (cut 3 per lb with bone):											
		Braised:											
9	1291	Lean and fat	1 ea	71	44	261	19	0	0	20	7.2	9.1	2.2
9	1292	Lean only	1 ea	55	51	150	18	0	0	8	2.8	3.6	.0
		Broiled:											
9	622	Lean and fat	3.1 oz	87	50	275	24	0	0	19	7	9	2
9	623	Lean only from #622	2.5 oz	72	57	166	23	0	0	8	2.6	3.4	.9

(Computer code number is for West Diet Analysis program)

GRP KEY: 1 = BEV 2 = DAIRY 3 = EGGS 4 = FAT/OIL 5 = FRUIT 6 = BAKERY 7 = GRAIN 8 = FISH **9 = BEEF** 10 = POULTRY 11 = SAUSAGE 12 = MIXED/FAST 13 = NUTS/SEEDS 14 = SWEETS 15 = VEG/LEG 16 = MISC 22 = SOUP/SAUCE

Chol (mg)	Calc (mg)	Iron (mg)	Magn (mg)	Phos (mg)	Pota (mg)	Sodi (mg)	Zinc (mg)	VT-A (RE)	Thia (mg)	Ribo (mg)	Niac (mg)	V-B6 (mg)	Fola (µg)	VT-C (mg)
71	7	2.3	21	156	302	52	3.98	<1	.09	.19	3.47	.29	6	0
68	6	2.55	25	177	346	56	4.59	<1	.09	.21	3.94	.33	7	0
1697	8	1.89	12	328	301	134	1.15	0	.11	.22	3.21	.33	5	3
164	5	6.39	21	213	198	54	2.66	0	.12	1.31	3.46	.18	2	1
410	9	5.34	20	392	310	90	4.63	9126[76]	.18	3.52	12.3	1.22	187	20
91	6	2.88	14	121	153	51	4.08	0	.03	.30	1.83	.14	4	<1
73	10	1.77	12	94	116	856	3.04	0	.02	.13	2.07	.11	8	1
12	2	1.28	9	49	126	984	1.49	0	.02	.06	1.6	1	3	4.2
84	18	1.7	18	145	216	51	4.28	2	.05	.18	4.7	.08	13	0
66	14	1.5	16	127	185	41	4.0	1	.04	.15	3.5	.07	12	0
64	13	1.15	15	125	209	49	2.22	2	.07	.16	4.5	.08	12	0
44	9	.93	13	105	175	39	1.91	1	.05	.13	3.2	.07	11	0
78	13	1.74	22	179	293	64	4.48	<1	.09	.24	5.37	.14	19	0
79	9	1.69	20	162	266	56	3.74	2	.09	.23	5.6	.13	17	0
76	7	1.81	22	175	287	58	4.2	1	.09	.25	5.4	.14	20	0
82	19	1.4	17	141	231	62	2.96	2	.07	.18	5.7	.10	13	0
74	18	1.5	20	165	268	69	3.8	<1	.08	.20	5.24	.13	19	0
78	15	1.72	19	155	220	55	3.81	<1	.08	.21	5.66	.10	17	0
73	14	1.9	22	172	236	57	4.46	<1	.08	.23	5.39	.12	21	0
2128	18	1.73	18	421	304	133	1.70	0	.14	.31	3.87	.20	6	20
212	12	4.70	21	216	160	54	3.13	0	.14	1.01	3.71	.25	2	6
347	29	1.53	20	357	221	179	1.79	0	.03	.2	1.79	.02	12	15
161	8	2.24	14	114	134	57	2.54	0	.07	.36	3.14	.14	2	6
16	2	.32	5	64	92	303	.62	0	.13	.05	1.39	.05	1	6[77]
36	5	.67	9	90	158	714	1.25	0	.25	.13	2.58	.12	1	15
27	5	.38	10	138	181	719	.79	0	.38	.09	3.22	.21	2	10[77]
53	6	.74	16	182	243	1009	1.97	0	.51	.19	3.8	.32	3	0
47	6	.8	19	193	269	1128	2.19	0	.58	.22	4.27	.4	3	0
35	6	.91	16	188	298	908	1.97	0	.82	.21	4.27	.33	4	19[77]
73	6	.82	14	141	245	46	2.15	2	.43	.21	4.24	.26	3	<1
58	5	.77	13	131	230	41	2.05	2	.38	.20	3.82	.25	3	<1
84	4	.71	22	184	312	61	1.68	3	.87	.24	4.35	.35	4	<1
71	4	.66	22	176	302	56	1.61	2	.83	.22	3.99	.34	4	<1

(76)Value varies widely.

(77)Values based on products containing added ascorbic acid or sodium ascorbate. If none added, ascorbic acid content would be negligible.

(For purposes of calculations, use "0" for t, <1, <.1, <.01, etc.)

Table F–1 Food Composition

Grp	Computer Code No.	Food Description	Measure	Wt (g)	H_2O (%)	Ener (cal)	Prot (g)	Carb (g)	Dietary Fiber (g)	Fat (g)	Fat Breakdown (g) Sat	Mono	Poly
		MEATS: BEEF, LAMB, PORK and others—Con.											
		PORK, fresh cooked—Con.											
		Pan fried:											
9	624	Lean and fat	3.1 oz	89	45	334	21	0	0	27	10	13	3
9	625	Lean only from #624	2.4 oz	67	54	178	19	0	0	11	3.7	4.8	1.3
		Leg, roasted:											
9	626	Lean and fat, piece 2½ × 2½ × ¾″	3 oz	85	53	250	21	0	0	18	6	8	2
9	627	Lean only from #626	3 oz	85	60	187	24	0	0	9	3.2	4.2	1.1
		Rib, roasted:											
9	628	Lean and fat, piece 2½ × 2½ × ¾″	3 oz	85	51	270	21	0	0	20	7	9	2
9	629	Lean only	3 oz	85	57	210	24	0	0	12	4.1	5.3	1.4
		Shoulder, braised:											
9	630	Lean and fat, 3 pieces 2½ × 2½ × ¼″	3 oz	85	47	293	23	0	0	22	8	10	2
9	631	Lean only	3 oz	85	54	208	27	0	0	10	4	5	1.3
9	1088	Spareribs, cooked, yield from 1 lb raw with bone	6.25 oz	177	40	703	51	0	0	54	20.8	25.1	6.2
9	1095	Rabbit, roasted (1 cup meat = 140g)	3 oz	85	59	175	26	0	0	7	2.1	1.9	1.4
		VEAL, cooked:											
9	632	Veal cutlet, braised or broiled, 4⅛ × 2¼ × ½″	3 oz	85	60	166	27	0	0	6	1.6	2.0	.5
9	633	Veal rib roasted, lean, 2 pieces 4⅛ × 2¼ × ¼″	3 oz	85	65	151	22	0	0	6	1.8	2.3	.6
9	634	Veal liver, pan-fried	3 oz	85	53	208	25	3	0	10	3.6	1.6	1.5
9	1096	Venison (Deer meat) roasted	3.5 oz	100	65	158	30	0	0	3	1.3	.9	.6
		MEATS: POULTRY and POULTRY PRODUCTS											
		CHICKEN, cooked:											
		Fried, batter dipped:[78]											
10	635	Breast (5.6 oz with bones)	1 ea	140	52	364	35	13	<1	19	5	8	4
10	636	Drumstick (3.4 oz with bones)	1 ea	72	53	193	16	6	<1	11	3	5	3
10	637	Thigh	1 ea	86	52	238	19	8	<1	14	4	6	3
10	638	Wing	1 ea	49	46	159	10	5	<1	11	3	4	3
		Fried, flour coated:[78]											
10	639	Breast (4.2 oz with bones)	1 ea	98	57	218	31	2	<1	9	2.4	3.4	1.9
10	1212	Breast, without skin	1 ea	86	60	161	29	<1	0	4	1.1	1.5	.9
10	640	Drumstick (2.6 oz with bones)	1 ea	49	57	120	13	1	<1	7	1.8	2.7	1.6
10	641	Thigh	1 ea	62	54	162	17	2	<1	9	2.5	3.6	2.1
10	1099	Thigh, without skin	1 ea	52	59	113	15	1	<1	5	1.5	2.0	1.3
10	642	Wing	1 ea	32	49	103	8	1	<1	7	1.9	2.8	1.6
		Roasted:											
10	643	All types of meat	1 c	140	64	266	41	0	0	10	2.9	3.7	2.4
10	644	Dark meat	1 c	140	63	286	38	0	0	14	3.7	5.0	3.2
10	645	Light meat	1 c	140	65	242	43	0	0	6	1.8	2.2	1.4
10	646	Breast, without skin	½ ea	86	65	142	27	0	0	3	.9	1.1	.7
10	647	Drumstick	1 ea	44	67	76	13	0	0	2	.7	.8	.6
10	648	Thigh	1 ea	62	59	153	16	0	0	10	2.9	3.8	2.1
10	1100	Thigh, without skin	1 ea	52	63	109	14	0	0	6	1.6	2.2	1.3
10	649	Stewed, all types:	1 c	140	67	248	38	0	0	9	2.6	3.3	2.2
10	656	Canned, boneless chicken	5 oz	142	69	235	31	0	0	11	3.1	4.5	2.5
10	1102	Chicken gizzards, simmered	1 ea	22	67	34	6	<1	0	1	.2	.2	.2
10	1101	Chicken hearts, simmered	1 ea	3.3	65	6	1	<1	0	<1	.1	.1	.1
10	650	Chicken liver, simmered	1 ea	20	68	30	5	2	0	1	.4	.3	.2

(78)Fried in vegetable shortening.

GRP KEY: 1 = BEV 2 = DAIRY 3 = EGGS 4 = FAT/OIL 5 = FRUIT 6 = BAKERY 7 = GRAIN 8 = FISH **9 = BEEF** 10 = POULTRY 11 = SAUSAGE 12 = MIXED/FAST 13 = NUTS/SEEDS 14 = SWEETS 15 = VEG/LEG 16 = MISC 22 = SOUP/SAUCE

Chol (mg)	Calc (mg)	Iron (mg)	Magn (mg)	Phos (mg)	Pota (mg)	Sodi (mg)	Zinc (mg)	VT-A (RE)	Thia (mg)	Ribo (mg)	Niac (mg)	V-B6 (mg)	Fola (µg)	VT-C (mg)
92	4	.75	23	190	323	64	1.74	3	.91	.25	4.58	.35	4	<1
71	3	.67	21	178	305	57	1.61	2	.84	.22	4.03	.34	4	<1
79	5	.85	18	210	280	50	2.43	2	.54	.27	3.89	.33	9	<1
80	6	.95	21	239	317	54	2.77	2	.59	.3	4.2	.38	10	<1
69	9	.76	16	190	313	37	1.67	3	.5	.24	4.17	.3	7	<1
67	10	.85	18	218	360	40	1.9	3	.54	.26	4.6	.34	7	<1
93	6	1.4	16	162	286	74	3.43	3	.46	.26	4.43	.23	3	<1
95	6	1.64	19	189	339	85	4.16	3	.5	.3	5	.35	4	<1
214	83	3.27	43	462	566	165	8.14	5	.72	.68	9.69	.62	7	0
73	17	2.02	17	192	255	31	2.02	2	.05	.14	6.09	.29	8	0
100	20	.99	24	213	288	76	4.33	t	.05	.29	7.16	.28	13	0
97	10	.82	20	176	264	82	3.81	t	.05	.25	6.4	.23	12	0
280	10	4.45	22	373	372	112	6.69	4784[79]	.21	2.86	14.4	.73	272	18
112	7	4.47	24	226	335	54	2.75	0	.18	.60	6.71	.32[80]	4[80]	0
119	28	1.75	34	258	282	385	1.33	28	.16	.2	14.7	.6	8	0
62	12	.97	14	106	134	194	1.67	19	.08	.16	3.67	.2	6	0
80	16	1.24	18	134	165	248	1.75	25	.1	.2	4.92	.23	8	0
39	10	.63	8	59	68	157	.67	17	.05	.07	2.58	.15	3	0
88	16	1.17	29	228	253	74	1.07	15	.08	.13	13.5	.57	4	0
78	14	.98	27	212	237	68	.93	6	.07	.11	12.7	.55	4	0
44	6	.66	11	86	112	44	1.42	12	.04	.11	2.96	.17	4	0
60	8	.93	15	116	147	55	1.56	18	.06	.15	4.31	.21	5	0
53	7	.76	14	103	134	49	1.45	11	.05	.13	3.70	.20	4	0
26	5	.4	6	48	57	25	.56	12	.02	.04	2.14	.13	1	0
125	21	1.69	35	273	340	120	2.94	22	.1	.25	12.8	.65	8	0
130	21	1.86	33	250	336	130	3.92	30	.1	.32	9.17	.5	11	0
118	21	1.49	38	302	345	108	1.73	12	.09	.16	17.4	.84	5	0
73	13	.89	25	196	220	64	.86	5	.06	.1	11.8	.52	3	0
41	5	.57	11	81	108	42	1.4	8	.03	.1	2.67	.17	4	0
58	8	.83	14	108	137	52	1.46	30	.04	.13	3.95	.19	4	0
49	6	.68	12	95	124	46	1.34	10	.04	.12	3.39	.18	4	0
116	20	1.63	29	210	252	98	2.79	21	.07	.23	8.56	.37	8	0
88	20	2.2	17	158	196	714	2.13	48	.02	.18	8.99	.5	4	3
43	2	.91	4	34	39	15	.96	12	.01	.05	.87	.03	12	<1
8	1	.30	1	7	4	2	.24	<1	<.01	.02	.09	.01	3	<1
126	3	1.7	2	62	28	10	.87	983	.03	.35	.89	.12	154	3

(79) Value varies widely.
(80) Values estimated from other game meat.

(For purposes of calculations, use "0" for t, <1, <.1, <.01, etc.)

Table F–1 Food Composition

Grp	Computer Code No.	Food Description	Measure	Wt (g)	H_2O (%)	Ener (cal)	Prot (g)	Carb (g)	Dietary Fiber (g)	Fat (g)	Fat Breakdown (g) Sat	Mono	Poly
		MEATS: POULTRY and POULTRY PRODUCTS—Con.											
		DUCK, roasted:											
10	1293	Meat with skin, about 2.7 cups	½ duck	382	52	1287	73	0	0	108	37	49	14
10	651	Meat only, about 1.5 cups	½ duck	221	64	445	52	0	0	25	9.2	8.2	3.2
		GOOSE, domesticated, roasted:											
10	1294	Meat only, 4.2 cups	½ goose	591	57	1406	171	0	0	75	27	26	9
10	1295	Meat w/skin, about 5.5 cups	½ goose	774	52	2362	195	0	0	170	53	79	20
		TURKEY, roasted, meat only:											
10	652	Dark meat	3 oz	85	63	159	24	0	0	6	2.1	1.4	1.8
10	653	Light meat	3 oz	85	66	133	25	0	0	3	.9	.5	.7
10	654	All types, chopped or diced	1 c	140	65	238	41	0	0	7	2.3	1.5	2.0
10	655	All types, sliced	3 oz	85	65	145	25	0	0	4	1.4	.9	1.2
10	1103	Ground turkey, cooked	3.5 oz	100	60	229	24	0	0	14	3.8	5.0	3.3
		Turkey breast:											
10	1104	Barbecued	1 oz	28	70	40	6	0	0	1	.4	.5	.3
10	1105	Hickory smoked	1 oz	28	70	35	6	1	0	1	.3	.3	.3
10	1106	Gizzard, cooked	1 ea	67	65	109	20	<1	0	3	.7	.5	.7
10	1107	Heart, cooked	1 ea	16	64	28	4	<1	0	1	.3	.2	.3
10	1108	Liver, cooked	1 ea	75	66	127	18	3	0	4	1.4	1.1	1.1
		Poultry food products (see also items in sausages and lunchmeats section):											
10	658	Chicken roll, light meat	2 pce	57	69	90	11	1	0	4	1.2	1.7	.9
10	659	Gravy and turkey, frozen package	5 oz	142	85	95	8	7	<1	4	1.2	1.4	.7
10	660	Turkey loaf, breast meat	2 pce	42	72	46	10	0	0	1	.2	.2	.1
10	661	Turkey patties, breaded, fried	1 ea	64	50	181	9	10	<1	12	3	4.8	3
10	662	Turkey, frozen, roasted, seasoned	3 oz	85	68	130	18	3	0	5	1.6	1	1.4
		MEATS: SAUSAGES and LUNCHMEATS (see also Poultry food products)											
		Beerwurst/beer salami:											
11	1072	Beef	1 pce	23	54	75	3	<1	0	7	2.8	3.3	.2
11	1074	Pork	1 pce	23	62	55	3	<1	0	4	1.4	2.1	.5
11	1075	Berliner	1 pce	23	61	53	4	1	0	4	1.4	1.8	.4
		Bologna:											
11	1297	Beef	1 pce	23	55	72	3	<1	0	7	2.7	3.1	.2
11	663	Beef and pork	1 pce	28	54	89	3	1	0	8	3.0	3.8	.7
11	1298	Pork	1 pce	23	61	57	4	<1	0	5	1.6	2.3	.5
11	664	Turkey	1 pce	28	66	56	4	<1	0	4	1.5	1.9	1.2
11	665	Braunschweiger sausage	2 pce	57	48	205	8	2	0	18	6.2	8.5	2.1
11	1073	Brotwurst, link	1 ea	70	51	226	10	2	0	20	7.0	9.3	2.0
11	666	Brown-and-serve sausage links, cooked	1 ea	13	45	50	2	<1	0	5	1.7	2.2	.5
11	1089	Cheesefurter/cheese smokie	1 ea	43	53	141	6	1	0	13	4.5	5.9	1.3
11	1090	Corned beef loaf, jellied	1 pce	28	67	46	7	0	0	2	.8	.9	.1
		Frankfurters (see also #657):											
11	1077	Beef, large link, 8/pkg.	1 ea	57	54	184	6	1	0	17	6.8	8.2	.7
11	1078	Beef and pork, large link, 8/pkg.	1 ea	57	54	183	6	1	0	17	6.1	7.8	1.6
11	667	Beef and pork, smaller link, 10/pkg.	1 ea	45	54	145	5	1	0	13	4.8	6.2	1.2
10	657	Chicken frankfurter, 10/pkg.	1 ea	45	58	115	6	3	0	9	2.5	3.8	1.8
11	668	Turkey, smaller link, 10/pkg.	1 ea	45	63	102	6	1	0	8	2.7	3.3	2.1
		Ham:											
11	669	Ham lunchmeat, canned, 3 x 2 x ½″	1 pce	21	52	70	3	<1	0	6	2.3	3.0	.8
11	670	Chopped ham, packaged	2 pce	22	61	98	7	<1	0	8	2.6	3.9	.9

(Computer code number is for West Diet Analysis program)

GRP KEY: 1=BEV 2=DAIRY 3=EGGS 4=FAT/OIL 5=FRUIT 6=BAKERY 7=GRAIN 8=FISH 9=BEEF **10=POULTRY** 11=SAUSAGE 12=MIXED/FAST 13=NUTS/SEEDS 14=SWEETS 15=VEG/LEG 16=MISC 22=SOUP/SAUCE

Chol (mg)	Calc (mg)	Iron (mg)	Magn (mg)	Phos (mg)	Pota (mg)	Sodi (mg)	Zinc (mg)	VT-A (RE)	Thia (mg)	Ribo (mg)	Niac (mg)	V-B6 (mg)	Fola (µg)	VT-C (mg)
320	43	10.3	62	595	780	227	7.12	241	.67	1.03	18.4	.70	25	0
198	26	5.97	44	449	557	143	5.75	51	.57	1.04	11.3	.55	22	0
569	84	17.0	148	1828	2291	447	16.0	71	.54	2.31	24.1	2.75	13	0
708	104	21.9	169	2091	2546	543	16.0	162	.60	2.50	32.3	2.89	17	0
72	27	1.99	21	174	247	67	3.8	0	.05	.21	3.1	.3	8	0
59	16	1.14	24	186	259	54	1.73	0	.05	.12	5.81	.46	5	0
107	35	2.49	37	298	418	99	4.34	0	.09	.26	7.62	.64	10	0
64	21	1.51	23	181	254	60	2.64	0	.05	.16	4.63	.39	6	0
69	25	1.93	24	196	270	83	2.86	0	.05	.17	4.82	.39	7	0
16	2	.12	7	74	57	156	.35	0	.01	.03	2.73	.11	1	<1
13	1	.20	7	79	59	208	.30	0	.01	.03	2.75	.11	1	<1
155	10	3.64	13	86	141	37	2.79	37	.02	.22	2.06	.08	36	1
36	2	1.10	4	33	29	9	.84	1	.01	.14	.52	.05	13	<1
469	8	5.85	11	204	146	48	2.32	2806	.04	1.07	4.46	.39	499	1
28	24	.55	10	89	129	331	.41	14	.04	.07	3	.31	2	0
26	20	1.32	11	115	87	787	.99	18	.03	.18	2.55	.14	2	0
17	3	.17	9	97	118	608	.48	0	.02	.05	3.54	.15	2	0[81]
40	9	1.41	12	173	176	512	1.5	7	.06	.12	1.47	.13	3	0
45	4	1.4	20	207	253	578	2.37	0	.04	.14	5.3	.24	5	0
13	2	.31	3	24	42	214	.61	0	.03	.03	.66	.05	1	3
13	2	.17	3	24	58	285	.40	0	.13	.04	.75	.08	1	7
11	3	.27	3	30	65	298	.57	0	.09	.05	.72	.05	1	2
13	3	.32	2	19	36	230	.46	0	.01	.03	.61	.04	1	4
16	3	.43	3	26	51	289	.55	0	.05	.04	.73	.05	1	6[82]
14	3	.18	3	33	65	272	.47	0	.12	.04	.90	.06	1	8
28	23	.43	4	37	56	248	.49	0	.02	.05	1.04	.05	1	<1
89	6	5.32	6	96	113	652	1.62	2406	.14	.87	4.78	.19	57	5[82]
44	34	.72	11	94	197	778	1.47	0	.18	.16	2.31	.09	2	20
9	1	.1	2	14	25	105	.15	0	.05	.02	.40	.03	1	0
29	25	.46	5	76	89	465	.97	3	.11	.07	1.25	.05	1	8
12	3	.58	3	18	25	294	1.08	0	<.01	.03	.46	.04	1	2
27	7	.76	7	47	90	584	1.21	0	.03	.06	1.44	.06	2	14
29	6	.66	7	49	95	639	1.05	0	.11	.07	1.50	.08	2	15
23	5	.52	6	39	75	504	.83	0	.09	.05	1.18	.06	2	12[82]
45	43	.9	8	48	38	616	1	17	.03	.05	1.39	.09	2	0
39	58	.77	8	83	88	454	1	17	.04	.08	1.7	.10	2	<1
13	1	.15	2	17	45	271	.31	0	.08	.04	.66	.04	1	<1
21	3	.4	5	58	119	573	.77	0	.23	.07	1.4	.13	2	1[82]

(81) If sodium ascorbate is added, product contains 11 mg ascorbic acid.

(82) Values based on products containing added ascorbic acid or sodium ascorbate. If none added, ascorbic acid content would be negligible.

Table F–1 Food Composition

Grp	Computer Code No.	Food Description	Measure	Wt (g)	H_2O (%)	Ener (cal)	Prot (g)	Carb (g)	Dietary Fiber (g)	Fat (g)	Fat Breakdown (g) Sat	Mono	Poly
		MEATS: SAUSAGES and LUNCHMEATS—Con.											
		Ham—Con.											
11	671	Ham lunchmeat, regular	2 pce	57	65	103	10	2	0	6	1.9	2.8	.7
11	672	Ham lunchmeat, extra lean	2 pce	57	70	75	11	1	0	3	.9	1.3	.3
11	673	Turkey ham	2 pce	57	72	73	11	1	0	3	1.0	.8	.8
11	1091	Keilbasa sausage	1 pce	26	54	81	3	1	0	7	2.6	3.4	.8
11	1092	Knockwurst sausage-link	1 ea	68	56	209	8	1	0	19	6.9	8.7	2.0
11	1093	Mortadella lunchmeat	1 pce	15	52	47	2	<1	0	4	1.4	1.7	.5
11	1097	Olive loaf lunchmeat	2 pce	57	58	133	7	5	<1	9	3.3	4.5	1.1
11	1080	Pastrami, turkey	2 pce	57	72	74	11	1	0	4	1.0	1.2	.9
11	1081	Pepperoni sausage, small slices	4 pce	22	27	109	5	1	0	10	3.6	4.6	1
11	1094	Pickle & pimento loaf	2 pce	57	57	149	7	3	<1	12	4.5	5.4	1.5
11	1082	Polish sausage	1 oz.	28	53	92	4	<1	0	8	2.9	3.8	.9
		Pork sausage, cooked:[83]											
11	674	Link, small	1 ea	13	45	48	3	<1	0	4	1.4	1.8	.5
11	1079	Patty	1 pce	27	45	100	5	<1	0	8	2.9	3.8	1.0
		Salami:											
11	675	Pork and beef	2 pce	57	60	143	8	1	0	11	4.6	5.2	1.1
11	676	Turkey	2 pce	57	66	111	9	<1	0	8	2.3	2.6	2.0
11	677	Dry, beef and pork	2 pce	20	35	85	5	1	0	7	2.4	3.4	.6
		Sandwich spreads:											
11	1300	Ham salad	1 c	240	63	518	21	26	<1	37	12.1	17.3	6.5
11	678	Pork and beef	1 tbsp	15	60	35	1	2	0	3	.9	1.1	.4
10	1296	Poultry sandwich spread	1 tbsp	13	60	25	2	1	0	2	.5	.4	.8
		Smoked link sausage:											
11	1083	Beef and pork	1 ea	68	39	265	15	1	0	22	7.7	10.0	2.6
11	1084	Pork	1 ea	68	52	229	9	1	0	21	7.2	9.7	2.2
11	1085	Summer sausage	1 pce	23	48	80	4	1	0	7	2.8	3.2	.4
11	1076	Turkey breakfast sausage	1 pce	28	60	65	6	0	0	4	1.6	1.8	1.2
11	679	Vienna sausage, canned	1 ea	16	60	45	2	<1	0	4	1.5	2.0	.3
		MIXED DISHES and FAST FOODS											
		MIXED DISHES:											
		Beef stew with vegetables:											
12	680	Homemade	1 c	245	82	220	16	15	3	11	4.4	4.5	.5
12	1109	Canned	1 c	245	83	194	14	18	1	8	3.1	3.1	.4
12	1116	Beef, macaroni & tomato sauce casserole	1 c	226	80	189	10	25	2	6	2.1	2.3	.4
12	681	Beef pot pie, homemade[84]	1 pce	210	55	515	21	39	1	30	8	13	7
12	682	Chicken à la king, home recipe	1 c	245	68	470	27	12	1	34	13	13	6
12	683	Chicken and noodles, home recipe	1 c	240	71	365	22	26	1	18	5	7	4
12	684	Chicken chow mein, canned	1 c	250	89	95	7	18	5	1	.1	.1	.8
12	685	Chicken chow mein, home recipe	1 c	250	78	255	23	10	4	11	4	4	3
12	686	Chicken pot pie, home recipe[84]	1 pce	232	57	545	23	42	2	31	10	16	7
12	1112	Chicken salad w/celery	.5 c	78	53	266	11	1	<1	25	4.1	7.2	12.0
12	687	Chili with beans, canned	1 c	255	76	286	15	30	8	14	6	6	1
12	688	Chop suey with beef and pork	1 c	250	75	300	26	13	2	17	4	7	4
12	689	Corn pudding[85]	1 c	250	76	271	11	32	9	13	6.3	4.3	1.7
12	690	Cole slaw[86]	1 c	120	82	84	2	15	2	3	.5	.9	1.6
12	1110	Corned beef hash-canned	1 c	220	67	382	18	22	1	10	4.2	4.9	.5
12	1113	Egg salad	1 c	183	66	438	19	3	<1	39	8.4	13.2	13.5

(83)Cooked weight is half the weight of raw sausage.

(84)Crust made with vegetable shortening and enriched flour.

(85)Recipe: 55% yellow corn, 23% whole milk, 14% egg, 4% sugar, 3% salt, and 1% pepper.

(86)Recipe: 41% cabbage; 12% celery; 12% table cream; 12% sugar; 7% green pepper; 6% lemon juice; 4% onion; 3% pimento; 3% vinegar; 2% each for salt, dry mustard, and white pepper.

GRP KEY: 1=BEV 2=DAIRY 3=EGGS 4=FAT/OIL 5=FRUIT 6=BAKERY 7=GRAIN 8=FISH 9=BEEF 10=POULTRY **11=SAUSAGE**
12=MIXED/FAST 13=NUTS/SEEDS 14=SWEETS 15=VEG/LEG 16=MISC 22=SOUP/SAUCE

Chol (mg)	Calc (mg)	Iron (mg)	Magn (mg)	Phos (mg)	Pota (mg)	Sodi (mg)	Zinc (mg)	VT-A (RE)	Thia (mg)	Ribo (mg)	Niac (mg)	V-B6 (mg)	Fola (μg)	VT-C (mg)
32	4	.56	11	140	188	746	1.21	0	.49	.14	2.98	.19	2	16[82]
27	4	.43	10	124	198	810	1.09	0	.53	.13	2.74	.26	2	15[82]
32	5	1.56	12	138	163	548	1.58	0	.04	.15	2.72	.16	4	0
17	11	.38	4	38	70	280	.52	0	.06	.06	.75	.05	1	6
39	7	.62	8	67	136	687	1.13	0	.23	.10	1.86	.11	2	18
8	3	.21	2	15	24	187	.32	0	.02	.02	.40	.02	<1	4
22	62	.31	11	72	169	842	.78	0	.17	.15	1.04	.13	1	5
30	5	.81	10	142	155	569	1.46	0	.05	.15	2.48	.16	4	<1
8	2	.31	4	26	76	449	.55	0	.07	.06	1.09	.06	—	<1
21	54	.58	10	79	193	787	.79	<1	.17	.14	1.16	.11	1	8
20	3	.41	4	39	67	248	.55	0	.14	.04	.98	.05	1	0
11	4	.16	2	24	47	168	.33	0	.1	.03	.59	.04	1	<1
22	9	.34	5	50	97	349	.68	0	.20	.07	1.22	.09	2	<1
37	7	1.51	9	65	112	604	1.21	0	.14	.21	2.02	.12	1	7[82]
46	11	.93	9	73	125	535	1.25	0	.06	.15	2.23	.14	5	<1
16	2	.3	4	28	76	372	.64	0	.12	.06	.97	.1	0	6[82]
88	19	1.42	23	286	359	2187	2.64	42	1.04	.29	5.02	.36	3	14
6	2	.12	1	9	16	152	.15	1	.03	.02	.26	.02	<1	0
4	1	.08	3	4	24	49	.25	6	<.01	.01	.22	.01	1	<1
46	20	.79	13	110	228	1020	1.92	0	.48	.18	3.08	.24	2	1
48	7	.99	8	73	129	642	1.44	0	.18	.12	2.19	.12	2	13
16	2	.47	3	23	53	334	.47	0	.04	.07	.94	.07	1	5
23	5	.52	6	52	76	191	.97	0	.03	.08	1.42	.08	1	—
8	2	.14	1	8	16	152	.26	0	.01	.02	.26	.02	<1	0
71	29	2.9	40	184	613	292	5.3	569	.15	.17	4.7	.28	37	17
15	23	3.18	39	56	417	992	4.23	262	.07	.12	2.43	.20	31	7
22	30	2.39	37	118	562	974	2.07	111	.19	.17	3.51	.30	23	16
42	29	3.8	6	149	334	596	3.17	517	.29	.29	4.8	.24	29	6
221	127	2.5	20	358	404	760	1.8	272	.1	.42	5.4	.23	11	12
103	26	2.4	37	247	211	600	2.14	130	.05	.17	4.3	.16	9	1
8	45	1.3	14	85	418	725	1.3	28	.05	.1	1	.09	12	13
75	58	2.50	28	293	473	718	2.12	50	.08	.23	4.3	.41	19	10
56	70	3.0	25	232	343	594	2.0	735	.32	.32	4.9	.46	29	5
48	16	.66	11	80	137	199	.80	31	.03	.08	3.25	.17	4	1
43	119	8.75	115	393	932	1330	5.10	86	.12	.27	.91	.34	41	4
68	60	4.80	32	248	425	1053	3.58	60	.28	.38	5.0	.32	22	33
230	100	1.40	38	143	402	138	1.26	89	1.03	.32	2.47	.30	63	7
10[87]	54	.70	12	38	218	28	.24	98	.08	.07	.33	.18	32	39
132	29	4.40	3	147	440	1354	4.38	0	.12	.40	4.60	.41	15	8
629	94	3.39	21	282	211	428	2.24	300	.12	.45	.16	.18	74	0

(82)Values based on products containing added ascorbic acid or sodium ascorbate. If none added, ascorbic acid content would be negligible.
(87)From dairy cream in recipe.

(For purposes of calculations, use "0" for t, <1, <.1, <.01, etc.)

Table F–1 Food Composition

Grp	Computer Code No.	Food Description	Measure	Wt (g)	H_2O (%)	Ener (cal)	Prot (g)	Carb (g)	Dietary Fiber (g)	Fat (g)	Fat Breakdown (g) Sat	Mono	Poly
		MIXED DISHES and FAST FOODS—Con.											
		MIXED DISHES—Con.											
12	691	French toast, home recipe[88]	1 pce	65	53	123	5	15	1	4	1.1	1.4	1.1
12	1355	Green pepper, stuffed	1 ea	172	76	217	10	16	1	13	5.3	5.2	.6
		Lasagna:											
12	1346	With meat	1 pce	245	64	398	26	30	2	20	9.2	7.2	1.5
12	1111	Without meat	1 pce	218	64	316	20	30	2	14	6.9	4.7	1.3
12	1117	Frozen entree	1 pce	205	73	275	17	19	1	12	6.3	4.2	1.2
		Macaroni and cheese:											
12	692	Canned[89]	1 c	240	80	230	9	26	1	10	5	3	1
12	693	Home recipe[90]	1 c	200	58	430	17	40	1	22	10	7	4
12	1115	Macaroni salad-no cheese	1 c	141	61	371	3	18	1	33	5.1	9.5	17.2
		Meat loaf:											
12	1120	Beef	1 pce	87	62	193	16	4	<1	12	4.8	5.2	.6
12	1119	Beef and pork (1/3)	1 pce	87	59	212	15	5	<1	15	5.5	6.3	1.2
12	1303	Moussaka (lamb and eggplant)	1 c	250	79	250	21	16	6	11	3.6	4.3	1.9
12	715	Potato salad with mayonnaise and egg[91]	1 c	250	76	358	7	28	4	21	4	6	9
12	694	Quiche lorraine, ⅛ of 8″ quiche[84]	1 pce	176	47	600	13	29	1	48	23	18	4
		Spaghetti (enriched) in tomato sauce:											
		With cheese:											
12	695	Canned	1 c	250	80	190	6	39	3	2	.4	.4	.5
12	696	Home recipe	1 c	250	77	260	9	37	3	9	3	3.6	1.2
		With meatballs:											
12	697	Canned	1 c	250	78	260	12	39	3	10	2	4	3
12	698	Home recipe	1 c	248	70	330	19	39	3	12	4	4	2
12	716	Spinach soufflé[92]	1 c	136	74	218	11	3	4	18	7	7	3
12	717	Tuna salad[93]	1 c	205	63	383	33	19	2	19	3	6	9
12	1121	Tuna noodle casserole, recipe	1 c	202	73	251	21	24	<1	7	2.0	1.5	3.2
12	1270	Waldorf salad	1 c	142	58	424	4	13	4	42	5.6	11.2	23.1
		FAST FOODS and SANDWICHES: see end of this appendix for additional Fast Foods.											
		Burrito:[94]											
12	699	Beef and bean	1 ea	175	54	390	21	40	5	18	7	7	2
12	700	Bean	1 ea	174	55	322	13	47	8	10	4	3	2
		Cheeseburger:											
12	701	Regular	1 ea	112	46	300	15	28	1	15	7	6	1
12	702	4-oz patty	1 ea	194	46	524	30	40	2	31	15	12	1
12	703	Chicken patty sandwich	1 ea	157	52	436	25	34	1	22	6	10	5
12	704	Corn dog	1 ea	111	45	330	10	27	<1	20	8	10	1
12	705	Enchilada, cheese	1 ea	163	63	320	10	29	3	19	11	6	.8
12	706	English muffin with egg, cheese, bacon	1 ea	138	49	360	18	31	2	18	8	8	.7
		Fish sandwich:											
12	707	Regular, with cheese	1 ea	140	43	420	16	39	1	23	6	7	8
12	708	Large, without cheese	1 ea	170	48	470	18	41	1	27	6	9	10

(84)Crust made with vegetable shortening and enriched flour.
(88)Recipe: 35% whole milk, 32% white bread, 29% egg, and cooked in 4% margarine.
(89)Made with corn oil.
(90)Made with margarine.
(91)Recipe: 62% potatoes; 12% egg; 8% mayonnaise; 7% celery; 6% sweet pickle relish; 2% onion; 1% each for green pepper, pimiento, salt, and dry mustard.
(92)Recipe: 29% whole milk, 26% spinach, 13% egg white, 13% cheddar cheese, 7% egg yolk, 7% butter, 4% flour, 1% salt and pepper.
(93)Made with drained chunk light tuna, celery, onion, pickle relish, and mayonnaise-type salad dressing.
(94)Made with a 10½″-diameter flour tortilla.

GRP KEY: 1 = BEV 2 = DAIRY 3 = EGGS 4 = FAT/OIL 5 = FRUIT 6 = BAKERY 7 = GRAIN 8 = FISH 9 = BEEF 10 = POULTRY 11 = SAUSAGE **12 = MIXED/FAST** 13 = NUTS/SEEDS 14 = SWEETS 15 = VEG/LEG 16 = MISC 22 = SOUP/SAUCE

Chol (mg)	Calc (mg)	Iron (mg)	Magn (mg)	Phos (mg)	Pota (mg)	Sodi (mg)	Zinc (mg)	VT-A (RE)	Thia (mg)	Ribo (mg)	Niac (mg)	V-B6 (mg)	Fola (µg)	VT-C (mg)
73	79	1.08	12	82	96	189	.47	57	.15	.17	1.09	.04	18	<1
38	15	2.32	23	91	227	210	2.58	29	.11	.10	2.96	.22	14	83
56	460	3.08	41	393	507	783	3.23	168	.22	.33	3.64	.35	16	7
30	457	2.38	35	345	424	760	1.93	168	.21	.28	2.01	.22	14	7
90	246	2.48	52	253	437	967	1.25	97	.19	.33	2.70	.29	25	6
24	199	1.0	31	182	139	730	1.20	72	.12	.24	1.0	.02	8	<1
24	27	1.14	23	50	162	315	.34	40	.10	.07	.67	.07	7	3
98	29	1.90	19	123	227	340	3.50	26	.06	.18	3.19	.18	8	1
97	33	1.39	18	128	238	392	2.86	26	.19	.19	3.07	.19	8	1
143	129	2.75	44	245	695	485	3.29	125	.25	.32	4.78	.35	44	7
170	48	1.63	39	130	635	1323	.78	83	.19	.15	2.23	.35	17	25
44	362	1.8	37	322	240	1086	1.20	232	.20	.40	1.8	.05	10	1
285	211	1.4	23	276	283	653	1.95	454	.11	.32	1.2	.15	17	<1
3	40	2.8	21	88	303	955	1.12	120	.35	.28	4.5	.13	6	10
8	80	2.3	26	135	408	955	1.3	140	.25	.18	2.3	.20	8	13
23	53	3.3	20	113	245	1220	2.39	100	.15	.18	2.3	.12	5	5
89	124	3.7	40	236	665	1009	2.45	159	.25	.30	.4	.20	10	22
184	230	1.34	37	231	202	763	1.29	675	.09	.31	.48	.12	62	3
27	35	2.0	40	365	365	824	1.15	55	.06	.14	13.3	.17	15	5
52	37	1.94	31	182	224	869	.97	34	.14	.17	8.59	.24	13	1
22	44	.98	41	88	279	246	.69	41	.10	.06	.37	.16	19	6
52	165	2.7	61	274	388	516	3.30	58	.26	.29	4.36	.73	48	5
15	181	2.53	76	243	427	1030	2.37	58	.26	.23	2.40	1.01	55	5
44	135	2.30	22	174	219	672	2.53	65	.26	.24	3.70	.11	20	1
104	236	4.45	43	320	407	1224	5.27	128	.33	.49	7.37	.23	23	3
68	44	1.87	30	173	194	2732	1.00	16	.29	.26	9.21	.37	18	4
37	34	1.94	22	303	164	1252	1.44	<1	.28	.17	3.27	.11	2	3
44	324	1.31	50	133	240	784	2.51	186	.09	.42	1.91	.39	34	1
213	197	3.10	28	290	201	832	1.86	160	.46	.50	3.71	.15	35	1
56	132	1.85	29	223	274	667	.95	25	.32	.27	3.30	.10	24	3
90	61	2.23	34	246	375	621	.88	15	.35	.24	3.52	.12	43	1

(For purposes of calculations, use "0" for t, <1, <.1, <.01, etc.)

• *Table F–1* Food Composition

Grp	Computer Code No.	Food Description	Measure	Wt (g)	H_2O (%)	Ener (cal)	Prot (g)	Carb (g)	Dietary Fiber (g)	Fat (g)	Fat Breakdown (g) Sat	Mono	Poly
		MIXED DISHES and FAST FOODS—Con.											
		FAST FOODS and SANDWICHES—Con.											
		Hamburger with bun:											
12	709	Regular	1 ea	98	46	245	12	28	1	11	4	5	1
12	710	4-oz patty	1 ea	174	50	445	25	38	1	21	7	12	1
12	711	Hotdog/frankfurter and bun	1 ea	85	53	260	8	21	1	15	5	7	2
12	712	Cheese pizza, ⅛ of 15″ round[95]	1 pce	120	46	290	15	39	2	9	4	3	1
		SANDWICHES:											
		Avocado, cheese, tomato & lettuce:											
12	1276	On white bread, firm	1 ea	205	59	464	15	39	7	29	9.1	11.8	6.0
12	1278	On part whole wheat	1 ea	195	60	432	14	33	8	29	8.7	11.8	6.0
12	1277	On whole wheat	1 ea	209	58	459	16	39	13	29	9.1	11.9	6.2
		Bacon, lettuce & tomato sandwich:											
12	1137	On white bread, soft	1 ea	135	54	333	11	30	2	19	5.2	7.4	5.5
12	1139	On part whole wheat	1 ea	135	54	327	12	28	3	19	4.9	7.5	5.5
12	1138	On whole wheat	1 ea	149	53	355	13	34	8	20	5.4	7.7	5.7
		Cheese sandwich, grilled:											
12	1140	On white bread, soft	1 ea	117	37	399	17	28	1	24	12.7	7.6	2.3
12	1142	On part whole wheat	1 ea	117	37	393	18	27	3	24	12.5	7.7	2.3
12	1141	On whole wheat	1 ea	131	38	420	20	33	7	25	12.9	7.9	2.6
		Chicken salad sandwich:											
12	1143	On white bread, soft	1 ea	99.7	44	300	10	28	1	16	3.0	4.9	7.5
12	1145	On part whole wheat	1 ea	99.7	44	294	11	27	3	16	2.8	5.0	7.5
12	1144	On whole wheat	1 ea	114	44	321	12	33	8	17	3.2	5.2	7.8
12	1146	Corned beef & swiss cheese on rye	1 ea	147	45	429	27	25	5	24	9.4	8.2	5.0
		Egg salad sandwich:											
12	1147	On white bread, soft	1 ea	111	47	325	9	28	1	19	3.9	6.2	7.7
12	1149	On part whole wheat	1 ea	111	47	319	10	27	3	19	3.7	6.3	7.7
12	1148	On whole wheat	1 ea	125	47	346	12	33	7	20	4.1	6.4	8.0
		Ham sandwich:											
12	1279	On rye bread	1 ea	116	55	242	16	25	5	9	1.9	3.2	2.8
12	1151	On white bread, soft	1 ea	122	54	262	16	28	1	9	2.2	3.4	2.7
12	1153	On part whole wheat	1 ea	122	54	256	17	27	3	9	2.0	3.5	2.7
12	1152	On whole wheat	1 ea	136	53	283	18	33	7	10	2.4	3.7	3.0
		Ham & cheese sandwich:											
12	1280	On soft white bread	1 ea	151	51	369	22	29	1	18	7.8	6.0	3.0
12	1282	On part whole wheat bread	1 ea	151	51	363	23	28	3	18	7.6	6.1	3.0
12	1281	On whole wheat	1 ea	165	50	390	25	33	7	19	8.0	6.2	3.3
12	1150	Ham & swiss on rye	1 ea	145	51	350	24	26	5	17	7.0	5.3	3.1
		Ham salad sandwich:											
12	1154	On white bread, soft	1 ea	125	48	345	10	34	1	19	4.8	7.2	5.9
12	1156	On part whole wheat	1 ea	125	48	339	11	33	3	19	4.6	7.3	6.0
12	1155	On whole wheat	1 ea	139	47	366	12	38	7	20	5.0	7.5	6.2
12	1157	Patty melt sandwich: ground beef & cheese on rye:	1 ea	177	45	567	32	25	5	38	14.1	13.9	6.5
		Peanut butter & jam sandwich:											
12	1158	On soft white bread	1 ea	100	27	347	12	45	3	15	2.8	6.8	4.3
12	1160	On part whole wheat	1 ea	100	27	341	12	44	5	15	2.5	6.9	4.3
12	1159	On whole wheat	1 ea	114	29	368	14	50	9	16	3.0	7.1	4.6
12	1161	Reuben sandwich, grilled: corned beef, swiss cheese, sauerkraut on rye:	1 ea	233	61	480	28	29	7	28	10.2	10.0	6.2
		Roast beef sandwich:											
12	713	On a bun	1 ea	150	52	345	22	34	1	13	4	7	2
12	1162	On soft white bread	1 ea	122	51	286	17	28	1	11	2.5	3.7	4.4

(95)Crust made with vegetable shortening and enriched flour.

GRP KEY: 1=BEV 2=DAIRY 3=EGGS 4=FAT/OIL 5=FRUIT 6=BAKERY 7=GRAIN 8=FISH 9=BEEF 10=POULTRY 11=SAUSAGE **12=MIXED/FAST** 13=NUTS/SEEDS 14=SWEETS 15=VEG/LEG 16=MISC 22=SOUP/SAUCE

Chol (mg)	Calc (mg)	Iron (mg)	Magn (mg)	Phos (mg)	Pota (mg)	Sodi (mg)	Zinc (mg)	VT-A (RE)	Thia (mg)	Ribo (mg)	Niac (mg)	V-B6 (mg)	Fola (μg)	VT-C (mg)
32	56	2.20	19	107	202	463	2.0	14	.23	.24	3.80	.12	16	1
71	75	4.84	38	225	404	763	5.01	28	.38	.38	7.85	.28	24	2
23	59	1.71	13	83	113	745	1.19	<1	.29	.19	2.48	.07	17	12
56	220	1.60	36	216	230	699	1.81	106	.34	.29	4.20	.04	40	2
32	312	3.02	54	242	557	556	1.69	160	.41	.43	3.98	.25	74	11
32	299	3.09	66	274	562	518	1.87	160	.36	.40	4.02	.29	76	11
32	279	3.52	105	353	608	660	2.46	160	.35	.37	4.18	.36	91	11
21	81	2.22	22	138	253	647	1.06	50	.42	.25	3.71	.10	35	13
21	80	2.57	36	181	269	661	1.30	50	.42	.26	4.13	.15	41	13
21	60	3.00	76	260	315	803	1.89	50	.41	.23	4.29	.21	55	13
55	424	1.82	25	489	158	1155	2.24	214	.28	.38	2.14	.06	25	<1
55	424	2.17	39	531	174	1169	2.49	214	.28	.38	2.56	.10	30	<1
55	404	2.61	78	610	219	1311	3.07	214	.26	.35	2.72	.17	45	<1
25	80	1.94	18	102	136	401	.76	18	.28	.21	3.73	.11	22	1
25	79	2.30	32	144	152	415	.00	18	.28	.22	4.15	.15	28	1
25	59	2.73	71	223	197	557	1.59	18	.27	.19	4.31	.22	43	1
85	331	3.98	32	310	174	1045	4.37	85	.23	.41	3.65	.14	25	0
164	96	2.49	17	133	119	447	.92	90	.29	.29	2.14	.07	38	<1
164	95	2.85	31	176	135	461	1.16	90	.29	.29	2.56	.11	44	<1
164	75	3.28	71	255	180	603	1.75	90	.28	.26	2.72	.18	59	<1
29	49	1.94	25	203	311	1261	1.91	4	.74	.30	4.50	.32	23	14
29	80	2.17	25	191	271	1199	1.50	4	.80	.31	4.94	.29	23	14
29	79	2.52	39	234	287	1213	1.74	4	.80	.32	5.36	.33	29	14
29	59	2.96	78	313	333	1355	2.33	4	.79	.29	5.52	.40	44	14
56	256	2.28	31	405	318	1610	2.44	88	.81	.42	4.96	.31	26	14
56	256	2.64	45	447	334	1624	2.69	88	.81	.42	5.38	.35	31	14
56	236	3.07	84	526	379	1766	3.27	88	.79	.39	5.54	.42	46	14
55	325	1.99	35	376	342	1336	3.03	77	.75	.40	4.52	.34	25	14
27	77	2.00	18	134	156	887	1.02	19	.52	.25	3.36	.11	21	4
27	77	2.36	32	177	172	901	1.26	19	.52	.25	3.78	.15	26	4
27	57	2.79	71	256	217	1043	1.85	19	.51	.22	3.94	.22	41	4
107	228	3.33	40	423	410	923	6.63	139	.25	.45	6.08	.31	26	<1
0	83	2.23	55	153	246	403	1.06	1	.30	.21	5.39	.12	42	<1
0	82	2.59	69	195	262	417	1.30	1	.30	.21	5.81	.16	47	<1
0	62	3.02	108	274	308	559	1.89	1	.28	.18	5.97	.23	62	<1
85	358	5.20	44	328	313	1642	4.55	133	.25	.43	3.80	.24	27	12
55	60	4.04	38	222	338	757	3.66	32	.39	.33	6.02	.28	42	2
30	80	2.86	23	157	298	757	2.63	8	.31	.29	5.10	.21	23	<1

(For purposes of calculations, use "0" for t, <1, <.1, <.01, etc.)

Table F–1 Food Composition

Grp	Computer Code No.	Food Description	Measure	Wt (g)	H_2O (%)	Ener (cal)	Prot (g)	Carb (g)	Dietary Fiber (g)	Fat (g)	Fat Breakdown (g) Sat	Mono	Poly
		MIXED DISHES and FAST FOOD—Con.											
		SANDWICHES—Con.											
		Roast Beef—Con.											
12	1164	On part whole wheat bread	1 ea	122	51	280	18	27	3	11	2.3	3.8	4.4
12	1163	On whole wheat bread	1 ea	136	50	307	19	32	7	12	2.7	3.9	4.7
		Tuna salad sandwich:											
12	1165	On soft white	1 ea	116	47	309	13	32	2	14	2.6	4.1	6.6
12	1167	On part whole wheat bread	1 ea	116	47	303	14	31	3	14	2.4	4.2	6.7
12	1166	On whole wheat bread	1 ea	130	47	331	15	37	8	15	2.8	4.4	6.9
		Turkey sandwich:											
12	1168	On soft white bread	1 ea	122	52	277	18	28	1	10	2.1	3.2	4.5
12	1170	On part whole wheat	1 ea	122	52	271	18	26	3	11	1.9	3.3	4.5
12	1169	On whole wheat	1 ea	136	51	298	20	32	7	11	2.3	3.4	4.8
		Turkey ham sandwich:											
12	1272	On rye bread	1 ea	116	55	239	15	25	5	9	1.9	2.6	3.3
12	1273	On soft white bread	1 ea	122	55	259	16	29	1	9	2.2	2.8	3.2
12	1275	On part whole wheat	1 ea	122	54	253	16	28	3	9	2.0	2.9	3.2
12	1274	On whole wheat	1 ea	136	53	281	18	33	7	10	2.4	3.1	3.5
12	714	Taco, corn tortilla, beef filling	1 ea	78	52	207	14	10	1	13	5	5	2
		Tostada:											
12	1114	With refried beans	1 ea	157	69	212	10	26	7	9	3.6	2.5	2.3
12	1118	With beans & beef	1 ea	192	67	332	18	20	4	21	9.4	7.2	2.6
12	1354	With beans & chicken	1 ea	157	67	249	19	19	4	11	4.4	3.5	2.9
		Vegetarian Foods:											
12	1175	Nuteena	1 ea	34	52	89	7	3	1	6	—	—	—
12	1171	Proteena	1 pce	67	58	160	8	5	1	12	—	—	—
12	1172	Redi-burger	1 pce	71	56	140	17	5	2	6	—	—	—
12	1173	Vege-Burger	1 pce	68	57	130	14	5	1	6	—	—	—
12	1174	Breakfast links	.5 c	108	73	110	22	4	1	1	—	—	—
		NUTS, SEEDS and PRODUCTS											
		Almonds:											
13	1365	Dry roasted, salted	1 c	138	3	810	23	33	18	71	6.8	46.2	15.0
13	718	Slivered, packed, unsalted	1 c	135	4	795	27	28	15[96]	70	7	46	15
		Whole, dried, unsalted:											
13	719	Cup	1 c	142	4	837	28	29	17[96]	74	7	48	16
13	720	Ounce	1 oz	28	4	167	6	6	3[96]	15	1	10	3
13	721	Almond butter	1 tbsp	16	1	101	2	3	1	9	1	6	2
13	722	Brazil nuts, dry (about 7)	1 oz	28	3	186	4	4	3	19	5	7	7
		Cashew nuts:											
		Dry roasted, salted											
13	723	Cup	1 c	137	2	787	21	45	8	63	13	37	11
13	724	Ounce	1 oz	28	2	163	4	9	2	13	3	8	2
		Oil roasted, salted:											
13	725	Cup	1 c	130	4	748	21	37	8	63	12	37	11
13	726	Ounce	1 oz	28	4	163	5	8	2	14	3	8	2

(96) Values reported for dietary fiber in almonds vary from 7.0 to 14.3g/100g.

GRP KEY: 1 = BEV 2 = DAIRY 3 = EGGS 4 = FAT/OIL 5 = FRUIT 6 = BAKERY 7 = GRAIN 8 = FISH 9 = BEEF 10 = POULTRY 11 = SAUSAGE **12 = MIXED/FAST** 13 = NUTS/SEEDS 14 = SWEETS 15 = VEG/LEG 16 = MISC 22 = SOUP/SAUCE

Chol (mg)	Calc (mg)	Iron (mg)	Magn (mg)	Phos (mg)	Pota (mg)	Sodi (mg)	Zinc (mg)	VT-A (RE)	Thia (mg)	Ribo (mg)	Niac (mg)	V-B6 (mg)	Fola (μg)	VT-C (mg)
30	79	3.22	37	200	314	771	2.87	8	.31	.29	5.52	.25	29	<1
30	59	3.65	76	279	359	912	3.46	8	.29	.26	5.68	.32	44	<1
25	80	2.27	23	133	199	559	.65	22	.28	.21	5.43	.14	30	2
25	80	2.63	37	176	215	573	.89	22	.28	.22	5.85	.19	36	2
25	60	3.06	76	255	260	715	1.48	22	.26	.19	6.01	.25	51	2
29	76	1.87	23	192	223	1151	1.00	8	.29	.24	6.82	.23	23	<1
29	76	2.23	37	235	239	1165	1.24	8	.28	.24	7.24	.27	28	<1
29	56	2.66	77	314	285	1307	1.83	8	.27	.21	7.40	.34	43	<1
35	50	3.04	27	214	273	986	2.37	4	.25	.32	4.46	.21	24	0
35	81	3.28	26	203	233	924	1.96	5	.31	.34	4.90	.18	24	<1
35	80	3.63	40	245	249	938	2.20	5	.30	.34	5.32	.23	29	<1
35	60	4.06	80	324	295	1080	2.79	5	.29	.31	5.48	.29	44	<1
45	85	1.29	23	141	183	141	2.89	27	.03	.13	2.49	.16	13	1
15	177	1.93	62	195	422	618	1.55	74	.06	.14	.85	1.01	47	6
62	186	2.16	52	247	442	483	3.57	132	.08	.24	2.94	.67	37	6
53	162	1.69	48	242	358	474	1.94	81	.07	.19	4.53	.73	34	3
<1	11	1.96	—	—	43	203	—	<1	1.65	.17	3.77	.20	—	<1
0	21	1.20	40	111	200	120	.87	10	.47	.58	.14	.45	60	—
0	22	1.60	31	99	280	460	1.20	26	.64	.50	7.80	.50	23	—
0	19	1.40	13	56	120	370	1.20	10	.60	.40	6.70	.80	17	—
0	32	2.70	24	105	110	190	1.10	10	.53	.68	5.00	.56	27	—
0	389	5.25	419	756	1063	1076	6.76	0	.18	.83	3.89	.10	88	1
0	359	4.94	400	702	988	15	3.94	0	.28	1.05	4.54	.15	79	1
0	378	5.20	420	738	1034	15[97]	4.15	0	.30	1.11	4.77	.16	83	1
0	75	1.04	84	147	208	3[97]	.83	0	.06	.22	.96	.03	17	<1
0	43	.59	49	84	121	2[98]	.49	0	.02	.1	.46	.01	0	<1
0	50	.97	64	170	170	<1	1.30	t	.28	.04	.46	.07	1	<1
0	62	8.22	356	671	774	877[99]	7.67	0	.27	.27	1.92	.35	95	0
0	13	1.70	74	139	160	181[99]	1.59	0	.06	.06	.4	.07	20	0
0	53	5.33	332	554	689	814[100]	6.18	0	.55	.23	2.34	.33	88	0
0	12	1.16	72	121	151	177[100]	1.35	0	.12	.05	.51	.07	19	0

(97)Salted almonds contain 1108 mg sodium per cup, 221 mg per ounce.
(98)Salted almond butter contains 72 mg sodium per tablespoon.
(99)Dry-roasted cashews without salt contain 21 mg sodium per cup, or 4 mg per ounce.
(100)Oil-roasted cashews without salt contain 22 mg sodium per cup, or 5 mg per ounce.

(For purposes of calculations, use "0" for t, <1, <.1, <.01, etc.)

Table F–1 Food Composition

Grp	Computer Code No.	Food Description	Measure	Wt (g)	H_2O (%)	Ener (cal)	Prot (g)	Carb (g)	Dietary Fiber (g)	Fat (g)	Fat Breakdown (g) Sat	Mono	Poly
NUTS, SEEDS and PRODUCTS—Con.													
		Cashew nuts, unsalted:											
13	1366	Dry roasted	1 c	137	2	787	21	45	8	64	12.6	37.4	10.7
13	1367	Oil roasted	1 c	130	4	748	21	37	8	63	12.4	36.9	10.6
13	727	Cashew butter	1 tbsp	16	3	94	3	4	1	8	2	5	1
13	728	European chestnuts, roasted, 1 c = approx 17 kernels	1 c	143	40	350	5	76	19	3	.6	1.1	1.2
		Coconut:											
		Raw:											
13	729	Piece 2 × 2 × ½″	1 pce	45	47	159	2	7	5	15	13	.6	.2
13	730	Shredded/grated, unpacked[101]	1 c	80	47	283	3	12	9	27	24	1	.3
		Dried, shredded/grated:											
13	731	Unsweetened	1 c	78	3	515	5	19	12	50	45	2	.6
13	732	Sweetened	1 c	93	16	466	3	44	9	33	29	1	.4
		Filberts (hazelnuts), chopped:											
13	733	Cup	1 c	115	5	727	15	18	7	72	5	57	7
13	734	Ounce	1 oz	28	5	179	4	4	2	18	1	14	2
		Macadamia nuts, oil roasted:											
		Salted:											
13	735	Cup	1 c	134	2	962	10	17	7	103	15	81	2
13	736	Ounce	1 oz	28	2	204	2	4	1	22	3	17	.4
13	1368	Unsalted	1 c	134	2	962	10	17	7	103	15.4	80.9	1.8
		Mixed nuts:											
13	737	Dry roasted, salted	1 c	137	2	814	24	35	12	70	10	43	15
13	738	Oil roasted, salted	1 c	142	2	876	24	30	13	80	12	45	19
13	1369	Oil roasted, unsalted	1 c	142	2	876	24	30	13	80	12.4	45.0	18.9
		Peanuts:											
		Oil roasted, salted:											
13	739	Cup	1 c	144	2	837	38	27	13	71	10	35.2	22.4
13	740	Ounce	1 oz	28	2	163	7	5	2	14	2	7	4
13	1370	Oil roasted, unsalted	1 c	144	2	837	38	27	13	71	9.9	35.2	22.4
		Dried, unsalted:											
13	741	Cup	1 c	146	7	827	38	24	13	72	10	36	23
13	742	Ounce	1 oz	28	7	161	7	5	3	14	2	7	4
13	743	Peanut butter	1 tbsp	16	2	94	4	3	1	8	1.5	4.0	2.3
		Pecans, halves:											
		Dried, unsalted:											
13	744	Cup	1 c	108	5	720	8	20	7[102]	73	6	46	18
13	745	Ounce	1 oz	28	5	190	2	5	2[102]	19	1.5	12	5
13	1372	Dry roasted, salted	¼ c	28	1	187	2	6	2	18	1.5	11.5	4.6
13	746	Pine nuts/piñons, dried	1 oz	28	6	161	3	5	2	17	3	7	7
		Pistachio nuts:											
13	747	Dried, shelled	1 oz	28	4	164	6	7	1	14	2	9	2
13	1373	Dry roasted, salted, shelled	1 c	128	2	776	19	35	14	68	8.6	45.7	10.3

(101) 1 c packed = 130 g.
(102) Dietary fiber data calculated/derived from data on other nuts.

GRP KEY: 1=BEV 2=DAIRY 3=EGGS 4=FAT/OIL 5=FRUIT 6=BAKERY 7=GRAIN 8=FISH 9=BEEF 10=POULTRY 11=SAUSAGE 12=MIXED/FAST **13=NUTS/SEEDS** 14=SWEETS 15=VEG/LEG 16=MISC 22=SOUP/SAUCE

Chol (mg)	Calc (mg)	Iron (mg)	Magn (mg)	Phos (mg)	Pota (mg)	Sodi (mg)	Zinc (mg)	VT-A (RE)	Thia (mg)	Ribo (mg)	Niac (mg)	V-B6 (mg)	Fola (µg)	VT-C (mg)
0	62	8.22	356	671	774	21	7.67	0	.27	.27	1.92	.35	95	0
0	53	5.33	332	554	689	22	6.18	0	.55	.23	2.34	.33	88	0
0	7	.09	41	73	87	2[103]	.83	0	.05	.03	.26	.04	11	0
0	42	1.30	47	153	846	3	.82	4	.35	.25	1.92	.71	100	37
0	6	1.09	14	51	160	9	.50	0	.03	.01	.24	.02	12	2
0	12	1.94	26	90	285	16	.88	0	.05	.02	.43	.04	21	3
0	20	2.59	70	161	423	29	1.57	0	.05	.08	.47	2.34	7	1
0	14	1.79	47	100	313	244	1.69	0	.03	.02	.44	.29	9	1
0	216	3.76	328	359	512	3	2.76	8	.57	.13	1.31	.7	83	1
0	53	.93	81	89	126	1	.68	2	.14	.03	.32	.17	20	<1
0	60	2.41	157	268	441	348[104]	1.47	1	.28	.15	2.71	.33	79	0
0	13	.51	33	57	94	74[104]	.31	<1	.06	.03	.57	.07	17	0
0	60	2.41	157	268	441	9	1.47	1	.28	.15	2.71	.33	79	0
0	96	5.07	308	596	817	917[105]	5.21	2	.27	.27	6.44	.41	69	1
0	153	4.56	334	659	825	926[105]	7.22	3	.71	.32	7.19	.34	118	1
0	153	4.56	334	659	825	16	7.22	3	.71	.32	7.19	.34	118	1
0	126	2.63	266	744	982	624[106]	9.55	0	.364	.156	20.6	.367	181	0
0	24	.51	52	145	191	121[106]	1.86	0	.07	.03	4	.07	35	0
0	126	2.63	266	744	982	8.6	9.55	0	.364	.156	20.6	.367	181	0
0	85	4.72	263	559	1047	23	4.78	0	.97	.19	20.7	.43	153	0
0	17	.92	51	109	204	5	.93	0	.19	.04	4.02	.08	30	0
0	5.5	.27	25	52	115	77[107]	.4	0	.02	.02	2.1	.06	13	0
0	39	2.30	138	314	423	1[108]	5.91	14	.92	.14	.96	.20	42	1
0	10	.61	36	83	111	<1	1.55	4	.24	.04	.25	.05	11	1
0	10	.62	38	86	105	221	1.61	4	.09	.04	.26	.05	12	1
0	2	.87	67	10	178	20	1.22	1	.35	.06	1.24	.08	19	<1
0	38	1.93	45	143	310	2[109]	.38	7	.22	.05	.31	.06	17	<1
0	90	4.06	166	609	1242	998	1.74	30	.54	.32	1.80	.27	74	0

(103) Salted cashew butter contains 98 mg sodium per tablespoon.
(104) Macadamia nuts without salt contain 9 mg sodium per cup, or 2 mg per ounce.
(105) Mixed nuts without salt contain about 15 mg sodium per cup.
(106) Peanuts without salt contain 22 mg sodium per cup, or 4 mg per ounce.
(107) Peanut butter without added salt contains 3 mg sodium per tablespoon.
(108) Salted pecans contain 816 mg sodium per cup, or 214 mg per ounce.
(109) Salted pistachios contain approx 221 mg sodium per ounce.

• *Table F–1* Food Composition

Grp	Computer Code No.	Food Description	Measure	Wt (g)	H_2O (%)	Ener (cal)	Prot (g)	Carb (g)	Dietary Fiber (g)	Fat (g)	Fat Breakdown (g) Sat	Mono	Poly
NUTS, SEEDS and PRODUCTS—Con.													
		Pumpkin kernels:											
13	748	Dried, unsalted	1 oz	28	7	154	7	5	2	13	2.5	4	6
13	1374	Roasted, salted	1 c	227	7	1185	75	31	9	96	18.1	29.7	43.6
13	749	Sesame seeds, hulled, dried	¼ c	38	5	221	10	4	6	21	3	8	9
		Sunflower seed kernels:											
13	750	Dry	¼ c	36	5	205	8	7	2	18	2	3	12
13	751	Oil roasted	¼ c	34	3	208	7	5	2	19	2	4	13
13	752	Tahini (sesame butter)	1 tbsp	15	3	91	3	3	2	8	1	3	4
		Black walnuts, chopped:											
13	753	Cup	1 c	125	4	759	30	15	7	71	5	16	47
13	754	Ounce	1 oz	28	4	172	7	3	2	16	1	4	11
		English walnuts, chopped:											
13	755	Cup	1 c	120	4	770	17	22	7	74	7	17	47
13	756	Ounce	1 oz	28	4	182	4	5	2	18	2	4	11
SWEETENERS and SWEETS: see also Dairy (milk desserts) and Baked Goods													
14	757	Apple butter	2 tbsp	35	52	66	<1	17	<1	<1	.1	<.1	.1
14	1124	Butterscotch topping	3 tbsp	50	33	156	1	41	0	<1	—	—	—
		Cake frosting:											
14	1127	Canned, average of all types	2.5 tbsp	39	15	160	0	24	0	7	1.7	2.9	1.7
14	1123	Prepared from mix	2.5 tbsp	39	15	167	0	28	0	6	—	—	—
		Candy:											
14	1128	Almond Joy® candy bar	1 oz	28	7	151	2	19	1.9	8	6.7	.6	.1
14	758	Caramel, plain or chocolate	1 oz	28	8	115	1	22	<1	3	2.2	.3	.1
		Chocolate (see also, #784, 785, 971):											
		Milk chocolate:											
14	759	Plain	1 oz	28	1	145	2	16	1	9	5.4	3	.3
14	760	With almonds	1 oz	28	2	150	3	15	1	10	4.4	4.7	1.0
14	761	With peanuts	1 oz	28	1	155	5	10	2	12	3.5	5.2	2.7
14	762	With rice cereal	1 oz	28	2	140	2	18	1	7	4.4	2.5	.2
14	763	Semisweet chocolate chips	1 c	170	1	860	7	97	5	61	36	20	2
14	764	Sweet dark chocolate	1 oz	28	1	150	1	16	1	10	5.9	3.3	.3
14	1133	English toffee candy bar	1 ea	32	2	220	1	11	<1	19	7	7	2
14	765	Fondant candy, uncoated (mints, candy corn, other)	1 oz	28	3	105	0	27	0	0	0	0	0
14	766	Fudge, chocolate	1 oz	28	8	115	1	21	2	3	2.1	1	.1
14	767	Gum drops	1 oz	28	12	98	0	25	0	<1	t	t	.1
14	768	Hard candy, all flavors	1 oz	28	1	109	0	28	0	0	0	0	0
14	769	Jelly beans	1 oz	28	6	104	t	26	0	<.1	t	t	.1
14	1134	M&M's Plain choc. candies®	48 grm	48	1	237	3	33	<1	10	5	3	3
14	1135	M&M's Peanut choc. candies®	47 grm	47.3	2	240	5	28	1	12	5	5	2
14	1130	MARS® bar	1 ea	50	7	240	4	30	1	11	4.8	4.4	.8
14	1129	MILKY WAY® candy bar	1 ea	60	7	260	3	43	<1	9	5.4	3.0	.3
14	1132	REESE's® peanut butter cup	2 ea	45	4	240	6	22	2	14	5.2	5.4	2.4
14	1131	SNICKERS® candy bar, 2.2oz size	1 ea	61.2	7	290	7	37	2	14	—	—	—
14	1125	Caramel topping	3 tbsp	50	31	155	1	39	<1	—	—	—	—
14	771	Gelatin salad/dessert	½ c	120	84	70	2	17	<1	0	0	0	0
		Honey:											
14	772	Cup	1 c	339	17	1030	1	279	0	0	0	0	0
14	773	Tablespoon	1 tbsp	21	17	65	<.1	17	0	0	0	0	0

(Computer code number is for West Diet Analysis program)

GRP KEY: 1=BEV 2=DAIRY 3=EGGS 4=FAT/OIL 5=FRUIT 6=BAKERY 7=GRAIN 8=FISH 9=BEEF 10=POULTRY 11=SAUSAGE 12=MIXED/FAST **13=NUTS/SEEDS** 14=SWEETS 15=VEG/LEG 16=MISC 22=SOUP/SAUCE

Chol (mg)	Calc (mg)	Iron (mg)	Magn (mg)	Phos (mg)	Pota (mg)	Sodi (mg)	Zinc (mg)	VT-A (RE)	Thia (mg)	Ribo (mg)	Niac (mg)	V-B6 (mg)	Fola (µg)	VT-C (mg)
0	12	4.25	152	333	229	5[110]	2.12	11	.06	.09	.50	.03	26	<1
0	98	33.9	1212	2600	1830	1305	16.9	88	.25	.66	3.60	.20	115	0
0	49	2.93	130	291	153	15	2.23	<1	.27	.03	1.76	.30	38	0
0	42	2.44	128	254	248	1	1.82	2	.83	.10	1.62	.46	85	<1
0	19	2.26	43	385	163	205[111]	1.76	2	.11	.10	1.40	.40	79	<1
0	21	.83	53	119	69	5	1.57	1	.24	.02	.85	.06	15	1
0	73	3.84	253	580	655	1	4.28	37	.27	.14	.86	.70	83	1
0	16	.87	57	132	149	0	.97	8	.06	.03	.20	.16	19	<1
0	113	2.93	203	380	602	12	3.28	15	.46	.18	1.25	.67	79	4
0	27	.69	48	90	142	3	.78	4	.11	.04	.30	.16	19	1
0	5	.25	2	13	89	1	.01	0	<.01	.01	.08	.01	<1	1
14	56	.10	3	23	34	66	.12	<1	0	.04	0	<.01	.06	0
0	—	—	—	—	—	91	—	0	—	—	—	—	—	—
0	—	—	—	—	—	84	—	0	—	—	—	—	—	—
0	20	.5	16	42	92	48	.43	3	.01	.05	.14	.05	2.1	.1
1	42	.4	6	35	54	64	.15	<1	.01	.05	.1	<.01	0	t
6	50	.4	16	61	96	23	.37	10	.02	.1	.1	.02	<1	t
5	61	.56	33	77	125	23	.48	8	.03	.13	.31	.02	4	t
3	32	.68	35	87	155	19	.68	8	.11	.07	2.2	.05	16	t
6	48	.2	13	57	100	46	.29	8	.01	.08	.1	.01	<1	t
0	51	5.8	230	178	593	24	2.39	3	.1	.14	.9	.04	22	t
0	7	.6	32	41	86	5	.42	1	.01	.04	.1	.01	5	t
0	0	.20	11.5	0	50	90	.24	5	.053	.05	.10	.04	1	0
0	2	.1	—	2	1	57	.1	0	<.01	<.01	.01	.01	0	0
1	22	.3	14	24	42	54	.16	16	.01	.03	.1	.01	2	t
0	2	.1	—	—	1	10	0	5	0	<.01	.01	0	0	0
0	6	.1	<1	2	1	7	0	0	0	0	0	0	0	0
0	1	.30	—	1	11	7	0	0	0	<.01	.01	—	0	0
0	79	.76	30	65	171	41	.57	13	.03	.12	.27	.01	5	—
0	59	.67	38	64	162	29	.66	<1	.03	.09	1.48	.03	5	—
0	85	.55	37	63	176	85	.59	<1	.02	.16	.48	.01	5	—
14	86	.49	22	80	167	140	.45	25	.03	.15	.20	.01	7	1
3	35	.68	47	87	168	92	.9	8	.03	.05	2.12	.06	17	—
0	70	.49	39	75	209	170	.69	5	.03	.11	1.84	.02	6	—
0	28	.10	3	23	33	152	—	<1	0	.05	0	—	—	0
0	2	.10	<1	23	91	55	.03	0	.01	.01	.20	<.01	0	0
0	17	1.70	7	20	173	17	.40	0	.02	.14	1.0	.06	32	3
0	1	.11	<1	1	11	1	.02	0	<.01	.01	.06	<.01	2	<1

(110)Salted pumpkin/squash kernels contain approximately 163 mg sodium per ounce.
(111)Unsalted sunflower seeds contain 1 mg sodium per ¼ cup.

Table F–1 Food Composition

Grp	Computer Code No.	Food Description	Measure	Wt (g)	H_2O (%)	Ener (cal)	Prot (g)	Carb (g)	Dietary Fiber (g)	Fat (g)	Fat Breakdown (g)		
											Sat	Mono	Poly
		SWEETENERS and SWEETS—Con.											
		Jams or preserves:											
14	774	Tablespoon	1 tbsp	20	29	54	<1	14	<1	<.1	0	t	t
14	775	Packet	1 ea	14	29	38	<.1	10	<1	<.1	0	t	t
		Jellies:											
14	776	Tablespoon	1 tbsp	18	28	49	<.1	13	<1	<.1	t	t	t
14	777	Packet	1 ea	14	28	39	<.1	10	<1	<.1	t	t	t
14	1136	Marmalade	1 tbsp	20	29	52	<1	14	<1	0	0	0	0
14	770	Marshmallows	4 ea	28	17	90	t	23	0	0	0	0	0
14	1126	Marshmallow creme topping	3 tbsp	50	20	158	<1	40	0	0	0	0	0
14	778	Popsicles, 3 oz when fluid	1 ea	95	80	70	0	18	0	0	0	0	0
		Sugars:											
14	779	Brown sugar	1 c	220	2	820	0	212	0	0	0	0	0
		White sugar, granulated:											
14	780	Cup	1 c	200	1	770	0	199	0	0	0	0	0
14	781	Tablespoon	1 tbsp	12	1	45	0	12	0	0	0	0	0
14	782	Packet	1 ea	6	1	25	0	6	0	0	0	0	0
14	783	White sugar, powdered, sifted	1 c	100	<1	385	0	99	0	0	0	0	0
		Syrups:											
		Chocolate:											
14	784	Thin type	2 tbsp	38	37	85	1	22	1	<1	.2	.1	.1
14	785	Fudge type	2 tbsp	38	25	125	2	21	1	5	3	2	.2
14	786	Molasses, blackstrap[112]	2 tbsp	40	24	85	0	22	0	0	0	0	0
14	787	Pancake table syrup (corn and maple)	¼ c	84	25	244	0	64	0	0	0	0	0
		VEGETABLES and LEGUMES											
15	788	Alfalfa seeds, sprouted	1 c	33	91	10	1	1	1	<1	t	t	.1
15	789	Artichokes, cooked globe (300 g with refuse)	1 ea	120	84	60	4	13	10	<1	<.1	t	.1
		Artichoke hearts:											
15	1177	Cooked from frozen	9 oz	240	87	108	7	22	18	1	.3	<.1	.5
15	1176	Marinated	6 oz	170	59	168	4	13	11	14	2.0	3.0	7.7
		Asparagus, green, cooked:											
		From raw:											
15	790	Cuts and tips	½ c	90	92	23	2	4	2	<1	.1	t	.1
15	791	Spears, ½″ diam at base	4 spears	60	92	15	2	3	1	<1	<.1	t	.1
		From frozen:											
15	792	Cuts and tips	1 c	180	91	50	5	9	3	1	.2	t	.3
15	793	Spears, ½″ diam at base	4 spears	60	91	17	2	3	1	<1	.1	t	.1
15	794	Canned, spears, ½″ diam at base	4 spears	80	95	11	2	2	1	1	.1	t	.2
15	795	Bamboo shoots, canned, drained slices	1 c	131	94	25	2	4	3	1	.1	t	.2
		Beans (see also Great northern, #855; Kidney beans, #860; Navy beans, #876; Pinto beans, #898; Refried beans, #921; Soybeans, #925):											
15	796	Black beans, cooked	1 c	172	66	227	15	41	15	1	.2	.1	.4
		Canned beans (white/navy):											
15	803	Beans w/pork and tomato sauce	1 c	253	73	247	13	49	14	3	1.0	1.1	.3
15	804	Beans w/pork and sweet sauce	1 c	253	71	282	13	53	14	4	1.4	1.6	.5
15	805	Beans with frankfurters	1 c	257	70	366	17	40	18	17	6	7	2
		Lima beans:											
15	797	Thick seeded (Fordhooks), cooked from frozen	½ c	85	74	85	5	16	5	<1	.1	t	.1

(112)Light molasses would contain about 66 mg calcium, 2.1 mg iron, 18 mg magnesium, and 366 mg potassium for 2 tbsp.

GRP KEY: 1 = BEV 2 = DAIRY 3 = EGGS 4 = FAT/OIL 5 = FRUIT 6 = BAKERY 7 = GRAIN 8 = FISH 9 = BEEF 10 = POULTRY 11 = SAUSAGE 12 = MIXED/FAST 13 = NUTS/SEEDS **14 = SWEETS** 15 = VEG/LEG 16 = MISC 22 = SOUP/SAUCE

Chol (mg)	Calc (mg)	Iron (mg)	Magn (mg)	Phos (mg)	Pota (mg)	Sodi (mg)	Zinc (mg)	VT-A (RE)	Thia (mg)	Ribo (mg)	Niac (mg)	V-B6 (mg)	Fola (μg)	VT-C (mg)
0	4	.20	1	2	18	2	.01	t	<.01	.01	.04	<.01	2	<1
0	3	.14	<1	1	13	1	<.01	t	<.01	.01	.03	<.01	1	<1
0	2	.12	<1	1	16	4	0	t	<.01	<.01	.04	<.01	2	1
0	1	.09	<1	1	12	3	0	t	<.01	<.01	.03	<.01	2	1
0	7	.12	1	3	12	4	—	1	<.01	<.01	.02	<.01	1	1.2
0	1	.45	1	2	2	25	<.01	0	0	<.01	.01	<.01	0	0
0	16	.8	2	6	16	29	<.01	0	0	<.01	.02	—	0	2
0	0	.01	—	0	4	11	0	0	0	0	0	0	0	0
0	187	4.80	135	56	757	97	.08	0	.02	.07	.20	0	0	0
0	3	.10	<1	.1	7	5	.04	0	0	0	0	0	0	0
0	<1	.01	<1	t	t	t	<.01	0	0	0	0	0	0	0
0	<1	<.01	<1	t	t	t	<.01	0	0	0	0	0	0	0
0	0	.08	<1	0	4	2	<.01	0	0	0	0	0	0	0
0	6	.75	26	49	85	36	.39	1	.02	.02	.11	<.01	3	0
0	38	.50	18	60	82	42	.39	13	.08	.08	.08	<.01	3	0
0	274[112]	10.1[112]	103[112]	34	1171[112]	38	0	0	.08	.08	.80	.11	6	0
0	2	.06	2	8	14	38	.08	0	0	0	0	t	<1	0
0	11	.32	9	23	26	2	.30	5	.03	.04	.16	.01	12	3
0	54	1.55	72	103	425	114	.59	22	.08	.08	1.20	.13	61	12
0	50	1.34	74	146	634	127	.86	39	.15	.38	2.20	.21	285	12
0	39	1.62	48	102	438	900	.54	28	.06	.17	1.38	.15	149	52
0	22	.59	17	55	279	4	.43	75	.09	.11	.95	.13	88	25
0	14	.4	11	37	186	2	.29	50	.06	.07	.63	.09	59	16
0	41	1.15	23	99	392	7	1.01	147	.12	.19	1.87	.16	176	44
0	14	.38	8	33	131	2	.34	49	.04	.06	.62	.06	59	15
0	11	.5	8	30	122	278[113]	.32	38	.05	.07	.7	.04	69	13
0	10	.42	6	33	105	9	.30	1	.03	.03	.18	—	40	1
0	47	3.60	121	241	611	1	1.92	1	.42	.10	.87	.12	256	0
17	141	8.30	88	297	759	45	2.60	31	.13	.12	1.26	.18	57	8
17	155	4.20	87	266	673	1113	3.80	29	.12	.15	.89	.22	95	8
15	123	4.45	71	267	604	849	4.79	40	.15	.14	2.32	.12	77	6
0	19	1.16	29	54	347	1105	.37	16	.06	.05	.91	.10	55	11

(112)Light molasses would contain about 66 mg calcium, 2.1 mg iron, 18 mg magnesium, and 366 mg potassium for 2 tbsp.
(113)Special dietary pack contains 3 mg sodium.

(For purposes of calculations, use "0" for t, <1, <.1, <.01, etc.)

Table F–1 Food Composition

Grp	Computer Code No.	Food Description	Measure	Wt (g)	H_2O (%)	Ener (cal)	Prot (g)	Carb (g)	Dietary Fiber (g)	Fat (g)	Fat Breakdown (g) Sat	Mono	Poly
		VEGETABLES and LEGUMES—Con.											
		Lima Beans—Con.											
15	798	Thin seeded (baby), cooked from frozen	½ c	90	72	94	6	18	8	<1	.1	t	.1
15	799	Cooked from dry, drained	1 c	188	70	217	15	39	18	1	.2	.1	.3
		Snap beans/green beans, cuts and french style:											
15	800	Cooked from raw	1 c	125	89	44	2	10	3	<1	.1	t	.2
15	801	Cooked from frozen	1 c	135	92	36	2	8	4	<1	<.1	t	.1
15	802	Canned, drained	1 c	136	93	26	2	6	2	<1	<.1	t	.1
		Bean sprouts (mung):											
15	806	Raw	1 c	104	90	31	3	6	3	<1	<.1	t	.1
15	807	Cooked, stir fried	1 c	124	84	62	5	13	3	<1	<.1	.1	.1
15	808	Cooked, boiled, drained	1 c	124	93	26	3	5	3	<1	<.1	t	<.1
		Beets:											
		Cooked from fresh:											
15	809	Sliced or diced	½ c	85	91	26	1	6	2	<.1	t	t	t
15	810	Whole beets, 2″ diam	2 beets	100	91	31	1	7	2	<.1	t	t	t
		Canned:											
15	811	Sliced or diced	½ c	85	91	27	1	6	2	<1	t	t	<.1
15	812	Pickled slices	½ c	114	82	74	1	19	2	<1	t	t	<.1
15	813	Beet greens, cooked, drained	1 c	144	89	40	4	8	3	<1	<.1	.1	.1
		Black-eyed peas: see Peas											
		Broccoli:											
15	817	Raw, chopped	1 c	88	91	24	3	5	3	<1	.1	t	.1
15	818	Raw, spears	1 spear	151	91	42	5	8	6	1	.1	<.1	.3
		Cooked from raw:											
15	819	Spears	1 spear	180	91	50	5	9	7	<1	.1	<.1	.3
15	820	Chopped	1 c	156	91	44	5	8	6	<1	.1	<.1	.3
		Cooked from frozen:											
15	821	Spear, small piece	1 spear	30	91	8	1	2	1	<.1	t	t	t
15	822	Chopped	1 c	184	91	51	6	10	6	<1	<.1	t	<.1
		Brussels sprouts:											
15	823	Cooked from raw	1 c	156	87	60	6	14	6	1	.2	.1	.4
15	824	Cooked from frozen	1 c	155	87	65	6	13	5	1	.1	.1	.3
		Cabbage, common varieties:											
15	825	Raw, shredded or chopped	1 c	70	92	16	1	4	2	<1	t	t	.1
15	826	Cooked, drained	1 c	150	94	32	1	7	4	<1	.1	<.1	.2
		Chinese cabbage:											
15	1178	Bok-choy, raw, shredded	1 c	70	95	9	1	2	1	<1	t	t	.1
15	827	Bok choy, cooked, drained	1 c	170	96	20	3	3	3	<1	<.1	t	.1
15	828	Pe-Tsai, raw, chopped	1 c	76	94	11	1	2	2	<1	<.1	t	.1
		Cabbage, red, coarsely chopped:											
15	829	Raw	1 c	70	92	19	1	4	2	<1	t	t	.1
15	830	Cooked	½ c	75	94	16	1	3	4	<1	t	t	.1
15	831	Savoy cabbage, coarsely chopped, raw	1 c	70	91	20	1	4	2	<.1	t	t	<.1

(Computer code number is for West Diet Analysis program)

GRP KEY: 1=BEV 2=DAIRY 3=EGGS 4=FAT/OIL 5=FRUIT 6=BAKERY 7=GRAIN 8=FISH 9=BEEF 10=POULTRY 11=SAUSAGE 12=MIXED/FAST 13=NUTS/SEEDS 14=SWEETS **15=VEG/LEG** 16=MISC 22=SOUP/SAUCE

Chol (mg)	Calc (mg)	Iron (mg)	Magn (mg)	Phos (mg)	Pota (mg)	Sodi (mg)	Zinc (mg)	VT-A (RE)	Thia (mg)	Ribo (mg)	Niac (mg)	V-B6 (mg)	Fola (µg)	VT-C (mg)
0	25	1.76	50	101	370	26	.50	15	.06	.05	.69	.11	58	5
0	32	4.50	82	208	955	4	1.79	0	.30	.10	.79	.3	156	0
0	58	1.60	32	48	373	4	.45	83[114]	.09	.12	.77	.07	42	12
0	61	1.11	29	33	151	17	.84	71[115]	.07	.10	.56	.08	42	11
0	36	1.22	18	26	147	339[116]	.39	47[117]	.02	.08	.27	.05	43	6
0	14	.95	22	56	154	6	.43	2	.09	.13	.78	.09	63	14
0	16	2.40	38	70	200	14	1.12	3	.17	.22	1.49	.10	72	20
0	15	.81	18	34	125	12	.58	2	.06	.13	1.01	.05	35	14
0	9	.53	31	26	266	42	.21	1	.03	.01	.23	.03	49	5
0	11	.62	37	31	312	49	.25	1	.03	.01	.27	.03	86	6
0	13	1.55	13	15	126	233[118]	.18	1	.01	.04	.15	.05	22	4
0	13	.47	17	19	169	301	.30	1	.03	.06	.29	.03	35	3
0	165	2.74	97	58	1308	346	.72	734	.17	.42	.72	.19	47	36
0	42	.78	22	58	286	24	.36	136[119]	.06	.10	.56	.14	62	82
0	72	1.33	38	99	490	41	.60	233[119]	.10	.18	.96	.24	107	141
0	83	1.51	43	106	525	47	.68	250[119]	.10	.2	1.03	.26	90	134
0	72	1.24	37	92	456	40	.59	217[119]	.09	.18	.90	.22	78	116
0	15	.18	6	16	54	7	.09	57[119]	.02	.02	.14	.04	9	12
0	94	1.12	37	101	331	44	.55	348[119]	.10	.15	.84	.19	55	74
0	56	1.88	32	87	491	17	.50	112	.17	.12	.95	.31	94	97
0	38	1.15	37	84	504	36	.55	91	.16	.18	.83	.27	157	71
0	32	.40	10	16	172	12	.12	9	.04	.02	.21	.07	40	33
0	50	.59	23	38	308	29	.24	13	.09	.08	.34	.10	31	36
0	74	.56	13	26	176	<1	.29	210	.03	.05	.35	.07	57	32
0	158	1.77	18	49	630	57	.43	437	.05	.11	.73	.30	32	44
0	59	.23	10	22	181	7	.17	91	.03	.04	.30	.18	60	21
0	36	.35	11	29	144	8	.15	3	.05	.02	.21	.15	19	40
0	28	.27	8	21	105	6	.11	2	.03	.01	.15	.11	9	26
0	25	.28	20	29	161	20	.26	70	.05	.02	.21	.13	32	22

(114)Data is for green varieties; yellow beans contain 10 RE per cup.
(115)Data is for green varieties; yellow beans contain 15 RE per cup.
(116)Dietary pack contains 3 mg sodium per cup.
(117)For green varieties; yellow beans contain 14 RE per cup.
(118)Dietary pack contains 39 mg sodium.
(119)Vitamin A for whole plant: leaves are 1600 RE/100 g raw; flower clusters are 300/100 g raw; stalks are 40 RE/100 g raw.

(For purposes of calculations, use "0" for t, <1, <.1, <.01, etc.)

Table F–1 Food Composition

Grp	Computer Code No.	Food Description	Measure	Wt (g)	H_2O (%)	Ener (cal)	Prot (g)	Carb (g)	Dietary Fiber (g)	Fat (g)	Fat Breakdown (g) Sat	Mono	Poly
		VEGETABLES and LEGUMES—Con.											
		Carrots:											
		Raw:											
15	832	Whole, 7½ × 1⅛″	1 carrot	72	88	31	1	7	2	<1	t	t	.1
15	833	Grated	½ c	55	88	24	1	6	2	<1	t	t	<.1
		Cooked, sliced, drained:											
15	834	Cooked from raw	½ c	78	87	35	1	8	3	<1	<.1	t	.1
15	835	Cooked from frozen	½ c	73	90	26	1	6	3	<.1	t	t	<.1
15	836	Canned, sliced, drained	½ c	73	93	17	<1	4	1	<1	<.1	t	.1
15	837	Carrot juice	½ c	123	89	49	1	11	2	<1	<.1	t	.1
		Cauliflower:											
15	838	Raw, flowerets	½ c	50	92	12	1	2	1	<.1	t	t	<.1
		Cooked, drained, flowerets:											
15	839	From raw	½ c	62	92	15	1	3	1	<1	t	t	.1
15	840	From frozen	1 c	180	94	34	3	7	3	<1	.1	<.1	.2
		Celery, pascal type, raw:											
15	841	Large outer stalk, 8 × 1½″ (at root end)	1 stalk	40	95	6	<1	1	1	<.1	t	t	t
15	842	Diced	½ c	60	95	11	<1	2	1	<.1	t	t	<.1
		Chard, swiss:											
15	1179	Raw, chopped	1 c	36	93	7	1	1	1	<1	t	t	<.1
15	1180	Cooked	1 c	175	93	35	3	7	4	<1	<.1	t	.1
		Chick-peas (see Garbanzo, #854)											
		Collards, cooked, drained:											
15	843	From raw	1 c	128	92	35	2	8	4	<1	.1	<.1	.1
15	844	From frozen	1 c	170	88	63	3	14	6	1	.1	.1	.3
		Corn:											
		Cooked, drained:											
15	845	From raw, on cob, 5″ long	1 ear	77	70	83	3	19	3	1	.2	.3	.5
15	846	From frozen, on cob, 3½″ long	1 ear	63	73	59	2	14	3	<1	.1	.1	.2
15	847	Kernels, cooked from frozen	½ c	82	76	67	2	17	3	<.1	t	t	<.1
		Canned:											
15	848	Cream style	½ c	128	79	93	2	23	2	<1	.1	.2	.3
15	849	Whole kernel, vacuum pack	1 c	210	77	166	5	41	3	1	.2	.3	.5
		Cowpeas; (see Black-eyed peas, #814–816)											
15	850	Cucumbers with peel, ⅛″ thick, 2⅛″ diam	6 slices	28	96	4	<1	1	<1	<.1	t	t	t
		Dandelion greens:											
15	851	Raw	1 c	55	86	25	1	5	1	<1	<.1	<.1	.2
15	852	Chopped, cooked, drained	1 c	105	90	35	2	7	1	1	.2	<.1	.4
15	853	Eggplant, cooked	1 c	160	92	45	1	11	6	<1	.1	<.1	.2
15	854	Garbanzo beans (chick-peas), cooked	1 c	164	60	269	15	45	11	4	.4	1.0	2.0
15	855	Great northern beans, cooked	1 c	177	69	210	15	37	11	1	.3	<.1	.3
15	856	Escarole/curly endive, chopped	1 c	50	94	9	1	2	1	<1	t	t	<.1
15	857	Jerusalem artichokes, raw slices	1 c	150	78	114	3	26	2	<.1	—	t	t
		Kale, cooked, drained:											
15	858	From raw	1 c	130	91	42	3	7	4	1	.1	<.1	.3
15	859	From frozen	1 c	130	90	39	4	7	3	1	.1	<.1	.3
15	860	Kidney beans, canned	1 c	256	77	216	13	39	19	<1	.1	.1	.4
		Kohlrabi:											
15	1181	Raw slices	1 c	140	91	38	2	9	2	<1	t	t	.1
15	861	Cooked	1 c	165	90	48	3	11	2	<1	t	t	.1

(Computer code number is for West Diet Analysis program)

GRP KEY: 1 = BEV 2 = DAIRY 3 = EGGS 4 = FAT/OIL 5 = FRUIT 6 = BAKERY 7 = GRAIN 8 = FISH 9 = BEEF 10 = POULTRY 11 = SAUSAGE 12 = MIXED/FAST 13 = NUTS/SEEDS 14 = SWEETS **15 = VEG/LEG** 16 = MISC 22 = SOUP/SAUCE

Chol (mg)	Calc (mg)	Iron (mg)	Magn (mg)	Phos (mg)	Pota (mg)	Sodi (mg)	Zinc (mg)	VT-A (RE)	Thia (mg)	Ribo (mg)	Niac (mg)	V-B6 (mg)	Fola (µg)	VT-C (mg)
0	19	.36	11	32	233	25	.14	2025	.07	.04	.67	.11	10	7
0	15	.28	8	24	178	19	.11	1547	.05	.03	.51	.08	8	5
0	24	.48	10	24	177	52	.23	1915	.03	.04	.40	.19	11	2
0	21	.35	7	19	115	43	.18	1292	.02	.03	.32	.09	8	2
0	19	.47	6	17	131	176[120]	.19	1006	.01	.02	.40	.08	7	2
0	29	.56	17	51	358	36	.22	3159	.11	.07	.47	.27	5	11
0	14	.29	7	23	178	7	.09	1	.04	.03	.32	.12	33	36
0	17	.26	7	22	200	4	.15	1	.04	.04	.34	.13	32	34
0	31	.74	16	43	250	33	.23	4	.07	.10	.56	.16	74	56
0	16	.16	5	10	115	35	.05	5	.02	.02	.13	.04	11	3
0	25	.25	7	15	170	55	.08	8	.03	.03	.19	.06	13	4
0	18	.65	29	17	136	77	.16	259	.01	.03	.14	.03	20	11
0	102	3.96	150	58	961	313	.59	1198	.06	.15	.63	.12	57	32
0	29	.21	9	10	168	21	.14	349	.03	.07	.37	.07	8	16
0	54	.38	16	19	307	37	.26	638	.05	.12	.68	.12	129	28
0	2	.47	25	79	192	13	.37	17[121]	.17	.06	1.24	.18	36	5
0	2	.38	18	47	158	3	.40	13[121]	.11	.04	.96	.14	19	3
0	2	.25	15	39	114	4	.29	20[121]	.06	.06	1.05	.18	19	2
0	4	.49	22	65	172	365[122]	.68	12[121]	.03	.07	1.23	.08	57	6
0	11	.88	48	134	390	572[123]	.97	51[121]	.09	.15	2.46	.12	104	17
0	4	.08	3	5	42	1	.07	1	.01	.01	.09	.02	4	1
0	103	1.71	20	36	218	42	.62	770	.11	.14	.39	.02	64	19
0	147	1.89	26	44	244	46	.80	1229	.14	.18	.50	.04	82	19
0	10	.56	21	35	397	5	.24	10	.12	.03	.96	.14	23	2
0	80	4.74	78	275	477	11	2.51	4	.19	.10	.86	.23	282	2
0	121	3.77	88	293	692	4	1.55	<1	.28	.10	1.21	.21	181	2
0	26	.42	8	14	157	11	.40	103	.04	.04	.20	.01	71	3
0	21	5.10	26	117	644	6	.11	3	.30	.09	1.95	.11	15	6
0	94	1.17	23	36	296	30	.31	962	.07	.09	.70	.18	30	53
0	179	1.22	23	36	417	20	.23	826	.06	.15	.87	.11	31	33
0	62	3.22	73	240	658	873	1.41	0	.27	.23	1.17	.06	129	3
0	34	.56	27	64	490	28	.32	5	.07	.03	.56	.21	14	87
0	41	.66	31	74	561	34	.32	6	.07	.03	.64	.18	13	89

(120) Dietary pack contains 31 mg sodium.
(121) For yellow varieties; white varieties contain only a trace of vitamin A.
(122) Dietary pack contains 4 mg sodium per ½ cup.
(123) Dietary pack contains 6 mg sodium per cup.

Table F–1 **Food Composition**

Grp	Computer Code No.	Food Description	Measure	Wt (g)	H_2O (%)	Ener (cal)	Prot (g)	Carb (g)	Dietary Fiber (g)	Fat (g)	Fat Breakdown (g) Sat	Mono	Poly
		VEGETABLES and LEGUMES—Con.											
		Leeks:											
15	1183	Raw, chopped	1 c	104	83	63	2	15	2	<1	.1	<.1	.4
15	1182	Cooked, chopped	.5 c	52	91	16	<1	4	2	<1	t	t	.1
15	862	Lentils, cooked from dry	1 c	198	70	230	18	40	10	1	.1	.1	.4
		Lentils, sprouted:											
15	1288	Stir fried	3.5 oz	100	69	101	9	21	4	<1	.1	.1	.2
15	1289	Raw	1 c	77	67	81	7	17	3	<1	<.1	.1	.2
		Lettuce:											
		Butterhead/Boston types:											
15	863	Head, 5″ diam	1 head	163	96	21	2	4	3	<1	<.1	t	.2
15	864	Leaves, 2 inner or outer	2 leaves	15	96	2	<1	<1	<1	<.1	t	t	t
		Iceberg/crisphead:											
15	865	Head, 6″ diam	1 head	539	96	70	5	11	9	1	.1	<.1	.5
15	866	Wedge, ¼ of head	1 wedge	135	96	18	1	3	2	<1	<.1	t	.1
15	867	Chopped or shredded	1 c	56	96	7	1	1	1	<1	t	t	.1
15	868	Loose leaf, chopped	1 c	56	94	10	1	2	1	<1	t	t	.1
		Romaine:											
15	869	Chopped	1 c	56	95	9	1	1	1	<1	t	t	.1
15	870	Inner leaf	1 leaf	10	95	2	<1	<1	<1	<.1	t	t	t
		Mushrooms:											
15	871	Raw, sliced	½ c	35	92	9	1	2	1	<1	t	t	.1
15	872	Cooked from raw, pieces	½ c	78	91	21	2	4	2	<1	<.1	t	.1
15	873	Canned, drained	½ c	78	91	19	1	4	2	<1	<.1	t	.1
		Mustard greens:											
15	874	Cooked from raw	1 c	140	94	21	3	3	3	<1	t	.2	.1
15	875	Cooked from frozen	1 c	150	94	29	3	5	3	<1	t	.2	.1
15	876	Navy beans, cooked from dry	1 c	182	63	259	16	43	16	1	.3	.1	.4
		Okra, cooked:											
15	877	From fresh pods	8 pods	85	90	27	2	6	2	<1	<.1	t	<.1
15	878	From frozen slices	½ c	92	91	34	2	8	2	<1	.1	.1	.1
		Onions:											
15	879	Raw, chopped	1 c	160	90	61	2	14	3	<1	<.1	<.1	.1
15	880	Raw, sliced	1 c	115	90	44	1	10	2	<1	<.1	<.1	.1
15	881	Cooked, drained, chopped	½ c	105	88	46	1	11	2	<1	<.1	<.1	.1
15	882	Dehydrated flakes	¼ c	14	4	45	1	12	1	<.1	t	t	<.1
		Spring onions:											
15	883	Chopped, bulb and top	½ c	50	90	16	1	4	1	.1	t	t	<.1
15	1185	Green tops only, chopped	1 c	100	92	34	2	6	3	<1	.1	.1	.2
15	1184	White part only, chopped	1 c	100	92	50	1	10	3	<1	<.1	t	.1
15	884	Onion rings, breaded, prepared f/frozen	2 rings	20	29	81	1	8	<1	5	1.7	2.2	1
		Parsley:											
15	885	Raw, chopped	½ c	30	88	10	1	2	2	<.1	t	t	<.1
15	886	Raw, sprigs	10 sprigs	10	88	3	<1	1	1	<.1	t	t	t
15	887	Freeze dried	¼ c	1	2	4	<1	1	1	<.1	t	t	<.1
15	888	Parsnips, sliced, cooked	1 c	156	78	125	2	30	5	1	.1	.2	.1
		Peas:											
		Black-eyed peas, cooked:											
15	814	From dry, drained	1 c	171	70	198	13	36	21	1	.2	.1	.4
15	815	From fresh, drained	1 c	165	76	160	5	33	12	1	.2	<.1	.3
15	816	From frozen, drained	1 c	170	66	224	14	40	14	1	.3	.1	.5
15	889	Edible-pod, peas, cooked	1 c	160	89	67	5	11	4	<1	.1	<.1	.2

(Computer code number is for West Diet Analysis program)

GRP KEY: 1=BEV 2=DAIRY 3=EGGS 4=FAT/OIL 5=FRUIT 6=BAKERY 7=GRAIN 8=FISH 9=BEEF 10=POULTRY 11=SAUSAGE 12=MIXED/FAST 13=NUTS/SEEDS 14=SWEETS **15=VEG/LEG** 16=MISC 22=SOUP/SAUCE

Chol (mg)	Calc (mg)	Iron (mg)	Magn (mg)	Phos (mg)	Pota (mg)	Sodi (mg)	Zinc (mg)	VT-A (RE)	Thia (mg)	Ribo (mg)	Niac (mg)	V-B6 (mg)	Fola (μg)	VT-C (mg)
0	61	2.18	29	36	187	21	.17	10	.06	.03	.42	.24	67	13
0	16	.57	7	9	45	5	.12	2	.01	.01	.10	.08	16	2
0	37	6.59	71	356	731	4	2.50	2	.34	.14	2.10	.35	358	3
0	14	3.10	35	153	284	9	1.60	4	.22	.09	1.20	.16	84	13
0	19	2.47	28	133	248	8	1.16	4	.18	.10	.87	.15	77	13
0	52	.49	18	38	419	8	.42	158	.10	.10	.49	.11	119	13
0	5	.05	2	3	39	1	.04	15	.01	.01	.05	.01	11	1
0	102	2.70	49	108	852	48	1.19	178	.25	.16	1.01	.22	302	21
0	26	.68	12	27	213	12	.30	45	.06	.04	.25	.05	76	5
0	11	.28	5	11	89	5	.12	19	.03	.02	.11	.02	31	2
0	38	.78	6	14	148	5	.19	106	.03	.04	.22	.03	60	10
0	20	.62	3	25	162	4	.19	146	.06	.06	.28	.03	76	13
0	4	.11	1	5	29	1	.03	26	.01	.01	.05	.06	14	2
0	2	.43	4	36	130	1	.30	0	.04	.16	1.44	.03	7	1
0	5	1.36	9	68	278	2	.68	0	.06	.23	3.48	.07	14	3
0	9	.62	6	52	101	332	.56	0	.05	.17	1.25	.06	10	0
0	104	1.56	21	57	283	22	.30	424	.06	.09	.61	.18	20	35
0	152	1.68	20	36	209	38	.30	671	.06	.08	.39	.16	20	21
0	128	4.5	107	285	669	2	1.93	<1	.37	.11	.97	.30	255	1
0	54	.38	48	48	274	4	.47	49	.11	.05	.74	.16	39	14
0	88	.62	47	42	215	3	.57	47	.09	.11	.72	.04	134	11
0	32	.35	16	53	251	5	.30	0	.07	.03	.24	.19	30	10
0	23	.25	12	38	181	3	.22	0	.05	.02	.17	.13	22	7
0	23	.25	12	37	174	3	.22	0	.04	.02	.17	.14	16	5
0	36	.22	13	42	227	3	.26	0	.01	.01	.03	.22	23	11
0	36	.74	10	19	138	8	.20	20	.03	.04	.26	.03	32	9
0	56	2.20	21	39	260	7	.22	400	.07	.10	.60	0	80	51
0	40	.89	16	40	230	7	.25	<1	.07	.03	.33	.10	36	27
0	6	.34	4	16	26	75	.08	5	.06	.03	.72	.02	3	<1
0	39	1.86	13	12	161	12	.22	156	.02	.03	.21	.05	55	27
0	13	.62	4	4	54	4	.07	52	.01	.01	.07	.02	18	9
0	2	.75	5	8	88	5	.09	89	.02	.03	.15	.02	22	2
0	58	.90	46	108	573	16	.40	0	.13	.08	1.10	.15	91	20[124]
0	42	4.30	91	266	476	6	2.20	3	.35	.1	.85	.17	356	1
0	211	1.85	86	84	690	7	1.7	131	.17	.24	2.3	.11	210	4
0	40	3.60	85	208	638	9	2.42	13	.42	.11	1.24	.16	240	5
0	67	3.15	42	89	383	6	.60	30	.21	.12	.86	.23	48	77

(124)Value for Vitamin C is highest right after harvest and drops after that.

(For purposes of calculations, use "0" for t, <1, <.1, <.01, etc.)

● *Table F–1* Food Composition

Grp	Computer Code No.	Food Description	Measure	Wt (g)	H_2O (%)	Ener (cal)	Prot (g)	Carb (g)	Dietary Fiber (g)	Fat (g)	Fat Breakdown (g) Sat	Mono	Poly
VEGETABLES and LEGUMES—Con.													
		Peas—Con.											
		Green peas:											
15	890	Canned, drained	½ c	85	82	59	4	11	4	<1	.1	<.1	.1
15	891	Cooked from frozen	½ c	80	80	63	4	11	4	<1	<.1	t	.1
15	892	Split, green, cooked from dry	1 c	196	69	231	16	41	10	1	.1	.2	.3
		Peas and carrots:											
15	1187	Cooked from frozen	½ c	80	86	38	2	8	3	<1	.1	<.1	.2
15	1186	Canned, with liquid	½ c	128	88	48	3	11	4	<1	.1	<.1	.2
		Peppers, hot:											
15	893	Hot green chili, canned	½ c	68	92	17	1	4	1	<.1	t	t	<.1
15	894	Hot green chili, raw	1 pepper	45	88	18	1	4	1	<.1	t	t	<.1
15	895	Jalapenos, chopped, canned	½ c	68	90	17	1	3	2	<1	.4	t	.2
		Peppers, sweet, green:											
15	896	Whole pod (90 g with refuse), raw	1 pod	74	92	20	1	5	1	<1	.1	t	.1
15	897	Cooked, chopped (1 pod cooked = 73 g)	½ c	68	92	19	1	5	1	<1	<.1	t	.1
		Peppers, sweet, red:											
15	1286	Raw, chopped	½ c	50	92	14	<1	3	1	<1	<.1	t	.1
15	1287	Cooked, chopped	½ c	68	92	19	1	5	1	<1	<.1	t	.1
15	898	Pinto beans, cooked from dry	1 c	171	64	235	14	44	20	1	.2	.2	.3
15	1191	Poi - two finger	1 c	240	72	269	1	65	6	<1	.1	<.1	.1
		Potatoes:[125]											
		Baked in oven, 4¾ × 2⅓" diam:											
15	899	With skin	1 potato	202	71	220	5	51	5	<1	.1	t	.1
15	900	Flesh only	1 potato	156	75	145	3	34	2	<1	<.1	t	.1
15	901	Skin only	1 ea	58	47	115	2	27	2	<.1	t	t	<.1
		Baked in microwave, 4¾ × 2⅓" diam:											
15	902	With skin	1 potato	202	72	212	5	49	5	<1	.1	t	.1
15	903	Flesh only	1 potato	156	74	156	3	36	2	<1	<.1	t	.1
15	904	Skin only	1 ea	58	64	77	3	17	2	<.1	t	t	<.1
		Boiled, about 2½" diam:											
15	905	Peeled after boiling	1 potato	136	77	119	3	27	2	<1	<.1	t	.1
15	906	Peeled before boiling	1 potato	135	78	116	2	27	2	<1	<.1	t	.1
		French fried, strips 2-3½" long, frozen:											
15	907	Oven heated	10 strips	50	53	111	2	17	1	4	2.1	1.8	.3
15	908	Fried in veg oil	10 strips	50	38	158	2	20	1	8	2.5	1.6	3.8
15	1188	Fried in veg. and animal oil	10 strips	50	38	158	2	20	1	8	3.4	4.0	.5
15	909	Hashed brown, from frozen	1 c	156	56	340	5	44	3	18	7	8	2
		Mashed:											
15	910	Home recipe with milk[126]	1 c	210	78	162	4	37	3	1	.7	.3	.1
15	911	Home recipe with milk and margarine	1 c	210	76	222	4	35	3	9	2.2	3.7	2.5
15	912	Prepared from flakes; water, milk, margarine, salt added	1 c	215	76	239	4	28	2	13	3.0	5.4	3.7
		Potato products, prepared:											
		Au gratin:											
15	913	From dry mix	1 c	245	79	228	6	32	4	10	6.3	3	.3
15	914	From home recipe[127]	1 c	245	74	322	12	28	4	19	12	5	1

(125) Vitamin C varies with length of storage. After 3 months of storage approximately two-thirds of the ascorbic acid remains; after 6 to 7 months, about one-third remains.

(126) Recipe: 84% potatoes, 15% whole milk, 1% salt.

(127) Recipe: 55% potatoes, 30% whole milk, 9% cheddar cheese, 3% butter, 2% flour, 1% salt.

GRP KEY: 1 = BEV 2 = DAIRY 3 = EGGS 4 = FAT/OIL 5 = FRUIT 6 = BAKERY 7 = GRAIN 8 = FISH 9 = BEEF 10 = POULTRY 11 = SAUSAGE 12 = MIXED/FAST 13 = NUTS/SEEDS 14 = SWEETS **15 = VEG/LEG** 16 = MISC 22 = SOUP/SAUCE

Chol (mg)	Calc (mg)	Iron (mg)	Magn (mg)	Phos (mg)	Pota (mg)	Sodi (mg)	Zinc (mg)	VT-A (RE)	Thia (mg)	Ribo (mg)	Niac (mg)	V-B6 (mg)	Fola (µg)	VT-C (mg)
0	17	.81	15	57	147	186[128]	.60	65	.10	.07	.62	.05	38	8
0	19	1.25	23	72	134	70	.75	77	.23	.14	1.18	.09	47	8
0	26	2.52	71	195	710	4	1.96	1	.37	.11	1.74	.09	127	1
0	18	.75	13	39	127	55	.36	621	.18	.06	.92	.07	21	7
0	29	.97	18	58	128	332	.74	739	.10	.07	.74	.11	24	8
0	5	.34	8	12	143	10	.02	42[129]	.01	.03	.54	.08	35	46
0	8	.54	11	21	153	3	.14	35[129]	.04	.04	.43	.13	11	109
0	18	1.90	8	12	92	995	.13	116	.02	.03	.34	.14	35	9
0	7	.34	7	14	131	1	.09	47	.05	.02	.38	.18	16	66
0	6	.31	7	12	113	1	.08	40	.04	.02	.32	.16	10	51
0	5	.23	5	10	89	1	.06	285	.03	.02	.26	.12	11	95
0	6	.31	7	12	113	1	.08	256	.04	.02	.32	.16	11	116
0	82	4.47	95	273	800	3	1.85	<1	.32	.16	.68	.27	294	4
0	37	2.11	58	94	439	28	2.04	5	.31	.10	2.64	—	—	10
0	20	2.75	55	115	844	16	.65	0	.22	.07	3.32	.70	22	26
0	8	.55	39	78	610	8	.45	0	.16	.03	2.18	.47	14	20
0	20	2.20	25	59	332	12	.28	0	.07	.07	1.78	.35	13	8
0	22	2.50	54	212	903	16	.73	0	.24	.07	3.46	.70	24	31
0	8	.64	39	170	641	11	.51	0	.20	.04	2.54	.50	19	24
0	27	3.44	22	48	377	9	.30	0	.04	.04	1.29	.28	10	9
0	7	.42	30	60	515	6	.41	0	.14	.03	1.96	.41	14	18
0	10	.42	26	54	443	7	.37	0	.13	.03	1.77	.36	12	10
0	4	.67	11	43	229	15	.21	0	.06	.02	1.15	.12	8	6
0	10	.38	17	47	366	108	.19	0	.09	.01	1.63	.12	15	5
0	10	.38	17	47	366	108	.19	0	.09	.01	1.63	.12	15	5
0	24	2.36	27	112	680	53	.50	0	.17	.03	3.78	.20	26	10
4	55	.57	39	100	628	636	.60	12	.19	.08	2.35	.49	17	14
4[130]	54	.55	37	97	607	619	.58	41	.18	.11	2.27	.47	17	13
4[130]	92	.40	30	108	428	733	.51	176	.30	.14	1.91	.26	15	25
12	203	.78	37	233	537	1076	.59	76	.05	.20	2.30	.10	3	8
56[131]	292	1.56	48	277	970	1064	1.69	93	.16	.28	2.43	.43	25	24

(128) Dietary pack contains 1.7 mg sodium.
(129) Data is for green chili peppers; red varieties contain 809 RE vitamin A per ½ cup; 484 RE per whole pepper.
(130) Data is for margarine; if butter is used, cholesterol = 25 mg for 29 total mg.
(131) Data is for butter; if margarine is used, cholesterol = 37 mg.

Table F–1 Food Composition

Grp	Computer Code No.	Food Description	Measure	Wt (g)	H_2O (%)	Ener (cal)	Prot (g)	Carb (g)	Dietary Fiber (g)	Fat (g)	Fat Breakdown (g) Sat	Mono	Poly
		VEGETABLES and LEGUMES—Con.											
		Potato Products—Con.											
		Potato salad (see Mixed Dishes #715)											
		Scalloped:											
15	915	From dry mix	1 c	245	79	228	5	31	3	11	6.5	3.0	.5
15	916	Home recipe[132]	1 c	245	81	210	7	26	3	9	5.5	2.6	.4
15	1192	Potato puffs, cooked from frozen	.5 c	62	53	138	2	19	1	7	3.2	2.7	.5
15	917	Potato chips (14 chips = about 1 oz)	14 chips	28	2	148	2	15	1	10	2.6	1.8	5.2
		Pumpkin:											
15	918	Cooked from raw, mashed	1 c	245	94	50	2	12	4	<1	.1	t	t
15	919	Canned	1 c	245	90	83	3	20	5	1	.4	.1	<.1
15	920	Red radishes	10 radishes	45	95	7	<1	2	1	<1	t	t	t
15	921	Refried beans, canned	1 c	253	72	270	16	47	22	3	1	1.2	.4
15	1375	Rutabaga, cooked cubes	.5 c	85	90	29	1	7	1	<1	<.1	<.1	.1
15	922	Sauerkraut, canned with liquid	1 c	236	92	44	2	10	4	<1	.1	<.1	.1
		Seaweed:											
15	923	Kelp, raw	1 oz	28	82	12	1	3	1	<1	.1	<.1	t
15	924	Spirulina, dried	1 oz	28	5	82	16	7	1	2	.8	.2	.6
15	925	Soybeans, cooked from dry	1 c	172	63	298	29	17	5	15	2.2	3.4	8.7
		Soybean products:											
15	926	Miso	½ c	138	46	283	16	39	7	8	1.2	1.9	4.7
15	927	Tofu	½ c	124	85	94	10	2	2	6	.9	1.3	3.4
		Spinach:											
15	928	Raw, chopped	1 c	56	92	12	2	2	2	<1	<.1	t	.1
		Cooked, drained:											
15	929	From raw	1 c	180	91	41	5	7	4	<1	.1	t	.2
15	930	From frozen (leaf)	1 c	190	90	53	6	10	5	<1	.1	t	.2
15	931	Canned, drained solids	1 c	214	92	50	6	7	6	1	.2	<.1	.5
		Spinach soufflé (Mixed Dishes)											
		Squash, summer varieties, cooked slices:											
15	932	Varieties averaged	1 c	180	94	36	2	8	3	1	.1	<.1	.2
15	933	Crookneck	1 c	180	94	36	2	8	3	1	.1	<.1	.2
15	934	Zucchini	1 c	180	95	29	1	7	4	<.1	t	t	<.1
		Squash, winter varieties, cooked:											
		Average of all varieties, baked:											
15	935	Mashed	1 c	245	89	96	2	21	7	2	.3	.1	.7
15	936	Baked cubes	1 c	205	89	79	2	18	6	1	.3	.1	.5
		Acorn squash:											
15	937	Baked, mashed	1 c	245	83	137	3	36	7	<1	<.1	t	.1
15	1218	Boiled, mashed	1 c	245	90	83	2	22	6	<1	<.1	t	.1
15	938	Butternut, baked cubes	1 c	205	88	83	2	22	6	<1	<.1	t	.1
		Butternut squash:											
15	1219	Baked, mashed	1 c	245	88	99	2	26	7	<1	<.1	t	.1
15	1193	Cooked from frozen	1 c	240	88	94	3	24	7	<1	<.1	t	.1
		Hubbard squash:											
15	1194	Baked, mashed	1 c	240	85	120	6	26	6	1	.3	.1	.6
15	1195	Boiled, mashed	1 c	236	91	70	4	15	7	1	.2	.1	.4
15	1196	Spaghetti squash, baked or boiled	1 c	155	92	45	1	10	4	<1	.1	<.1	.2
15	1189	Succotash, cooked from frozen	1 c	170	74	158	7	34	9	2	.3	.3	.7

(132)Recipe: 59% potatoes, 36% whole milk, 2% butter, 2% flour, 1% salt.

GRP KEY: 1=BEV 2=DAIRY 3=EGGS 4=FAT/OIL 5=FRUIT 6=BAKERY 7=GRAIN 8=FISH 9=BEEF 10=POULTRY 11=SAUSAGE 12=MIXED/FAST 13=NUTS/SEEDS 14=SWEETS **15=VEG/LEG** 16=MISC 22=SOUP/SAUCE

Chol (mg)	Calc (mg)	Iron (mg)	Magn (mg)	Phos (mg)	Pota (mg)	Sodi (mg)	Zinc (mg)	VT-A (RE)	Thia (mg)	Ribo (mg)	Niac (mg)	V-B6 (mg)	Fola (µg)	VT-C (mg)
27	88	.93	34	137	497	835	.61	51	.05	.14	2.52	.10	3	8
29[133]	140	1.41	46	154	926	821	.98	46	.17	.23	2.58	.44	21	26
0	19	.97	12	30	236	462	.19	1	.12	.05	1.34	.14	.10	4
0	7	.34	17	43	369	133[134]	.30	0	.04	.01	1.19	.14	13	12
0	37	1.40	22	74	564	3	.45	265	.08	.19	1.01	.16	33	12
0	64	3.41	56	85	504	12	.42	5404	.06	.13	.9	.14	30	10
0	9	.13	4	8	104	11	.13	t	<.01	.02	.14	.03	12	10
0	118	4.5	99	214	994	1071	3.45	0	.12	.14	1.23	.28	150	15
0	36	.40	18	42	244	15	.26	0	.06	.03	.54	.08	13	19
0	72	3.47	31	46	401	1561	.44	4	.05	.05	.34	.31	4	35
0	48	.81	34	12	25	66	.35	3	.01	.04	.13	—	51	—
0	34	8.08	55	33	386	297	—	16	.68	1.04	3.63	.10	—	3
0	175	8.84	148	421	886	1	1.98	2	.27	.49	.69	.40	93	3
0	92	3.78	58	211	226	5032	4.58	12	.13	.35	1.19	.3	46	0
0	130	6.65	127	120	150	9	1.00	11	.10	.06	.24	.06	19	<1
0	55	1.52	44	27	312	44	.30	448	.04	.11	.41	.11	109	16
0	244	6.42	157	100	838	126	1.37	1750	.17	.43	.88	.44	262	40
0	277	2.89	131	91	566	163	1.33	1756	.11	.32	.80	.28	204	23
0	271	4.92	162	94	740	683[135]	.99	1878	.03	.30	.83	.21	209	31
0	48	.64	44	69	346	2	.71	52[136]	.08	.07	.92	.12	36	9
0	48	.64	44	69	346	2	.71	52[136]	.09	.09	.92	.17	36	10
0	23	.63	40	72	455	5	.32	43[136]	.07	.07	.77	.14	30	8
0	34	.81	20	49	1071	2	.64	872	.21	.06	1.72	.18	69	24
0	28	.67	16	41	895	3	.54	730	.17	.05	1.43	.15	57	20
0	108	2.28	104	111	1071	11	.42	105	.41	.03	2.16	.48	46	26
0	65	1.37	63	67	645	6	.27	63	.25	.02	1.30	.29	28	16
0	84	1.23	59	55	582	7	.27	1435	.15	.04	1.99	.25	39	31
0	100	1.47	71	66	697	8	.32	1715	.18	.04	2.38	.30	47	37
0	46	1.40	22	34	319	4	.29	801	.12	.09	1.11	.17	29	8
0	41	1.13	53	55	859	19	.36	1450	.18	.11	1.34	.41	39	23
0	23	.67	32	33	504	12	.22	945	.10	.07	.79	.24	23	15
0	33	.52	17	21	182	28	.31	17	.06	.03	1.26	.15	12	6
0	25	1.51	39	119	451	77	.76	39	.13	.12	2.22	.16	57	10

(133)Data is for butter; if margarine is used cholesterol = 15 mg.
(134)If no salt added, sodium = 2 mg.
(135)Dietary pack contains 58 mg sodium.
(136)Applies to squash including skin; flesh has no appreciable vitamin A value.

Table F–1 Food Composition

Grp	Computer Code No.	Food Description	Measure	Wt (g)	H_2O (%)	Ener (cal)	Prot (g)	Carb (g)	Dietary Fiber (g)	Fat (g)	Fat Breakdown (g) Sat	Mono	Poly
VEGETABLES and LEGUMES—Con.													
		Sweet potatoes:											
		Cooked, 5 × 2″ diam:											
15	939	Baked in skin, peeled	1 potato	114	73	118	2	28	3	<1	<.1	t	.1
15	940	Boiled without skin	1 potato	151	73	160	2	37	5	<1	.1	t	.2
15	941	Candied, 2½ × 2″	1 pce	105	67	144	1	29	2	3	1.4	.7	.2
		Canned:											
15	942	Solid pack, mashed	1 c	265	74	258	5	59	6	<1	.1	t	.2
15	943	Vacuum pack, mashed	1 c	255	76	233	4	54	5	1	.1	t	.2
15	944	Vacuum pack, 2¾ × 1″	1 pce	40	76	36	1	8	1	<1	t	t	<.1
		Tomatoes:											
15	945	Raw, whole, 2⅗″ diam	1 tomato	123	94	26	1	6	2	<1	<.1	<.1	.2
15	946	Raw, chopped	1 c	180	94	38	2	8	3	<1	.1	.1	.2
15	947	Cooked from raw	1 c	240	92	65	3	14	4	1	.1	.2	.4
15	948	Canned, solids and liquid	1 c	240	94	47	2	10	3	1	.1	.1	.2
15	949	Tomato juice, canned	1 c	244	94	42	2	10	2	<1	t	t	.1
		Tomato products, canned:											
15	950	Paste	1 c	262	74	220	10	49	11	2	.3	.4	.9
15	951	Puree	1 c	250	87	102	4	25	6	<1	<.1	<.1	.1
15	952	Sauce	1 c	245	89	74	3	18	4	<1	.1	.1	.2
15	953	Turnips, cubes, cooked from raw	½ c	78	94	14	1	4	2	<1	t	t	<.1
		Turnip greens, cooked:											
15	954	From raw (leaves and stems)	1 c	144	94	29	2	6	4	<1	.1	t	.1
15	955	From frozen (chopped)	½ c	82	90	24	3	4	4	<1	.1	t	.1
15	956	Vegetable juice cocktail, canned	1 c	242	94	46	2	11	2	<1	<.1	<.1	.1
		Vegetables, mixed:											
15	957	Canned, drained	1 c	163	87	77	4	15	6	<1	.1	<.1	.2
15	958	Frozen, cooked, drained	1 c	182	83	107	5	24	7	<1	.1	t	.1
		Water chestnuts, canned:											
15	959	Slices	½ c	70	86	35	1	9	2	<.1	t	t	t
15	960	Whole	4 ea	28	86	14	<1	4	1	<1	t	t	t
15	1190	Watercress, fresh, chopped	.5 c	17	95	2	<1	<1	<1	<1	t	t	t
MISCELLANEOUS													
		Baking powders for home use:											
		Sodium aluminum sulfate:											
16	962	With monocalcium phosphate monohydrate	1 tsp	3	2	5	t	1	0	0	0	0	0
16	963	With monocalcium phosphate monohydrate, calcium sulfate	1 tsp	3	1	5	t	1	0	0	0	0	0
16	964	Straight phosphate	1 tsp	4	2	5	t	1	0	0	0	0	0
16	965	Low sodium	1 tsp	4	1	5	t	1	0	0	0	0	0
16	1204	Baking soda	1 tsp	3	1	0	0	0	0	0	0	0	0
16	966	Basil, ground	1 tbsp	5	6	11	1	3	1	<1	—	—	—
16	961	Carob flour	1 c	103	3	185	5	92	34	1	.1	.2	.2

(Computer code number is for West Diet Analysis program)

GRP KEY: 1=BEV 2=DAIRY 3=EGGS 4=FAT/OIL 5=FRUIT 6=BAKERY 7=GRAIN 8=FISH 9=BEEF 10=POULTRY 11=SAUSAGE 12=MIXED/FAST 13=NUTS/SEEDS 14=SWEETS **15=VEG/LEG** 16=MISC 22=SOUP/SAUCE

Chol (mg)	Calc (mg)	Iron (mg)	Magn (mg)	Phos (mg)	Pota (mg)	Sodi (mg)	Zinc (mg)	VT-A (RE)	Thia (mg)	Ribo (mg)	Niac (mg)	V-B6 (mg)	Fola (µg)	VT-C (mg)
0	32	.52	23	63	397	12	.33	2488	.08	.14	.7	.28	26	28
0	32	.8	15	41	278	20	.4	2575	.08	.21	1	.36	22	26
0[137]	27	1.2	12	27	198	73	.16	440	.02	.04	.41	.17	12	7
0	77	3.4	61	133	536	191	.54	3857	.07	.23	2.4	.48	42	13
0	56	2.27	57	125	796	136	.46	2036	.09	.14	1.89	.49	42	67
0	9	.36	9	20	125	21	.07	319	.02	.02	.3	.08	7	11
0	6	.55	14	30	273	11	.11	77	.07	.06	.77	.10	18	22[138]
0	9	.81	20	43	400	16	.16	112	.11	.09	1.13	.14	27	34[138]
0	14	1.34	34	74	670	26	.26	178	.17	.14	1.80	.23	31	55
0	63[139]	1.45	29	46	529	390[140]	.38	145	.11	.07	1.76	.22	35	36
0	22	1.41	27	46	537	881[141]	.34	136	.12	.08	1.64	.27	49	45
0	92	7.84	134	207	2442	170[142]	2.1	647	.41	.5	8.44	1	40	111
0	37	2.32	60	99	1051	49[143]	.54	340	.18	.14	4.29	.38	39	88
0	34	1.88	46	78	908	1481[144]	.6	240	.16	.14	2.82	.33	39	32
0	18	.17	6	15	106	39	.16	0	.02	.02	.23	.05	7	9
0	198	1.15	32	41	293	41	.29	792	.07	.1	.59	.26	171	40
0	125	1.59	21	27	184	12	.34	654	.04	.06	.38	.06	32	18
0	27	1.02	27	41	467	883	.48	283	.1	.07	1.76	.34	38	67
0	44	1.71	26	68	474	243	.67	1899	.07	.08	.94	.13	39	8
0	46	1.49	40	93	308	64	.89	779	.13	.22	1.55	.14	35	6
0	3	.61	3	14	82	6	.27	t	.01	.02	.25	—	8	1
0	1	.25	1	5	33	2	.11	t	<.01	.01	.1	—	3	<1
0	20	.03	4	10	56	7	.03	80	.02	.02	.03	.02	34	7
0	58	0	t	87	5	329	0	0	0	0	0	0	0	0
0	183	0	—	45	4	290	0	0	0	0	0	0	0	0
0	239	0	—	359	6	312	0	0	0	0	0	0	0	0
0	207	0	—	314	891	t	0	0	0	0	0	0	0	0
0	0	—	—	—	—	821	—	0	0	0	0	0	0	0
0	95	1.89	18	22	154	2	.26	42	.01	.01	.31	—	—	3
0	359	3.03	56	81	852	36	.94	2	.06	.48	1.95	.38	30	<1

(137)For recipe using margarine; if butter is used, cholesterol = 8 mg.

(138)Year-round average. From June through October, ascorbic acid is approximately 32 mg and 47 mg, respectively, for one tomato and 1 c chopped tomato. From November through May, market samples average around 12 and 18 mg, respectively.

(139)Calcium is added as a firming agent.

(140)Dietary pack contains 31 mg sodium.

(141)If no salt is added, sodium content is 24 mg.

(142)If salt is added, sodium content is 2070 mg.

(143)If salt is added, sodium content is 998 mg.

(144)With salt added.

(For purposes of calculations, use "0" for t, <1, <.1, <.01, etc.)

Table F–1 Food Composition

Grp	Computer Code No.	Food Description	Measure	Wt (g)	H_2O (%)	Ener (cal)	Prot (g)	Carb (g)	Dietary Fiber (g)	Fat (g)	Fat Breakdown (g) Sat	Mono	Poly
MISCELLANEOUS—Con.													
		Catsup:											
16	967	Cup	1 c	245	67	255	4	67	4	1	.2	.2	.4
16	968	Tablespoon	1 tbsp	15	67	16	<1	4	<1	<.1	t	t	t
16	1200	Cayenne (red pepper)	1 tbsp	5.3	8	17	1	3	2	1	.2	.2	.4
16	969	Celery seed	1 tsp	2	6	9	<1	1	<1	1	<.1	.3	.1
16	970	Chili powder	1 tsp	3	8	8	<1	1	1	<1	.1	.1	.2
		Chocolate:											
16	971	Baking, unsweetened	1 oz	28	2	145	4	7	4	15	9	5	.5
		For other chocolate items, see Sweeteners and Sweets											
16	972	Coriander, fresh	¼ c	4	93	<1	<1	<1	<1	<.1	<.01	<.01	.01
16	1197	Cornstarch	1 tbsp	8	8	20	<.1	5	<.1	<.1	t	t	t
16	973	Cinnamon	1 tsp	2	10	6	<1	2	1	<.1	t	t	t
16	974	Curry powder	1 tsp	2	10	6	<1	1	<1	<1	t	.2	<.1
16	1202	Dill weed, dried	1 tbsp	3.1	7	8	1	2	<1	<1	—	—	—
		Garlic:											
16	975	Cloves	4 cloves	12	59	18	1	4	<1	<.1	t	t	<.1
16	976	Powder	1 tsp	3	6	9	<1	2	<1	<.1	t	t	t
16	977	Gelatin, dry, plain	1 envelope	7	13	25	6	0	1	0	0	0	0
16	978	Ginger root, raw, sliced	5 slices	11	87	8	<1	2	<1	<.1	t	t	t
16	1198	Horseradish, prepared	1 tbsp	15	87	6	<1	1	<1	<1	t	t	t
16	1199	Hummous/Humous	1 c	246	65	420	33	50	4	21	3.1	8.8	7.8
16	979	Mustard, prepared, (1 packet = 1 tsp)	1 tsp	5	80	4	<1	<1	<1	<1	t	.2	t
		Miso (see #926 under Vegetables and Legumes, Soybean products)											
		Olives:											
16	980	Green	10 olives	39	78	45	<1	<1	1	6	.6	3.6	.3
16	981	Ripe, pitted	10 olives	45	80	52	<1	3	1.5	5	.6	3.6	.4
16	982	Onion powder	1 tsp	2.1	5	5	<1	2	<1	<.1	t	t	t
16	983	Oregano, ground	1 tsp	2	7	5	<1	1	<1	<1	t	t	.1
16	984	Paprika	1 tsp	2	10	6	<1	1	<1	<1	t	t	.2
16	985	Pepper, black	1 tsp	2	11	5	<1	1	<1	<.1	<.1	<.1	<.1
		Pickles:											
16	986	Dill, medium, 3¾ × 1¼″ diam	1 pickle	65	92	12	<1	3	1	<1	<.1	t	<.1
16	987	Fresh pack, slices, 1½″ diam × ¼″	4 slices	30	79	20	<1	5	<1	<.1	t	t	t
16	988	Sweet, medium	1 pickle	35	65	41	<1	11	<1	.1	t	t	<.1
16	989	Pickle relish, sweet	1 tbsp	15	63	20	<.1	5	<1	<.1	t	t	<.1
16	1201	Sage, ground	1 tbsp	2	8	6	<1	1	<1	<1	.1	<.1	<.1
		Popcorn (see Grain Products, #539-541)											
22	1347	Salsa, from recipe	.85 c	184	91	79	2	9	3	5	.7	3.4	.5
16	990	Salt	1 tsp	6	0	0	0	0	0	0	0	0	0
		Salt substitute:											
16	1205	Morton Salt Substitute	1 tbsp	6	0	0	0	<1	0	0	0	0	0
16	1206	No Salt, packet, Norcliff Thayer	1 packet	.75	0	0	0	0	0	0	0	0	0
16	1207	Light Salt, Morton	1 tsp	6	0	0	0	0	0	0	0	0	0
16	991	Vinegar, cider	1 tbsp	15	94	2	0	1	0	0	0	0	0
		Yeast:											
16	992	Baker's, dry, active, package	1 package	7	5	20	3	3	2	<1	t	.1	t
16	993	Brewer's, dry	1 tbsp	8	5	25	3	3	3	<.1	t	t	0

GRP KEY: 1=BEV 2=DAIRY 3=EGGS 4=FAT/OIL 5=FRUIT 6=BAKERY 7=GRAIN 8=FISH 9=BEEF 10=POULTRY 11=SAUSAGE 12=MIXED/FAST 13=NUTS/SEEDS 14=SWEETS 15=VEG/LEG **16=MISC** 22=SOUP/SAUCE

Chol (mg)	Calc (mg)	Iron (mg)	Magn (mg)	Phos (mg)	Pota (mg)	Sodi (mg)	Zinc (mg)	VT-A (RE)	Thia (mg)	Ribo (mg)	Niac (mg)	V-B6 (mg)	Fola (µg)	VT-C (mg)
0	47	1.72	54	96	1178	2906	.56	250	.22	.18	3.3	.44	37	37
0	3	.11	3	6	72	178	.04	15	.01	.01	.21	.03	2	2
0	8	.41	8	16	107	7	.13	221	.02	.05	.46	—	—	4
0	38	.90	10	11	30	4	.14	<1	.01	.01	.1	—	—	<1
0	7	.37	4	8	50	26	.07	91	.01	.02	.21	—	1	2
0	22	1.9	82	109	235	1	1.01	1	.02	.1	.38	.01	18	0
0	4	.08	1	1	22	1	—	11	<.01	<.01	.03	<.01	.4	<1
0	.12	.08	.16	.7	.16	.5	<.01	0	0	0	0	0	0	0
0	28	.86	1	1	11	1	.05	1	<.01	<.01	.03	.02	—	1
0	10	.59	5	7	31	1	.08	2	<.01	<.01	.07	—	—	<1
0	50	1.50	13	16	110	6	.10	—	.01	.01	.09	.05	—	—
0	22	.2	3	18	48	2	1.06	0	.02	.01	.08	.40	<1	4
0	2	.08	2	12	31	1	.07	0	.01	<.01	.02	.57	2	<1
0	1	0	2	0	2	6	0	0	0	0	0	<.01	0	0
0	2	.05	5	3	46	1	.22	0	<.01	<.01	.08	.02	2	1
0	9	.10	4	5	44	14	.18	0	.01	<.01	.06	.01	2	1
0	124	3.87	71	275	427	599	2.70	6	.23	.13	1.01	.98	146	19
0	4	.1	3	4	7	63	.03	0	<.01	.01	.07	<.01	0	<1
0	24	.6	9	6	21	936	.03	12	<.01	<.01	.01	.01	<1	<1
0	40	1.49	2	1	4	392	.10	18	<.01	<.01	.02	<.01	.3	.4
0	8	.06	3	7	20	1	.05	0	.01	<.01	.01	.03	3	<1
0	24	.66	4	3	25	<1	.07	10	<.01	t	.09	—	—	1
0	4	.50	4	7	49	1	.09	127	.01	.04	.32	—	—	2
0	9	.61	4	4	26	1	.03	<1	<.01	<.01	.02	0	—	0
0	6	.34	7	14	199	833	.09	21	.01	.02	.04	<.01	1	1
0	3	.20	2	6	20	201	.02	4	t	.01	.02	<.01	0	1
0	1	.21	1	4	11	329	.03	4	<.01	.01	.06	.01	<1	<1
0	3	.13	1	2	30	107	.01	2	t	t	<.01	0	0	1
0	33	.56	9	2	21	0	.09	12	.02	.01	.11	—	—	1
0	18	.86	19	41	347	191	.20	150	.09	.07	.93	.16	28	39
0	14	<.01	2	3	.3	2132	t	0	0	0	0	0	0	0
0	30	0	t	28	2800	t	0	0	0	0	0	0	0	0
0	—	—	—	—	385	0	—	0	0	0	0	0	0	0
0	<1	0	4	0	1500	1100	0	0	0	0	0	0	0	0
0	1	.09	<1	1	15	t	.02	0	0	0	0	0	0	0
0	4	1.1	16	90	140	4	.43	t	.17	.38	2.7	.14	266	t
0	17[145]	1.39	18	140	152	10	.63	t	1.25	.34	3.16	.4	313	t

(145) Value varies from 6 to 60 mg.

• *Table F–1* Food Composition

Grp	Computer Code No.	Food Description	Measure	Wt (g)	H_2O (%)	Ener (cal)	Prot (g)	Carb (g)	Dietary Fiber (g)	Fat (g)	Fat Breakdown (g) Sat	Mono	Poly
		SOUPS, SAUCES, AND GRAVIES											
		SOUPS, canned, condensed:											
		Unprepared, condensed:											
22	1210	Cream of celery	1 c	251	85	180	3	18	1	11	2.8	2.6	5.0
22	1215	Cream of chicken	1 c	251	82	233	7	19	<1	15	4.2	.8	3.0
22	1216	Cream of mushroom	1 c	251	81	257	4	19	<1	19	5.2	3.6	8.9
22	1220	Onion	1 c	246	86	114	8	16	1	3	.5	1.5	1.3
		Prepared with equal volume of whole milk:											
22	994	Clam chowder, New England	1 c	248	85	163	9	17	1	7	3.0	2.3	1.1
22	1209	Cream of celery	1 c	248	87	165	6	15	<1	10	4.0	2.5	2.7
22	995	Cream of chicken	1 c	248	85	191	7	15	<1	12	5	4	2
22	996	Cream of mushroom	1 c	248	85	205	6	15	<1	14	5	3	5
22	1214	Cream of potato	1 c	248	87	148	6	17	<1	6	3.8	1.7	.6
22	1213	Oyster stew	1 c	245	89	134	6	10	0	8	5.1	2.1	.3
22	997	Tomato	1 c	248	85	160	6	22	<1	6	2.9	1.6	1.1
		Prepared with equal volume of water:											
22	998	Bean with bacon	1 c	253	84	173	8	23	3	6	1.5	2.2	1.8
22	999	Beef broth, bouillon, consommé	1 c	240	98	16	3	<1	0	1	.3	.2	t
22	1000	Beef noodle	1 c	244	92	84	5	9	<1	3	1.2	1.2	.5
22	1001	Chicken noodle	1 c	241	92	75	4	9	1	2	.7	1.1	.6
22	1002	Chicken rice	1 c	241	94	60	4	7	1	2	.5	.9	.4
22	1208	Chili beef soup	1 c	250	85	169	7	22	1	7	3.3	2.8	.3
22	1003	Clam chowder, Manhatten	1 c	244	92	78	2	12	1	2	.4	.4	1.3
22	1004	Cream of chicken	1 c	244	91	115	3	9	<1	7	2.1	3.3	1.5
22	1005	Cream of mushroom	1 c	244	90	130	2	9	1	9	2.4	1.7	4.2
22	1006	Minestrone	1 c	241	91	80	4	11	1	3	.5	.7	1.1
22	1211	Onion soup	1 c	241	93	57	4	8	<1	2	.3	.8	.7
22	1007	Split pea with ham	1 c	253	82	189	10	28	1	4	1.8	1.8	.6
22	1008	Tomato	1 c	244	90	86	2	17	<1	2	.4	.4	1.0
22	1009	Vegetable beef	1 c	244	92	79	6	10	1	2	.9	.8	.1
22	1010	Vegetarian vegetable	1 c	241	92	70	2	12	2	2	.3	.8	.7
		SOUPS, dehydrated:											
		Unprepared, dry products:											
22	1011	Bouillon	1 packet	6	3	14	1	1	<1	1	.3	.2	t
22	1012	Onion	1 packet	7	4	20	1	4	<1	<1	.1	.2	.1
		Prepared with water:											
22	1299	Beef broth/bouillon	1 c	244	97	20	1	2	<1	1	.3	.3	<.1
22	1376	Chicken broth/bouillon	1 c	244	97	21	1	1	<1	1	.3	.4	.4
22	1013	Chicken noodle	¾ c	188	94	40	2	6	<1	1	.2	.4	.3
22	1122	Cream of chicken	1 c	261	91	107	2	13	1	5	3.4	1.2	.4
22	1014	Onion	¾ c	184	96	20	1	4	<1	<1	.1	.3	.1
22	1217	Split pea	1 c	255	87	133	8	23	1	2	.4	.7	.3
22	1015	Tomato vegetable	¾ c	189	94	41	1	8	<1	1	.3	.3	.1
		SAUCES											
		From dry mixes, prepared with milk:											
22	1016	Cheese sauce	1 c	279	77	305	16	23	<1	17	9	5	2
22	1017	Hollandaise	1 c	259	84	240	5	14	—	20	12	6	1
22	1019	White sauce	1 c	264	81	240	10	21	<1	13	6	5	2
		From home recipe:											
22	1019	White sauce, medium[146]	1 c	250	73	395	10	24	<1	30	9	12	7
		Ready to serve:											
22	1020	Barbeque sauce	1 tbsp	16	81	10	<1	2	<1	<1	<.1	.1	.1
22	1021	Soy sauce	1 tbsp	18	71	9	1	2	0	t	0	0	0

(146)Made with enriched flour, margarine, and whole milk.

(Computer code number is for West Diet Analysis program)

GRP KEY: 1 = BEV 2 = DAIRY 3 = EGGS 4 = FAT/OIL 5 = FRUIT 6 = BAKERY 7 = GRAIN 8 = FISH 9 = BEEF 10 = POULTRY 11 = SAUSAGE 12 = MIXED/FAST 13 = NUTS/SEEDS 14 = SWEETS 15 = VEG/LEG 16 = MISC **22 = SOUP/SAUCE**

Chol (mg)	Calc (mg)	Iron (mg)	Magn (mg)	Phos (mg)	Pota (mg)	Sodi (mg)	Zinc (mg)	VT-A (RE)	Thia (mg)	Ribo (mg)	Niac (mg)	V-B6 (mg)	Fola (µg)	VT-C (mg)
28	80	1.25	13	75	246	1899	.30	61	.06	.10	.67	.03	5	<1
20	68	1.21	5	75	174	1973	1.26	112	.06	.12	1.64	.03	3	<1
3	64	1.05	9	84	167	2032	1.19	0	.06	.17	1.62	.03	7	2
0	53	1.35	5	22	138	2116	1.23	0	.07	.05	1.21	.10	31	3
22	187	1.48	23	157	300	992	1.3	40	.07	.24	1.03	.13	12	4
32	186	.69	22	151	309	1010	.20	68	.07	.25	.44	.06	9	1
27	180	.67	18	152	273	1046	.68	94	.07	.26	.92	.07	8	1
20	178	.59	20	156	270	1076	.64	38	.08	.28	.81	.06	15	2
22	166	.54	17	160	323	1060	.68	67	.08	.24	.64	.09	9	1
32	167	1.04	21	162	235	1040	10.3	45	.07	.23	.34	.06	7	4
17	159	1.82	23	148	450	932	.29	109	.13	.25	1.52	.16	21	68
3	81	2.05	44	132	403	952	1.03	89	.09	.03	.57	.04	32	2
1	15	.41	9	31	130	782	.6	0	<.01	.05	1.87	.07	2	0
5	15	1.1	6	46	100	952	1.54	63	.07	.06	1.07	.04	4	<1
7	17	.78	7	36	55	900	.55	71	.05	.06	1.39	.01	2	<1
7	17	.75	1	22	101	815	.26	66	.02	.02	1.13	.02	1	<1
12	43	2.40	30	148	525	1035	1.40	503	.06	.08	1.07	.16	10	4
2	27	1.64	10	41	188	578	.98	98	.03	.04	.82	.10	10	4
10	34	.61	3	37	88	986	.63	56	.03	.06	.82	.02	2	<1
2	46	.5	5	49	100	1032	.59	0	.05	.09	.7	.02	3	1
2	34	.92	7	56	312	911	.74	234	.05	.04	.94	.10	16	1
0	26	.67	2	11	69	1053	.61	0	.03	.02	.60	.05	15	1
8	22	2.28	48	213	399	1008	1.32	44	.15	.08	1.48	.07	3	1
0	13	1.76	8	34	263	872	.24	69	.09	.05	1.42	.11	15	67
5	17	1.11	6	41	173	956	2	189	.04	.05	1.03	.08	11	2
0	21	1.08	7	35	209	823	.46	301	.05	.05	.92	.06	11	1
1	4	.06	3	19	27	1019	0	<1	<.01	.02	.27	.01	2	0
<1	10	.14	3	23	47	627	.06	<1	.02	.04	.4	.01	2	<1
0	10	.02	7	24	37	1362	.07	.5	<.01	.02	.36	0	0	.01
1	15	.08	4	13	25	1484	.01	4	.01	.03	.20	.02	—	<1
2	24	.37	5	24	23	957	.15	5	.05	.04	.66	.01	1	<1
3	76	—	—	96	215	1184	—	—	—	.20	—	.05	—	—
0	9	.14	6	22	48	635	.06	<1	.02	.04	.36	<.01	2	<1
3	22	1.01	46	134	238	1220	.59	5	.22	.15	1.34	.05	15	—
0	6	.47	15	23	78	856	.13	15	.04	.03	.59	.04	2	5
53	569	.3	32	438	552	1565	.95	117	.15	.56	.3	.1	12	2
52	124	.9	—	127	124	1564	—	220	.05	.18	.1	.5	—	t
34	425	.3	30	256	444	797	1.15	92	.08	.45	.5	.06	16	3
32	292	.9	35	238	381	888	1.05	340	.15	.43	.8	.1	12	2
0	3	.13	1	3	27	128	.03	14	<.01	<.01	.06	.02	1	1
0	3	.36	6	20	32	1029	.07	0	.01	.02	.61	.03	3	0

(For purposes of calculations, use "0" for t, <1, <.1, <.01, etc.)

Table F–1 Food Composition

Grp	Computer Code No.	Food Description	Measure	Wt (g)	H_2O (%)	Ener (cal)	Prot (g)	Carb (g)	Dietary Fiber (g)	Fat (g)	Fat Breakdown (g) Sat	Mono	Poly
SOUPS, SAUCES and GRAVIES—Con.													
		SAUCES—Con.											
		Spaghetti sauce: canned:											
22	1377	Plain	1 c	249	75	272	5	40	3	12	1.7	6.1	3.3
22	1378	With meat	.8 c	206	75	220	8	27	1	10	2.5	4.5	1.5
22	1379	With mushrooms	.75 c	185	75	162	2	9	2	5	.6	2.3	1.2
22	1380	Teriyaki sauce	1 tbsp	18	84	15	1	3	0	<1	t	t	<.1
		GRAVIES:											
		Canned:											
22	1022	Beef	1 c	233	87	123	9	11	<1	5	2.7	2.2	.2
22	1023	Chicken	1 c	238	85	189	5	13	<1	14	3.4	6.1	3.6
22	1024	Mushroom	1 c	238	89	120	3	13	<1	6	1	3	2.4
		From dry mix:											
22	1025	Brown	1 c	258	92	75	2	13	<1	2	.8	.7	.1
22	1026	Chicken	1 c	260	91	85	3	14	<1	2	.5	.9	.4

GRP KEY: 1=BEV 2=DAIRY 3=EGGS 4=FAT/OIL 5=FRUIT 6=BAKERY 7=GRAIN 8=FISH 9=BEEF 10=POULTRY 11=SAUSAGE 12=MIXED/FAST 13=NUTS/SEEDS 14=SWEETS 15=VEG/LEG 16=MISC **22=SOUP/SAUCE**

Chol (mg)	Calc (mg)	Iron (mg)	Magn (mg)	Phos (mg)	Pota (mg)	Sodi (mg)	Zinc (mg)	VT-A (RE)	Thia (mg)	Ribo (mg)	Niac (mg)	V-B6 (mg)	Fola (µg)	VT-C (mg)
0	70	1.62	60	90	957	1236	.53	306	.14	.15	3.75	.40	39	28
17	36	2.80	15	106	444	1045	1.05	189	.20	.16	3.40	.27	13	2
0	22	1.50	22	45	500	744	.51	362	.12	.12	1.40	.24	19	14
0	4	.31	11	28	41	690	.02	0	<.01	.01	.23	.02	4	0
7	14	1.63	5	70	189	1305	2.33	0	.07	.08	1.54	.02	5	0
5	48	1.1	5	69	260	1375	1.91	264	.04	.1	1.06	.02	3	0
0	17	1.6	—	36	252	1357	1.66	0	.08	.15	1.6	.05	0	0
3	67	.2	10	44	57	1076	.31	0	.04	.09	.8	0	0	0
3	39	.3	—	47	62	1134	.32	0	.05	.15	.8	.03	—	3

Table F–1 Food Composition

Grp	Computer Code No.	Food Description	Measure	Wt (g)	H_2O (%)	Ener (cal)	Prot (g)	Carb (g)	Dietary Fiber (g)	Fat (g)	Fat Breakdown (g) Sat	Mono	Poly
ARBY'S													
12	1402	Bac'n Cheddar, deluxe	1 ea	229	56	532	29	35	<1	33	8	14	11
		Roast beef sandwiches:											
12	1403	Regular	1 ea	147	51	353	22	32	<1	15	7	5	2
12	1404	Junior	1 ea	85	48	218	13	21	<1	11	4	5	2
12	1405	Super	1 ea	246	58	529	33	46	<1	28	3	11	9
12	1406	Deluxe	1 ea	247	62	486	26	43	<1	23	9	8	5
12	1407	Beef 'n Cheddar	1 ea	198	57	451	25	42	<1	20	7	8	4
		Chicken sandwiches:											
12	1408	Chicken breast sandwich	1 ea	184	52	489	23	48	<1	26	4	8	14
12	1409	Chicken salad sandwich	1 ea	156	53	386	18	33	<1	20	—	—	—
12	1410	Chicken salad & croissant	1 ea	150	50	472	22	16	<1	36	—	—	—
12	1411	Roast Chicken club sandwich	1 ea	234	44	513	31	40	<1	29	5	8	14
12	1412	Hot ham and cheese sandwich	1 ea	162	62	330	23	33	<1	15	4	7	3
12	1413	Turkey deluxe sandwich	1 ea	221	61	399	27	36	<1	20	4	4	12
		Baked potatoes:											
12	1414	Plain	1 ea	241	75	240	6	50	6	2	.06	.01	.1
12	1415	Deluxe, w/butter & sour cream	1 ea	312	74	463	8	53	6	25	12	8	3
12	1416	W/broccoli & cheese	1 ea	340	70	417	11	55	6	18	7	7	8
12	1417	W/mushrooms & cheese	1 ea	347	70	515	15	58	6	27	6	11	9
12	1418	Taco	1 ea	425	70	619	23	73	6	27	11	9	3
		Milkshakes:											
12	1419	Chocolate	1 ea	340	74	451	10	77	<1	12	3	7	2
12	1420	Jamocha	1 ea	326	75	368	9	59	0	11	3	6	2
12	1421	Vanilla	1 ea	312	75	330	11	46	0	12	4	5	2
Source: Arby's Inc., Atlanta Georgia for the basic nutrients. Values for dietary fiber, magnesium, phosphorus, potassium, zinc, vitamin A (in RE's), B6, folacin, some of the fatty acids, and percent water are estimates calculated from known values for major ingredients.													
BURGER KING													
		Croissant sandwiches:											
12	1422	With egg, bacon & cheese	1 ea	119	49	335	15	20	<1	24	13	8	2
12	1423	With egg, sausage & cheese	1 ea	163	49	538	19	20	<1	41	20	12	3
12	1424	With egg, ham & cheese	1 ea	145	58	335	18	20	<1	20	12	7	1
		Whopper sandwiches:											
12	1425	Whopper	1 ea	265	57	640	27	42	<1	41	16	19	4
12	1426	Whopper w/cheese	1 ea	289	57	723	31	43	<1	48	20	20	3
12	1427	Double beef	1 ea	351	56	850	46	52	<1	52	20	24	5
12	1428	Double w/cheese	1 ea	374	55	950	51	54	<1	60	24	28	4
12	1429	Whopper, Junior	1 ea	136	52	370	15	31	<1	17	6	8	1
12	1430	Whopper, Junior w/cheese	1 ea	158	55	420	17	32	<1	20	9	8	1
12	1431	Hamburger	1 ea	109	46	275	15	29	<1	12	5	6	<1
12	1432	Cheeseburger	1 ea	120	45	317	17	30	<1	15	7	6	1
12	1433	Bacon double cheeseburger	1 ea	159	41	510	33	27	<1	31	14	15	2
12	1434	Chicken sandwich	1 ea	230	46	688	26	56	<1	40	11	17	10
12	1435	Chicken tenders	1 ea	95	50	204	20	10	0	10	3	4	2
12	1436	Ham & cheese sandwich	1 ea	230	59	471	24	44	<1	23	10	8	4
12	1437	Whaler fish sandwich	1 ea	189	45	488	19	45	<1	27	6	9	10
12	1438	Whaler sandwich w/cheese	1 ea	201	45	530	21	46	<1	30	7	9	10
12	1439	French fries, regular	1 svg	74	37	227	3	24	<1	13	5	4	1
12	1440	Onion rings, regular	1 svg	79	37	274	4	28	<1	16	5	7	4
		Milkshakes:											
12	1441	Chocolate, medium	1 ea	273	76	320	8	46	<1	12	—	—	—
12	1442	Vanilla, medium	1 ea	273	74	321	9	49	<1	10	—	—	—

GRP KEY: 1 = BEV 2 = DAIRY 3 = EGGS 4 = FAT/OIL 5 = FRUIT 6 = BAKERY 7 = GRAIN 8 = FISH 9 = BEEF 10 = POULTRY 11 = SAUSAGE **12 = MIXED/FAST** 13 = NUTS/SEEDS 14 = SWEETS 15 = VEG/LEG 16 = MISC 22 = SOUP/SAUCE

Chol (mg)	Calc (mg)	Iron (mg)	Magn (mg)	Phos (mg)	Pota (mg)	Sodi (mg)	Zinc (mg)	VT-A (RE)	Thia (mg)	Ribo (mg)	Niac (mg)	V-B6 (mg)	Fola (μg)	VT-C (mg)
83	120	2.5	—	—	422	1672	3	85	.4	.48	7	—	—	1
39	32	2	16	120	368	588	3	t	.27	.43	6.23	.20	14	0
23	16	1	8	60	197	345	1.5	t	.13	.24	4	.10	7	0
47	48	2.5	25	190	503	798	3.8	60	.34	.4	7	.30	21	1.2
59	100	6.30	25	190	500	1288	3.8	10	.30	.34	5	.30	22	t
52	76	2	24	260	335	955	3	60	.27	.4	6	.22	19	0
45	64	2	30	180	330	1099	1.5	0	.20	.5	7	.38	18	5
30	—	—	—	—	—	630	—	—	—	—	—	—	—	—
12	—	—	—	—	—	725	—	—	—	—	—	—	—	—
75	120	2	—	—	430	1423	2.3	—	.47	.57	8	—	—	0
45	80	1.5	31	405	312	1350	.9	60	.4	.32	4	.31	26	24
39	64	1.5	30	250	346	1047	1.5	91	.27	.4	7	.52	20	5
0	0	1.80	80	175	1333	58	0	0	.08	.13	2.7	1.08	30	33
40	520	1.5	83	200	1420	203	0	60	.08	.13	2.7	1.10	33	33
22	80	1.5	97	400	1455	361	0	60	.08	.16	2.7	1.15	60	45
47	200	1.5	91	440	1445	923	.9	227	.13	.24	2.7	1.25	36	33
145	450	3.60	105	530	1425	1065	4.7	860	.38	.26	8	1.40	38	63
36	200	.4	48	350	410	341	1.5	91	.11	.65	.7	.14	14	0
35	200	0	36	350	525	262	1.5	91	.11	.65	.7	.14	14	0
32	240	0	36	350	686	281	1.5	91	.11	.65	0	.14	37	0
249	136	2.00	20	249	182	762	1.5	150	.32	.30	2	.06	24	t
293	145	2.90	19	292	284	1042	2.4	150	.36	.32	4	.06	24	t
262	136	2.20	24	317	256	987	1.9	150	.49	.32	3	.06	24	t
94	80	4.90	43	237	547	842	4.5	60	.33	.41	7	.40	35	14
117	210	4.90	47	360	570	1126	5.1	85	.34	.48	7	.40	35	14
188	91	7.30	60	387	760	1080	8.5	60	.34	.56	10	.50	45	14
211	222	7.30	65	510	730	1535	9.1	85	.35	.63	10	.50	45	14
41	40	2.80	24	127	275	486	2.3	30	.23	.25	4	.20	17	6
52	105	2.80	27	189	287	628	2.6	85	.23	.29	4	.20	17	6
37	37	2.70	23	124	235	509	2.4	15	.23	.25	4	.12	18	3
48	102	3.80	26	186	247	651	2.6	70	.23	.29	4	.13	24	3
104	168	3.80	37	328	363	728	5.1	85	.31	.42	6	.30	30	t
82	79	3.30	54	274	375	1423	1.2	13	.45	.31	10	.40	18	t
47	18	.70	24	236	200	636	.6	5	.08	.08	7	.34	10	t
70	195	3.20	42	384	419	1534	2.4	85	.87	.42	6	.31	25	7
84	t	2.20	40	249	366	592	.1	20	.28	.21	4	.13	3	t
95	112	2.20	43	311	378	734	1.1	40	.27	.24	4	.13	3	t
14	t	.50	21	114	360	160	.3	0	.10	.30	7.5	.23	20	t
0	124	.80	18	195	173	665	.4	—	t	t	t	.07	8	t
—	260	1.60	46	262	567	202	1.0	—	.13	.55	t	—	—	t
—	295	t	32	284	505	205	1.0	—	.11	.57	t	—	—	t

(For purposes of calculations, use "0" for t, <1, <.1, <.01, etc.)

Table F–1 Food Composition

Grp	Computer Code No.	Food Description	Measure	Wt (g)	H_2O (%)	Ener (cal)	Prot (g)	Carb (g)	Dietary Fiber (g)	Fat (g)	Fat Breakdown (g) Sat	Mono	Poly
		BURGER KING—Con.											
		Pies:											
12	1443	Apple pie	1 ea	125	51	305	3	44	<1	12	—	—	—
12	1444	Cherry pie	1 ea	128	42	357	4	55	<1	13	—	—	—
12	1445	Pecan pie	1 ea	113	20	459	5	64	1	20	3	11	5

Source: Burger King Corporation for basic nutrients. Values for dietary fiber and percent water, calculated from known values for major ingredients.

Grp	Computer Code No.	Food Description	Measure	Wt (g)	H_2O (%)	Ener (cal)	Prot (g)	Carb (g)	Dietary Fiber (g)	Fat (g)	Fat Breakdown (g) Sat	Mono	Poly
		DAIRY QUEEN											
		Ice cream cones:											
12	1446	Small	1 ea	85	65	140	3	22	0	4	2	1	<1
12	1447	Regular	1 ea	142	65	240	6	38	0	7	—	—	—
12	1448	Large	1 ea	213	65	340	9	57	0	10	—	—	—
		Dipped ice cream cones:											
12	1449	Small	1 ea	92	58	190	3	25	<1	9	—	—	—
12	1450	Regular	1 ea	156	58	340	6	42	<1	16	—	—	—
12	1451	Large	1 ea	234	58	510	9	64	<1	24	—	—	—
		Sundaes:											
12	1452	Small	1 ea	106	60	190	3	33	<1	4	—	—	—
12	1453	Regular	1 ea	177	60	310	5	56	<1	8	—	—	—
12	1454	Large	1 ea	248	60	440	8	78	<1	10	—	—	—
12	1455	Banana split	1 ea	383	67	540	9	103	<1	11	—	—	—
12	1456	Peanut buster parfait	1 ea	305	52	740	16	94	<1	34	—	—	—
12	1457	Hot fudge brownie delight	1 ea	266	55	600	9	85	<1	25	—	—	—
12	1458	Strawberry shortcake	1 ea	312	61	540	10	100	<1	11	—	—	—
12	1459	Buster bar	1 ea	149	45	460	10	41	<1	29	—	—	—
12	1460	Dilly bar	1 ea	85	55	210	3	21	<1	13	—	—	—
12	1461	DQ ice cream sandwich	1 ea	60	47	140	3	24	<1	4	—	—	—
		Milkshakes:											
12	1462	Small	1 ea	291	63	490	10	82	<1	13	—	—	—
12	1463	Regular	1 ea	418	63	710	14	120	<1	19	—	—	—
12	1464	Large	1 ea	489	63	831	16	140	<1	22	—	—	—
		Malted milkshakes:											
12	1465	Small	1 ea	291	60	520	10	91	<1	13	—	—	—
12	1466	Regular	1 ea	418	60	760	14	134	<1	18	—	—	—
12	1467	Large	1 ea	489	60	889	16	157	<1	21	—	—	—
12	1468	Float	1 ea	397	76	410	5	82	0	7	—	—	—
12	1469	Freeze	1 ea	397	72	500	9	89	0	12	—	—	—
		Mr. Misty:											
12	1470	Regular	1 ea	330	81	250	0	63	0	0	0	0	0
12	1471	Kiss	1 ea	89	81	70	0	17	0	0	0	0	0
12	1472	Freeze	1 ea	411	72	500	9	91	0	12	—	—	—
12	1473	Float	1 ea	411	78	390	5	74	0	7	—	—	—
12	1474	Chicken sandwich	1 ea	202	46	608	27	46	<1	34	8	15	17
12	1475	Fish fillet sandwich	1 ea	177	52	430	20	45	<1	18	4	6	6
12	1476	Fish fillet sandwich w/cheese	1 ea	191	51	483	23	46	<1	22	7	7	6
		Hamburgers:											
12	1477	Single	1 ea	148	51	360	21	33	<1	16	6	7	1
12	1478	Double	1 ea	210	52	530	36	33	<1	28	10	13	2
12	1479	Triple	1 ea	272	52	710	51	33	<1	45	17	21	4
		Cheeseburgers:											
12	1480	Single	1 ea	162	51	410	24	33	<1	20	8	8	1
12	1481	Double	1 ea	239	51	650	43	34	<1	37	15	14	2
12	1482	Triple	1 ea	301	52	820	58	34	<1	50	20	20	3

GRP KEY: 1=BEV 2=DAIRY 3=EGGS 4=FAT/OIL 5=FRUIT 6=BAKERY 7=GRAIN 8=FISH 9=BEEF 10=POULTRY 11=SAUSAGE **12=MIXED/FAST** 13=NUTS/SEEDS 14=SWEETS 15=VEG/LEG 16=MISC 22=SOUP/SAUCE

Chol (mg)	Calc (mg)	Iron (mg)	Magn (mg)	Phos (mg)	Pota (mg)	Sodi (mg)	Zinc (mg)	VT-A (RE)	Thia (mg)	Ribo (mg)	Niac (mg)	V-B6 (mg)	Fola (μg)	VT-C (mg)
4	t	1.20	t	31	122	412	.2	4	.27	.16	.6	.03	7	5
6	t	1.10	12	37	166	204	.2	15	.24	.16	.5	.03	4	8
4	24	1.10	16	84	204	374	<1	16	.28	.18	.6	.06	15	t
10	100	.40	13	100	134	45	.47	25	.03	.17	t	.04	2	t
15	150	.70	20	200	220	80	.49	49	.06	.34	t	.06	3	t
25	250	1.40	30	300	330	115	1.0	98	.12	.51	t	.09	4	t
10	100	.40	13	100	134	55	.47	25	.03	.17	t	.04	2	t
20	150	.70	20	200	220	100	.70	49	.06	.34	t	.06	3	t
30	250	1.40	30	300	330	145	1.0	98	.12	.51	t	.09	4	t
10	100	.40	13	150	145	75	.45	25	.03	.17	.17	.03	2	t
20	200	1.10	26	200	290	120	.90	49	.06	.34	.3	.06	4	t
30	250	1.40	40	300	435	165	1.35	98	.12	.43	.4	.09	6	t
30	250	1.80	60	350	670	150	2.1	160	.15	.51	.4	.80	9	15
30	250	1.80	50	450	500	250	1.5	74	.15	.43	2	.10	7	t
20	200	1.80	30	300	300	225	.90	74	.12	.34	.3	.06	4	t
25	250	1.80	—	300	—	215	—	98	.23	.51	t	—	—	12
10	100	1.10	—	250	—	175	—	25	.12	.17	2	—	—	t
10	100	.40	—	100	—	50	—	25	.03	.17	t	—	—	t
5	60	.04	—	60	—	40	—	15	.03	.07	.4	—	—	t
35	350	1.80	30	400	480	180	.10	123	.15	.60	.3	.14	3	t
50	450	2.70	43	500	690	260	.14	184	.23	.77	.4	.20	4	t
60	550	3.60	60	600	960	304	.20	200	.30	.94	.4	.28	6	t
35	350	2.70	30	400	480	180	.10	123	.15	.60	.4	.14	3	t
50	450	4.50	43	600	690	260	.14	184	.30	.85	.8	.20	4	t
60	550	5.40	60	700	960	304	.20	200	.37	.90	.8	.28	6	t
20	200	1.10	—	200	—	85	—	40	.06	.26	t	—	—	t
30	300	1.80	—	350	—	180	—	98	.15	.51	t	—	—	t
0	t	t	—	t	—	10	—	0	t	t	t	—	—	t
0	t	t	—	t	—	10	—	—	t	t	t	—	—	t
30	300	1.40	—	200	—	140	—	98	.12	.51	t	—	—	t
20	200	.70	—	200	—	95	—	49	.06	.26	t	—	—	t
78	150	5.4	15	250	200	725	.5	20	.6	.59	.8	.16	9	2.4
40	150	3.6	20	150	370	674	.3	<1	.6	.42	8	.16	40	<1
49	250	3.6	22	200	370	870	.3	100	.67	.51	8	.16	20	<1
45	100	3.60	33	150	290	630	4.5	10	.30	.17	5	.18	16	t
85	100	6.30	45	300	410	660	6.4	20	.45	.34	9	.28	23	t
135	100	9.00	60	450	532	690	8.2	28	.60	.51	14	.33	29	t
50	200	3.60	35	250	300	790	5.0	110	.30	.17	5	.20	20	t
95	350	6.30	50	500	443	980	7.3	160	.45	.43	9	.30	30	t
145	350	9.00	65	700	550	1010	9.2	200	.60	.60	14	.55	37	t

(For purposes of calculations, use "0" for t, <1, <.1, <.01, etc.)

• *Table F–1* Food Composition

Grp	Computer Code No.	Food Description	Measure	Wt (g)	H_2O (%)	Ener (cal)	Prot (g)	Carb (g)	Dietary Fiber (g)	Fat (g)	Fat Breakdown (g) Sat	Mono	Poly
DAIRY QUEEN—Con.													
		Hotdogs:											
12	1483	Regular	1 ea	100	50	280	11	21	<1	16	6	7	2
12	1484	With cheese	1 ea	114	49	330	15	21	<1	21	8	8	2
12	1485	With chili	1 ea	128	55	320	13	23	2	20	8	8	2
		Super hotdogs:											
12	1486	Regular	1 ea	175	48	520	17	44	<1	27	9	12	3
12	1487	With cheese	1 ea	196	48	580	22	45	<1	34	11	13	3
12	1488	With chili	1 ea	218	53	570	21	47	2	32	11	13	3
12	1489	French fries, small	1 svg	71	47	200	2	25	<1	10	4	3	<1
12	1490	French fries, large	1 svg	113	47	320	3	40	<1	16	7	5	1
12	1491	Onion Rings	1 svg	85	28	280	4	31	<1	16	5	7	4

Source: International Dairy Queen Inc., Minneapolis, MN for basic nutrients. Values for dietary fiber, magnesium, potassium, zinc, fatty acids, vitamin A (RE's), B6, folacin and percent water, calculated from known values for the major ingredients.

Grp	Computer Code No.	Food Description	Measure	Wt (g)	H_2O (%)	Ener (cal)	Prot (g)	Carb (g)	Dietary Fiber (g)	Fat (g)	Fat Breakdown (g) Sat	Mono	Poly
JACK IN THE BOX													
12	1492	Breakfast Jack sandwich	1 ea	126	49	307	18	30	<1	13	—	—	—
12	1493	Canadian crescent	1 ea	134	42	472	19	25	<1	31	—	—	—
12	1494	Sausage crescent	1 ea	156	38	584	22	28	<1	43	—	—	—
12	1495	Supreme crescent	1 ea	146	38	547	20	27	<1	40	—	—	—
12	1496	Pancakes breakfast platter	1 ea	231	45	612	15	87	<1	22	8.6	7.6	3.5
12	1497	Scrambled egg breakfast platter	1 ea	249	51	662	24	52	<1	40	17.1	16	4.7
12	1498	Hamburger	1 ea	98	44	276	13	30	<1	12	—	—	—
12	1499	Cheeseburger	1 ea	113	44	323	16	32	<1	15	—	—	—
12	1500	Jumbo Jack	1 ea	205	57	485	26	38	<1	26	—	—	—
12	1501	Jumbo Jack w/cheese	1 ea	246	56	630	32	45	<1	35	—	—	—
12	1502	Bacon cheeseburger supreme	1 ea	231	45	724	34	44	<1	46	—	—	—
12	1503	Swiss & baconburger	1 ea	231	52	643	33	31	<1	43	—	—	—
12	1504	Ham & swiss burger	1 ea	203	44	638	36	37	<1	39	—	—	—
12	1505	Chicken supreme	1 ea	228	52	601	31	39	<1	36	—	—	—
12	1506	Moby Jack sandwich	1 ea	137	40	444	16	39	<1	25	—	—	—
12	1583	Double cheeseburger	1 ea	149	64	467	21	33	—	27	12.3	11.6	3.1
		Tacos:											
12	1508	Regular	1 ea	81	57	191	8	16	<1	11	—	—	—
12	1509	Super	1 ea	135	63	288	12	21	<1	17	—	—	—
12	1513	Taco salad	1 ea	358	81	377	31	10	1	24	—	—	—
12	1516	French fries	1 svg	68	40	221	2	27	<1	12	—	—	—
12	1517	Hash brown potatoes	1 svg	62	60	116	2	11	<1	7	3.6	3.2	.4
12	1518	Onion rings	1 svg	108	28	382	5	39	<1	23	—	—	—
		Milkshakes:											
12	1519	Chocolate	1 ea	322	77	330	11	55	0	7	—	—	—
12	1520	Strawberry	1 ea	328	77	320	10	55	0	7	—	—	—
12	1521	Vanilla	1 ea	317	76	320	10	57	0	6	—	—	—
12	1522	Apple turnover	1 ea	119	38	410	4	45	<1	24	—	—	—

Source: Jack in the Box Restaurants, Foodmaker, Inc., San Diego, CA for basic nutrients. Some values for dietary fiber, magnesium, phosphorus, potassium, zinc, vitamin A (RE's), B6, folacin, and fatty acids calculated from known values for major ingredients.

GRP KEY: 1=BEV 2=DAIRY 3=EGGS 4=FAT/OIL 5=FRUIT 6=BAKERY 7=GRAIN 8=FISH 9=BEEF 10=POULTRY 11=SAUSAGE **12=MIXED/FAST** 13=NUTS/SEEDS 14=SWEETS 15=VEG/LEG 16=MISC 22=SOUP/SAUCE

Chol (mg)	Calc (mg)	Iron (mg)	Magn (mg)	Phos (mg)	Pota (mg)	Sodi (mg)	Zinc (mg)	VT-A (RE)	Thia (mg)	Ribo (mg)	Niac (mg)	V-B6 (mg)	Fola (µg)	VT-C (mg)
45	80	1.40	21	100	130	830	1.4	t	.12	.14	3	.08	20	<1
55	150	1.40	24	200	140	990	1.9	85	.12	.17	3	.08	24	<1
55	80	1.80	38	150	170	985	1.8	60	.15	.26	4	.17	30	<1
80	150	2.70	24	150	210	1365	2.8	t	.23	.26	5	.14	35	<1
100	250	1.40	38	300	220	1605	2.5	100	.23	.26	5	.16	39	<1
100	150	2.70	48	250	250	1595	2.5	60	.23	.43	6	.25	45	<1
10	t	.34	16	60	450	115	t	0	.06	t	.8	.16	15	9
15	t	1.08	24	100	700	185	.3	0	.09	.03	1.2	.30	25	15
15	20	.72	16	60	110	140	.3	15	.09	t	.4	.08	10	2
203	170	3.10	24	310	190	871	1.8	120	.47	.41	3	.11	—	<1
226	125	3.40	—	—	—	851	—	135	.50	.40	3.6	—	—	3
187	170	2.90	—	—	—	1012	—	—	.60	.51	4.6	—	—	t
178	150	2.70	—	—	—	1053	—	—	.64	.54	4.2	—	—	t
99	100	1.8	36	633	237	888	1.9	69	.03	.75	7	.19	3	6
354	200	5.4	55	483	635	1188	3.0	252	.3	.77	5	.34	30	4.8
29	70	2.70	20	115	165	521	1.8	9	.36	.24	3.2	.10	—	1
42	160	2.70	22	194	177	749	2.3	57	.36	.27	3.3	.10	—	1
64	97	6.90	35	208	390	905	3.7	—	.51	.21	7	.25	—	5
110	250	4.50	49	411	499	1665	4.8	—	.53	.34	12	.31	—	5
70	310	4.90	—	—	—	1307	—	—	.56	.51	8.8	—	—	3
99	230	4.70	—	—	—	1354	—	—	.45	.41	6.8	—	—	3
117	268	6.10	—	—	—	1330	—	—	.76	.48	7.6	—	—	10
60	240	3.00	—	—	—	1582	—	—	.52	.37	10.6	—	—	4
47	160	2.20	30	263	246	820	1.1	—	.40	.25	2.8	.08	—	<1
72	400	2.7	—	—	—	842	—	—	.15	.34	6	—	—	—
21	100	1.10	35	146	257	460	1.2	—	.07	.17	1.0	.13	—	<1
37	150	1.60	45	198	347	765	1.8	—	.12	.08	1.4	.18	—	2
102	280	4.30	—	—	—	1436	—	141	.18	.53	6	—	—	7
8	10	.50	23	75	360	164	.26	<1	.07	.03	1.20	.18	—	3
3	40	.36	—	—	—	211	—	0	.06	.03	1.2	—	—	4
27	30	1.40	16	69	109	407	.40	<1	.21	.12	1.80	.06	—	3
25	350	.70	55	330	650	270	1.20	—	.15	.59	.60	.18	—	3
25	350	.40	40	328	613	240	1.10	—	.15	.43	.40	.16	—	3
25	350	.30	38	312	599	230	1.00	<1	.15	.34	.40	.20	—	<1
15	11	1.40	10	33	69	350	.20	—	.23	.12	2.50	.03	—	<1

Table F–1 Food Composition

Grp	Computer Code No.	Food Description	Measure	Wt (g)	H_2O (%)	Ener (cal)	Prot (g)	Carb (g)	Dietary Fiber (g)	Fat (g)	Fat Breakdown (g) Sat	Mono	Poly
		KENTUCKY FRIED CHICKEN											
		Original Recipe:											
12	1253	Center breast	1 ea	95	52	236	24	7	<1	14	4	7	2
12	1251	Side breast	1 ea	69	39	199	16	7	<1	12	3	5	3
12	1250	Drumstick	1 ea	47	53	117	12	3	<1	7	2	3	2
12	1252	Thigh	1 ea	88	49	257	18	7	<1	18	4	7	4
12	1249	Wing	1 ea	42	44	136	10	4	<1	9	2	4	2
		Dinners:											
12	1254	2 pce dinner, white	1 ea	322	64	604	30	48	1	32	7	12	10
12	1255	2 pce dinner, dark	1 ea	346	65	643	35	46	1	35	8	13	11
12	1256	2 pce dinner, combination	1 ea	341	63	661	33	48	1	38	8	14	11
		Extra crispy recipe:											
12	1261	Center breast	1 ea	104	39	297	24	14	<1	16	4	7	4
12	1259	Side breast	1 ea	84	39	286	17	14	<1	18	5	7	4
12	1258	Drumstick	1 ea	58	51	155	13	5	<1	9	2	4	2
12	1260	Thigh	1 ea	107	45	343	20	13	<1	23	6	10	6
12	1257	Wing	1 ea	53	36	201	11	9	<1	14	4	6	3
		Dinners:											
12	1262	2 pce dinner, white	1 ea	348	60	755	33	60	1	43	10	16	12
12	1263	2 pce dinner, dark	1 ea	375	62	765	38	55	1	54	11	16	13
12	1264	2 pce dinner, combination	1 ea	371	60	902	36	58	1	48	12	18	14
12	1265	Mashed potatoes	⅓ c	80	81	60	2	12	<1	1	<1	<1	<1
12	1266	Chicken gravy	⅓ c	78	76	59	2	4	<1	4	1	2	<1
12	1267	Dinner roll	1 ea	21	31	61	2	11	<1	1	<1	<1	<1
12	1268	Corn on the cob	1 ea	143	70	176	5	32	2	3	<1	1	1
12	1269	Coleslaw	⅓ c	79	76	103	1	12	<1	6	1	2	3
12	1381	Kentucky nuggets	1 ea	16	44	46	3	2	<1	3	1	2	<1
		Kentucky nugget sauces:											
12	1382	Barbeque	2 tbsp	30	51	35	<1	7	—	1	<1	<1	<1
12	1383	Sweet & sour	2 tbsp	30	50	58	<1	13	—	1	<1	<1	<1
12	1384	Honey	1 tbsp	15	50	49	0	12	—	<1	—	—	—
12	1385	Mustard	2 tbsp	30	52	36	1	6	—	1	—	—	—
12	1386	Kentucky fries	1 svg	119	45	268	5	33	<1	13	3	8	1
12	1387	Mashed potatoes & gravy	⅓ c	86	80	62	2	10	<1	1	<1	<1	<1
12	1388	Buttermilk biscuit	1 ea	75	27	269	5	32	<1	14	4	8	1
12	1389	Potato salad	⅓ c	90	76	141	2	13	1	9	1	3	5
12	1390	Baked beans	⅓ c	89	71	105	5	18	6	1	<1	<1	<1
12	1391	Chicken Little sandwich	1 ea	57	52	177	6	17	1	9	2	3	3

Source: Kentucky Fried Chicken Corporation

Grp	Computer Code No.	Food Description	Measure	Wt (g)	H_2O (%)	Ener (cal)	Prot (g)	Carb (g)	Dietary Fiber (g)	Fat (g)	Fat Breakdown (g) Sat	Mono	Poly
		LONG JOHN SILVER'S											
		Fish, batter fried:											
12	1523	Fish & fryes, 3 pce	1 ea	350	55	853	43	64	<1	48	—	—	—
12	1524	Fish & fryes, 2 pce	1 ea	260	53	651	30	53	<1	36	—	—	—
12	1525	Fish dinner, 3 pce	1 ea	540	60	1180	47	93	<1	70	—	—	—
		Fish, breaded & fried:											
12	1526	Fish dinner, 3 pce	1 ea	450	60	940	35	84	<1	52	—	—	—
12	1527	Fish dinner, 2 pce	1 ea	400	60	818	26	76	<1	46	—	—	—
		Chicken:											
12	1528	Chicken plank dinner, 3 pce	1 ea	370	60	885	32	72	<1	51	—	—	—
12	1529	Chicken plank dinner, 4 pce	1 ea	440	60	1037	41	82	<1	59	—	—	—
12	1530	Chicken nugget dinner, 6 pce	1 ea	300	60	699	23	54	<1	45	—	—	—
12	1531	Clam chowder	1 svg	185	85	128	7	15	<1	5	—	—	—
12	1532	Clam dinner	1 ea	460	60	955	22	100	<1	58	—	—	—
12	1533	Fish & chicken dinner	1 ea	460	60	935	36	73	<1	55	—	—	—

GRP KEY: 1 = BEV 2 = DAIRY 3 = EGGS 4 = FAT/OIL 5 = FRUIT 6 = BAKERY 7 = GRAIN 8 = FISH 9 = BEEF 10 = POULTRY 11 = SAUSAGE **12 = MIXED/FAST** 13 = NUTS/SEEDS 14 = SWEETS 15 = VEG/LEG 16 = MISC 22 = SOUP/SAUCE

Chol (mg)	Calc (mg)	Iron (mg)	Magn (mg)	Phos (mg)	Pota (mg)	Sodi (mg)	Zinc (mg)	VT-A (RE)	Thia (mg)	Ribo (mg)	Niac (mg)	V-B6 (mg)	Fola (µg)	VT-C (mg)
87	30	1.17	28	205	267	631	.72	6	.08	.11	7.57	.31	8	2
70	50	.98	19	151	176	558	.77	4	.06	.08	5.66	.20	6	1
63	12	.80	13	95	122	207	1.29	3	.04	.09	2.38	.09	4	1
109	34	1.45	22	169	217	566	1.65	5	.08	.16	4.03	.17	9	2
55	22	.68	10	76	86	302	.58	3	.03	.04	2.28	.10	4	1
133	142	3.31	61	326	643	1528	1.88	77	.22	.19	10.0	.50	39	37
180	116	3.90	66	363	720	1441	3.47	77	.25	.32	8.46	.46	42	37
172	126	3.78	64	344	684	1536	2.76	77	.24	.27	8.36	.47	41	37
79	62	1.29	29	218	244	584	.77	6	.11	.11	7.89	.30	11	2
65	57	1.12	21	157	188	564	.88	5	.12	.13	5.37	.24	9	2
66	11	.95	14	100	147	263	1.32	4	.07	.11	3.07	.16	6	1
109	49	1.49	24	185	228	549	1.73	7	.12	.19	5.35	.17	11	2
59	16	.65	12	77	100	312	.67	3	.06	.09	2.94	.11	5	1
132	143	6.03	65	333	689	1544	2.08	77	.31	.29	10.4	.56	43	37
183	130	4.09	70	383	776	1480	3.58	77	.32	.38	10.4	.54	46	37
176	135	6.40	68	361	729	1529	2.93	77	.31	.35	10.3	.49	45	37
<1	21	.28	14	41	218	228	.16	5	.01	.04	.96	.11	7	5
2	9	.48	2	10	21	398	.04	1	.01	.03	.47	<.01	2	<1
1	21	.53	6	28	29	118	.20	1	.10	.04	.98	.01	7	<1
<1	7	.79	53	134	323	12	.99	27	.14	.11	1.80	.22	71	2
4	29	.19	9	20	115	171	.13	28	.03	.03	.20	.07	10	19
12	2	.13	4	29	33	140	.22	30	.02	.03	1.00	.04	1	2
1	6	.24	5	10	75	450	.05	37	.01	.01	.19	.02	3	<1
1	5	.16	2	5	39	148	.02	6	.01	.02	.04	.01	1	<1
t	1	.11	<1	<1	6	10	<.01	0	.01	<.01	.04	t	1	3
1	10	.26	6	15	23	346	.09	1	.02	.01	.16	.02	3	1
1	24	.94	28	78	606	81	.31	0	.17	.06	2.70	.18	20	3
1	19	.35	9	28	137	297	.11	5	.01	.04	1.00	.08	8	1
1	77	1.22	9	264	95	521	.29	30	.28	.13	1.80	.03	8	<1
11	10	.32	15	32	256	396	.29	27	.07	.02	.60	.19	7	3
1	54	1.43	29	90	229	387	1.29	10	.06	.04	.50	.07	32	2
20	39	1.40	10	105	114	398	.93	6	.15	.14	1.65	.07	11	<1

106	—	—	—	—	—	2025	—	—	—	—	—	—	—	—
75	—	—	—	—	—	1352	—	—	—	—	—	—	—	—
119	—	—	—	—	—	2797	—	—	—	—	—	—	—	—
101	—	—	—	—	—	1900	—	—	—	—	—	—	—	—
76	—	—	—	—	—	1526	—	—	—	—	—	—	—	—
25	—	—	—	—	—	1918	—	—	—	—	—	—	—	—
25	—	—	—	—	—	2433	—	—	—	—	—	—	—	—
25	—	—	—	—	—	853	—	—	—	—	—	—	—	—
17	—	—	—	—	—	611	—	—	—	—	—	—	—	—
27	—	—	—	—	—	1543	—	—	—	—	—	—	—	—
56	—	—	—	—	—	2076	—	—	—	—	—	—	—	—

(For purposes of calculations, use "0" for t, <1, <.1, <.01, etc.)

Table F–1 Food Composition

Grp	Computer Code No.	Food Description	Measure	Wt (g)	H_2O (%)	Ener (cal)	Prot (g)	Carb (g)	Dietary Fiber (g)	Fat (g)	Fat Breakdown (g) Sat	Mono	Poly
		LONG JOHN SILVER'S—Con.											
12	1534	Oyster dinner	1 ea	360	60	789	17	78	<1	45	—	—	—
12	1535	Scallop dinner	1 ea	320	60	747	17	66	<1	45	—	—	—
12	1536	Seafood platter	1 ea	410	60	976	29	85	<1	58	—	—	—
12	1537	Batter fried shrimp dinner	1 ea	300	60	711	17	60	<1	45	—	—	—
12	1538	Fish sandwich platter	1 ea	400	60	835	30	84	<1	42	—	—	—
		Salads:											
12	1539	Ocean chef	1 ea	320	85	229	27	13	2	8	—	—	—
12	1540	Seafood	1 ea	480	85	426	19	22	2	30	—	—	—
12	1541	Cole slaw	1 svg	98	70	182	1	11	<1	15	—	—	—
12	1542	Fries	1 svg	85	42	247	4	31	<1	12	—	—	—
12	1543	Hush puppies	1 ea	47	37	145	3	18	<1	7	—	—	—
		Source: Long John Silver's Inc., Lexington, KY.											
		McDONALD'S											
		Sandwiches:											
12	1221	Big Mac	1 ea	215	48	560	25	43	1	32	10	21	2
12	1591	McDLT Sandwich	1 ea	234	59	580	26	36	1.4	37	12	17	9
12	1222	Quarter Pounder	1 ea	166	49	410	23	34	1	21	8	11	1
12	1223	Quarter Pounder w/cheese	1 ea	194	48	520	29	35	1	29	11	16	1
12	1224	Filet-O-Fish sandwich	1 ea	142	44	440	14	38	<1	26	5	10	11
12	1225	Hamburger	1 ea	102	46	260	12	31	<1	10	4	5	1
12	1226	Cheeseburger	1 ea	116	45	310	15	31	<1	14	5	8	1
12	1227	French fries	1 svg	68	37	220	4	26	1	12	3	8	.5
12	1228	Chicken McNuggets	6 ea	112	49	270	20	17	<1	15	4	10	2
		Sauces:											
12	1229	Hot Mustard	1 ea	30	53	70	.5	8	<1	4	<1	1	1
12	1230	Barbecue	1 ea	30	51	50	.3	12	<1	<1	<1	<1	<1
12	1231	Sweet & sour	1 ea	32	50	60	<1	14	<1	<1	<1	<1	<1
		Lowfat Milkshakes:											
12	1232	Chocolate	10 fl oz	293	70	320	12	66	<1	2	.8	.9	<1
12	1233	Strawberry	10 fl oz	293	72	320	11	67	<1	1	.6	.6	<1
12	1234	Vanilla	10 fl oz	293	73	290	11	60	<1	1	.63	.67	<1
		Sundaes:											
12	1235	Hot fudge	1 ea	169	60	240	7	51	<1	3	2	1	<1
12	1236	Strawberry	1 ea	171	62	210	6	49	<1	1	1	4	<1
12	1237	Hot Caramel	1 ea	174	57	270	7	59	<1	3	2	1	<1
12	1238	Vanilla cone	1 ea	80	65	100	4	22	<1	1	<1	<1	<1
		Pies:											
12	1239	Apple pie	1 ea	83	45	260	2	30	<1	15	5	9	1
12	1240	Apple Bran Muffin	1 ea	85	44	190	5	46	3	0	0	0	0
		Cookies, package:											
12	1241	McDonaldland cookies	1 pkg	56	3	290	4	47	<1	9	2	7	<1
12	1242	Chocolate chip cookies	1 pkg	56	3	330	4	42	2	16	5	10	<1
		Breakfast items:											
12	1243	English muffin, w/butter	1 ea	59	42	170	5	27	<1	5	2	2	1
12	1244	Egg McMuffin	1 ea	138	51	290	8.2	28	<1	11	4	6	1
12	1245	Hot cakes w/butter & syrup	1 ea	176	46	410	8	74	<1	9	4	3	3
12	1246	Scrambled eggs	1 ea	100	70	140	12	1	<1	10	3	5	1
12	1247	Pork Sausage	1 svg.	48	43	180	8	0	<1	16	6	9	2
12	1248	Hash brown potato patty	1 ea	53	56	130	1	15	1	7	3	4	<1
12	1392	Sausage McMuffin	1 ea	117	38	370	17	27	<1	22	8	12	2
12	1393	Sausage McMuffin w/egg	1 ea	167	47	440	23	28	<1	27	9	15	3
12	1394	Biscuit with spread	1 ea	75	27	260	5	32	<1	13	3	9	1

GRP KEY: 1=BEV 2=DAIRY 3=EGGS 4=FAT/OIL 5=FRUIT 6=BAKERY 7=GRAIN 8=FISH 9=BEEF 10=POULTRY 11=SAUSAGE **12=MIXED/FAST** 13=NUTS/SEEDS 14=SWEETS 15=VEG/LEG 16=MISC 22=SOUP/SAUCE

Chol (mg)	Calc (mg)	Iron (mg)	Magn (mg)	Phos (mg)	Pota (mg)	Sodi (mg)	Zinc (mg)	VT-A (RE)	Thia (mg)	Ribo (mg)	Niac (mg)	V-B6 (mg)	Fola (μg)	VT-C (mg)
55	—	—	—	—	—	763	—	—	—	—	—	—	—	—
37	—	—	—	—	—	1579	—	—	—	—	—	—	—	—
95	—	—	—	—	—	2161	—	—	—	—	—	—	—	—
127	—	—	—	—	—	1297	—	—	—	—	—	—	—	—
75	—	—	—	—	—	1402	—	—	—	—	—	—	—	—
64	—	—	—	—	—	986	—	—	—	—	—	—	—	—
113	—	—	—	—	—	1086	—	—	—	—	—	—	—	—
12	—	—	—	—	—	367	—	—	—	—	—	—	—	—
13	—	—	—	—	—	.6	—	—	—	—	—	—	—	—
—	—	—	—	—	—	405	—	—	—	—	—	—	—	—
103	256	4	41	338	268	950	5.04	88	.48	.41	6.81	.285	23	2
109	225	4	45	321	414	990	6	188	.39	.36	7	.26	30	7
86	142	4	38	258	334	660	5.3	45	.36	.29	6.7	.28	24	3
118	296	3.7	42	315	356	1150	6	190	.37	.39	6.7	.24	24	3
50	165	1.8	27	227	149	1030	.88	36	.30	.15	3.00	.10	20	.1
37	122	2.29	20	129	145	500	2.13	15	.28	.16	3.84	.12	17	2
53	197	2.3	23	205	157	750	2.60	112	.30	.21	3.86	.12	21	2
0	9	.61	27	101	564	70	.32	0	.13	0	1.8	.22	19	2
56	14	1	27	293	313	580	.923	0	.12	.12	8.3	.394	11	0
5	15	.22	6	15	23	250	.09	1.6	.01	.01	.15	.01	3	.45
0	13	.31	5	10	75	340	.05	15	.01	.01	.17	.02	3	2.34
0	11	.17	2	5	39	190	.02	32	0	.01	.08	.01	.6	.64
10	322	.84	47	319	555	240	1.21	92	.13	.52	.41	.148	15	0
10	327	.1	36	302	509	170	1.07	92	.13	.48	.31	.148	11	0
10	327	.10	35	339	521	170	1.09	92	.13	.48	.31	.148	36	0
6	235	.48	36	243	422	170	1.01	65	.08	.35	.30	.138	11	0
5	191	.16	29	188	302	95	.838	65	.07	.29	.25	.056	21	1
13	222	.1	31	243	356	180	.916	88	.08	.35	.26	.054	14	0
3	112	.23	13	120	136	70	.482	87	.04	.18	.37	.046	2	0
0	11	.71	6	26	38	240	.16	0	.06	.02	.32	.02	5	11
0	31	.6	—	—	—	230	—	.7	.02	.08	.4	—	—	.7
0	9	2.1	11	72	50	300	.325	0	.25	.18	2.54	.03	6	0
4	24	2.2	27	102	160	280	.50	0	.18	.21	2.47	.03	6	0
9	151	1.61	13	69	66	270	.50	31	.33	.14	2.47	.04	16	0
226	256	2.77	26	322	168	740	1.92	151	.47	.33	3.71	.21	30	0
21	114	2.08	23	412	154	640	.56	52	.32	.33	2.82	.099	7	0
399	57	2.08	13	269	138	290	1.69	157	.07	.26	.05	.20	66	0
48	8	.67	8	86	115	350	1.33	0	.27	.10	2.31	.165	1	0
9	6	.27	13	65	238	330	.164	0	.06	.02	.85	.124	6	2
64	235	2.3	24	189	219	830	1.71	72	.60	.29	4.8	.15	23	0
263	263	3.34	30	291	298	980	2.39	150	.64	.42	4.8	.20	33	0
1	75	1.31	9	264	95	730	.292	0	.23	.11	1.65	.03	8	0

Table F–1 Food Composition

Grp	Computer Code No.	Food Description	Measure	Wt (g)	H_2O (%)	Ener (cal)	Prot (g)	Carb (g)	Dietary Fiber (g)	Fat (g)	Fat Breakdown (g) Sat	Mono	Poly
		McDONALD'S—Con.											
		Breakfast Items—Con.											
12	1395	Biscuit w/sausage	1 ea	123	32	440	13	32	<1	29	9	17	3
12	1396	Biscuit w/sausage & egg	1 ea	180	43	529	20	33	<1	35	11	20	3
12	1397	Biscuit w/bacon, egg & cheese	1 ea	156	41	440	18	33	<1	26	8	16	2
		Salads:											
12	1398	Chef salad	1 ea	283	84	230	21	8	2	13	6	7	1
12	1399	Shrimp salad	1 ea	262	88	104	14	6	2	3	1	2	<1
12	1400	Garden salad	1 ea	213	91	110	7	6	2	7	3	3	<1
12	1401	Chunky Chicken salad	1 ea	250	88	140	23	5	2	3	1	2	1

Source: McDonald's Corporation, Oak Brook, Illinois. Some values for Salads estimated from known values for major ingredients.

Grp	Computer Code No.	Food Description	Measure	Wt (g)	H_2O (%)	Ener (cal)	Prot (g)	Carb (g)	Dietary Fiber (g)	Fat (g)	Sat	Mono	Poly
		TACO BELL											
		Burritos:											
12	1544	Bean	1 ea	191	58	357	13	54	8	10	3	5	2
12	1545	Beef	1 ea	191	58	403	22	39	2	17	7	7	2
12	1546	Bean & beef	1 ea	191	58	381	17	46	5	14	7	6	1
12	1547	Burrito supreme	1 ea	241	66	413	18	46	5	18	8	8	2
12	1548	Double beef supreme	1 ea	255	66	457	24	42	2	22	10	10	2
12	1549	Enchirito	1 ea	213	61	382	20	31	5	20	9	8	1
12	1550	Fajita (steak taco)	1 ea	135	65	234	15	20	2	11	5	4	1
		Tacos:											
12	1551	Regular	1 ea	78	55	183	10	11	1	11	5	3	1
12	1552	Taco bellgrande	1 ea	163	63	355	18	18	2	23	11	6	1
12	1553	Taco light	1 ea	170	59	410	19	18	2	29	12	8	5
12	1554	Soft taco	1 ea	92	52	228	12	18	2	12	5	4	1
		Tostadas:											
12	1555	Regular	1 ea	156	67	243	10	27	7	11	4	4	1
12	1556	Beefy tostada	1 ea	198	69	322	15	22	4	20	10	8	1
12	1557	Bellbeefer	1 ea	177	63	312	17	32	<1	13	6	4	2
12	1558	Mexican pizza	1 ea	223	55	575	21	40	5	48	31	14	2
12	1559	Taco salad with salsa	1 ea	595	73	941	36	63	5	61	19	18	12
		Nachos:											
12	1560	Regular	1 ea	106	40	356	7	38	<1	19	12	5	1
12	1561	Bellgrande	1 ea	287	58	649	22	61	6	35	12	20	3
12	1562	Pintos & cheese	1 ea	128	69	190	9	19	7	9	4	4	1
12	1563	Taco sauce	1 ea	3.7	96	2	<1	<1	<1	<1	<1	<1	<1
12	1564	Salsa	1 ea	9.7	95	18	1	4	1	<1	<1	<1	<1
12	1565	Cinnamon Crispas	1 ea	47.3	1	259	3	27	<1	15	4	2	1

Source: Taco Bell Corporation, California for most nutrient values. Values for Dietary fiber, mono-unsaturated fat, magnesium, phosphorus, zinc, folacin, Vitamin B6, Vitamin A in REs, and percentage water are estimates calculated from known values of major ingredients.

Grp	Computer Code No.	Food Description	Measure	Wt (g)	H_2O (%)	Ener (cal)	Prot (g)	Carb (g)	Dietary Fiber (g)	Fat (g)	Sat	Mono	Poly
		WENDY's											
		Hamburgers:											
12	1566	Single, on white bun, no toppings	1 ea	119	41	350	21	29	<1	16	7	9	1
12	1568	Double, on white bun, no toppings	1 ea	197	44	560	41	32	<1	34	7	13	8
12	1569	Big classic	1 ea	241	63	470	26	36	2	25	7	10	5
		Cheeseburgers:											
12	1570	Bacon cheeseburger	1 ea	147	46	460	29	23	<1	28	13	13	2
12	1571	Single, w/all toppings	1 ea	215	50	548	30	32	2	33	13	12	5
12	1572	Double, w/all toppings	1 ea	291	50	735	48	27	2	48	18	18	6

GRP KEY: 1=BEV 2=DAIRY 3=EGGS 4=FAT/OIL 5=FRUIT 6=BAKERY 7=GRAIN 8=FISH 9=BEEF 10=POULTRY 11=SAUSAGE **12=MIXED/FAST** 13=NUTS/SEEDS 14=SWEETS 15=VEG/LEG 16=MISC 22=SOUP/SAUCE

Chol (mg)	~~Calc~~ (mg)	~~Iron~~ (mg)	Magn (mg)	Phos (mg)	Pota (mg)	Sodi (mg)	Zinc (mg)	VT-A (RE)	Thia (mg)	Ribo (mg)	Niac (mg)	V-B6 (mg)	Fola (μg)	VT-C (mg)
49	83	1.98	18	359	235	1080	1.33	0	.49	.21	3.96	.12	12	0
275	116	3.16	25	490	321	1250	3.16	88	.53	.35	3.99	.199	36	0
253	185	2.56	21	496	250	1230	1.67	162	.36	.33	2.47	.11	47	0
128	256	1.51	35	200	400	490	1.40	514	.31	.29	3.6	.04	60	14
193	65	1.33	60	180	420	480	1.90	372	.13	.10	1.08	.06	60	13
83	149	1.26	18	80	280	160	.40	391	.10	.16	.59	.06	60	14
78	24	1	20	140	350	230	.66	458	.22	.17	8.5	.34	61	20
9	147	3.47	65	210	428	888	2.05	65	.037	2.02	1.98	1.00	55	53
57	114	3.73	35	225	313	1051	4.00	100	.398	2.14	3.44	.23	27	2
36	111	2.15	50	220	370	958	2.67	80	.49	.42	3.09	.59	38	2
33	153	3.6	50	227	432	921	3.00	185	.41	2.12	2.89	.52	40	27
57	145	4	52	230	431	1053	4.00	200	.43	2.2	3.68	.30	30	9
54	269	2.84	61	263	423	1243	3.51	157	.256	.418	2.3	.61	29	28
14	117	3.03	24	150	207	485	3.18	133	.403	.341	3.71	.17	15	3
32	84	1.10	16	100	159	276	2.12	42	.05	.142	1.07	.12	10	1
56	182	1.91	18	100	334	472	2.12	132	.11	.29	2.02	.12	13	5
56	155	2.4	18	100	316	594	2.12	128	.2	.33	2.5	.12	13	5
32	116	2.27	18	100	178	516	2.12	42	.39	.22	2.74	.12	10	1
16	179	1.53	62	195	401	596	1.55	84	.061	.169	.626	1.01	47	45
40	185	1.96	43	206	408	764	2.97	152	.24	.29	1.61	.56	31	6
39	174	2.36	22	125	299	855	2.10	121	.16	.30	1.73	.12	<1	5
81	453	3.08	80	400	449	1364	5.40	355	.36	.39	2.00	1.11	60	7
80	398	7.1	130	460	1212	1662	5.59	450	.51	.75	4.8	1.30	140	77
9	178	.99	40	200	158	423	.80	27	.03	.16	.09	.14	4	2
36	297	3.48	100	400	674	997	4.30	280	.104	.34	2.17	.98	33	58
16	156	1.42	110	156	385	642	2.17	87	.05	.146	.396	.21	68	52
0	2	.07	—	—	13	126	—	19	<.01	<.01	.06	—	—	<1
0	36	.60	—	—	376	376	—	112	.02	.14	—	—	—	2
1	37	1.26	—	—	36	127	—	<1	.138	.084	.966	—	—	<1
65	100	4.50	20	118	265	420	2.10	—	.38	.34	6	.12	<1	<1
125	48	6.30	42	339	431	575	8.35	—	.22	.43	9.00	.47	29	<1
80	40	4.55	34	200	470	900	5.11	60	.26	.25	4.80	.25	30	12
65	136	3.60	33	296	332	860	5.14	82	.27	.28	5.70	.24	25	1
84	177	4.00	33	339	430	864	4.41	111	.34	.35	5.29	.25	28	6
165	180	5.40	50	470	620	883	8.80	112	.36	.53	10.0	.46	31	6

(For purposes of calculations, use "0" for t, <1, <.1, <.01, etc.)

● *Table F–1* Food Composition

Grp	Computer Code No.	Food Description	Measure	Wt (g)	H_2O (%)	Ener (cal)	Prot (g)	Carb (g)	Dietary Fiber (g)	Fat (g)	Fat Breakdown (g) Sat	Mono	Poly
WENDY'S—Con.													
		Baked potatoes:											
12	1573	Plain	1 ea	250	75	250	6	52	5	<1	<1	<1	<1
12	1574	W/bacon & cheese	1 ea	350	71	570	19	57	5	30	12	11	6
12	1575	W/broccoli & cheese	1 ea	365	74	500	13	54	5	25	9	8	5
12	1576	W/cheese	1 ea	350	71	590	17	55	5	34	13	13	7
12	1577	W/chili & cheese	1 ea	400	72	510	22	63	8	20	13	7	<1
12	1578	W/sour cream & chives	1 ea	310	71	460	7	53	5	24	10	8	3
12	1579	Chili	1 c	256	77	230	21	16	5	9	3	4	<1
12	1580	French fries	1 svg	106	43	306	4	38	<1	15	7	5	2
12	1581	Frosty dairy dessert	1 c	216	35	354	7	53	0	13	5	3	2
12	1582	Chocolate chip cookie	1 ea	64	5	320	3	40	1	17	6	6	5

Source: Wendy's International, for most nutrient values. Some of the values for Dietary fiber, the types of fatty acids, magnesium, phosphorus, zinc, Vitamin B6, Vitamin A in REs, and percentage water for estimates calculated from known values of major ingredients.

GRP KEY: 1 = BEV 2 = DAIRY 3 = EGGS 4 = FAT/OIL 5 = FRUIT 6 = BAKERY 7 = GRAIN 8 = FISH 9 = BEEF 10 = POULTRY 11 = SAUSAGE **12 = MIXED/FAST** 13 = NUTS/SEEDS 14 = SWEETS 15 = VEG/LEG 16 = MISC 22 = SOUP/SAUCE

Chol (mg)	Calc (mg)	Iron (mg)	Magn (mg)	Phos (mg)	Pota (mg)	Sodi (mg)	Zinc (mg)	VT-A (RE)	Thia (mg)	Ribo (mg)	Niac (mg)	V-B6 (mg)	Fola (μg)	VT-C (mg)
0	40	2.7	67	169	1360	60	.65	0	.28	.10	3.82	.70	68	36
22	200	3.7	80	406	1380	180	2.53	150	.225	.17	4.64	.866	33	36
22	250	3.6	83	373	1550	2.19	.865	350	.31	.255	4	.861	66	90
22	350	3.6	78	49.7	1380	2.22	.609	200	.225	.255	3.3	.80	33	36
22	250	6.1	111	498	1590	810	3.78	172	.32	.26	4.1	.9	50	36
15	40	2.7	70	185	1420	230	.9	100	.225	.13	3	.79	32	36
30	60	4.50	60	320	565	960	3.78	200	.12	.17	3.00	.26	40	9
15	13	1.02	45	197	689	105	.51	0	.15	.04	2.96	.27	33	12
45	257	.86	43	238	518	194	.92	143	.11	.45	.31	.12	17	<1
5	10	1.09	15	62	100	235	.46	0	.06	.07	.4	.03	6	0

Index

Boldface type indicates pages with marginal definitions.

D

E

F

Q

R

S

T

U

V

Photo Credits—Continued

171 Ray Stanyard; **173** Ray Stanyard; **Chapter 7** **180** Courtesy of Gjon Mill; © *Nutrition Today*; **182** Felicia Martinez/Photo Edit; **185** Courtesy of the U.S. Department of Agriculture; **191** Charles Feil/Stock, Boston; Felicia Martinez/Photo Edit; **194** Ray Stanyard; **198** © Camera M.D. Studios, Inc.; **Chapter 8** **203** © Tony Freeman/Photo Edit; **204** © Tony Freeman/Photo Edit; © Frank Siteman 1989/Stock, Boston; © David Young-Wolff/Photo Edit; **231** ©Tony Freeman/Photo Edit; **237** © George S. Zimbel/Monkmeyer Press; **238** © Felicia Martinez/Photo Edit; **Chapter 9** **243** © Richard Hutchings/Info Edit; **244** © Tony Freeman/Photo Edit; **247** Photo by Elena Rooraid/Photo Edit; **256** © Tony Freeman/Photo Edit; **258** © David Young-Wolff/Photo Edit; **264** John Bahlik; **274** © David Young-Wolff/Photo Edit; **Chapter 10** **282** © Richard Hutchings/InfoEdit; **283** (far left and far right) Streissguth, A. P., Clarren, S. K. & Jones, K L. (1985, July). Natural History of the Fetal Alcohol Syndrome: A ten-year follow-up of eleven patients. *Lauret, II,* 89–92; (center left and center right) Photos courtesy of Ann Pytkowicz Streissguth, University of Washington. Reprinted by permission of CIBA Foundation; **284** © Tony Freeman/Photo Edit; **285** © Myrleen Ferguson/Photo Edit; **287** © Mary Kate Denny/Photo Edit; **289** © Robert Brenner/Photo Edit; **291** © Robert Brenner/Photo Edit; **292** © Anthony Vannelli; **299** © Tony Freeman/Photo Edit; **Chapter 11** **326** © Phil Borden/Photo Edit; **339** © Tony Freeman/Photo Edit; **351** (top) © Rick Browne/Stock, Boston; (bottom) ©Cary Wolinsky/Stock, Boston; **354** © Alan Oddie/Photo Edit.